Skin, Mucosa and Menopause

Miranda A. Farage · Kenneth W. Miller
Nancy Fugate Woods
Howard I. Maibach
Editors

Skin, Mucosa and Menopause

Management of Clinical Issues

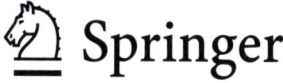

Editors
Miranda A. Farage, MSc, PhD
Procter and Gamble Company
Cincinnati, OH
USA

Kenneth W. Miller, PhD
Procter and Gamble Company
Cincinnati, OH
USA

Nancy Fugate Woods, PhD, BSN, MN
School of Nursing
University of Washington
Seattle, WA
USA

Howard I. Maibach, MD
Department of Dermatology
University of California
School of Medicine
San Francisco, CA
USA

ISBN 978-3-662-44079-7   ISBN 978-3-662-44080-3 (eBook)
DOI 10.1007/978-3-662-44080-3
Springer Heidelberg New York Dordrecht London

Library of Congress Control Number: 2014956097

© Springer-Verlag Berlin Heidelberg 2015

This work is subject to copyright. All rights are reserved by the Publisher, whether the whole or part of the material is concerned, specifically the rights of translation, reprinting, reuse of illustrations, recitation, broadcasting, reproduction on microfilms or in any other physical way, and transmission or information storage and retrieval, electronic adaptation, computer software, or by similar or dissimilar methodology now known or hereafter developed. Exempted from this legal reservation are brief excerpts in connection with reviews or scholarly analysis or material supplied specifically for the purpose of being entered and executed on a computer system, for exclusive use by the purchaser of the work. Duplication of this publication or parts thereof is permitted only under the provisions of the Copyright Law of the Publisher's location, in its current version, and permission for use must always be obtained from Springer. Permissions for use may be obtained through RightsLink at the Copyright Clearance Center. Violations are liable to prosecution under the respective Copyright Law.

The use of general descriptive names, registered names, trademarks, service marks, etc. in this publication does not imply, even in the absence of a specific statement, that such names are exempt from the relevant protective laws and regulations and therefore free for general use.

While the advice and information in this book are believed to be true and accurate at the date of publication, neither the authors nor the editors nor the publisher can accept any legal responsibility for any errors or omissions that may be made. The publisher makes no warranty, express or implied, with respect to the material contained herein.

Printed on acid-free paper

Springer is part of Springer Science+Business Media (www.springer.com)

Foreword

Skin, Mucosa, and Menopause: Management of Clinical Issues is a unique volume that brings together experts from around the world to focus on two very important parts of the body – skin and mucosa.

Skin aging begins at birth, and with life expectancy increasing in most countries, skin demands our attention. Most people would like a healthy and inoffensive exterior enveloping their bodies. Aging affects the skin of both men and women, but women experience a major shift in hormones at midlife that adds to the complexity of skin, mucosa and physiological changes associated with aging.

The respected contributors selected by the editors bring their global expertise and perspective to a wide variety of topics from physiologic changes of menopause and aging to genital symptoms associated with low estrogen, hair and nail changes, autoimmune effects on skin, the effects of appearance and function on quality of life and self-esteem, as well as health policy implications. There is an effective blend of clinical issues and research findings that will appeal to both the clinician and the researcher.

The latest research on oxidative stress and cytokines and their role in skin damage and healing are presented. The effects of genetics, the immune system, the environment, and the decline in many sex steroids are explored.

From a clinical perspective, symptoms are of utmost importance, and for postmenopausal women, vaginal dryness is an almost universal symptom. The changes in vaginal mucosa related to low estrogen levels can be severe enough to adversely affect quality of life.

Many options for women are discussed, including the roles of hormone therapy, cosmeceuticals and cosmetic surgery. Healthy aging and quality of life go hand in hand. Understanding skin, mucosa and physiology as they relate to menopause will improve both.

This comprehensive volume should broaden the perspectives of researchers and clinicians and motivate ongoing interest in skin and mucosa to the benefit of midlife women.

Mayfield Heights, OH, USA   Margery L.S. Gass, MD

Preface

The global population is aging. One in eight people worldwide will be over the age of 65 by year 2030. For the first time in history, the elderly will outnumber younger generations.

What was previously thought of as "old" (i.e., age 40) is no longer considered old. Indeed, people aged 70 often do not consider themselves old. This population remains intellectually vibrant and will contribute broad experience, a wiser perspective, and more mature judgment to society. We should embrace this change.

Our societal institutions must address the implications of this demographic shift. The medical and public health communities can make a positive contribution in this regard. Of the many challenges ahead, three significant areas come to mind. The first is our outlook and attitudes. We can shift the paradigm from being considered "old" toward respecting the value of maturity. Second, we must help society recognize and better accommodate age-related changes in physiology, sensory perception, mobility, reflexes and cognitive abilities, and assist our social institutions to adapt to the physical, emotional and social needs of older adults. Third, notwithstanding considerable popular and commercial interest given to the health issues of aging men, the fact is that women generally live longer and will comprise a more substantial portion of the older population. The experience of the older woman will gain prominence and must be addressed in a thoughtful and comprehensive way.

This volume focuses on the older woman and specifically on the major life transition of menopause. This transition is accompanied by changes in urogenital morphology, physiology, tissue atrophy, sexuality, susceptibility to infection, and urinary continence and function. Because menopause is defined by the cessation of menstruation, with attendant connotations of decline, it is traditionally seen as a loss. Moreover, because of its association with sexuality, the challenges of menopause also remain somewhat taboo. We must redefine the experience of menopause from being a "loss" to being a life transition in which the health and helping professions can offer support. This volume compiles a breadth of fundamental understanding about postmenopausal health and well being. It is our hope that the information provided herein will contribute to better health outcomes and a thriving quality of life for the older woman. Armed with this knowledge and a positive perspective, let us affirm menopause as the transition through which our mothers, partners, sisters, and friends come of age as wise and wonderful elders of society.

Researchers and clinicians who have contributed to this volume hope to promote a better understanding to women's menopausal state. We hope that this compilation will be valuable to its intended audience. Your editors welcome comments and suggestions.

Cincinnati, OH, USA	Miranda A. Farage, MSc, PhD
Cincinnati, OH, USA	Kenneth W. Miller, PhD
Seattle, WA, USA	Nancy Fugate Woods, PhD, BSN, MN
San Francisco, CA, USA	Howard I. Maibach, MD

Acknowledgments

Deep appreciation and grateful thank-yous are extended to the many people who contributed both knowingly and indirectly to this book.

A special thank you and our heartfelt gratitude go to Dr. Pamela Schofield, who encouraged and supported this book from the start. She has our heartfelt and deepest gratitude.

Many thanks go to the significant efforts of all the contributors of this book and the valuable time they dedicated to preparing their chapters. This book represents the fruits of a jointly conceived and executed venture and has benefited from global and diverse partners.

We would also like to single out Diane Lamsback (Developmental Editor, Springer) for a special recognition. Her great efforts, time, discipline and dedication helped moved this book forward in a timely and organized manner. In addition, we would like to thank both Sverre Klemp and Ellen Blasig (Springer) for their help in moving this book forward.

In addition, Dr. Deborah A. Hutchins, Ms. Zeinab Schwen, Ms. Gayle Entrup and Dr. T. L. Nusair have all assisted and given input to vastly improve the texts.

Above all, our everlasting gratitude, thanks and love go to our parents, who inspired us, and to our families and children, who supported, helped and encouraged us all the way with their incredible patience. Your continuous care, unconditional love and sacrifice made all this possible, and easier to achieve.

Miranda A. Farage, MSc, PhD
Kenneth W. Miller, PhD
Nancy Fugate Woods, PhD, BSN, MN
Howard I. Maibach, MD

Abbreviations

3′ UTR	3 prime Untranslated region
5-meC	5-Methylcytosine
AA	Alopecia areata
AAB	Autoantibody
AFC	Antral follicle counts
AGA	Androgenetic alopecia
AGE	Advanced glycosylation end-products
AID	Autoimmune disease
AIH	Autoimmune hepatitis
ANA	Anti-nuclear antibody
APC	Antigen presenting cell
Ar	Androgen receptor
AS	Ankylosing spondylitis
AVF	Altered vaginal flora
BMI	Body mass index
BP	Base pair
CAD	Coronary artery disease
CBT	Cognitive behavioral therapy
CI	Confidence interval
CLA	Cutaneous lymphocyte antigen
CML	N^{ε}-[Carboxymethyl-]lysine
CNS	Central nervous system
CPA	Cyproterone acetate
CS	Cervantes Scale
CVD	Cardiovascular disease
CVE	Cardiovascular events
DC	Dendritic cell
DEJ	Dermal epidermal junction
DHEA	Dehydroepiandrosterone
DHT	Dihydrotestosterone
DIV	Desquamative inflammatory vaginitis
DS	Down syndrome
dsDNA	Double-strand deoxyribonucleic acid
E1	Estrone
E2	Estradiol
E3	Estriol
EAE	Experimental autoimmune encephalomyelitis

ECG	Electrocardiogram
EPT	Estrogen and Progesterone therapy
ER	Estrogen receptor
ERE	Estrogen responsive element
FFA	Frontal fibrosing alopecia
FL	Fructosalysine
FMP	Final menstrual period
FPHL	Female pattern hair loss
FR	Free radicals
FSH	Follicle-stimulating hormone
GM-CSF	Granulocyte macrophage colony stimulating factors
GPx	Glutathione peroxidase
HapMap	Halotype map
HAT	Histone-acetylation enzyme histonacetyl transferase
HERS	Heart and Estrogen/Progestin Replacement Study
HRT	Hormone-replacement therapy
HT	Hormone therapy
ICC	Intraclass correlation coefficient
IFNGR	Interferon gamma receptor
IFN-γ	Interferon-gamma
Ig	Immunoglobulin
IGF	Insulin-like growth factor
IL	Interleukin
IKβ	Inhibitory Kβ
JAK	Janus kinase
LH	Luteinizing hormone
LP	Lichen planus
LPP	Lichen planopilaris
LPPAI	Lichen Planopilaris Activity Index
LPS	Lipopolysaccharide
LPV	Localized provoked vestibulodynia
LS	Lichen sclerosus
LSC	Lichen simplex chronicus
LUMINA	Lupus in Minorities: Nature vs. Nature
meC	Methylcytosine
MENQOL	The Menopause-Specific Quality of Life Questionnaire
MHC	Major histocompatibility complex
MIF	Macrophage inhibitory factor
miRNA	Micro ribonucleic acid
MMP	Matrix metalloproteinase
MPA	Medroxyprogesterone acetate
MQOL	The Menopause Quality of Life Scale
mRNA	Messenger ribonucleic acid
MRS	Menopause Rating Scale
MS	Multiple sclerosis
mtDNA	Mitochondrial DNA
$\Delta\Psi m$	Mitochondrial membrane potential
MZ	Monozygotic

NADPH	Nicotine adenine dinucleotide phosphate
NF-Kβ	Nuclear factor kappa-light-chain enhancer
NGFs	Non-growing follicles
NK	Natural killer
NO·	Nitric oxide radical
NOS	Nitric oxide synthase
NVA	National Vulvodynia Association
$O_2^{·-}$	Superoxide anion
OC	Oral contraceptives
·OH	Hydroxyl radical
$ONOO^-$	Peroxynitrite radical
OS	Oxidative stress
PBMC	Peripheral blood mononuclear cells
PCR	Polymerase chain reaction
PMA	Post-menopausal aging
PMNs	Polymorphonuclear leukocytes
POF	Premature ovarian failure
PPAR	Peroxisome-proliferator activated receptor
PR	Progesterone receptor
PTPN	Protein tyrosine phosphatase
PUFA	Polyunsaturated fatty acids
PUPPP	Pruritic urticarial papules and plaques of pregnancy
QoL	Quality of life
QST	Quantitative sensory testing
QWB	Quality of well-being
RA	Rheumatoid arthritis
RC	Respiratory control
RCS	Reactive chlorine species
RNP	Ribonucleoprotein
RNS	Reactive nitrogen species
$ROO^{·-}$	Peroxyl radical
ROS	Reactive oxygen species
RR	Relative risk
RSS	Reactive sulfur species
RVVC	Recurrent vulvovaginal candidiasis
SASP	Senescence-associated phenotype
SCC	Squamous cell carcinoma
SERMs	Selective estrogen receptor modulators
SHBG	Sex hormone-binding globulin
SLE	Systemic lupus erythematosus
SLEDAI	SLE Disease Activity Index
SM	Sphingomyelin
SNP	Single nucleotide polymorphisms
SNRIs	Selective norepinephrine reuptake inhibitor
SOD	Superoxide dismutase
SS	Sjögren's syndrome
SSRIs	Selective serotonin reuptake inhibitor
STAT4	Signal transducer and activator of transcription 4

STS	Skin tensile strength
SWAN	Study of Woman's Health Across the Nation
T1DM	Type 1 diabetes mellitus
TA	Traction alopecia
TBG	Thyroid binding globulin
TDA	Transdermal administration
TET	Transdermal estrogen therapy
TEWL	Trans-epidermal water loss
Tfh cell	Follicular helper T cell
Th	T helper cell
TIMP	Tissue inhibitors of metalloproteinases
TLR	Toll-like receptors
TMD	Temporomandibular joint and muscle disorder
TNF-α	Tumor necrosis factor-alpha
TNF-β	Tumor necrosis factor-beta
TPO	Thyroid peroxidase autoantibody
Treg	Regulatory T cells
TSECs	Tissue selective estrogen complexes
UC	Ulcerative colitis
UDCA	Ursodeoxycholic acid
UQOL	Utian Quality of Life
UTR	Untranslated region
UV	Ultraviolet
VMI	Vaginal Maturation Index
VMS	Vasomotor symptoms
VTE	Venous thromboembolism
VVA	Vulvovaginal atrophy
VVC	Vulvovaginal candidiasis
VVS	Vulvar vestibular syndrome
WCA	Women climacteric aging
WHI	Women's Health Initiative
WHO	World Health Organization
WHOQOL	World Health Organization Quality of Life
WHQ	Women's Health Questionnaire

Contents

Part I Skin, Physiological Changes, and Menopause

1. **What Is Menopause? An Overview of Physiological Changes** 3
   Aikaterini E. Deliveliotou

2. **Skin and Menopause** 15
   Elisangela S.P. Pereira, Stéphanie Barros Langen,
   Maria C. Fidelis, Margareth O. Pereira, and Adilson Costa

3. **Skin Changes in Menopause** 25
   Renata Saucedo, Arturo Zárate,
   and Marcelino Hernández-Valencia

4. **Menopause and Oxidative Stress** 33
   Martha A. Sánchez-Rodríguez, Mariano Zacarías-Flores,
   and Víctor Manuel Mendoza-Núñez

5. **The Effect of Cytokines on Skin During Menopause** 53
   Marika Borg and Jean Calleja-Agius

6. **The Role of Estrogen Deficiency in Skin Aging and Wound Healing** 71
   Charis R. Saville and Matthew J. Hardman

7. **Skin and Effect of Hormones and Menopause** 89
   Miranda A. Farage, Kenneth W. Miller, Ghebre E. Tzeghai,
   Enzo Berardesca, and Howard I. Maibach

8. **Effects of Hormone Replacement Therapy on Skin Viscoelasticity During Climacteric Aging** 97
   Gérald E. Piérard, Trinh Hermanns-Lê, Sébastien Piérard,
   and Claudine Piérard-Franchimont

9. **Frontal Fibrosing Alopecia** 105
   Alexandra Katsarou-Katsari and Konstantina M. Papagiannaki

10. **Female-Specific Pruritus from Childhood to Postmenopause: Clinical Features, Hormonal Factors, and Treatment Considerations** 111
    Lauren P. Rimoin, Gil Yosipovitch, and Marilynne McKay

11 **Gender Differences in Production and Circulating Levels of Sex Hormones and Their Impact on Aging Skin** 125
Miranda A. Farage, Kenneth W. Miller, Christos C. Zouboulis, Gérald E. Piérard, and Howard I. Maibach

12 **Hair Changes Caused by Aging** 151
Caroline Romanelli, Ellem T.S. Weimann, Felipe B.C. Santos, and Adilson Costa

13 **Changes in Nails Caused by Aging** 163
Ana Carolina B.B. Arruda, Aline S. Talarico, Felipe B.C. Santos, and Adilson Costa

Part II Hormonal Change and Therapy

14 **Atrophic Vaginitis in the Menopause** 175
Ryan Sobel and Jack D. Sobel

15 **Sensory Perception on the Vulva and Extragenital Sites** 181
Miranda A. Farage, Kenneth W. Miller, Denniz A. Zolnoun, and William J. Ledger

Part III Menopause and Genital Health

16 **Gynaecological Problems Associated with Menopause** 199
Aikaterini E. Deliveliotou

17 **Changes to Skin with Aging and the Effects of Menopause and Incontinence** 209
Miranda A. Farage, Kenneth W. Miller, Enzo Berardesca, Nabil A.M. Naja, Ghebre E. Tzeghai, and Howard I. Maibach

18 **Current and Emerging Treatment Options for Vulvovaginal Atrophy** 229
Jill M. Krapf, Zoe Belkin, Frank Dreher, and Andrew T. Goldstein

19 **Implications of the Vulvar Sensitive Skin Syndrome After Menopause** 237
Paul R. Summers

20 **Vulval Disease in Postmenopausal Women** 249
Allan B. MacLean and Maxine Chan

21 **Vulvodynia in Menopause** 275
Miranda A. Farage, Kenneth W. Miller, Nancy Phillips, Micheline Moyal-Barracco, and William J. Ledger

22 **Dermatologic Conditions of the Vulva During Menopause** ... 285
Caroline D. Lynch and Nancy Phillips

Part IV Menopause and Autoimmune Disease

23 The Effects of Menopause on Autoimmune Diseases 299
Miranda A. Farage, Kenneth W. Miller, and Howard I. Maibach

24 Genes, Hormones, Immunosenescence, and Environmental Agents: Toward an Integrated View of the Genesis of Autoimmune Disease 319
Miranda A. Farage, Kenneth W. Miller, and Robert G. Lahita

25 Menopause and Aging Skin in the Elderly 345
Camil Castelo-Branco and Jhery Davila

26 Autoimmune Skin Diseases: Role of Sex Hormones, Vitamin D, and Menopause 359
DeLisa Fairweather

Part V Menopause, Quality of Life, and Healthy Aging

27 Postmenopausal Vulva and Vagina 385
Miranda A. Farage, Kenneth W. Miller, and Howard I. Maibach

28 Physical Activity and Quality of Life During Menopausal Transition and Postmenopause 397
Kirsi Mansikkamäki and Riitta M. Luoto

29 Quality of Life 405
Maria Celeste O. Wender and Patrícia Pereira de Oliveira

30 Vasomotor Symptoms 415
Maria Celeste O. Wender and Patrícia Pereira de Oliveira

31 The Menopausal Transition and Women's Health 433
Nancy Fugate Woods and Ellen Sullivan Mitchell

Part VI Menopause and Cosmetic Procedures

32 Menopause and Cosmeceuticals 455
Estela G. de Nóvoa, Raquel Fávaro, Thaísa S.T. Silvino,
Fernanda C.N. Ribeiro, Raissa M. Santos, and Adilson Costa

33 Cosmetic Procedures in Menopause 479
Renan Lage, Maria da Glória Samartin Sasseron, Elisa Moraes,
Erica B. Botero, Lissa S. De Matos, and Adilson Costa

Part VII Menopause and Global Considerations

34 Menopause: Cross-Cultural Considerations 495
Paula R. DeCola

Contributors

Ana Carolina B.B. Arruda, MD Department of Dermatology, Pontifical Catholic University of Campinas, Campinas, São Paulo, Brazil

Zoe Belkin Department of Obstetrics and Gynecology, George Washington University School of Medicine and Health Sciences, Washington, DC, USA

Enzo Berardesca, MD Clinical Dermatology, San Gallicano Dermatological Institute, Rome, Italy

Marika Borg Department of Anatomy, Faculty of Medicine and Surgery, University of Malta, Msida, Malta

Erica B. Botero, MD Department of Dermatology, Pontifical Catholic University of Campinas, Campinas, São Paulo, Brazil

Jean Calleja-Agius, MD, MRCOG, MRCPI, PhD Department of Anatomy, Faculty of Medicine and Surgery, University of Malta, Msida, Malta

Camil Castelo-Branco, MD, PhD Faculty of Medicine, Clinic Institute of Gynecology, Obstetrics and Neonatology, University of Barcelona, Hospital Clinic, Institut D'Investigacions Biomèdiques August Pi Sunyer, Barcelona, Spain

Maxine Chan, MB, BS, BSc Department of Obstetrics and Gynaecology, University College Hospital, London, UK

Adilson Costa, MD, MSc, PhD Department of Dermatology, Pontifical Catholic University of Campinas, Campinas, São Paulo, Brazil

Paula R. DeCola, RN, MSc External Medical Affairs, Pfizer Inc, New York, NY, USA

Aikaterini E. Deliveliotou, MD, PhD Department of Obstetrics and Gynaecology, "Aretaieion" University Hospital of Athens' Medical School, Athens, Greece

Lissa S. De Matos, MD Department of Dermatology, Pontifical Catholic University of Campinas, Campinas, São Paulo, Brazil

Frank Dreher NEOGYN Inc., Troy, MI, USA

DeLisa Fairweather, PhD Department of Environmental Health Sciences, Johns Hopkins Bloomberg School of Public Health, Baltimore, MD, USA

Miranda A. Farage, MSc, PhD Clinical Innovative Sciences, The Procter and Gamble Company, Cincinnati, OH, USA

Raquel Fávaro, MD Department of Dermatology, Pontifical Catholic University of Campinas, Campinas, São Paulo, Brazil

Maria C. Fidelis, MD Department of Dermatology, Pontifical Catholic University of Campinas, Campinas, São Paulo, Brazil

Claudine Piérard-Franchimont, MD, PhD Department of Dermatopathology, University Hospital of Liege, Liege, Belgium

Nancy Fugate Woods, PhD, BSN, MN Biobehavioral Nursing, University of Washington, Seattle, WA, USA

Margery L.S. Gass, MD Department of Obstetrics and Gynecology, Cleveland Clinic Lerner College of Medicine of Case Western Reserve University, Mayfield Heights, OH, USA

Andrew T. Goldstein, MD Department of Obstetrics and Gynecology, Center for Vulvovaginal Diseases, Washington, DC, USA

Jhery O. Davila Guardia, MD Faculty of Medicine, Clinic Institute of Gynecology, Obstetrics and Neonatology, University of Barcelona, Hospital Clinic, Institut D'Investigacions Biomèdiques August Pi Sunyer, Barcelona, Spain

Matthew J. Hardman, PhD The Healing Foundation Centre, Faculty of Life Sciences, University of Manchester, Manchester, UK

Trinh Hermanns-Lê, MD, PhD Department of Dermatopathology, University of Liege, Liege, Belgium

Marcelino Hernández-Valencia, MD, PhD Endocrine Research Unit, Instituto Mexicano Seguro Social, Mexico City, Mexico

Alexandra Katsarou-Katsari, MD, PhD Department of Dermatology, University Clinic, "A. Syggros" Hospital, National Kapodistian University of Athens, Athens, Greece

Jill M. Krapf, MD Department of Obstetrics and Gynecology, George Washington University, Washington, DC, USA

Renan Lage, MD Department of Dermatology, Pontifical Catholic University of Campinas, Campinas, São Paulo, Brazil

Robert G. Lahita, MD, PhD Department of Medicine, Newark Beth Israel Medical Center, Newark, NJ, USA

Stéphanie Barros Langen, MD Department of Dermatology, Pontifical Catholic University of Campinas, Campinas, São Paulo, Brazil

William J. Ledger, MD Department of Obstetrics and Gynecology, Weill Medical College, New York, NY, USA

Riitta M. Luoto, MD, PhD UKK Institute for Health Promotion, Tampere, Finland

Caroline D. Lynch, MD Department of Obstetrics, Gynecology, and Reproductive Sciences, Rutgers-Robert Wood Johnson Medical School, New Brunswick, NJ, USA

Marilynne McKay, MD Department of Dermatology, Emory University School of Medicine, Atlanta, GA, USA

Allan B. MacLean, BMedSc, MD, FRCOG, FRCP Edin Department of Obstetrics and Gynaecology, Royal Free Campus, University College London, London, UK

Howard I. Maibach, MD Department of Dermatology, University of California, School of Medicine, San Francisco, CA, USA

Kirsi Mansikkamäki, MS UKK Institute for Health Promotion, Tampere University of Applied Sciences, Tampere, Finland

Víctor Manuel Mendoza-Núñez, PhD Unidad de Investigación en Gerontología, Facultad de Estudios Superiores Zaragoza, Universidad Nacional Autónoma de México, México City, Mexico

Kenneth W. Miller, PhD Global Product Stewardship, The Procter and Gamble Company, Cincinnati, OH, USA

Ellen Sullivan Mitchell, PhD, BSN, MN Family and Child Nursing, University of Washington, Seattle, WA, USA

Elisa Moraes, MD Department of Dermatology, Pontifical Catholic University of Campinas, Campinas, São Paulo, Brazil

Micheline Moyal-Barracco, MD Department of Dermatology, Hôpital Tarnier Cochin, Paris, France

Nabil A.M. Naja, MD Department of Geriatrics, Dar Alajaza Hospital, Beirut, Lebanon

Estela G. de Nóvoa, MD Department of Dermatology, Pontifical Catholic University of Campinas, Campinas, São Paulo, Brazil

Patrícia Pereira de Oliveira, PhD Department of Medicine, University Unochapecó, Chapecó, Santa Catarina, Brazil

Konstantina M. Papagiannaki, MD Dermatology Department, Sismanoglio General Hospital, Athens, Greece

Elisangela S.P. Pereira, MD Department of Dermatology, Pontifical Catholic University of Campinas, Campinas, São Paulo, Brazil

Margareth O. Pereira, MD Department of Dermatology, Pontifical Catholic University of Campinas, Campinas, São Paulo, Brazil

Nancy Phillips, MD Department of Obstetrics, Gynecology and Reproductive Science, Rutgers-Robert Wood Johnson Medical School, New Brunswick, NJ, USA

Gérald E. Piérard, MD, PhD Department of Dermatopathology, University Hospital of Liege, Liege, Belgium

Sébastien Piérard, MD, PhD Telecommunications and Imaging Laboratory, Montefiore Institute, Intelsig, University of Liege, Liege, Belgium

Fernanda C.N. Ribeiro, MD Dermatology Research, KOLderma Clinical Trials Institute, Campinas, São Paulo, Brazil

Lauren P. Rimoin, MD Department of Dermatology, Emory University, Atlanta, GA, USA

Maria Glória da Samartin Sasseron Department of Dermatology, Pontifical Catholic University of Campinas, Campinas, São Paulo, Brazil

Martha A. Sánchez-Rodríguez, PhD Unidad de Investigación en Gerontología, Facultad de Estudios Superiores Zaragoza, Universidad Nacional Autónoma de México, Mexico City, Mexico

Caroline Romanelli, MD Department of Dermatology, Pontifical Catholic University of Campinas, Campinas, São Paulo, Brazil

Felipe B.C. Santos, MD Department of Dermatology, Pontifical Catholic University of Campinas, Campinas, São Paulo, Brazil

Raíssa M. Santos, MD Dermatology Research, KOLderma Clinical Trials Institute, Campinas, São Paulo, Brazil

Renata Saucedo, PhD Endocrine Research Unit, Instituto Mexicano Seguro Social, Mexico City, Mexico

Charis R. Saville, BSc, PhD The Healing Foundation Centre, Faculty of Life Sciences, University of Manchester, Manchester, UK

Thaísa S.T. Silvino, MD Department of Dermatology, Pontifical Catholic University of Campinas, Campinas, São Paulo, Brazil

Jack D. Sobel, MD Division of Infectious Diseases, Department of Internal Medicine, Wayne State University School of Medicine, Detroit Medical Center, Detroit, MI, USA

Ryan Sobel, MD Department of Obstetrics and Gynecology, Jefferson Medical College, Jefferson University Hospitals, Philadelphia, PA, USA

Paul R. Summers, MD Department of Obsterics and Gynecology, University of Utah School of Medicine, Salt Lake City, UT, USA

Aline S. Talarico, MD Department of Dermatology, Pontifical Catholic University of Campinas, Campinas, São Paulo, Brazil

Ghebre E. Tzeghai, PhD Quantitative Sciences and Innovation, Corporate R&D, The Procter and Gamble Company, Mason, OH, USA

Ellem T.S. Weimann, MD Department of Dermatology, Pontifical Catholic University of Campinas, Campinas, Sao Paulo, Brazil

Maria Celeste O. Wender, MD, PhD Department of Obstetrics and Gynecology, Menopause Clinic of Hospital de Clinicas de Porto Alegre, Federal University of Rio Grande do Sul, Porto Alegre, Rio Grande do Sul, Brazil

Gil Yosipovitch, MD Department of Dermatology, Itch Center, Temple University, Philadelphia, PA, USA

Mariano Zacarías-Flores, MD Obstetrics-Gynecology Department, Hospital Gustavo Baz Prada, Instituto de Salud del Estado de México, Mexico City, Mexico

Arturo Zárate, MD, PhD Endocrine Research Unit, Instituto Mexicano Seguro Social, Mexico City, Mexico

Denniz A. Zolnoun, MD, MPH Department of Obstetrics and Gynecology, Clinical Core and Pelvic Pain Research Center, The Center for Neurosensory Disorder, The University of North Carolina at Chapel Hill, Chapel Hill, NC, USA

Christos C. Zouboulis, MD Departments of Dermatology, Venereology, Allergology and Immunology, Dessau Medical Center, Dessau, Saxony-Anhalt, Germany

Part I

Skin, Physiological Changes, and Menopause

What Is Menopause? An Overview of Physiological Changes

Aikaterini E. Deliveliotou

Contents

1.1	Introduction	3
1.2	**Definitions: Terminology**	3
1.2.1	Menopause	4
1.2.2	Perimenopause	4
1.2.3	Menopausal Transition	4
1.2.4	Postmenopausal Period	5
1.2.5	Time of Natural Menopause	5
1.2.6	Induced Menopause	5
1.2.7	Premature Menopause	6
1.3	**Physiology of the Normal Menopause**	6
1.4	**Endocrinology of the Normal Menopause**	8
1.4.1	Estrogens	10
1.4.2	Progesterone	10
1.4.3	Androgens	10
1.4.4	Diagnosis of Menopause	11
1.5	**Stages of Reproductive Aging**	11
1.5.1	Late Reproductive Stage (Stage −3)	11
1.5.2	Early Menopausal Transition (Stage −2)	12
1.5.3	Late Menopausal Transition (Stage −1)	12
1.5.4	Early Postmenopause (Stage +1a, +1b, +1c)	12
1.5.5	Late Postmenopause (Stage +2)	13
1.6	**Summary**	13
	References	13

A.E. Deliveliotou, MD, PhD
Department of Obstetrics and Gynaecology,
"Aretaieion" University Hospital of Athens'
Medical School, 121, Vasilissis Sofias Avenue,
Athens Gr-11521, Greece
e-mail: kdeliveliotou@hotmail.com

1.1 Introduction

The extension of life and population aging are world-changing events that will have profound impacts on generations to come. In 1990 there were an estimated 467 million women aged 50 years and over in the world. This number is expected to increase to 1,200 million by the year 2030 [1]. More than 30 % of the female population of the United States is currently postmenopausal, and this percentage is predicted to increase in the next decades [2]. These demographic trends will exacerbate the economic and social challenges as well as the medical and psychological implications posed by a growing female, elderly population [3]. But if the extension of life achieved in the coming decades can be converted into healthy productive years, then these challenges could be counterbalanced by an equal measure of opportunity and the emergence of a dynamic and equitable aging society.

Because the loss of ovarian function has profound impact on the hormonal milieu in women and on the subsequent risk for the development of disease via the loss of estrogen production, improving our understanding of reproductive aging is critical to care for all women.

1.2 Definitions: Terminology

Reproductive aging is a continuum beginning in utero and ending with menopause. The stages along this continuum have been difficult to define.

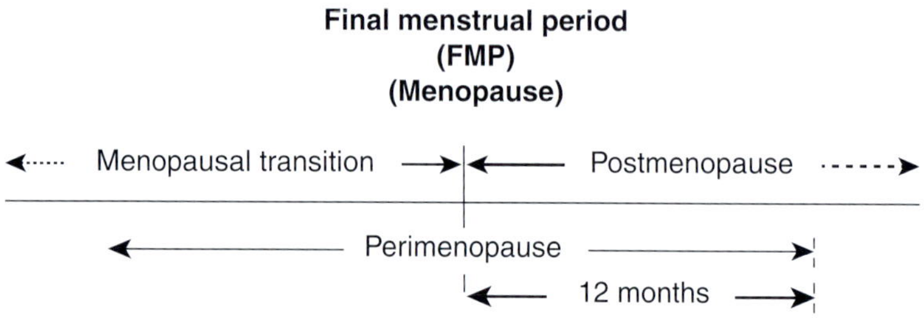

Fig. 1.1 Relationship between different time periods surrounding the menopause. (Reproduced, with permission of the publisher, from World Health Organization Scientific Group. Research on the menopause in the 1990s [5])

Numerous terms have been used clinically, including perimenopause, menopausal transition, climacteric, menopause, and postmenopause, to describe the various nodal points surrounding the menopause. In 1980, a WHO Scientific Group on Research on the Menopause proposed some definitions, in order to be used in studies and reports on the menopause and to extract comparable findings, and there are shown in Fig. 1.1 [4].

1.2.1 Menopause

Menopause is the most identifiable event of the perimenopausal period and should be characterized as an event rather than a period of time. The most widely used definition for natural menopause is as defined by the World Health Organization as at least 12 consecutive months of amenorrhea not because of surgery or other obvious causes [5]. When referring to menopausal age or onset of menopause in this chapter, we mean natural menopause as defined above. This cessation of menses resulting from the loss of ovarian function is a natural event, a part of the normal process of aging, and is physiologically correlated with the decline in estrogen production resulting from the loss of ovarian follicular function and therefore represents the end of a woman's reproductive life.

1.2.2 Perimenopause

The perimenopausal period includes the time before, during, and after menopause, when the endocrinological, biological, and clinical features of approaching menopause commence. The years immediately preceeding and the decades afterward, however, are of far greater clinical significance. The length of this period varies, but it is usually considered to last approximately 7 years, beginning with the decline in ovarian function in a woman's 40s and continuing until she has not had a menstrual period for 1 year [6]. Perimenopause usually begins in the mid- to late 40s; it is often uneventful but may be abrupt and symptomatic. The term "climacteric" should be abandoned to avoid confusion. Symptoms that begin with the menopausal transition usually continue into the postmenopausal period.

1.2.3 Menopausal Transition

The period of hormonal transition that precedes menopause is sometimes known as the menopausal transition period and is characterized by a varying degree of somatic changes that reflect alterations in the normal functioning of the ovary. Early recognition of the symptoms and the use of appropriate screening tests can minimize the impact of this potentially disruptive period [6]. In many cases, however, it is difficult to differentiate stress-related symptoms from those associated with decreasing levels of estrogen. For this reason, both stress and relative estrogen deficiency should be considered when managing problems associated with the menopausal transition.

In some women, menstrual irregularity is the most significant symptom of the menopausal transition [7]. Because abnormal bleeding is one of the most common symptoms of uterine problems, menstrual irregularity during the perimenopause should be evaluated carefully. Often uterine bleeding associated with this transition period is secondary to normal physiologic estrogen fluctuations rather than underlying pathology and may be treated medically [8].

1.2.4 Postmenopausal Period

The postmenopausal period is one of relative ovarian quiescence following menopause [4, 6]. Given the current lifespan of women in the United States, this period can comprise more than one-third of the average woman's life. During this prolonged period, women are susceptible to health problems associated with estrogen deficiency that tend to be chronic rather than acute. First of all osteoporosis is not clinically apparent until decades after menopause, when unfortunately it becomes harder to treat. Additionally, the impact of estrogen deficiency on cardiovascular disease is often confused with age-related changes, while, because of the peripheral conversion of both ovarian and adrenal androgens to estrogen, the loss of ovarian function does not result in an acute estrogen deficiency in all women.

1.2.5 Time of Natural Menopause

Natural menopause occurs at a median age of 51.4 years and is more or less normally distributed with a range roughly between 42 and 58 years [7, 9, 10]. However, there is no way to predict when an individual woman will have menopause or begin having symptoms suggestive of menopause. The average age of menopause has remained invariable during the last decades.

Environmental factors explain only a small part of the age variance at which menopause commences [11]. The variation in natural menopause is a trait predominantly determined by interaction of multiple genes, whose identity and causative genetic variation remains to be determined. Based on the fact that there is a strong association between age at menopause between mothers and daughters, it is suggested that there might be a largely genetically determined trait [12]. Furthermore, the onset of menopause does not appear to be related significantly to race, parity, height, weight, socioeconomic status, nutritional status, or age at menarche [13]. On the other hand the interaction among environmental factors such as smoking (known to accelerate the age of menopause by 1.5–2 years), body mass index (BMI), alcohol use, and socioeconomic status and genetic risk may be important [14]. As a result, it has been noticed that menopause occurs earlier in nulliparous women, in tobacco smokers, and in some women who have had hysterectomies [11, 15].

1.2.6 Induced Menopause

There are some medical and surgical conditions that can influence the timing of menopause. The term induced menopause is defined as the cessation of menstruation which follows either surgical removal of both ovaries or iatrogenic ablation of ovarian function by chemotherapy or radiation.

1.2.6.1 Surgical Menopause
It is called the surgical removal of the ovaries (oophorectomy) throughout reproductive period and results in an immediate cessation of estrogen production. In more than 40 % of women who have hysterectomies, both ovaries are removed, and this is usually performed at a significantly younger age than the age of natural menopause. In this case, there is no perimenopause, and after surgery, hot flashes and other acute symptoms associated with the perimenopausal period often become especially intense [15]. In addition, long-term surgical menopause has been associated with significantly higher risk for osteoporosis than has natural menopause [16]. On the other hand, recent data suggest that surgical menopause is not a key determinant of cardiovascular disease (CVD) risk factor status either before or after elective surgery in midlife [17]. These results should provide reassurance to women and their clinicians that hysterectomy in midlife is

unlikely to accelerate the CVD risk of women, in contrast to older reports that women with a hysterectomy had a worse risk profile and higher prevalence and incidence of CVD [18]. If a hysterectomy is not accompanied by the removal of both ovaries in a woman who has not yet reached menopause, the remaining ovary or ovaries are still capable of normal hormone production. In this case, a woman cannot menstruate but hormonal production from the ovaries can continue up until the normal time when menopause would naturally occur. At that time women could report the other symptoms of menopause such as mood swings and hot flashes, which are not therefore associated with the cessation of menstruation.

1.2.6.2 Cancer Chemotherapy and Radiation Therapy

Chemotherapy and/or radiation therapy in a woman of reproductive age can result in menopause. The effect of such a treatment on ovarian function is directly depended on the type and location of the cancer as well as the toxicity of the medications used [19]. In this case, the symptoms of menopause may begin during the cancer treatment or may develop in the months following the treatment, independently of the woman's age.

1.2.7 Premature Menopause

Premature menopause or premature ovarian failure (POF) is defined as the spontaneous occurrence of menopause before the age of 40, occurring in 0.1 % of women under 30 years of age and 1 % of women by age 40 [20, 21]. This definition is rather arbitrary, because it is based on age only. POF is a collective term for which proposed causes include autoimmune disease, syndromes such as fragile X, or inherited (genetic) factors [22]. Genetic factors are thought to have a strong association with POF. Among patients with idiopathic POF, a higher incidence of family history of early menopause and infertility has been noted so that a familial transmission is observed in 30–40 % [23]. Although inheritance appears to be either X-linked or autosomal dominant sex limited, paternal transmission cannot be excluded. Furthermore, women with POF have a genetic pattern similar to whose with idiopathic early menopause (between the ages of 40 and 45), suggesting the existence of common underlying causal factors in both entities. Women with premature menopause are at risk of premature death, neurological diseases, psychosexual dysfunction, mood disorders, osteoporosis, ischemic heart disease, and infertility. Public enlightenment and education is important tool to save those at risk [24].

1.3 Physiology of the Normal Menopause

The ovary is unique in that the age associated with decline in function (to complete failure) appears to have remained relatively constant despite the increase in longevity experienced by women over the last century [25]. The primary determinant of reproductive age in women is the number of ovarian nongrowing (primordial, intermediate and primary) follicles (NGFs). The leading theory regarding the onset of menopause relates to a critical threshold in oocyte number and particularly the number of ovarian follicles present in the ovary. Therefore, the number of ovarian granulosa cells available for hormone secretion appears to be the most critical determinant of age at menopause, steroid hormone secretion, and gonadotrophin levels [26].

Human follicles begin their development during the fourth gestational month. Approximately 1,000–2,000 germ cells migrate to the gonadal ridge and multiply, reaching a total of five to seven million around the fifth month of intrauterine life [27, 28]. In female fetus, between the 12th and 18th week, the germ cells will enter meiosis and differentiate so that all germ stem cells have differentiated prior to birth. At this point, replication stops and follicle loss begins so that the population of NGFs is estimated to be approximately 500,000–1 million at birth, which represents the initial NGF endowment in women. At menarche 500,000–600,000 follicles exist, while in the adult woman through a combination of recruitment toward dominant follicle development and ovulation or atresia, the stock of NGFs is depleted [29, 30]. The pioneering work of these investigators led to the understanding that ovarian follicle number decreases with increasing age and that ultimately few, if any, follicles remain following menopause [31, 32].

Using the combined data from these studies, it has been suggested that the decline in ovarian follicles associated with aging was best described by a biphasic-exponential model, which was better fitted to the data than either a linear or single exponential model, as shown in Fig. 1.2 [33]. In this model, the total follicular endowment at birth is estimated to be 952,000, with an initial rate of decay of −0.097. At the age of 38 years and a follicle count of 25,000, a sudden increase in decay occurs to over twofold the initial rate (−0.237).

At this point, the rate of follicular atresia accelerates. In the absence of this acceleration, the model suggests menopause would be delayed until age 71. The unexpectedly faster rate of ovarian aging afterwards lowers the follicle population to 1,000 at approximately 51 years and is adopted as the menopausal threshold as it corresponds to the median age of menopause. The cause of this accelerated depletion is not well defined. It is also clear that if the factor influencing the rate of decline is follicle number and not age, other factors which might account for a diminished follicle number (genetic risk and possible toxic exposure) would lead to an earlier rate of accelerated decline and an earlier age of menopause.

Realizing the biological implausibility of a sudden acceleration in follicular depletion, a

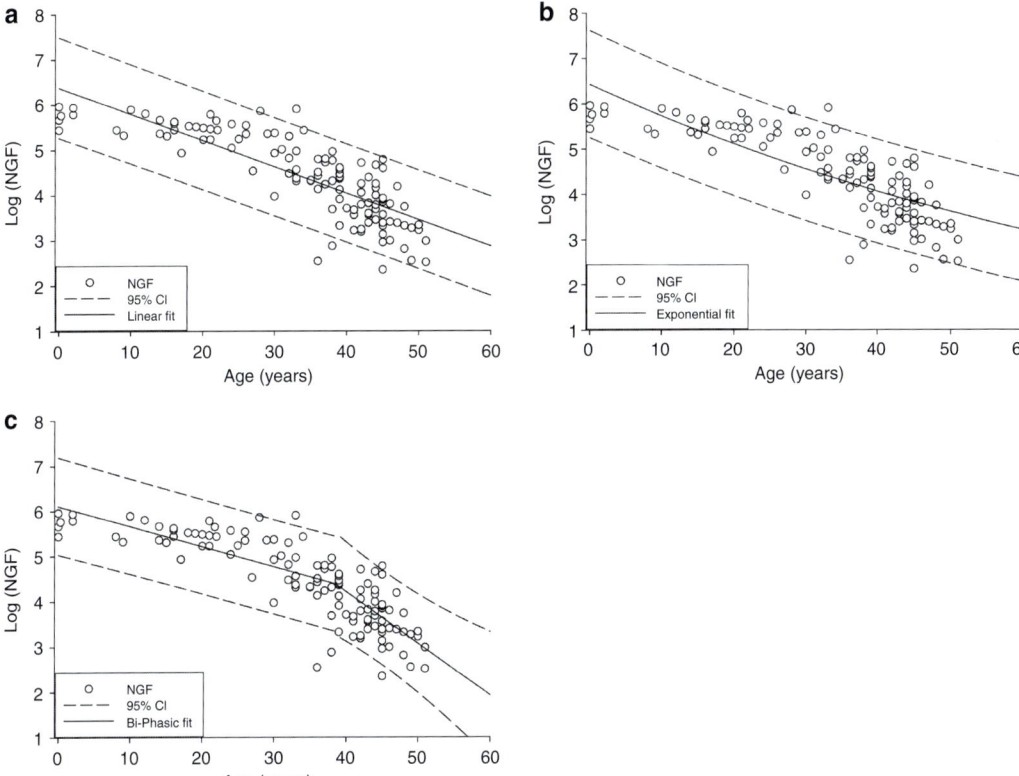

Fig. 1.2 Models of ovarian NGF decay. The log of the ovarian NGF number is plotted versus age (years). (**a**) Linear model, (**b**) exponential model, and (**c**) biphasic-exponential model. *Solid lines* indicate the fitted model with *dashed lines* representing the 95 % confidence interval ($n = 122$) (Reprinted from Hansen et al. [26], by permission of Oxford University Press)

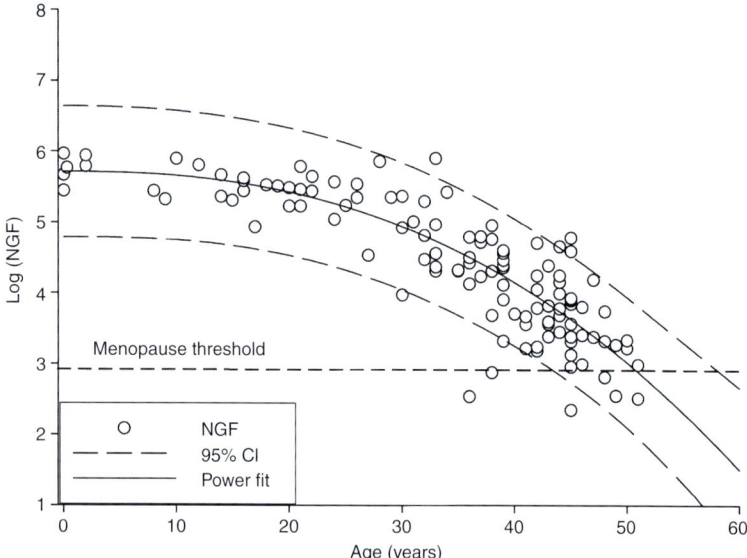

Fig. 1.3 Power model of ovarian NGF decay. The log of the ovarian NGF number is plotted versus age (years). The *solid line* indicates the fitted model with *dashed lines* representing the 95 % CI (Reprinted from Hansen et al. [26], by permission of Oxford University Press)

newer power model has been proposed [26]. This power model suggests that the decay of NGFs is constantly accelerating rather than suddenly increasing at 38 years as shown in Fig. 1.3. It suggests that age accounts for approximately 84 % of the variation in NGF count at different ages and agrees well with the known distribution of menopausal age but also is more biologically plausible than previous models.

The biology underlying the transition to menopause includes not only the profound decline in follicle numbers of the ovary but also a significant increase in random genetic damage within the ovaries. This is supported by the fact that in women over 40 years old, oocytes harvested for in vitro fertilization are karyotypically abnormal approximately 40 % of the time [34]. At the same time an increase in aneuploidy in the offspring of older mothers confirms the potential role of a genetic ovarian defect, while new information will have to accumulate before the factors governing human oocyte atresia are elucidated more clearly.

1.4 Endocrinology of the Normal Menopause

Menopause and the years preceding are characterized by cessation of ovarian function, concomitant hormonal changes, and monthly menstruation and are associated with the end of reproductive capability. The biological basis for these events is well established, being dependent on changes in ovarian structure and function. During the menopause, there is a reciprocal relationship between ovarian hormone levels, which decline, and pituitary gonadotrophins, which increase (Fig. 1.4) [35].

The ovarian hormones are divided into two classes: the steroids, primarily estradiol and progesterone and secondary androgens, and the peptides, primarily inhibins and activins. Estradiol and the peptide hormones are secretory products of the ovarian granulosa cells, the major cell type of ovarian follicle, whereas progesterone is a product of the corpus luteum. The primary biological properties of the peptide hormones are implied by their names; inhibin suppresses synthesis and secretion of pituitary follicle-stimulating hormone (FSH), whereas activin stimulates FSH secretion. In addition to FSH, the other relevant pituitary hormone is luteinizing hormone (LH), whose secretion is controlled primarily by the steroid hormones, whereas FSH is regulated by both the steroids and the peptide hormones [36].

FSH is an established indirect marker of follicular activity. In studies of groups of women, its concentration, particularly in the early follicular phase of the menstrual cycle, begins to increase some years before there are any clinical

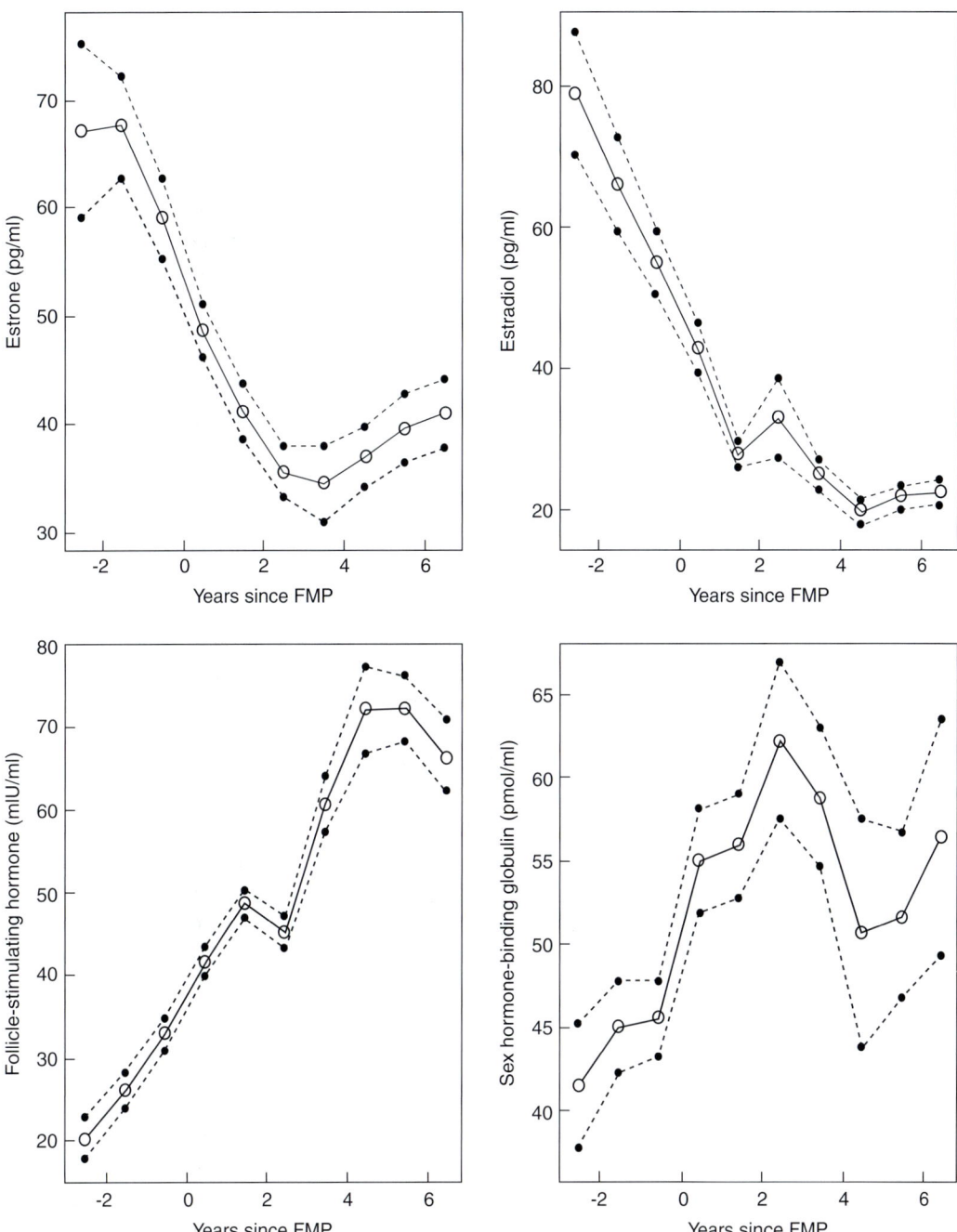

Fig. 1.4 Selected serum hormone levels versus years since final menstrual period (*FMP*). The *dotted lines* indicate the mean levels ± the standard error (Reprinted from Maturitas, 23/2, McKinlay [35], with permission from Elsevier)

indications of approaching menopause [37]. The rise in FSH is the result of declining levels of inhibin B (INH-B), a dimeric protein that reflects the fall in ovarian follicle numbers, with or without any change in the ability of the lining granulosa cells to secrete INH-B. Early on, there is also a decline in luteal phase progesterone levels. As ovarian aging progresses, estradiol levels may be quite variable, with chaotic patterns and, occasionally, very high and very low levels.

This dramatic variability may lead to an increase in symptomatology during the perimenopause. As peripheral gonadotrophin levels rise, LH pulsatile patterns become abnormal. There is an increase in pulse frequency with a decrease in opioid inhibition. As a result, during the transition, hormone levels frequently vary markedly – hence, measures of FSH and estradiol are unreliable guides to menopausal status.

1.4.1 Estrogens

The main circulating estrogen during the reproductive years is 17β-estradiol. Estradiol levels range from 50 to 300 pg/mL and are controlled by the developing follicle and resultant corpus luteum. It is estimated that 95 % of circulating estradiol is derived from the ovary, based on the fact that surgical removal of the ovaries reduces peripheral estradiol levels from 120 to 18 pg/mL. Additionally small amounts of estradiol are produced by the adrenal gland as well as by the peripheral conversion of testosterone and estrone [25].

Even though the amount of estrogen secreted by the postmenopausal ovary is insignificant, postmenopausal women continue to have measurable amounts of both estrone and estradiol [38]. Estrone and estradiol production rates in postmenopausal women are 40 and 6 μg/day, compared to 80 and 500 μg/day, respectively, during the reproductive years. After menopause the main circulating estrogen is estrone, which has a biologic activity approximately less than 30 % of estradiol activity and is mostly derived from peripheral conversion of androstenedione. Extraglandular aromatase is found in liver, fat, and some hypothalamic nuclei, and its activity increases with aging as well as with a higher fat content. Estradiol in the postmenopausal women is derived mainly from conversion of estrone.

1.4.2 Progesterone

Given that progesterone is produced by of the corpus luteum, its levels decline postmenopausally [39]. During the reproductive years, progesterone protects the endometrium from excess estrogen stimulation by directly regulating estrogen receptors, while exerts a direct intranuclear effect by inhibiting the trophic effects of estrogen on the endometrium [6]. Because circulating levels of estrogen can remain relatively high enough to stimulate the endometrium both pre- and postmenopausally, this unopposed stimulation of the endometrium just prior to and after menopause may explain the higher risk of endometrial hyperplasia and cancer reported during this time.

1.4.3 Androgens

The third class of steroids produced by the ovaries is androgens, particularly testosterone and androstenedione. During the reproductive years, the ovaries produce approximately 50 % of the circulating androstenedione, which is the predominant androgen at that period, and 25 % of the testosterone produced by a woman's body. After menopause, total androgen production decreases, mainly because ovarian production decreases but also because adrenal production decreases [38]. Androstenedione production declines from 1,500 to 800 pg/mL in postmenopausal women. The postmenopausal ovary contributes only 20 % to the circulating androstenedione. Testosterone levels also decline after menopause, but not to the same extent as estradiol levels. Postmenopausal testosterone is derived from the ovary (25 %), the adrenal gland (25 %), and extraglandular conversion from androstenedione (50 %). The postmenopausal ovary produces a larger percentage of testosterone (50 %) than does the premenopausal ovary.

Dehydroepiandrosterone (DHEA) and its sulfated conjugate, DHEA-S, have been shown to decrease, along with adrenal corticotropin responsiveness, with aging [6]. DHEA-S levels decrease in both men and women, but this decline is greater in women and may be due to the relative estrogen deprivation. Ovarian failure, at any age, accelerates this decline. Evidence suggests physiologic levels of DHEA may protect against neoplasia, enhance insulin action, protect against osteoporosis, increase immune competency, and offer some cardio protection. Changes in DHEA levels also have been associated with alterations in body composition which, in themselves, appear to impact cardiac and breast cancer risk. DHEA-S levels may also have an impact on "sense of mental well-being."

1.4.4 Diagnosis of Menopause

Traditionally, menopause has been diagnosed retrospectively based on the lack of menstrual periods for a 6-month period. With the advent of modern laboratory testing, menopause may now be more precisely defined as amenorrhea, with signs of hypoestrogenemia, and an elevated serum FSH level of greater than 40 IU/L. Menopause can also be diagnosed on the basis of subjective symptoms, such as hot flashes, or on the basis of provocative studies such as the progesterone withdrawal test. Hot flashes and other acute symptoms associated with the perimenopausal period often become more intense near menopause when the levels of circulating estrogen suddenly drop. These symptoms are especially intense in patients who experience premature ovarian failure or surgical menopause, which are accompanied by gradual drops in circulating estrogens.

1.5 Stages of Reproductive Aging

To address the lack of a pertinent reproductive staging system which takes into account endocrinology, menstrual cyclicity and symptomatology beginning with menarche and ending with a woman's demise, the Stages of Reproductive Aging Workshop (STRAW) was convened in July 2001 [40]. This workshop proposed a consistent reproductive aging system including menstrual and qualitative hormonal criteria to define each stage in order to be used as a nomenclature and guidelines, for health practitioners, the medical research community, and the public [41–44]. The foundation of the staging system is the final menstrual period (FMP). The STRAW staging system is widely considered the gold standard for characterizing reproductive aging through menopause, just as the Marshall-Tanner Stages characterize pubertal maturation [45]. Although this staging system was said to include endocrinologic aspects of ovarian aging, it was still dependent largely on menstrual cyclicity as a key indicator of ovarian aging, and it did not include measurement of FSH; however, by the time FSH is elevated, even with cyclic menstrual cycles, oocyte depletion already has proceeded to such an extent that fertility (as a marker of reproductive aging) is diminished significantly. Research conducted during the past 10 years has advanced knowledge of the critical changes in hypothalamic-pituitary and ovarian function that occur before and after the final menstrual period.

STRAW + 10 revised extended the STRAW recommendations to include additional criteria for defining specific stages of reproductive life [46]. The revised staging system provides a more comprehensive basis for classification and assessment, from the late reproductive stage through the menopausal transition and into postmenopause. Its application improves comparability of studies of midlife women by establishing clear criteria for ascertaining women's reproductive stage. According to STRAW + 10, five stages precede the FMP and two follow it, for a total of seven stages. Stages −5 to −3 are called the reproductive interval, stages −2 to −1 are termed the menopausal transition, and stages +1 and +2 are known as the postmenopause, as shown in Table 1.1.

1.5.1 Late Reproductive Stage (Stage −3)

The time when fecundability begins to decline and during which a woman may begin to notice changes in her menstrual cycles. It is subdivided into two substages (−3b and −3a). In Stage −3b, menstrual cycles remain regular without change in length or early follicular phase FSH levels; however, AMH, inhibin B, and antral follicle counts (AFC) are low. In Stage −3a, slightly

Table 1.1 The stages of reproductive aging in women

	Stage	Duration	Menstrual pattern	FSH	AMH	Inhibin B	Antral follicle count	Symptoms
Postmenopause	Late +2	Remaining lifespan						Urogenital atrophy
	Early +1c	3–6 years		Stabilize	Very low	Very low		
	Early +1b	1 year		High	Low	Low	Very low	Vasomotor symptoms most likely
	Early +1a	1 year		High	Low	Low	Very low	
Final menstrual period								
Menopausal transition	Late −1	1–3 years	Intervals of amenorrhea >60 days	High >25 iu/l	Low	Low	Low	Vasomotor symptoms likely
	Early −2	Variable	Variable length	High	Low	Low	Low	
Reproductive years	Late −3a		Slight changes in length flow	Low	Low	Low		
	Late −3b		Regular	Low	Low			
	Peak −4		Regular					
	Early −5		Variable regular					
Menarche								

shorter menstrual cycles are noticed. Early follicular phase FSH increases and becomes more variable, with the other three markers of ovarian aging being low.

1.5.2 Early Menopausal Transition (Stage −2)

The stage with variable menstrual cycle length, defined as a persistent difference of 7 days or more in the length of consecutive cycles. Persistence is defined as recurrence within 10 cycles of the first variable length cycle. During this stage elevated but variable early follicular phase FSH levels and low AMH levels and AFC are noticed.

1.5.3 Late Menopausal Transition (Stage −1)

This stage is marked by the occurrence of amenorrhea of 60 days or longer, with an increased variability in cycle length, extreme variation in hormonal levels, and increased prevalence of anovulation. Quantitative FSH criteria, with levels greater than 25 IU/L in a random blood draw, are characteristic of this stage. Symptoms, most notably vasomotor symptoms, are likely to occur during this stage. The duration of this stage is estimated to be, on average, 1–3 years.

1.5.4 Early Postmenopause (Stage +1a, +1b, +1c)

FSH continues to increase and estradiol continues to decrease until approximately 2 years after the FMP, after which the levels of each of these hormones stabilize. It is subdivided into three substages (+1a, +1b, and +1c).

Stage +1a marks the end of the 12-month period of amenorrhea required to define that the FMP has occurred and corresponds to the end of "perimenopause." "Perimenopause" is a term still in common usage that means the time around menopause and begins at Stage −2 and ends 12 months after the FMP.

Stage +1b includes the rest of the period of rapid changes in mean FSH and estradiol levels. Symptoms, most notably vasomotor symptoms, are most likely to occur during this stage. Each one of Stages +1a and +1b last 1 year and end at the time point at which FSH and estradiol levels stabilize.

Stage +1c is the period of stabilization of high FSH and low estradiol levels that is estimated to last 3–6 years; therefore, the entire early postmenopause lasts approximately 5–8 years.

1.5.5 Late Postmenopause (Stage +2)

The period in which further alterations in reproductive endocrine function are limited and somatic symptoms like urogenital atrophy and vaginal dryness become increasingly prevalent at this time. Nevertheless, many years after menopause, it has been observed that there may be a further decline in levels of FSH in very old persons.

1.6 Summary

1. Age at menopause is determined by the number of NGFs present in the ovary. The number of NGFs decreases from late fetal life onward and few, if any, remain in the ovary after menopause.
2. Granulosa cells in the ovarian follicle are the source of estrogens and inhibins, which have a reciprocal relationship through feedback mechanisms with FSH secretion and serum concentrations.
3. Estrogen levels decline and FSH levels rise during the menopausal transition and stabilize 3–6 years after the FMP.
4. Levels of steroid and peptide hormones and of gonadotrophins are unpredictable and variable during the menopausal transition and cannot be used to predict fertility or timing of menopause.
5. Serum testosterone and androstenedione decline at the time of menopause as the ovarian function declines, while DEHA-S levels decrease linearly with increasing age.

References

1. United Nations. World population ageing: 1950–2050. New York: Population Division, Department of Economic and Social Affairs; 2001. Available at http://www.un.org/esa/population/publications/worldageing19502050/accessed. 22 Sept 2009.
2. Kingkade WW, Torrey BB. The evolving demography of aging in the United States of America and the former USSR. World Health Stat Q. 1992;45:15–28.
3. Olshansky SJ, Goldman DP, Zheng Y, Rowe JW. Aging in America in the Twenty-first Century: demographic forecasts from the MacArthur Foundation Research Network on an Aging Society. Milbank Q. 2009;87(4):842–62.
4. Research on the menopause. Report of a WHO Scientific Group. Geneva: World Health Organization; 1981 (WHO Technical Report Series, No 670).
5. World Health Organization Scientific Group. Research on the menopause in the 1990s. World Health Organ Tech Rep Ser. 1996;866:1–107.
6. Berek JS. Chapter 29. In: Novac's gynecology. 13th ed. Baltimore: Lippincott Williams & Wilkins; 2002.
7. McKinlay SM, Brambilla DJ, Posner JG. The normal menopause transition. Maturitas. 1992;14:103–15.
8. McKinlay SM. The normal menopause transition. Maturitas. 1996;23:137–45.
9. Whelan EA, Sandler DP, McConnaughey DR, Weinberg CR. Menstrual and reproductive characteristics and age at natural menopause. Am J Epidemiol. 1990;131:625–8.
10. Morabia A, Costanza MC. International variability in ages at menarche, first livebirth, and menopause. World Health Organization Collaborative Study of Neoplasia and Steroid Contraceptives. Am J Epidemiol. 1998;148:1195–205.
11. Brambilla DJ, McKinlay SM. A prospective study of factors affecting age at menopause. J Clin Epidemiol. 1989;42:1031–9.
12. de Bruin JP, Bovenhuis H, van Noord PA, Pearson PL, van Arendonk JA, te Velde ER, Kuurman WW, Dorland M. The role of genetic factors in age at natural menopause. Hum Reprod. 2001;16(9):2014–8.
13. Meschia M, Pansini F, Modena AB, de Aloysio D, Gambacciani M, Parazzini F, et al. Determinants of age at menopause in Italy: results from a large cross-sectional study. ICARUS Study Group Italian Climacteric Res Group Study. Maturitas. 2000;34:119–25.
14. Midgette AS, Baron JA. Cigarette smoking and the risk of natural menopause. Epidemiology. 1990;1:474–80.
15. Siddle N, Sarrel P, Whitehead M. The effect of hysterectomy on the age at ovarian failure: identification of a subgroup of women with premature loss of ovarian function and literature review. Fertil Steril. 1987;47:94–100.
16. Hreshchyshyn MM, Hopkins A, Zylstra S, Anbar M. Effects of natural menopause, hysterectomy, and

16. oophorectomy on lumbar spine and femoral neck bone densities. Obstet Gynecol. 1988;72:631–8.
17. Matthews KA, Gibson CJ, El Khoudary SR, Thurston RC. Changes in cardiovascular risk factors by hysterectomy status with and without oophorectomy: study of Women's Health Across the Nation. J Am Coll Cardiol. 2013;62(3):191–200.
18. Howard BV, Kuller L, Langer R, Manson JE, Allen C, Assaf A, Cochrane BB, Larson JC, Lasser N, Rainford M, Van Horn L, Stefanick ML, Trevisan M, Women's Health Initiative. Risk of cardiovascular disease by hysterectomy status, with and without oophorectomy: the Women's Health Initiative Observational Study. Circulation. 2005;111(12):1462–70.
19. Meng K, Tian W, Zhou M, Chen H, Deng Y. Impact of chemotherapy-induced amenorrhea in breast cancer patients: the evaluation of ovarian function by menstrual history and hormonal levels. World J Surg Oncol. 2013;11:101.
20. Coulam CB, Anderson SC, Annegan JF. Incidence of premature ovarian failure. Obstet Gynecol. 1986;67:604–6.
21. Nelson LM. Clinical practice. Primary ovarian insufficiency. N Engl J Med. 2009;360:606–14.
22. Tibiletti MG, Testa G, Vegetti W, Alagna F, Taborelli M, Dalpra L, Bolis PF, Crosignani PG. The idiopathic forms of premature menopause and early menopause show the same genetic pattern. Hum Reprod. 1999;14:2731–4.
23. Vegetti W, Marozzi A, Manfredini E, Testa G, Alagna F, Nicolosi A, et al. Premature ovarian failure. Mol Cell Endocrinol. 2000;161:53–7.
24. Okeke T, Anyaehie U, Ezenyeaku C. Premature menopause. Ann Med Health Sci Res. 2013;3(1):90–5.
25. Scott JR, Gibbs RS, Karlan BY, Haney AF, Danforth DN. Chapter 41. In: Danforth's obstetrics and gynecology. 9th ed. Baltimore: Lippincott Williams & Wilkins; 2003.
26. Hansen KR, Knowlton NS, Thyer AC, Charleston JS, Soules MR, Klein NA. A new model of reproductive aging: the decline in ovarian non-growing follicle number from birth to menopause. Hum Reprod. 2008;23(3):699–708.
27. Forabosco A, Sforza C, DePol A, Vizzotto L, Marzona L, Ferrario VF. Morphometric study of the human neonatal ovary. Anat Rec. 1991;231:201–8.
28. Block E. A quantitative morphological investigation of the follicular system in newborn female infants. Acta Anat. 1953;17:201–6.
29. Block E. Quantitative morphological investigations of the follicular system in women: variations at different ages. Acta Anat. 1952;14 Suppl 16:108–23.
30. Gougeon A, Chainy GB. Morphometric studies of small follicles in ovaries of women at different ages. J Reprod Fertil. 1987;81:433–42.
31. Gougeon A, Ecochard R, Thalabard J. Age-related changes of the population of human ovarian follicles: increase in the disappearance rate of non-growing and early-growing follicles in aging women. Biol Reprod. 1994;50:653–63.
32. Richardson S, Senikas V, Nelson J. Follicular depletion during the menopausal transition: evidence for accelerated loss and ultimate exhaustion. J Clin Endocrinol Metab. 1987;65:1231–7.
33. Faddy M, Gosden R, Gougeon A, Richardson S, Nelson J. Accelerated disappearance of ovarian follicles in mid-life: implications for forecasting menopause. Hum Reprod. 1992;7:1342–6.
34. Liu J, Wang W, Sun X, Liu L, Jin H, Li M, et al. DNA microarray reveals that high proportions of human blastocysts from women of advanced maternal age are aneuploid and mosaic. Biol Reprod. 2012;87(6):148.
35. McKinlay SM. The normal menopause transition: an overview. Maturitas. 1996;23(2):137–45.
36. Burger HG. The endocrinology of the menopause. Maturitas. 1996;23(2):129–36.
37. Burger HG, Dudley EC, Robertson DM, Dennerstein L. Hormonal changes in the menopause transition. Recent Prog Horm Res. 2002;57:257–75.
38. Adashi EY. The climacteric ovary as a functional gonadotropin-driven androgen-producing gland. Fertil Steril. 1994;62:20–7.
39. Dennefors BL, Janson PO, Knutson F, Hamberger L. Steroid production and responsiveness to gonadotropin in isolated stromal tissue of human postmenopausal ovaries. Am J Obstet Gynecol. 1980;136:997–1002.
40. Soules MR, Sherman S, Parrott E, Rebar R, Santoro N, Utian W, et al. Stages of Reproductive Aging Workshop (STRAW). J Womens Gend Based Med. 2001;10:843–8.
41. Soules MR, Sherman S, Parrott E, Rebar R, Santoro N, Utian W, et al. Executive summary: Stages of Reproductive Aging Workshop (STRAW). Climacteric. 2001;4:267–72.
42. Soules MR, Sherman S, Parrott E, Rebar R, Santoro N, Utian W, et al. Stages of Reproductive Aging Workshop (STRAW). J Womens Health Gend Based Med. 2001;10:843–8.
43. Soules MR, Sherman S, Parrott E, Rebar R, Santoro N, Utian W, et al. Executive summary: Stages of Reproductive Aging Workshop (STRAW). Fertil Steril. 2001;76:874–8.
44. Soules MR, Sherman S, Parrott E, Rebar R, Santoro N, Utian W, et al. Executive summary: Stages of Reproductive Aging Workshop (STRAW) Park City, Utah, July, 2001. Menopause. 2001;8:402–7.
45. Marshall WA, Tanner JM. Variations in pattern of pubertal changes in girls. Arch Dis Child. 1969;44:291–303.
46. Harlow SD, Gass M, Hall JE, Lobo R, Maki P, Rebar RW, Sherman S, Sluss PM, de Villiers TJ. STRAW + 10 Collaborative Group. Executive summary of the Stages of Reproductive Aging Workshop + 10: addressing the unfinished agenda of staging reproductive aging. J Clin Endocrinol Metab. 2012;97(4):1159–68.

Skin and Menopause

Elisangela S.P. Pereira, Stéphanie Barros Langen, Maria C. Fidelis, Margareth O. Pereira, and Adilson Costa

Contents

2.1	The Postmenopause	15
2.2	The Skin	16
2.3	Estrogen	16
2.4	Estrogen and Postmenopause	17
2.5	Hormone Receptors and Skin	17
2.6	Skin Hydration	18
2.7	Skin Thickness and Postmenopause	18
2.8	Skin Collagen and Postmenopause	19
2.9	Skin Looseness and Wrinkling	19
2.10	Wound Healing in Postmenopause	19
2.11	Urogenital and Menopausal Problems	20
2.12	Atrophic Vaginitis	21
2.13	Menopausal Flushing	21
2.14	Hormone Replacement Therapy	22
References		22

E.S.P. Pereira, MD (✉) • S.B. Langen, MD
M.C. Fidelis, MD • M.O. Pereira, MD
A. Costa, MD, MSc, PhD
Department of Dermatology,
Pontifical Catholic University of Campinas,
Av. John Boyd Dunlop, Campinas,
São Paulo 13060-803, Brazil
e-mail: elisp7@gmail.com; the-langen@hotmail.com; carolfidelis@hotmail.com; margareth_med@yahoo.com.br; adilson_costa@hotmail.com

2.1 The Postmenopause

On average, women live about 30 years beyond postmenopause. Menopause is defined as the period of 12 months of amenorrhea after the last menstrual cycle. About 60–70 % of the visits to general practitioners and specialists are of people over the age of 60, mostly women [1]. Thus, hormonal influence in the skin aging process has drawn more and more attention. Several functions of the skin are known to be hormone dependent and, although the effects of estrogen on skin are not fully understood, the decline in estrogen is known to be associated with various skin disorders, many of which can be reversed through hormone replacement treatment [2, 3].

Studies involving postmenopausal women indicate that the decline in estrogen is associated with atrophy, fine wrinkles, scarring, and hot flushes. Other incidences may be the thinning of the epidermis, decrease of dermal collagen, sagging, and impaired wound healing [3]. The decline in estrogen reduces the mitotic activity of the basal layer of the epidermis and also modifies its lipid synthesis, causing xerosis [4]. Hormone replacement therapy (HRT) has beneficial effects on some of the lost properties of the skin and can slowdown the intrinsic aging process. The phenomenon of hormone-related skin aging has been demonstrated; however, to distinguish it from the effects of senescence, photoaging, and genetic and environmental aggressions is difficult [5]. It is our objective to present to you in this chapter some of the most important changes.

2.2 The Skin

The skin is the largest organ in the body, accounting for approximately 15 % of the total body weight of a human adult. It performs several vital functions to protect the body against environmental aggressions. This is made possible owing to the skin's elaborate structure, the ectodermal and mesodermal origin of its tissues, and its organization in three layers: the epidermis (and its appendages), the dermis, and the hypodermis [6].

Most dermal fibers (over 90 %) are made of interstitial collagen, mainly types I and III. The collagen fibers are responsible for the mechanical strength of the skin. Collagen is responsible for 98 % of the total dry weight of the dermis. On the other hand, the elastic fibers, which are responsible for the shrinking properties of the skin, are composed of elastin, an insoluble protein which is surrounded by a variable number of microfibrils. Viewed under electronic microscope, the elastic fibers show variations depending on age and exposure study area (whether exposed to the sun or not). The reticulin fibers consist of a group of biochemically fine collagen type I and III fibers, as well as fibronectin [6].

The effects of estrogen deficiency in postmenopausal women include: atrophy, decrease in collagen content and hydration, reduction in sebaceous secretions, loss of elasticity, and manifestations of hyperandrogenism (Fig. 2.1). The cumulative effects of estrogen deficiency contribute to poor wound healing in older patients and accelerated skin aging; however, it is difficult to distinguish between changes that occur specifically with age and those that occur as a result of estrogen deprivation [7].

2.3 Estrogen

Estrogen, the main steroid responsible for the secondary gender characteristics in females, affects most systems in the body. The skin is the largest nonreproductive estrogen target area [3].

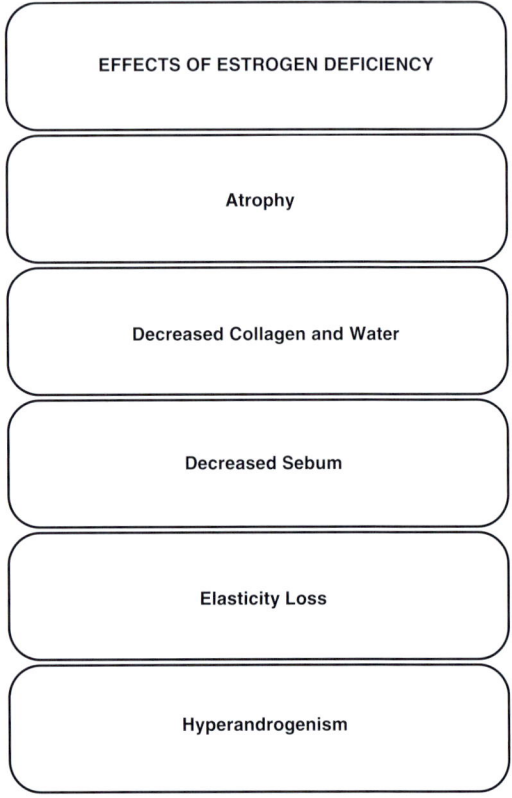

Fig. 2.1 Effects of estrogen deficiency

Estrogen production is regulated by the axle involving the hypothalamus, pituitary gland, and ovary. The pulsatile release of the gonadotropin-releasing hormone from the hypothalamus stimulates the pituitary gland to secrete luteinizing hormone (LH) and follicle-stimulating hormone (FSH). In the ovary, LH stimulates the theca cells to produce androstenedione, while FSH stimulates the follicular cells to convert androstenedione to estradiol (Fig. 2.2). The increase in serum estradiol results in the negative feedback to the production of LH and FSH from the hypothalamus, maintaining serum estradiol levels of around 10–20 mIU/mL. Consequently, with a decrease in estradiol production during postmenopause, negative feedback is lost, and there is an increase in serum levels of FSH and LH. The absence of menstruation associated with high levels of FSH and LH is a possible diagnosis of ovarian failure [3].

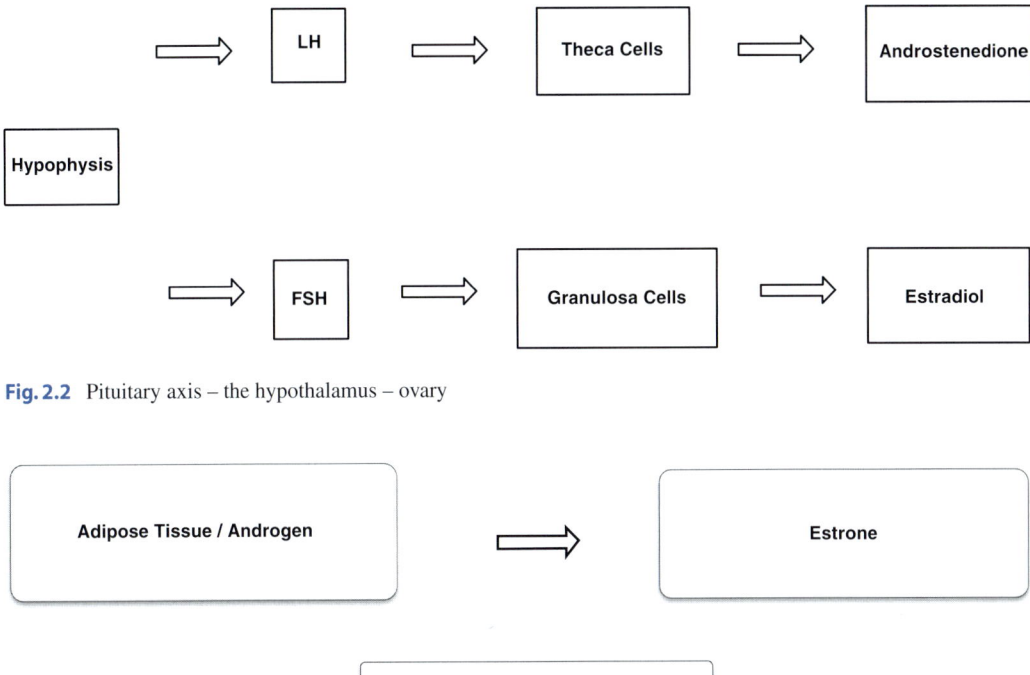

Fig. 2.2 Pituitary axis – the hypothalamus – ovary

Fig. 2.3 Peripheral conversion of androgen

2.4 Estrogen and Postmenopause

After postmenopause, estrogen production by the ovaries becomes negligible. However, women maintain detectable levels of estradiol (E2) and estrone (E1) throughout their lives. This occurs as a result of the ability of the peripheral tissues to convert (aromatize) androgens produced by the adrenal glands and ovaries [8, 9].

Estrone is the primary estrogen after postmenopause and is derived from the peripheral conversion of androgens in the muscle, liver, and brain tissue, as well as in the adipose tissue, since the aromatase enzyme displays greater expression in the adipose tissue [8, 9] (Fig. 2.3). Estradiol continues to be produced after postmenopause through the peripheral conversion of estrone; however, it presents in much lower levels than during reproductive life and also in levels lower than those of estrone. The changes in estrogen levels are responsible for most of the morbidity in women after postmenopause, such as osteoporosis, cardiovascular diseases, vulvovaginal atrophy (VVA), and sagging, among others [8, 9].

2.5 Hormone Receptors and Skin

Several functions of the skin have proved to be hormone dependent. Sex steroids clearly play a key role in the skin aging process, as evidenced by the rapid decline in skin appearance noticeable from onset of the premenopausal years. These changes have not been studied thoroughly, although the histological work has demonstrated the presence of estrogen and progesterone receptors in the skin and a relative decrease in expression from the onset of postmenopause [10].

The concentration of estrogen receptors in nuclear and cytoplasmic skin is relatively low. However, surgically induced hypoestrogenemia

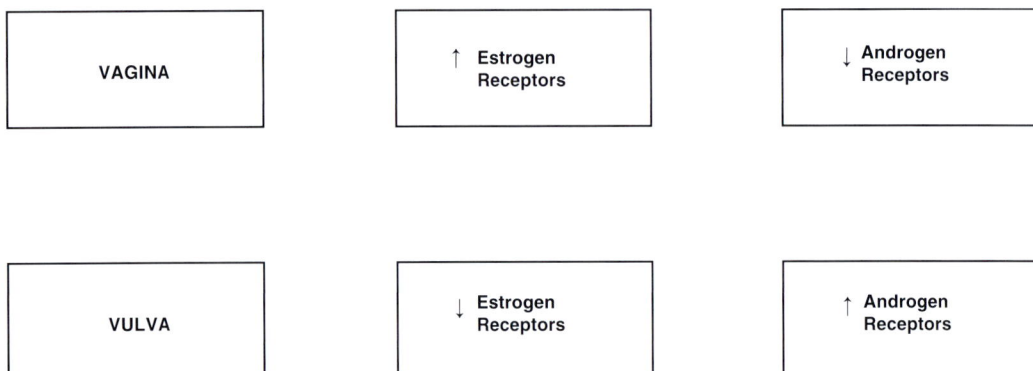

Fig. 2.4 Concentrations of estrogen and androgen receptors in the vagina and vulva

resulted in a significant decrease in the expression of these receptors [10]. Similarly, studies have revealed a gradient coloration of such specific receptors in the epidermis, with darker color in the granular layer. Similar staining has been observed in the hair follicles and sebaceous glands. Although the presence of estrogen receptors on the skin does not confirm their role on the skin, the even distribution of color suggests that the skin is a major target organ of sex steroids [10].

Based on the levels of the concentrations observed in the female genital tract, the highest concentration of estrogen receptors is found in the vaginal epithelium. Androgen receptors are also expressed on the skin of the external female genitalia. Immunohistochemistry studies identified a greater proportion of estrogen receptors in the vagina compared to androgen receptors, and this ratio in the vulva is reversed where an increased number of androgen receptors are found, with an accompanying decrease of estrogen receptors and progesterone [11] (Fig. 2.4).

During the postmenopausal period, changes occur in the following indexes; while the concentration of estrogen receptors in the pubic skin remains stable before and after postmenopause, the concentration of androgen receptors, in relation to estrogen receptors, decreases by almost 40 % in the postmenopausal period, and there is also a significant reduction in the level of progesterone receptors [2]. These changes may be relevant for purposes of treatment of dermatoses in the vulvovaginal region in postmenopausal women [10].

2.6 Skin Hydration

The dermis contributes to water retention by way of its hydrophilic content contained in the glycosaminoglycans. The glycosaminoglycans have a negative ionic charge, transporting water to the dermis and, therefore, contributing to skin turgor and tissue protection against excessive compression [12]. Glycosaminoglycans decrease with aging, and this contributes to skin dryness, atrophy, and rhytids [3].

Estrogen enhances the hygroscopic quality of the dermis, most probably by increasing the synthesis of the hyaluronic acid [12, 13]. Studies with animals confirm the hormonal role in skin hydration, showing a significant increase in glycosaminoglycans after estrogen-based therapies [13].

2.7 Skin Thickness and Postmenopause

The thinning of the dermis, clinically recognized by easy bruising and tearing, always occurs with aging. Most studies suggest that the loss of collagen is more closely linked to the postmenopausal period and less to the chronological age, hence hormonal influence [3].

The skin tends to become thinner as postmenopause progresses, and this can be confirmed by high-frequency ultrasound (22.5 MHz). Ultrasound can also be used to measure the thickness of the epidermis and dermis. Several studies using ultrasound have showed that the dermal skin thickness increases with estrogen replacement therapy, such as the finding in a double-blind placebo-controlled randomized study by Maheux et al. The aforementioned study displayed a significant increase in skin thickness, measured at the level of the greater trochanter in postmenopausal women who received conjugated estrogens. This finding was confirmed by both an ultrasound scan and a skin biopsy [14].

2.8 Skin Collagen and Postmenopause

In 1941, Albright et al. observed that postmenopausal women with osteoporosis had a remarkably thin skin, suggesting that the atrophy was more comprehensive than that found in the bone matrix [15]. Brincat et al. demonstrated a similar decrease in the skin thickness and collagen content, corresponding to a reduction of bone mineral density measured throughout the years following postmenopause [15]. In 1983, Brincat et al. concluded in their study that postmenopausal women on hormone replacement therapy with estrogen and testosterone had a collagen content 48 % higher compared to the content measured in untreated women, who were grouped by age [16].

The decrease in collagen levels on the skin occurs at an accelerated rate immediately after postmenopause and subsequently becomes more gradual. Approximately 30 % of skin collagen is lost during the first 5 years after postmenopause, with an average decrease of 2.1 % per year in postmenopausal women over a period of 20 years [10].

2.9 Skin Looseness and Wrinkling

The aging of the skin on the face is characterized by a progressive increase in stretch, associated with reduced elasticity. The loss of tonicity is accompanied by a progressive aggravation of facial wrinkles [17]. Bolognia et al., in a double-blind, placebo-controlled study, observed that young women in early menopause have an accelerated increase in degeneration of elastic fibers in the dermis [18]. Histologically, severe degenerative changes of elastic fibers have been noticed, including the coalescence of cystic spaces into lacunae, peripheral fragmentation, granular degeneration, and the splitting of the fibers into strands. These changes were noticed in individuals 20 years older than said patients. This suggests a close association between estrogen deprivation and changes in elastic fibers [18].

2.10 Wound Healing in Postmenopause

Healing of the skin is first characterized by an inflammation, followed by the formation of granulation tissue, after reepithelialization, and finally, the remodeling of tissues. Delayed wound healing usually occurs in the elderly, and estrogen has been shown to play a crucial role in wound healing [3].

Elastase is capable of degrading a wide range of functional and structural proteins, such as proteoglycans, fibronectin, and collagen. Fibronectin is essential for the healing process by influencing reepithelialization, collagen deposition, and wound contraction. With age, the amount of fibronectin decreases and is degraded secondary by elastase, which is high due to the increased number of neutrophils found in old wounds (Fig. 2.5). Therapies aimed at decreasing elastase, such as those aiming at reducing the number of neutrophils, can enhance the healing process [19, 20].

Ashcroft et al. in a randomized double-blind placebo-controlled study investigated the effects of topical estrogen on wound healing in healthy elderly men and women and reported the results of this therapy in terms of inflammatory response and elastase levels during the healing process. Compared to placebo, the treatment with estrogen increased the levels of collagen and fibronectin and resulted in a decrease in elastase levels, secondary to a reduction in the number of neutrophils, with consequent reduction in the degradation of fibronectin. The data thus obtained suggest that the delay in wound healing of the elderly can be improved by topical estrogen therapy [21]. Following the same reasoning, recent studies have shown that hormone replacement therapies prevent the onset of ulcers and venous stasis in postmenopausal women [14].

More recently, Ashcroft et al. conducted a study on mice, the results of which suggesting that estrogen also has a role in regulating the migratory inhibitory factor (MIF) of macrophages. Estrogen acts as a proinflammatory agent and has been implicated in the formation of aberrant scarring and in the alteration of inflammatory response in vivo. The estrogen-deficient mice showed a marked increase in the MIF in wound healing, while mice lacking the MIF gene showed no delayed wound healing, despite their estrogen deficiency. We may, therefore, confirm the role of estrogen in the regulation of the MIF and its role in wound healing [22].

2.11 Urogenital and Menopausal Problems

The epitheliums of the vulvar, vaginal, and urinary tracts show a relatively high number of estrogen receptors and are, therefore, sensitive to decreased levels of circulating estrogens. Usual urogenital changes that occur during postmenopause occur as the result of a combination of physiological aging and low estrogen levels [23].

Lower levels of estradiol lead to numerous adverse effects, including changes in the lower urinary tract. The main change is vaginal atrophy: the mucosa becomes thinner and drier. This may lead to vaginal discomfort, dryness, stinging, pruritus, and dyspareunia (Fig. 2.6). The vaginal epi-

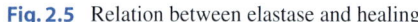

Fig. 2.5 Relation between elastase and healing

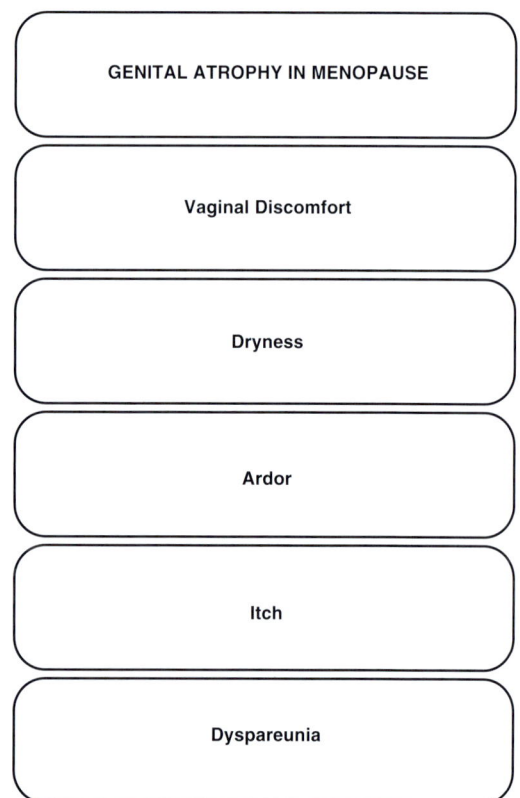

Fig. 2.6 Genital changes in menopause

thelium can become inflamed, thus contributing to urinary symptoms, such as increased urinary frequency and urgency, dysuria, incontinence, and recurring infections. Furthermore, it has been suggested that reduced estrogen levels can affect the periurethral tissues and contribute to loosening and pelvic incontinence. In association with hypoestrogenemia, these changes in pH and vaginal flora may predispose postmenopausal women to urinary tract infection [24, 25].

2.12 Atrophic Vaginitis

Atrophic vaginitis is inflammation of the vagina that develops when there is a significant decrease in estrogen levels. Estradiol plays a vital role in maintaining the vaginal tissue healthy and lubricated, and decreased levels of estradiol may cause the vaginal epithelium to become atrophic, thin, dry, and wrinkled. Common conditions of low estrogen levels that result in atrophic vaginitis include postmenopause, breastfeeding, surgical removal of the ovaries in young women, and medication used to decrease estrogen levels in conditions such as uterine fibroids or endometriosis [24, 25].

Diagnosis is possible by way of physical examination; however, the diagnosis has to be confirmed by cytological examination. Due to the fact that estrogen stimulates the maturation of the vaginal epithelium from basal to superficial cells, in general a postmenopausal smear will act initially and advance from a decreased number of superficial cells to being completely clear eventually. A predominance of basal cells associated with a relative absence of superficial cells is indicative of atrophy [5].

The treatment may be conducted topically with estrogen, and this method of treatment should not influence the success of treatment. The topical estrogen lowers the vaginal pH, induces the maturation of vaginal and urethral mucosa, and decreases the frequency of urinary tract infections (Fig. 2.7). Atrophy is quickly reversed after 1–2 weeks. Many treatments are suggested, and generally, those with estriol and estradiol creams are the treatments most frequently recommended. The appropriate duration of therapy is unknown [5, 23].

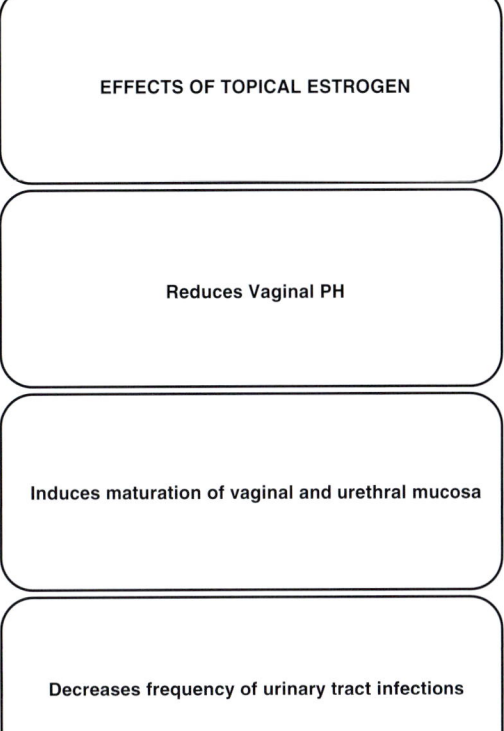

Fig. 2.7 Effects of topical estrogen

2.13 Menopausal Flushing

During postmenopause, 70–80 % of women experience transient flushing and sweating that may be associated with palpitations, anxiety symptoms, and sleep disorders and 25 % reported flushes by up to 5 years [5, 10]. The blush seems to cause vasodilatation in the papillary dermis and subcutaneous tissue and occurs mainly in the face, neck, chest, palms, and soles [10]. Rosacea is known to be a complication of flushing, which is more commonly detected in postmenopausal women than in men of the same age [26]. The prevalence of this condition during the early years of postmenopause may in part be explained by virtue of the loss of the peripheral vascular control seen in association with estrogen deficiency, which is correctable with hormone replacement therapy [27]. Studies show that low doses of a combination of androgen and estrogen are as effective as high doses of estrogen on its own. However, persistent flushing during the use of HRT may occur due to the increase of sex hormone-building globulin (SHBG), which decreases the bioavailability of testosterone. In this case, HRT can be exchanged from oral to patch, gel, or implant, leading to a reduction of SHBG in 6–8 weeks [28]. An empirical study conducted to analyze the changes in peripheral vascular control in postmenopausal women induced by topical estrogen cream suggested that both estrogen and its metabolites have a direct effect on neurotransmitters and their neurovascular control [29].

2.14 Hormone Replacement Therapy

Estrogen HRT, with or without progesterone, has been used to treat menopausal symptoms and prevent long-term illnesses such as osteoporosis and cardiovascular disease [3]. Observational studies have found lower rates of coronary heart disease in women taking estrogen after postmenopause, compared with women who did not receive this therapy. This association has been reported as a means of secondary prevention in women with coronary artery disease, with hormone users experiencing 35–80 % fewer recurring events than nonusers. If this association is causal, estrogen therapy may be an important method for the prevention of coronary heart disease in postmenopausal women. However, the observed association between estrogen therapy and the reduced risk of coronary events can be attributed to a selection bias, if the women who choose to take hormones are healthier and have a more favorable cardiovascular profile than those who do not. Observational studies have not been able to resolve this uncertainty [30]. In addition, the American Heart Association does not recommend the use of HRT for the secondary prevention of cardiovascular disease [31].

In 2002, the Women's Health Initiative reported results of a randomized controlled trial involving 16,608 postmenopausal women, comparing the effects of estrogen and progesterone with placebos with regard to the risk of chronic disease, and confirmed that the combination of estrogen and progesterone increases the risk of invasive breast cancer. However, this treatment did not alter the risk of endometrial cancer and decreased the chance/risk of colon cancer and osteoporosis [32]. In 2003, Rowan et al. confirmed the observation in relation to the risk of breast cancer, showing that estrogen combined with short-term progesterone relatively increased the incidence of breast cancer diagnosed at a more advanced stage, compared to the use of a placebo, and also substantially increased the percentage of women with abnormal mammograms. These results suggest that estrogen and progesterone can stimulate the growth of breast cancer and make its diagnosis more difficult [33].

With regard to the skin, the treatment with estrogen in postmenopausal women has been proved to increase, on several occasions, the content of collagen, dermal thickness, and elasticity. Studies also illustrated the role of estrogen in wound healing, showing its beneficial effects [34]. Topical estrogen creams applied locally on confined surface areas (such as facial and vaginal application) appear to be safe, without significant systemic absorption [3].

References

1. Al-Azzawi F. Endocrinological aspects of the menopause. BMJ. 1992;48:262–75.
2. Schmidt JB, Lindmaier A, Spona J. Hormone receptors in pubic skin of premenopausal and postmenopausal females. Gynecol Obstet Invest. 1990;30(2):97–100.
3. Hall G, Phillips TJ. Estrogen and skin: the effects of estrogen, menopause, and hormone replacement therapy on the skin. J Am Acad Dermatol. 2005;53:555–68.
4. Blume-Peytavi U, Atkin S, Gieler U, Grimalt R. Skin Academy: hair, skin, hormones and menopause – current status/knowledge on the management of hair disorders in menopausal women. Eur J Dermatol. 2012;22(3):310–8.
5. Wines N, Willsteed E. Menopause and skin. Australas J Dermatol. 2001;42:149–60.
6. Kanitakis J. Anatomy, histology and immunohistochemistry of normal human skin. Eur J Dermatol. 2002;12(4):390–401.
7. Calleja-Agius J, Brincat M. The effect of menopause on the skin and other connective tissues. Gynecol Endocrinol. 2012;28(4):273–7.

8. Nelson LR, Bulun SE. Estrogen production and action. J Am Acad Dermatol. 2001;45(Suppl):S116–24.
9. Edman CD, MacDonald PC. Effect of obesity on conversion of plasma androstenedione to estrone in ovulatory and anovulatory young women. Am J Obstet Gynecol. 1978;130:456–61.
10. Raine-Fenning NJ, Brincat MP, Muscat-Baron Y. Skin aging and menopause. Am J Clin Dermatol. 2003;4(6): 371–8.
11. MacLean AB, Nicol LA, Hodgins MB. Immunohistochemical localization of estrogen receptors in the vulva and vagina. J Reprod Med. 1990;35(11):1015–6.
12. Danforth DN, Veis A, Breen M, Weinstein HG, Buckingham JC, Manalo P. The effect of pregnancy and labor on the human cervix: changes in collagen, glycoproteins, and glycosaminoglycans. Am J Obstet Gynecol. 1974;120(5):641–51.
13. Grosman N, Hvidberg E, Schou J. The effect of estrogenic treatment on the acid mucopolysaccharide pattern in skin of mice. Acta Pharmacol Toxicol. 1971;30:458–64.
14. Maheux R, Naud F, Rioux M, Grenier R, Lemay A, Guy J, et al. A randomized, double-blind, placebo-controlled study on the effect of conjugated estrogens on skin thickness. Am J Obstet Gynecol. 1994;170(2):642–9.
15. Holland EF, Studd JW, Mansell JP, Leather AT, Bailey AJ. Changes in collagen composition and cross-links in bone and skin of osteoporotic postmenopausal women treated with percutaneous estradiol implants. Obstet Gynecol. 1994;83(2):180–3.
16. Brincat M, Moniz CF, Studd JW, Darby AJ, Magos A, Cooper D. Sex hormones and skin collagen content in postmenopausal women. Br Med J (Clin Res Ed). 1983;287(6402):1337–8.
17. Henry F, Pierard-Franchimont C, Cauwenbergh G, Pierard GE. Age-related changes in facial skin contours and rheology. J Am Geriatr Soc. 1997;45:220–2.
18. Bolognia JL, Braverman IM, Rousseau ME, Sarrel PM. Skin changes in menopause. Maturitas. 1989;11: 295–304.
19. Herrick SE, Ashcroft GS, Ireland G, Horan MA, McCollum C, Ferguson MWJ. Up-regulation of elastase in acute wounds of healthy aged humans and chronic venous leg ulcers is associated with matrix degradation. Lab Invest. 1996;77:281–8.
20. Ashcroft GS, Horan MA, Ferguson MWJ. Ageing is associated with reduced deposition of specific extracellular matrix components, an up-regulation of angiogenesis, and an altered inflammatory response in a murine incisional wound healing model. J Invest Dermatol. 1997;108:430–7.
21. Ashcroft GS, Greenwell-Wild T, Horan MA, Wahl SM, Ferguson MW. Topical estrogen accelerates cutaneous wound healing in aged humans associated with an altered inflammatory response. Am J Pathol. 1999;155:1137–46.
22. Ashcroft GS, Mills SJ, Lei KJ, Gibbons L, Jeong MJ, Taniguchi M, et al. Estrogen modulates cutaneous wound healing by downregulating macrophage migration inhibitory factor. J Clin Invest. 2003;111: 1309–18.
23. Schaffer J, Fantil JA. Urogenital effects of the menopause. Clin Obstet Gynaecol. 1996;10:401–17.
24. Castelo-Branco C, Cancelo MJ, Villero J, Nohales F, Juliá MD. Management of postmenopausal vaginal atrophy and atrophic vaginitis. Maturitas. 2005;52(Supp.1):S46–52.
25. Palacios S, Castelo-Branco C, Cancelo MJ, Vazquez F. Low-dose, vaginally administered oestrogens may enhance local benefits of systemic therapy in the treatment of urogenital atrophy in post-menopausal women on hormone therapy. Maturitas. 2005;50:98–104.
26. Bergfield WF. A lifetime of healthy skin: implications for women. Int J Fertil Womens Med. 1999;44(2): 83–95.
27. Ginsburg J, Hardiman P, O'Reilly B. Peripheral blood flow in menopausal women who have hot flushes and in those who do not. BMJ. 1989;298(6686):1488–90.
28. Simon J, Klaiber E, Wiita B, Bowen A, Yang HM. Differential effects of estrogen-androgen and estrogen-only therapy on vasomotor symptoms, gonadotropin secretion, and endogenous androgen bioavailability in postmenopausal women. Menopause. 1999;6:138–46.
29. Brincat M, de Trafford JC, Lafferty K, Studd JW. Peripheral vasomotor control and menopausal flushing: a preliminary report. Br J Obstet Gynaecol. 1984;91(11):1107–10.
30. Hulley S, Grady D, Bush T, Furberg C, Herrington D, Riggs B, et al. Randomized trial of estrogen plus progestin for secondary prevention of coronary heart disease in postmenopausal women. JAMA. 1998;280: 605–13.
31. Mosca L, Collins P, Herrington DM, Mendelsohn ME, Pasternak RC, Robertson RM, et al. Hormone replacement therapy and cardiovascular disease – a statement for healthcare professionals from the American Heart Association. Circulation. 2001;104(4):499–503.
32. Chlebowski RT, Hendrix SL, Langer RD, Stefanick ML, Gass M, Lane D, et al. Influence of estrogen plus progestin on breast cancer mammography in healthy postmenopausal women. JAMA. 2003;289(24):3243–53.
33. Rossouw JE, Anderson GL, Prentice RL, LaCroix AZ, Kooperberg C, Stefanick ML, et al. Risks and benefits of estrogen plus progestin in healthy postmenopausal women – principal results from the Women's Health Initiative. JAMA. 2002;288(3):321–33.
34. Brincat MP, Baron YM, Galea R. Estrogens and the skin. Climacteric. 2005;8:110–23.

Skin Changes in Menopause

Renata Saucedo, Arturo Zárate, and Marcelino Hernández-Valencia

Contents

3.1	Estrogens and Collagen	26
3.2	Estrogens and Skin Moisture	26
3.3	Estrogen Effect on Skin Wrinkling	26
3.4	Estrogen and Skin Elasticity	26
3.5	Estrogen Effect on Skin Pigmentation	26
3.6	Estrogen and Hair Growth	27
3.7	Selective Estrogen Receptor Modulators	27
3.8	Phytoestrogens	27
3.9	Effects of Estrogens in Skin	27
3.10	The Skin as an Independent Steroidogenic Organ	28
3.11	Skin Disorders in Menopause	28
3.11.1	Atrophic Vulvovaginitis	28
3.11.2	Lichen Sclerosis	29
3.11.3	Dysesthetic Vulvodynia	29
3.11.4	Keratoderma Climactericum	29
3.12	Melanoma and Nonmelanoma Skin Cancers	29
3.13	Quality of Life	29
References		30

R. Saucedo, PhD • A. Zárate, MD, PhD (✉)
M. Hernández-Valencia, MD, PhD
Endocrine Research Unit,
Instituto Mexicano Seguro Social,
Cuauhtemoc 330, Mexico City DF 06720, Mexico
e-mail: sgrenata@yahoo.com; zaratre@att.net.mx;
mhernandezvalencia@prodigy.net.mx

Human skin is a dynamic organ that normally serves as a protective barrier between the internal environment and the outside world. It plays an important barrier function against pathogens and other external factors, such as UV light. Although it is extremely durable, it undergoes aging, just like any other organ, in a process influenced by hormonal, environmental, and genetic factors of individuals [1, 2].

Estrogens have a profound influence on skin. The first study proving an effect of estrogens on skin was published in 1937 and showed an improvement of acne and eczema upon estrogen treatment [3]. In addition, several observational studies indicate that skin composition and integrity are altered during each menstrual cycle in response to cyclic variation of estrogen: it has been observed as a variation in skin thickness during the menstrual cycle, with skin thickness lowest at the start of the menstrual cycle, when estrogen and progesterone levels are low, which then increases with the rising levels of estrogen [4, 5]. However, many of the effects of estrogen on human skin are based on the changes that are seen in postmenopausal women. The relative hypoestrogenism that accompanies menopause exacerbates the deleterious effects of both intrinsic and environmental aging which results in thinner skin, an increase in number and depth of wrinkles, increased skin dryness, and decreased skin firmness and elasticity [6–10]. In postmenopausal women, skin thickness decreases by 1.13 % per postmenopausal year, with an associated decrease in collagen content (2 % per postmenopausal year) [11, 12].

Estrogen administration has been shown to have positive effects on the skin by delaying or preventing skin aging manifestations.

3.1 Estrogens and Collagen

Estrogen plays a critical role in maintaining collagen homeostasis. Callens et al. studied the influence of different hormone replacement therapy (HRT) regimens on postmenopausal women using skin echography and found an increase in skin thickness of 7–15 % in postmenopausal women utilizing an estradiol gel patch or estradiol transdermal system [13]. Castelo-Branco et al. showed by skin biopsies an increase in skin collagen content of 1.8–5.1 % with oral and transdermal HRT over 12 months [14]. Maheux et al. studied postmenopausal nuns utilizing a randomized, double-blind, placebo-controlled study and showed that in the group treated with oral conjugated estrogens, there was a significant increase in skin thickness and skin dermis at the level of the greater trochanter as measured by ultrasonography and skin biopsy, respectively [15]. Using computerized image analysis of skin samples, Sauerbronn et al. found an increase of 6.49 % of collagen fibers in the dermis after 6 months of topical treatment with estradiol valerate and cyproterone acetate [16]. Varila et al. showed that topical estrogen causes an increase in collagen synthesis [17].

3.2 Estrogens and Skin Moisture

It has been demonstrated that postmenopausal women who are not taking HRT are significantly more likely to experience dry skin compared with those postmenopausal women taking estrogen [18]. Denda et al. demonstrated changes in the stratum corneum sphingolipids with aging and suggested a possible hormonal influence [19]. Pierard-Franchimont et al. showed that transdermal estrogen therapy leads to significantly increased water-holding capacity of the stratum corneum suggesting that estrogen may play a role in the stratum corneum barrier function [20]. Estrogens also affect dermal water-holding capacity, increasing dermal hydroscopic qualities [21].

3.3 Estrogen Effect on Skin Wrinkling

Young et al. pointed out that hypoestrogenism increases the risk for wrinkling in Korean women [22]. Dunn et al. reported that postmenopausal women using estrogen were significantly less likely to develop skin wrinkles, and Creidi et al., in a double-blind, placebo-controlled study, showed that a conjugated estrogen cream applied to the facial skin of postmenopausal women resulted in significant improvement in fine wrinkles [23, 24]. However, smoking is a major risk factor for facial skin wrinkling, and hormone therapy cannot diminish this impact of smoking [25].

3.4 Estrogen and Skin Elasticity

Changes in the skin elastic fibers have been reported after application of estriol ointments to the skin of postmenopausal women. These changes included a thickening of the elastic fibers in the papillary dermis. The elastic fibers were also noted to be in better orientation and slightly increased in number [26]. Furthermore, conjugated equine estrogen has been shown to increase forearm skin elasticity in postmenopausal women [27].

3.5 Estrogen Effect on Skin Pigmentation

Estrogens regulate skin pigmentation. There are few reports on the effects of estrogens on pigmentary changes in photoaged skin. Creidi et al. reported no improvement in mottled pigmentation and lentigines [24]. Schmidt et al. also did not mention any improvement in dyspigmentation [28].

3.6 Estrogen and Hair Growth

Niiyama et al. have demonstrated the ability of estrogen to modify androgen metabolism in dermal papillae of hair follicle [29]. They showed that estradiol diminishes the amount of dihydrotestosterone (DHT) in human hair follicle by inducing aromatase activity. The induction of aromatase activity increases the conversion of testosterone to estradiol, thereby diminishing the amount of testosterone available for the conversion to DHT which might explain the beneficial effect of estrogen treatment of androgenetic alopecia (AGA).

Although systemic hormone replacement therapy has been used for many years, recent trials have reported a significant increased risk of breast cancer and other pathologies with this treatment [30, 31]. This has led to reconsider the risks and benefits of HRT.

3.7 Selective Estrogen Receptor Modulators

Selective estrogen receptor modulators (SERMs) are pharmaceutical compounds that bind to estrogen receptors (ERs), acting either as agonists to mimic positive estrogen effects or as antagonists to block negative estrogen effects, in a tissue-specific manner. There are two well-characterized SERMs, tamoxifen and raloxifene. Despite the well-characterized effects of SERMs on uterus, breast, and bone tissue, there is very limited data on the effect of SERMs on the skin. In vitro studies with human fibroblasts showed that raloxifene may exert stimulatory effects on skin collagen synthesis [32]. Also, raloxifene appears to improve skin elasticity in postmenopausal women [33].

3.8 Phytoestrogens

Phytoestrogens are plant derivatives that structurally resemble endogenous estrogens, isoflavones being the most widespread. Isoflavones, in particular, the genistein, have demonstrated beneficial effects to aging skin in terms of photoprotection, skin wrinkling, skin elasticity, and skin hydration [34].

3.9 Effects of Estrogens in Skin

Estrogens regulate hair growth, sebaceous gland function, proliferation and differentiation of epithelial cells of the epidermis and adnexa, functional activity of dermal fibroblasts and fibrocytes, wound healing, and skin immune cells activity [35]. However, the mechanisms of estrogen action on skin are still poorly understood. Estrogen receptors ERα and ERβ have been detected in keratinocytes, fibroblast, and melanocytes, and recent studies suggest that estrogens exert their effect in skin through the same molecular pathways used in other nonreproductive tissues, via a combination of genomic and non-genomic pathways [36–38].

In the genomic pathway, the estrogen receptor, unattached to its ligand and loosely bound in its cytoplasmic or nuclear location, is attached to receptor-associated proteins. These proteins serve as chaperones that stabilize the receptor in an unactivated state or mask the DNA-binding domain of the receptor. As free estrogen diffuses into the cell, it binds to the ligand-binding domain of the receptor, which dissociates from its cytoplasmic chaperones; the complex of estrogen and estrogen receptor then diffuses into the cell nucleus. These estrogen–estrogen receptor complexes bind to specific sequences of DNA called estrogen-response elements on the promoter regions of targeted genes and thereby enhances their expression. The estrogen–estrogen receptor complexes bind not only to the response elements but also to nuclear-receptor coactivators or repressors [39].

In the non-genomic pathways, estrogens have effects on cell membranes and are mediated by cell-surface forms of estrogen receptor. These receptors are thought to resemble their intracellular counterparts and modulate signal transduction through membrane-associated molecules, such as ion channels, G proteins, the tyrosine kinase c-Src, and growth factor receptors, leading to many downstream cellular activation cascades [40].

Table 3.1 Hormones produced in the skin

Vitamin D
PTHrP
Estrogens
Androgens
T3
MSH
ACTH
TRH
GH

3.10 The Skin as an Independent Steroidogenic Organ

The skin function extends beyond that of static barrier organ. In addition to separating the external environment from internal homeostasis, the skin also exerts important endocrine and exocrine activities. The exocrine function is performed by the adnexal structures that comprise eccrine, apocrine, and sebaceous glands and hair follicles. These are important in strengthening the epidermal barrier, in thermoregulation, and in the defense against microorganisms. The endocrine function of the skin is performed by cells compartmentally arranged into endocrine units. These units are composed of cells of epithelial, neural crest, mesenchymal, and bone marrow origin that form the epidermal, dermal, and adnexal structures [1]. These cutaneous cells and adnexal structures can concomitantly produce hormones and express the corresponding receptors (Table 3.1).

The skin cells contain the entire biochemical apparatus necessary for production of glucocorticoids, androgens, and estrogens either from precursors of systemic origin or, alternatively, through the conversion of cholesterol to pregnenolone and its subsequent transformation to biologically active steroids. The level of production and nature of the final steroid products are dependent on the cell type or cutaneous compartment, e.g., epidermis, dermis, adnexal structures, or adipose tissue [41].

The skin can transform the steroids dehydroepiandrosterone (DHEA) and its sulfate (DHEA-S) into active androgens and estrogens. Specifically, enzymatic activity corresponding to 3b-hydroxysteroid dehydrogenase/D5–D4 isomerase (3b-HSD) has been localized to the sebaceous glands and, to a lesser degree, in hair follicles, epidermis, and eccrine glands, while 17b-hydroxysteroid dehydrogenase (17b-HSD) has been localized to follicular and epidermal keratinocytes. 3b-HSD converts DHEA into 4-androstenedione and 5-androstene-3b,17b-diol into testosterone, while 17b-HSD converts DHEA into 5-androstene-3b,17b-diol, 4-androstenedione into testosterone, and androstenedione into DHT. Testosterone is also converted into DHT through the action of a 5a-reductase, detected in dermal and dermal papilla fibroblasts, follicular and epidermal keratinocytes, and sebaceous and apocrine glands. There are two isozymic forms of the 5a-reductase, but the skin expresses predominantly the type I in a highly specific cellular and regional distribution. Nevertheless, cutaneous expression of 5a-reductase type 2 has been also reported, but at much lower levels; this form has been immunodetected in hair follicles of the human scalp. The skin immune system can also convert DHEA into 5-androstene-3b,17b-diol and into 5-androstene-3b,7b,17b-triol. Cutaneous conversion of testosterone into estradiol is mediated by an aromatase expressed in dermal fibroblasts and adipocytes, but not in keratinocytes. However, in keratinocytes 17b-HSD can transform 17b-estradiol into estrone or estrone into 17bestradiol [41].

Locally produced glucocorticoids, androgens, and estrogens affect functions of the epidermis and adnexal structures as well as local immune activity. Malfunction of these steroidogenic activities can lead to inflammatory disorders or autoimmune diseases.

3.11 Skin Disorders in Menopause

Skin conditions that tend to occur more commonly in postmenopausal women include atrophic vulvovaginitis, lichen sclerosis, dysesthetic vulvodynia, and keratoderma climactericum [42].

3.11.1 Atrophic Vulvovaginitis

Hypoestrogenism leads to atrophy of the vagina and vulval vestibule. This thinned tissue is easily irritated and is also susceptible to secondary infection. The patient complains of vulvar burning, dysuria, pruritus, tenderness, and dyspareunia. Atrophy reverses rapidly and returns to premenopausal levels after 1–2 weeks of estrogen therapy [43].

3.11.2 Lichen Sclerosis

Lichen sclerosus is a rare inflammatory disease of unknown etiology. It mainly affects postmenopausal women in the anogenital area and only in 2.5 % cases it is found exclusively at an extragenital site. The inner thighs, submammary region, and upper arms are the most commonly affected sites [44]. Topical corticosteroids, such as betamethasone dipropionate or clobetasol propionate, are effective in improving symptoms and reversing the disease process [45].

3.11.3 Dysesthetic Vulvodynia

Patients present with chronic constant unremitting vulval burning that does not respond to topical applications and frequently have no abnormality detected on physical examination. The etiology of this condition is thought to be neurological. It may be related to abnormal cutaneous perception, either centrally or at nerve root level. The pain can be bilateral, may involve the inner thighs, and may be provoked by vaginal penetration [46]. Tricyclic antidepressants such as amitriptyline and nortriptyline, in low doses, as well as some anticonvulsants, such as carbamazepine and sodium valproate, are effective for the management of neuropathic pain. These drugs should be commenced at the lowest possible dose [47].

3.11.4 Keratoderma Climactericum

Keratoderma climactericum is a hyperkeratosis of the palms and soles affecting mainly obese women. Thickening first develops in weight-bearing areas such as plantar pressure points, making walking difficult. Patients also complain of painful fissures and itch. Involvement of the hands is often discrete [42]. Treatment with a low dose of etretinate has been demonstrated to lead effectively to partial or total remission of hyperkeratosis [48].

3.12 Melanoma and Nonmelanoma Skin Cancers

Preclinical and clinical findings suggest that estrogen may be involved in the development of skin cancer. Several studies have found an association between oral contraceptive use and an increased risk of nonmelanoma skin cancer [49, 50]. However, epidemiological studies of menopausal hormone therapy and the risk of melanoma have produced mixed findings; several studies reported that hormone use was associated with increased risk of melanoma [51–53]. In the recent large multiethnic Women's Health Initiative (WHI) clinical trials of estrogen plus progestin (E + P) vs. placebo and estrogen alone (E-alone) vs. placebo, the hormone therapy during 6 years did not affect overall incidence of nonmelanoma skin cancer or melanoma. The rates of incident nonmelanoma skin cancer and melanoma were similar between the active hormone (combined analysis of E + P and E-alone) and placebo groups (nonmelanoma skin cancer: HR = 0.98, 95 % CI = 0.89–1.07; melanoma: HR = 0.92, 95 % CI = 0.61–1.37) [54]. However, it cannot rule out a delayed effect of hormone therapy on risk of skin cancer.

3.13 Quality of Life

A variety of cutaneous changes with the menopause cause significant anxiety and may impact the quality of life. Estrogens can improve the changes in skin, and general lifestyle changes can be effective in reducing, in the long term, the signs of skin aging. The latter include the use of sun protection and over-the-counter moisturizers [55]. In addition, cosmetic interventions such as topical retinoids, facial peels, botulinum neurotoxin, soft tissue fillers, and surgical procedures can be employed to improve the appearance of the skin [56, 57].

References

1. Slominski A, Wortsman J. Neuroendocrinology of the skin. Endocr Rev. 2000;21:457–87.
2. Vierkötter A, Krutmann J. Environmental influences on skin aging and ethnic-specific manifestations. Dermatoendocrinol. 2012;4:227–31.
3. Loeser AA. The resorption and action of follicular hormone rubbed into the skin. J Obstet Gynaecol Br Emp. 1937;44:710–4.
4. Muizzuddin N, Marenus KD, Schnittger SF, Sullivan M, Maes DH. Effect of systemic hormonal cyclicity on skin. J Cosmet Sci. 2005;56:311–21.
5. Eisenbeiss C, Welzel J, Schmeller W. The influence of female sex hormones on skin thickness: evaluation using 20 MHz sonography. Br J Dermatol. 1998;139:462–7.
6. Wend K, Wend P, Krum SA. Tissue-specific effects of loss of estrogen during menopause and aging. Front Endocrinol. 2012;8:19.
7. Shu YY, Maibach HI. Estrogen and skin: therapeutic options. Am J Clin Dermatol. 2011;12:297–311.
8. Stevenson S, Thornton J. Effect of estrogens on skin aging and the potential role of SERMs. Clin Interv Aging. 2007;2:283–97.
9. Verdier-Sévrain S, Bonté F, Gilchrest B. Biology of estrogens in skin: implications for skin aging. Exp Dermatol. 2006;15:83–94.
10. Thornton MJ. Estrogens and aging skin. Dermatoendocrinol. 2013;5:264–70.
11. Brincat M, Moniz CJ, Studd JW, Darby A, Magos A, Emburey G, et al. Long-term effects of the menopause and sex hormones on skin thickness. Br J Obstet Gynaecol. 1985;92:256–9.
12. Affinito P, Palomba S, Sorrentino C, Di Carlo C, Bifulco G, Arienzo MP, et al. Effects of postmenopausal hypoestrogenism on skin collagen. Maturitas. 1999;33:239–47.
13. Callens A, Valliant L, Lecomte P, Berson M, Gall Y, Lorette G. Does hormonal skin aging exist? A study of the influence of different hormone therapy regimens on the skin of postmenopausal women using non-invasive measurement techniques. Dermatology. 1996;193:289–94.
14. Castelo-Branco C, Duran M, Gonzales-Merlo J. Skin collagen and bone changes related to age and hormone replacement therapy. Maturitas. 1992;14:113–9.
15. Maheux R, Naud F, Rioux M, Grenier R, Lemay A, Guy J, et al. A randomized, double-blind, placebo-controlled study on the effect of conjugated estrogens on skin thickness. Am J Obstet Gynecol. 1994;170:642–9.
16. Sauerbronn AVD, Fonseca AM, Bagnoli VR, Saldiva PH, Pinotti JA. The effects of systemic hormone replacement therapy on the skin of the postmenopausal women. Int J Gynecol Obstet. 2000;68:35–41.
17. Varila E, Rantala I, Oikarinen A, Risteli J, Reunala T, Oksanen H, et al. The effect of topical oestradiol on skin collagen of postmenopausal women. Br J Obstet Gynaecol. 1995;120(12):985–9.
18. Calleja-Agius J, Brincat M. The effect of menopause on the skin and other connective tissues. Gynecol Endocrinol. 2012;28:273–7.
19. Denda M, Koyama J, Hori J, Horii I, Takahashi M, Hara M, et al. Age- and sex-dependent change in stratum corneum sphingolipids. Arch Dermatol Res. 1993;285:415–7.
20. Pierard-Franchimont C, Letawe C, Goffin V, Piérard GE. Skin water-holding capacity and transdermal estrogen therapy for menopause/a pilot study. Maturitas. 1995;22:151–4.
21. Grosman N, Hvidberg E, Schou J. The effect of osteogenic treatment on the acid mucopolysaccharide pattern in skin of mice. Acta Pharmacol Toxicol. 1971;30:458–64.
22. Young CS, Kwon OS, Won CH, Hwang EJ, Park BJ, Eun HC. Effect of pregnancy and menopause on facial wrinkling in women. Acta Derm Venereol. 2003;83(6):419–24.
23. Dunn L, Damesyn M, Moore A, Reuben DB, Greendale GA. Does estrogen prevent skin aging? Results from the first National Health and Nutritional Examination Survey. Arch Dermatol. 1997;133:339–42.
24. Creidi P, Faivre B, Agache P, Richard E, Haudiquet V, Sauvanet JP. Effect of a conjugated estrogen (Premarin) cream on ageing facial skin. A comparative study with a placebo cream. Maturitas. 1994;19:211–23.
25. Castelo-Branco C, Figueras F, Martínez de Osaba MJ, Vanrell JA. Facial wrinkling in postmenopausal women. Effects of smoking status and hormone replacement therapy. Maturitas. 1998;29:75–86.
26. Punnonen R, Vaajalahti P, Teisala K. Local oestriol treatment improves the structure of elastic fibers in the skin of postmenopausal women. Ann Chir Gynaecol. 1987;202:39–41.
27. Sumino H, Ichikawa S, Abe M, Endo Y, Nakajima Y, Minegishi T, et al. Effects of aging and postmenopausal hypoestrogenism on skin elasticity and bone mineral density in Japanese women. Endocr J. 2004;51:159–64.
28. Schmidt JB, Binder M, Macheiner W, Kainz CH, Gitsch G, Bieglmayer CH. Treatment of skin ageing symptoms in perimenopausal females with estrogen compounds. A pilot study. Maturitas. 1994;20:25–30.
29. Niiyama R, Happle R, Hoffmann R. Influence of estrogens on the androgen metabolism in different subunits of human hair follicles. Eur J Dermatol. 2001;11:165–8.
30. Rossouw JE, Anderson GL, Prentice RL, LaCroix AZ, Kooperberg C, Stefanick ML, et al. Risk and benefits of estrogen plus progestin in healthy postmenopausal women: principal results from the women's health initiative randomized controlled trial. JAMA. 2002;288:321–33.
31. Soloman CG, Dluhy RG. Rethinking post-menopausal hormone therapy. N Engl J Med. 2003;348:579–80.
32. Surazynski A, Jarzabek K, Haczynski J, Laudanski P, Palka J, Wolczynski S. Differential effects of estradiol and raloxifene on collagen biosynthesis in cultured

human skin fibroblasts. Int J Mol Med. 2003;12: 803–9.
33. Verdier-Sévrain S. Effect of estrogens on skin aging and the potential role of selective estrogen receptor modulators. Climacteric. 2007;10:289–97.
34. Izumi T, Saito M, Obata A. Oral intake of soy isoflavone aglycone improves the aged skin of adult women. J Nutr Sci Vitaminol. 2007;53:57–62.
35. Hall G, Phillips TJ. Estrogen and skin: the effects of estrogen, menopause, and hormone replacement therapy on the skin. J Am Acad Dermatol. 2005;53:555–68.
36. Jee SH, Lee SY, Chiu HC, Chang CC, Chen TJ. Effects of estrogen and estrogen receptor in normal human melanocytes. Biochem Biophys Res Commun. 1994;199:1407–12.
37. Hughes SV, Robinson E, Bland R, Lewis HM, Stewart PM, Hewison M. 1,25-dihydroxyvitamin D regulates estrogen metabolism in cultured keratinocytes. Endocrinology. 1997;138:3711–8.
38. Haczynski J, Tarkowski R, Jarzabek K, Slomczynsk M, Wolczynski S, Magoffin DA, et al. Human cultured skin fibroblasts express estrogen receptor alpha and beta. Int J Mol Med. 2002;10:149–53.
39. Gruber CJ, Tschugguel W, Schneeberger C, Huber JC. Production and actions of estrogens. N Engl J Med. 2002;346:340–52.
40. Simoncini T, Genazzani AR. Non-genomic actions of sex steroid hormones. Eur J Endocrinol. 2003;148: 281–92.
41. Slominski A, Zbytek B, Nikolakis G, Manna PR, Skobowiat C, Zmijewski M, et al. Steroidogenesis in the skin: implications for local immune functions. J Steroid Biochem Mol Biol. 2013;137:107–23.
42. Wines N, Willsteed E. Menopause and the skin. Australas J Dermatol. 2001;42:149–8.
43. Schaffer J, Fantil JA. Urogenital effects of the menopause. Clin Obstet Gynaecol. 1996;10:401–17.
44. Meffert JJ, Davis BM, Grimwood RE. Lichen sclerosus. J Am Acad Dermatol. 1995;32:393–416.
45. Cattani P, Manfrin E, Presti F, Sartori R, Buffo L. Our experience in treating vulvar lichen sclerosus. Minerva Ginecol. 1997;49:207–12.
46. McKay M. Vulvodynia. A multifactorial problem. Arch Dermatol. 1989;125:256–62.
47. McKay M. Dysaesthetic (essential) vulvodynia: treatment with amitriptyline. J Reprod Med. 1993;38:9–13.
48. Deschamps P, Leary D, Pedalles S, Mandard JC. Keratoderma climactericum (Haxthausen's disease). Clinical signs, laboratory findings and etretinate treatment in 10 patients. Dermatologica. 1986;172:258–62.
49. Applebaum KM, Nelson HH, Zens MS, Stukel TA, Spencer SK, Karagas MR. Oral contraceptives: a risk factor for squamous cell carcinoma? J Invest Dermatol. 2009;129:2760–5.
50. Asgari MM, Efird JT, Warton EM, Friedman GD. Potential risk factors for cutaneous squamous cell carcinoma include oral contraceptives: results of a nested case-control study. Int J Environ Res Pub Health. 2010;7:427–42.
51. Gupta A, Driscoll MS. Do hormones influence melanoma? Facts and controversies. Clin Dermatol. 2010;28:287–92.
52. Mor Z, Caspi E. Cutaneous complications of hormonal replacement therapy. Clin Dermatol. 1997;15:147–54.
53. Koomen ER, Joosse A, Herings RMC, Casparie MK, Guchelaar HJ, Nijsten T. Estrogens, oral contraceptives and hormonal replacement therapy increase the incidence of cutaneous melanoma: a population-based case-control study. Ann Oncol. 2009;20:358–64.
54. Tang JY, Spaunhurst KM, Chlebowski RT, Wactawski-Wende J, Keiser E, Thomas F, et al. Menopausal hormone therapy and risks of melanoma and nonmelanoma skin cancers: women's health initiative randomized trials. J Natl Cancer Inst. 2011;103:1469–75.
55. Blume-Peytavi U, Atkin S, Gieler U, Grimalt R. Skin academy: hair, skin, hormones and menopause – current status/knowledge on the management of hair disorders in menopausal women. Eur J Dermatol. 2012;22:310–8.
56. Sator PG. Skin treatments and dermatological procedures to promote youthful skin. Clin Interv Aging. 2006;1:51–6.
57. Bonaparte JP, Ellis D, Quinn JG, Ansari MT, Rabski J, Kilty SJ. A comparative assessment of three formulations of botulinum toxin A for facial rhytides: a systematic review and meta-analyses. Syst Rev. 2013;2:40.

Menopause and Oxidative Stress

4

Martha A. Sánchez-Rodríguez,
Mariano Zacarías-Flores,
and Víctor Manuel Mendoza-Núñez

Contents

4.1	**Menopause and Aging**	34
4.2	**Oxidative Stress**	35
4.2.1	Oxidant Process	35
4.2.2	Antioxidant Process	38
4.2.3	Third Level of Antioxidant Defense	41
4.3	**Oxidative Damage from Biomolecules**	42
4.3.1	Lipid Oxidation	42
4.3.2	Proteins Oxidation	43
4.3.3	Carbohydrates Oxidation	43
4.3.4	DNA Oxidative Damage	44
4.4	**Skin and Oxidative Stress**	45
4.5	**Menopause as Risk Factor for Oxidative Stress**	47
References		48

M.A. Sánchez-Rodríguez, PhD (✉)
V.M. Mendoza-Núñez, PhD
Unidad de Investigación en Gerontología,
Facultad de Estudios Superiores Zaragoza,
Universidad Nacional Autónoma de México,
Av. Guelatao No. 66 Col. Ejército de Oriente,
09230 Mexico City, Distrito Federal, Mexico
e-mail: masanrod@yahoo.com.mx;
mendovic@servidor.unam.mx

M. Zacarías-Flores, MD
Obstetrics-Gynecology Department, Hospital Gustavo
Baz Prada, Instituto de Salud del Estado de México,
Mexico City, Distrito Federal, Mexico
e-mail: mzacariasf@yahoo.com

Aging is the process of morphological, physiological, biochemical, and psychological modifications over time in living organisms. For example, aging promotes a relative decrease in the homeostatic response, causes reversible damage when it exceeds the natural mechanisms of homeostasis, and generates disease. In this sense, the postmenopausal period may be considered the beginning of the aging process in women. Postmenopausal aging is produced by a series of endocrinological changes that are caused by the production of estrogens (mainly estradiol) and lead to low estrogen (E2) levels. Once women begin ovarian senescence and alterations of hypothalamic pituitary axis are manifest, E2 production becomes erratic, and many women develop a series of symptoms in a period known as perimenopause (Table 4.1). Some of these changes involve the skin.

In fact, associations between estrogen deprivation and skin changes such as dryness, the reduction of epidermal and dermal thickness, decreased collagen content, a reduction in elasticity, fragility, and poor healing have been shown in postmenopausal women [1, 2]. Additionally, changes in hair are commonly observed. Hirsutism (i.e., the appearance of unwanted facial hair), alopecia, skin atrophy, and weakness of facial skin beginning at this stage of a woman's life are results of the reduction in progesterone and the increasing impact of free and unopposed circulating androgens on the sebaceous glands and hair follicles [3, 4].

Table 4.1 Perimenopausal alterations in women

Physical symptoms and signs	Psychological	Systemic	Skin and hair
Hot flushes	Anxiety	Atherosclerosis	Dryness
Headache	Humor alterations	Cardiovascular disease	Decreased collagen content
Nocturnal wet	Sadness	Osteoporosis and osteopenia	Reduction in elasticity
Vaginal dryness	Loneliness sense	Increased body fat, mainly abdominal	Reduction of epidermal an dermal thickness
Dyspareunia	Sleep disturbances		Fragility and poor healing
Muscular and articular ache	Memory disturbances		Alopecia
Genitourinary changes	Concentration disturbances		Hirsutism

Many authors link the decline in estrogen to distinct cellular aging mechanisms involving oxidative damage and cellular senescence. This theory has been proposed mainly because estrogens function as sex hormones and antioxidant molecules that counterbalance oxidative damage, which is also called oxidative stress.

In this chapter, we review the general aspects of postmenopause that are linked to oxidative stress and the relationship of oxidative stress with skin aging.

4.1 Menopause and Aging

Ovarian aging is caused by a gradual decline in the quantity and quality of oocytes that are present in the ovarian tissue until the menstrual cycle reaches its end (i.e., last menstrual bleeding). This process is characterized by the gradual and erratic decrease of estrogen secretion and a consequent changes in gonadotrophins (FSH and LH) due to the failure of feedback signaling by estrogen and possible alterations of hypothalamic pituitary feedback mechanism [5, 6]. Estrogen depletion affects many tissues of the body and produces a wide range of signs and symptoms. However, in the Study of Woman's Health Across the Nation (SWAN), it has been observed that the symptoms reported frequently as being part of a menopausal syndrome such as hot flashes, night sweats, menstrual irregularities, vaginal dryness, depression, nervous tension, palpitations, headaches, insomnia, lack of energy, difficulty concentrating, and dizzy spells are not inherent manifestations to this process [7]. Indeed, several of these symptoms may be linked to the biological changes seen in aging; although, it is known that the aging is individualized and is determined by genetic and cultural factors [8–10]. It also greatly impacts female fertility related to aging. In fact, ovarian tissue ages much more rapidly than do the tissues of other body systems [5, 11].

In this context, the age-associated malfunction of human cells results from the physiological accumulation of irreparable damage to biomolecules, which is an unavoidable side effect of normal aerobic metabolism. As noted above, this process is termed oxidative stress (OS).

During aging, oxidative stress increases [12] and causes many of the normal and pathological characteristics that are found in the elderly. Moreover, symptoms and pathological findings that are associated with postmenopause may be related, at least in part, to OS, mainly because of estrogen deficiency; therefore, it is possible to say that this stage of life represents the beginning of the aging process in women.

From the cellular point of view, some researchers have found that the luteinizing granulosa cells in women aged >38 years contain higher numbers of mitochondrial DNA (mtDNA) deletions and exhibit reduced expression of antioxidant enzymes compared with those of younger women [11], which suggests oxidative damage. Other studies have shown that age-related changes in the female ovary could be due to a lowering of enzymatic antioxidant defenses and an increase in oxidant molecules production of possible multiple cellular origins (i.e., mitochondria, cytoplasm) [13].

Recently, it has been noted that the age at natural menopause reflects a complex interrelation of health and socioeconomic factors and might be a marker of aging and general health [14]. Similar to aging, premature and early menopause, either spontaneous or induced, are associated with long-term health risks such as premature death, cardiovascular disease, neurologic disease, osteoporosis, optic nerve aging, and glaucomatous neurodegeneration [15, 16]. However, some of these adverse outcomes may be prevented by hormone therapy with estrogens initiated after the onset of menopause. These effects were observed in women exposed to estrogen therapy and are most likely explained by a positive effect on oxidative damage [17]. Moreover, menopausal symptoms are associated with low biological antioxidant potential [18].

A biological model of premature aging is Down syndrome (DS). Individuals with this pathology experience premature aging and dementia with alterations in the oxidative metabolism of neutrophils, which contribute to alterations of physiological functions [19]. It is reported that persons with DS have excess Cu/Zn superoxide dismutase (SOD) activity, which causes an imbalance between the activity of antioxidant enzymes and leads to increased oxidative molecule levels and cellular senescence [19, 20]. In fact, women with DS experience the menopause at an earlier age than women in the general population [21], and this finding has health implications because early menopause is a risk factor for several age-related diseases, as we described previously.

Therefore, it is important to understand the oxidative process and place it in the context of perimenopause and the changes that estrogen deprivation causes in women.

4.2 Oxidative Stress

Oxidative stress, or redox imbalance, occurs when the balance between oxidant reactive species, free radicals (FRs), non-radicals, and antioxidants is disrupted because of an accumulation of reactive species or the depletion of antioxidants; this in turn leads to oxidative damage to biomolecules [22, 23]. This biochemical process was first described by Rebeca Gerschman et al. in 1954 [24], who noted that FRs are toxic agents that cause disease.

By 1956, Denham Harman [25] had linked FRs to aging and the most prevalent chronic conditions that plague this stage of life. This proposal was later reinforced by the discovery of the enzyme SOD by McCord and Fridovich in 1969 [26]. This enzyme lies at the axis of the antioxidant system. At present, it is recognized that the production of reactive species and oxidative stress occurs intracellularly and within the extracellular space. Oxidative damage can compromise cell metabolism, differentiation, proliferation, survival, and reproduction, and the long-term effects of oxidative damage are implicated in skin aging, cancer, and inflammation [27].

To better understand the biological process of oxidative stress, we will divide the topic into its two components: oxidant and antioxidant process.

4.2.1 Oxidant Process

Reactive species can be separated into four groups based in their main atom: oxygen (ROS), nitrogen (RNS), sulfur (RSS), and chlorine (RCS), with ROS being the most abundant [23, 28–30].

ROS are intermediate metabolites that are produced through the univalent reduction of oxygen in normal aerobic metabolism and are part of a group of FRs and non-radicals with highly oxidizing structures. FRs are chemical species that possess one unpaired electron in their last orbital; therefore, they are able to extract an electron from a neighboring atom or molecule to complete its orbit. When two FRs share their unpaired electrons, non-radical molecules are formed [22, 28, 30].

In living organisms, ROS are produced by various metabolic processes, such as the mitochondrial respiratory chain, phagocytosis, detoxification reactions in cytochrome P450, and prostaglandin synthesis, as well as various inflammatory and nonenzymatic reactions between oxygen and organic compounds that include nicotine adenine dinucleotide phosphate (NADPH) oxidase. ROS can be created by exposure to ionizing radiation but are formed mainly by oxidation-reduction (redox) reactions. It is known that ROS can interfere with cell differentiation, aging, and apoptosis [28, 31–34].

The main generator of ROS is the mitochondria, as a side effect of the electron transport system of the respiratory chain, whose principal function is ATP production. In this process, electrons are transferred by the tetravalent reduction of oxygen to form water (H_2O), but approximately 1–3 % of the electrons are lost in the system, producing the superoxide anion ($O_2^{\cdot-}$), the first FR molecule that is formed by the addition of one electron to oxygen, mediated by NADPH oxidase [23]. As a cascade of electron transfer reactions occurs, $O_2^{\cdot-}$ is produced in the union sites of the ubiquinone in the I (NADH:ubiquinone oxidoreductase) and III (ubiquinol:cytochrome c oxidoreductase) complexes. The $O_2^{\cdot-}$ is then converted to hydrogen peroxide (H_2O_2), which is a non-radical molecule with strong oxidant power, by the action of superoxide dismutase (SOD, EC 1.15.1.1); H_2O_2, in turn, is acted upon by catalases (EC 1.11.1.6), peroxidases, and peroxiredoxins. Glutathione peroxidase (GPx, EC 1.11.1.9) is the main enzyme that is responsible for producing H_2O. In the glutathione peroxidase reaction, glutathione is oxidized to glutathione disulfide, which can be reconverted to glutathione by glutathione reductase in an NADPH-consuming process [23, 35–37]. In the presence of transition metal cations such as iron (Fe^{2+}) and copper (Cu^{2+}), H_2O_2 is converted to a hydroxyl radical ($^{\cdot}OH$), which is the most reactive and dangerous FR, and the metal is reduced through the Fenton reaction during cellular metabolism. Moreover, $O_2^{\cdot-}$ can oxidize Fe^{3+}. This integrated reaction when produced by iron is named the Haber-Weiss reaction [38, 39]:

$$H_2O_2 + Fe^{2+} \rightarrow {}^{\cdot}OH + OH^- + Fe^{3+} \quad \text{Fenton reaction}$$

$$O_2^{\cdot-} + Fe^{3+} \rightarrow O_2 + Fe^{2+}$$

$$H_2O_2 + O_2^{\cdot-} \xrightarrow{Fe^{2+}} {}^{\cdot}OH + OH^- + O_2 \quad \text{Haber–Weiss reaction}$$

To balance the oxidation reactions, each oxygen atom generates one molecule of H_2O, but during intermediary reactions, three ROS are formed by the addition of four electrons (Fig. 4.1):

$$O_2 \rightarrow O_2^{\cdot-} \rightarrow H_2O_2 \rightarrow {}^{\cdot}OH \rightarrow H_2O$$

Importantly, it has been documented that $^{\cdot}OH$ can also be formed under reducing conditions, i.e., molecules that function as true antioxidants (reducers) may increase rather than decrease free radical stress [40].

Hydroxyl radicals react with biomolecules such as lipids, carbohydrates, proteins, and DNA to produce peroxyl radicals ($ROO^{\cdot-}$), which conduct a series of chain reactions that result in hydrogen abstraction during biomolecule oxidation. However, $O_2^{\cdot-}$ and H_2O_2 do not react with most biological molecules.

Recently, it has been noted that the production of ROS in mitochondria is based on its high membrane potential (mt$\Delta\Psi$) or high amounts of NADH/NAD^+. The mechanism that has been proposed is based on results from animal models and suggests a switch of oxidative phosphorylation between high efficiency at low mt$\Delta\Psi$ and low ROS formation, through a second mechanism of respiratory control (RC2 on) and the activated state with maximum rates of ATP synthesis (maximum output power) at lower efficiency accompanied by high mt$\Delta\Psi$ and ROS formation (RC2 off). This hypothesis proposes that health and long life in animals are, in part, dependent on RC2 to maintain low mt$\Delta\Psi$ values and low ROS formation [37].

ROS can also act through indirect mechanisms, and the cascade of effects reflects the changes in the level and function of redox-sensitive transcription factors and signaling proteins such as Nrf2, NF-κB, AP-1, p53, and MAP kinases. These mechanisms are complex and go beyond the scope of this review.

ROS production and release can be influenced by environmental factors such as UV radiation, air pollution, and exogenous toxins such as nitric oxide, cigarette smoke, alcohol intake, caffeine consumption, and exposure to drugs.

The second major group of reactive species in the oxidative stress process is nitrogen species

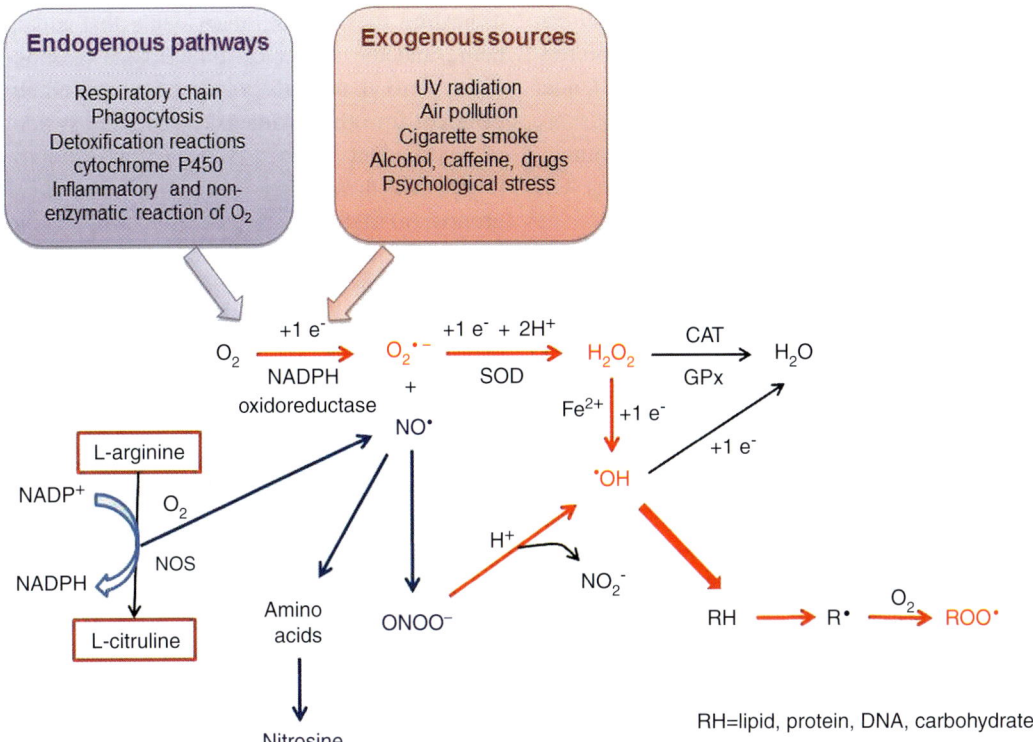

Fig. 4.1 Chain of reactions to produce ROS and RNS, both inside and outside of cells. The reactions begin with the addition of an electron to an oxygen atom either by the metabolic pathways (in *purple*) or exogenous sources (*pink*). The ROS formation is in *red* and the RNS in *blue*. See corresponding text to explain. *SOD* superoxide dismutase, *CAT* catalase, *GPx* glutathione peroxidase, *NOS* nitric oxide synthase

(RNS), which are also formed during intracellular metabolism. The most abundant RNS is the nitric oxide radical (NO•), which is a vasodilator with anti-inflammatory and anticoagulant properties. NO• is a gaseous FR derivate that results from the oxidation of the terminal guanido-nitrogen atom of L-arginine in a reaction that consumes molecular oxygen and reduces equivalents of nicotine adenine dinucleotide phosphate reduced coenzyme (NADPH) to form L-citrulline. This reaction is catalyzed by nitric oxide synthases (NOS). NO• can be rapidly inactivated by reacting with $O_2^{•-}$ to form the strong oxidant peroxynitrite (ONOO−), which, in an acidic environment, is converted to peroxynitric acid and subsequently decomposed to •OH and nitrite (NO_2^-) [36, 41, 42]. Additionally, under certain conditions, NO• can react with amino acid residues to produce nitrosine, which is a biochemical compound that inactivates enzymes [43]. It is important to note that NO• and its derivatives (RNS) inhibit mitochondrial respiration reactions and either stimulate or inhibit cell death depending on the prevailing conditions [44].

Reactive species of sulfur (RSS) form the third group, and these species have stressor properties that are similar to those found in ROS. Thiols and disulfides are easily oxidized to sulfur species such as thiyl radicals, disulfides, sulfenic acids, and disulfide-S-oxides. RSS are in turn oxidized and inhibit thiol proteins and enzymes, collaborating to exacerbate oxidative stress [30].

The last group of reactive species is composed of chlorine molecules (RCS) that are formed by the action of myeloperoxidase at the expense of H_2O_2 in a chloride ion-dependent reaction during phagocytosis. The reaction product, the hypochlorite ion (OCl⁻), is in balance with its protonated form, hypochlorous acid (HOCl). Under physiological conditions, both compounds are potent oxidizing agents that may attack biomolecules and produce ROS and RNS, as does ˙OH and ONOO⁻ [28, 45].

4.2.2 Antioxidant Process

Cells have effective mechanisms for the defense against oxidative damage. Because the main reactions involving reactive species take place in the intracellular compartment, these defense mechanisms are usually carried out by enzymes; however, in the extracellular compartment, antioxidant molecules and mechanisms of a different chemical nature are found. The antioxidant scavenging capability of cells varies according to the type of oxidants that attack them, and the ability of antioxidants to scavenge peroxyl radicals might be considerably different for other oxidants. Hence, the system of antioxidant protection occurs at different levels, and these levels are divided into three groups: (a) first level, the actions are directed to prevent the formation of reactive species or to intercept these molecules when they are formed; (b) second level, the mechanisms are directed to trap the reactive species that are formed, thus terminating or preventing the initiation of an oxidative chain reaction; and (c) third level, a group of enzymes that directly restore native biomolecules and other catabolic molecules that can specifically degrade nonfunctional molecules. This degradation can serve to remove oxidized molecules from the cytosol or to fill up the pool of precursors for resynthesis (Fig. 4.2) [36, 46–48].

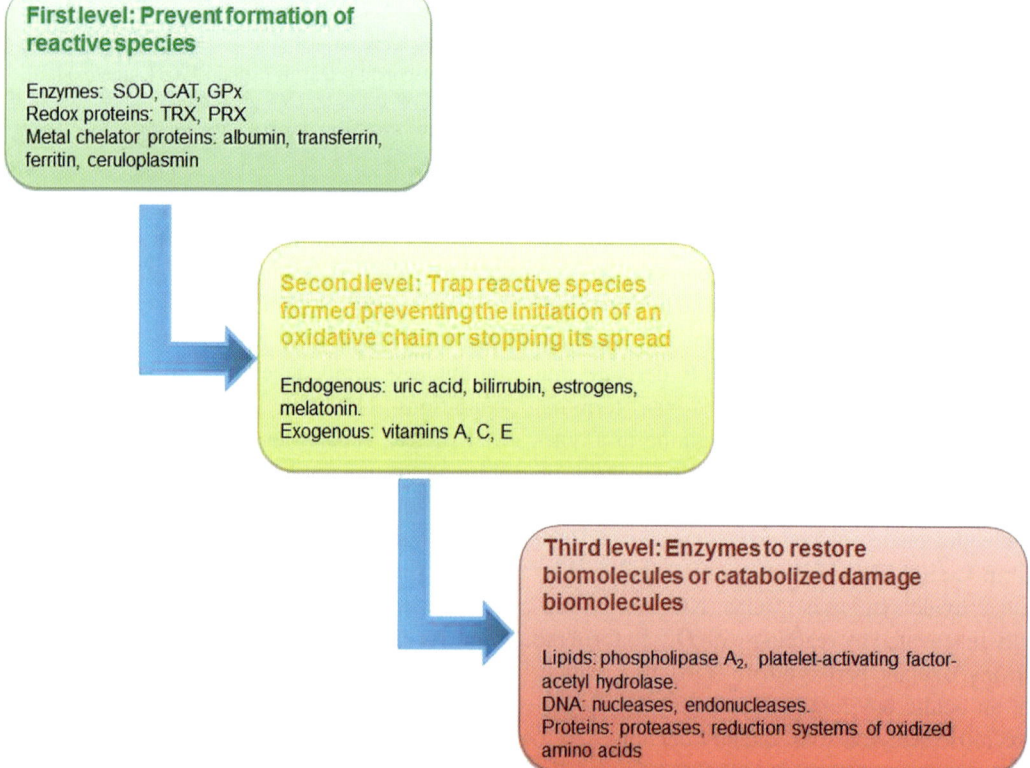

Fig. 4.2 Antioxidant systems by level of action versus oxidative damage. *SOD* superoxide dismutase, *CAT* catalase, *GPx* glutathione peroxidase, *TRX* thioredoxin, *PRX* peroxyredoxin

4.2.2.1 First Level of Antioxidant Defense

At this level, we find the major antioxidant enzymes, SOD (EC 1.15.1.11), catalase (EC 1.11.1.6), and GPx (EC 1.11.1.9), and to complete this line of defense, we can add other enzymes, including hemooxygenase-1 (EC 1.14.99.3) and redox proteins such as thioredoxins (TRXs, EC 1.8.4.10) and peroxiredoxins (PRXs, EC 1.11.1.15). All of these molecules are responsible for maintaining a redox steady state [28].

The superoxide dismutases are a group of tetrameric oxidoreductases that catalyze the dismutation of $O_2^{\cdot-}$ to H_2O_2 and O_2. Three isoforms that are located in different subcellular locations but catalyze the same reaction are included in this group: SOD1 (CuZnSOD) in the cytosol, SOD2 (MnSOD) in the mitochondrial matrix, and SOD3 (ecSOD) in the extracellular fluid. SOD2 is of particular interest because the mitochondrial matrix represents the first line of antioxidant defense against the $O_2^{\cdot-}$ that is produced as a byproduct of oxidative phosphorylation [28, 41]. Moreover, it has been reported that SOD1 has a CO_2-dependent peroxidase weak activity; this CO_2 dependence occurs by generating a strong oxidant in the copper site of the enzyme due to two sequential reactions with H_2O_2, followed by the oxidation of CO_2 to a carbonate radical, which is responsible of several oxidation reactions subsequent [49].

The H_2O_2 product of the dismutation reaction is more stable than $O_2^{\cdot-}$. It can traverse membranes and has been shown to be an essential signaling molecule in a variety of signaling cascades and cell matrix interactions [50]. This molecule, in turn, is converted into H_2O by the action of catalases, peroxiredoxins, and peroxidases. Catalase is a tetrameric hemoprotein with four heme groups at its active site and is located in the cytosol and peroxisomes. Its catalytic action resides in the iron within its structure that is actively involved in coordinately binding water or forming a complex with an atom of O_2 during the reaction. Likewise, catalase can also bind NADPH, which prevents its oxidative inactivation or the formation of complex II by the action of H_2O_2 because it is reduced to water [28, 51].

Glutathione peroxidases form a group of tetrameric enzymes that contain a molecule of selenium-cysteine in their active sites and use glutathione (GSSG) and other thiols to reduce H_2O_2 or organic hydroperoxides to water or alcohols, respectively. Four glutathione peroxidase isoforms have been identified in mammals: GPx1 (in the cytosol and mitochondria), GPx2 (in the intestinal epithelium), GPx3 (in the extracellular space), and GPx4 (in cellular membranes). The mechanism for reducing glutathione (GSH) or a thiol compound begins by reducing selenium. The reduced enzyme then reacts with H_2O_2, and H_2O is released. Subsequently, a second GSH molecule undergoes thiol-disulfide exchange, which releases GSSG and regenerates the enzyme [28, 52].

Metal chelator proteins are also considered part of the first level of defense against oxidation, and the principal proteins include albumin, α-lactalbumin, transferrin, ferritin, ceruloplasmin, β-lactoglobulin, and immunoglobulins. These enzymes act mainly to remove FR from the extracellular space, and their antioxidant mechanism involves amino acids such as tyrosine and cysteine, due to their structures, and the chelation of transition metals [53–55]. Albumin is the most abundant of the serum-circulating proteins, and its antioxidant function involves more than one mechanism of action. It is noted that more than 70 % of the serum FR-trapping activity is due to this protein [54]. The antioxidant capability of albumin can be attributed to two mechanisms: its ability to bind multiple ligands through its multiple binding sites and its propensity for FR trapping. However, this protein is also susceptible to oxidation, which diminishes its antioxidant activity [55]. Its FR trapping ability resides in its cysteine (Cys34) and methionine (Met) residues, but cysteine plays a more important role in this process [56].

Iron-binding proteins such as transferrin and ferritin are capable of preventing the Fenton reaction because they are iron chelators. This antioxidant action is possible because they bind iron, and once bound, they are not available to stimulate FR reactions or form ˙OH, which is an important part of the extracellular antioxidant defense system [53, 57, 58]. Another enzyme that avoids the Fenton reaction is ceruloplasmin. This enzyme has ferroxidase action, which inhibits the formation of ˙OH iron and is dependent on H_2O_2. This enzyme also has a synergic activity with ferritin, which inhibits superoxide-dependent iron release and limits its biodisponibility in vivo to reinstate iron to the enzyme when it is released [53, 59].

4.2.2.2 Second Level of Antioxidant Defense

When the first level of antioxidant defense is exceeded, organisms have a second level of protection. The role of these antioxidants is to "trap" FR once it is formed, thus terminating or preventing the initiation of an oxidative chain reaction. Exogenous and endogenous molecules are included in this group. Serum compound such as uric acid and bilirubin, and hormones such as estrogens and melatonin, are all endogens secondary antioxidants; vitamins A, C and E; poliphenolic compounds, and aromatic amines are all exogenous antioxidant compounds. An important characteristic of exogenous antioxidants is that they have the ability to become radical species; therefore, they are potentially prooxidants [39, 47].

Estrogens are linked to menopause; therefore, they will be emphasized here. Estrogens and their metabolites possess antioxidant capabilities due to the presence of an OH at C3 of the phenolic ring in the A position. The antioxidant activities of estrogen are carried out in different ways: estrogen molecules act as free radical scavengers, neutralize excess ROS, and increase the amount of antioxidant molecules such as thioredoxin and SOD [17, 60, 61]. As FR scavengers, estrogens can be considered polycyclic phenolic compounds, which are molecules that are capable of intercalating into the cellular and mitochondrial membranes, where they directly interrupt lipid peroxidation (lipid oxidation) or through poorly defined lipophilic derivatives [62]. Indeed, several in vivo and in vitro studies indicated that the oxidation of LDL isolated from postmenopausal women was differentially inhibited by various estrogens, and the most active were the unique, ring B unsaturated estrogens [63]. Moreover, estrogens can act in trapping transition metals, such as Fe^{2+} and Cu^+, reducing and maintaining low levels of these metals, and preventing them from acting as oxidants again. Thus, estrogens attenuate the ROS that are created by the Fenton reaction in vitro [64]. Because of its capability for incrementing antioxidant molecules, estradiol increases the transcription, expression, and activity of SOD2 and SOD3 without affecting GPx and catalase [65].

Additionally, estrogens can act as prooxidants because they are oxidized to 4-hydroxy-estrogens or catechol-estrogens by the action of a wide range of oxidative enzymes, such as cytochrome P450, and metallic ions in the presence of molecular O_2. The cytochrome P450 pathway generates reactive electrophilic estrogen *o*-quinones and ROS, through the redox cycling of the *o-quinones*, mainly by the TCDD-inducible P450 isozymes, P4501A1/1A2 and P4501B1, which selectively catalyze hydroxylation at the 2 and 4 positions of estrone and 17β-estradiol, respectively. In this redox cycling, the 4-hydroxy-estrogens are oxidized to semiquinones and quinones, which can be reduced by cytochome P450 NADPH-dependent reductase to generate $O_2^{˙-}$, which in turn reduces Fe^{3+} to Fe^{2+} by the Fenton reaction to produce ˙OH. These reactions are dependent on the levels of metallic ions in the given environment. Importantly, catechol-estrogen metabolites are likely contributors to the development of cancer [66, 67].

Antioxidant vitamins are also relevant during menopause. Recent research has focused on the antioxidant activity and possible anticancer properties of vitamins A, C, and E, which have been commonly thought to prevent or dampen the effect of chronic degenerative diseases. These vitamins have been effective antioxidants in vitro and in vivo [68, 69], and several studies have shown that vitamins C and E, when administered at different concentrations, exert antioxidant effects that prevent or reduce oxidative stress. Vitamin E or α-tocopherol is the major membrane-bound antioxidant in the cell. Vitamin E donates an electron to a peroxyl radical, which is produced during lipid peroxidation and acts as a chain-breaking antioxidant by scavenging chain-initiation and -propagation radicals. Vitamin E also reduces the consequences of oxidized LDL by decreasing the ability of monocytes to bind to endothelial cells [70–72]. Under such circumstances, vitamin E is considered a suppressor of LDL lipid oxidation because it is the main antioxidant molecule in human lipoproteins [73]. Vitamin C, when in its L-ascorbic acid form, acts as an antioxidant in the aqueous conditions of the plasma and cytoplasm and is converted to dehydroascorbic acid in the presence of oxidants. Ascorbic acid crosses the cytoplasmic membrane, directly scavenges ROS through the major antioxidant pathway and acts as an electron-donor by maintaining iron in its ferrous state. This ability to donate one or two electrons makes ascorbate an excellent reducing and antioxidant agent [74, 75]. Additionally, vitamin C acts synergistically with vitamin E because vitamin E protects membranes from lipid peroxidation by transforming itself into an α-tocoperoxyl radical once it captures free ROS in the membrane. Ascorbic acid reduces this radical form and makes it reactive for new, reducing lipid oxidation, which consequentially leads to a decrease in oxidative stress. The interaction between vitamins E and C has led to the idea of "vitamin E recycling," which is when the antioxidant function of oxidized vitamin E is continuously restored by other antioxidants, mainly vitamin C [76, 77]. Under normal physiological conditions, the α-tocopherol/ascorbic acid pair is the major antioxidant system that suppresses excess LDL oxidation in the plasma [78]. Another observed effect of vitamin C is in the modulation of DNA repair, although the impact of vitamin C on DNA damage is dependent on the background values of vitamin C in the individual and on the level of oxidative stress [79]. Moreover, vitamin C affects NO bioavailability due to its ability to prevent eNOS-related superoxide production by a mechanism that is not entirely known [77].

As described previously for estrogens, antioxidant vitamins also act as prooxidant agents. The α-tocoperoxyl radical is relatively nonreactive, although it can exert prooxidant activities in the absence of ascorbic acid and reduced coenzyme Q_{10}, thus acting on LDL as a chain-transfer agent rather than as a radical trap and oxidizing LDL via a free radical chain [73, 78]. Recent studies in yeast have suggested the potential prooxidant action of α-tocopherol and coenzyme Q_{10}, warning against antioxidant supplementation as an approach to increase longevity [72].

In the same way, ascorbic acid can cause serious oxidative damage because it reacts with free iron and produces the ascorbyl radical, and it can undergo pH-dependent autoxidation to form H_2O_2. The ascorbyl radical in turn reduces iron when it appears as a free ferric cation in biological fluids, thus accelerating the auto-oxidation reaction and favoring the Fenton reaction to produce an ˙OH, which causes oxidative damage to biomolecules [74, 75]. Additionally, it is feasible that the release of iron and the presence of vitamin C during acute inflammation could lead to the generation of ˙OH, ascorbyl, and thiyl radicals [80].

4.2.3 Third Level of Antioxidant Defense

There are some circumstances in which biomolecules are oxidized, necessitating a third level of antioxidant defense including repair enzymes such as phospholipases, nucleases, reductases, and proteases, which repair oxidative damage, remove the oxidized products, and reconstitute the lost function. Phospholipases, such as phospholipase A_2 or platelet-activating factor-acetyl hydrolase, remove oxidized fatty acids because they must be in a nonesterified form to be detoxified [81, 82].

Redoxy-endonucleases endogenously repair DNA damage that is generated by exposure to ionizing radiation [83]. The action of these enzymes is mediated by nucleotide excision repair (NER), which is a pathway of DNA repair that is responsible for eliminating diverse oxidative lesions. Approximately 30 proteins participate in this mechanism, but ERCC1-XPF and XPG are the major structure-specific endonucleases that make 5′ and 3′ excisions into damaged DNA, respectively, and release the damaged oligonucleotide [84]. Other smaller base adducts, such as hydroxyl or alkyl groups at different positions, and single-strand breaks serve as substrates for DNA base excision repair (BER) [85].

Finally, most oxidized proteins cannot be repaired by cells. An alternative method for preventing further damage is the catabolism of oxidatively modified proteins via proteases that are generated in latent proteolytic systems, which are activated when cells are challenged with ROS [54, 86, 87]. Two key proteases have been identified: a cytosolic, proteolytic system known as the 20S proteasome and a mitochondrial protease called the Lon protease, which is involved in the degradation of oxidized aconitase [88].

Together with degradation, specific enzyme systems contain proteins that reduce certain amino acid oxidation products that contain sulfur, cysteine, and methionine and are most susceptible to oxidation. The glutaredoxin/glutathione/glutathione reductase and thioredoxin/thioredoxin reductase systems reverse the oxidation of cysteine disulfide bonds and sulfonic acid, while the methionine sulfoxide reductase system (MSR) reduces methionine sulfoxide to methionine [88]. If FR damage to DNA is not repaired, it may lead to genetic instability, which has been proposed as the leading cause of disease processes such as carcinogenesis [89].

4.3 Oxidative Damage from Biomolecules

As explained above, the consequence of producing reactive species is the oxidation of biomolecules such as lipids, proteins, DNA, and carbohydrates. In this section, we will address the oxidation of each type of molecule.

4.3.1 Lipid Oxidation

Of all biomolecules that can be attacked by ROS, lipids are the most susceptible. Three different mechanisms for lipid oxidation exist: (1) enzymatic oxidation; (2) nonenzymatic, free radical-mediated oxidation; and (3) nonenzymatic, non-radical oxidation [90, 91].

Lipid oxidation reactions that are mediated by enzymes are carried out as part of the catalytic action of the enzyme; for example, lipoxygenases, cyclooxygenases, and cytochrome c use FRs as intermediaries in the reactions that form endoperoxides and hydroperoxides. In these cases, the FR is bound to the protein active site [43, 92], where it induces structural changes in the cells under different physiopathological conditions [93].

The nonenzymatic reactions are performed primarily in cell membranes because they are rich in polyunsaturated fatty acids (PUFA), which are easily oxidized by lipid peroxidation, and their products are referred to as lipoperoxides. This process directly damages the structure of the cell membrane and indirectly damages other cellular components by producing reactive aldehydes. Lipid peroxidation is carried out by five in-chain reactions [90–92]:

1. A PUFA is attacked by a FR ($^{\bullet}$OH or ROO$^{\bullet-}$), which abstracts one hydrogen atom (H$^{\bullet}$) from a methylene group with an adjacent double bound (—CH—), and this abstraction results in a pentadienyl carbon-centered lipid radical (—$^{\bullet}$CH—).
2. The carbon-centered lipid radical undergoes a molecular rearrangement to form a conjugated diene, which then combines with O_2 to form a lipidic peroxyl radical (ROO$^{\bullet}$).
3. The lipidic peroxyl radical is fragmented to give O_2 and a lipid radical (the reverse of reaction 2).
4. A rearrangement of the peroxyl radical occurs.
5. A cyclization of the peroxyl radical occurs, but this reaction is only carried out when PUFA has more than three double bonds.

These new peroxyl radicals are capable of extracting the hydrogen atom of other PUFAs and inducing further oxidation. Peroxidation is continued until the substrate is terminated or the sequence is interrupted by an antioxidant [43, 90, 91].

Extensive lipid peroxidation in biological membranes causes fluidity loss, loss of membrane potential, increased permeability to H$^+$ and other ions, and, eventually, the release of cell contents and organelles resulting in cell death, whether programmed (apoptosis) or unprogrammed [43, 92, 93]. Likewise, lipid peroxidation products such as malondialdehyde and unsaturated aldehydes inactivate cellular proteins by forming protein cross-linkages [23].

Lipid peroxidation by a nonenzymatic, nonradical mechanism is induced by singlet oxygen and ozone [90], but this process has not been well studied, and the mechanism is not fully understood.

4.3.2 Proteins Oxidation

Proteins are also direct targets of ROS/RNS because of their high concentrations in living organisms, and different reactions involving proteins occur, such as carboxylation, nitration, loss of sulfhydryls, backbone damage, side-chain damage, fragmentation, unfolding and conformational changes in tertiary and quaternary structures, alteration of electrical charge, oxidation of specific amino acids, spontaneous reactions with glucose (glycosylation), and covalent cross-links [83, 87, 94].

Protein, as well as lipid, oxidation by FRs is initiated by the abstraction of a hydrogen atom from the a-carbon site, resulting in a carbon-centered radical. This reaction can be carried out at the backbone or in the side chain, and in both cases, these species appear to have two major fates: reaction with O_2 to give a peroxyl radical or a reaction with another radical. The peroxyl radicals that are formed undergo different subsequent reactions that are dependent on if the reaction is with the backbone or side chain. When the reaction occurs with the backbone, an elimination reaction releases $HO_2^{\cdot}$ and generates an imine, which undergoes further hydrolysis and backbone fragmentation. When the reaction occurs with the side chain, peroxyl radicals undergo a range of radical–radical termination reactions that can generate alcohols and carbonyl compounds or, alternatively, alkoxyl radicals and O_2. When the reaction occurs with another radical, the carbon-centered radical is converted into a hydroperoxide, and if this reaction occurs with the backbone, the subsequent decomposition of the hydroperoxide to a radical can result in backbone fragmentation via an alkoxyl-radical-mediated process [85, 95].

All amino acids in the side chains of the proteins, but mainly methionine, cysteine, tyrosine, phenylalanine, tryptophan, and histidine, undergo attack by $^{\cdot}OH$. As we have explained previously, oxidized proteins are easily degraded by proteolytic enzymes due to carboxylation, thus creating new N-terminal groups or conformational changes. In this sense, $ONOO^-$ oxidizes membrane and cytoplasmic proteins, which affect their physical and chemical natures [83, 87, 94, 96].

Moreover, it is noted that decreased enzyme binding constants (increased K_m) for coenzymes or substrates can result from protein deformation and loss of function due to an age-related decline in membrane fluidity or to polymorphisms and/or mutation [97].

After the oxidation of sulfur centers by most radical oxidants, thiyl radicals (RSS) are formed, and the presence of these radicals and the loss of the -SH groups of the proteins can cause misfolding, catalytic inactivation, reduction in the antioxidant capability, and the loss of specific functions, for example, albumin binding to heavy metals and sulfur-containing amino acids [98].

4.3.3 Carbohydrates Oxidation

The best understood effects of FRs on carbohydrates are mediated by glycosylation reactions with proteins; its other effects are less well known. Glycation involves the nonenzymatic interaction between reducing sugars, mainly glucose, with the primary amino groups of proteins. The major product in tissue proteins is fructoselysine (FL), which is in balance with its Schiff base that is formed by glycation of the ε-amino groups on lysine residues. The subsequent Maillard reactions undergo molecular rearrangement to produce ketamines (or Amadori compounds) or intermediate glycation products. This process occurs after several weeks; therefore, it affects long-lived proteins and contributes to the cross-linking of tissue proteins. Amadori compounds form α–dicarbonyl or α-oxoaldehyde compounds, which are fragmentation products that are subsequently condensed and conformed to advanced glycosylation end products (AGE) or advanced Maillard products, principally Nε-[carboxymethyl]-lysine (CML) and pentosidine, through an oxidative pathway in the presence of $O_2^{\cdot-}$ and Fe^{2+}. This oxidation process accompanied by glycation is known as glycoxidation, and the molecules that are formed are called glycoxidation products. The extent of tissue protein glycation depends on the ambient glucose concentration and remains relatively constant with age; therefore, subjects with diabetes mellitus can have high AGE levels. An important consequence of the glycation of tissue proteins is a reduction in their susceptibility to catabolism [99–101].

Furthermore, a previous study described that ONOO⁻ could induce protein modification by oxidative cleavage of Amadori products and by generating reactive α-oxyaldehydes from glucose, thus forming CML [102].

4.3.4 DNA Oxidative Damage

Nuclear and mitochondrial DNA is not exempt from oxidative processes. Of the stresses that cells undergo, OS is an important cause of DNA damage.

Hydroxyl radicals can cause protein-DNA cross-linking, sister chromatid exchange, sugar bond modifications, and oxidation of heterocyclic DNA bases.

Oxidative DNA damage has been estimated at 1.5×10^5 oxidative adducts per human cell, if 8-oxo-desoxyguanosine represents 5 % of the total adducts. That is, for every 10^{12} oxygen molecules entering a cell each day, 1 in 200 will damage DNA. DNA oxidative damage can compromise cellular function, and it is most likely the major factor involved in mutagenesis, carcinogenesis, and aging [103, 104].

Covalent DNA-protein cross-links are formed in mammalian cells by reactions between ·OH and chromatin, which are induced by H_2O_2/metal ions, and thymine-tyrosine (Thy-Tyr) cross-links have been found to be major products in many experiments. The oxidative modification of deoxyribose can induce abasic sites and single- or double-stranded DNA breaks, and oxidative modifications of the bases can produce degradation, mutations, deletions, or translocations [23, 89, 104].

In general, ·OH can lead to multiple products of base oxidation through an 8-hydroxylation reaction. Of the DNA bases, guanine has the lowest reduction potential; therefore, it is the best electron donor and is preferentially oxidized. The main compounds that are formed by oxidation are 8-hydroxyguanine (8-OHG), 8-hydroxy-2′-deoxyguanosine (8-OHdG), 8-hydroxyadenine, and thymine glycol. Of these, 8-OHdG is the principal biomarker that is used due its mutagenicity and correlation with aging and different chronic diseases such as cancer because it induces a guanine to thymine base transversion [23, 105, 106]. Moreover, ONOO⁻ is produced by the transition metal-catalyzed formation of ·OH or during the production of 8-oxo-guanosine in the inflammation process [104].

The reactivity of ·OH towards deoxyribose varies considerably. The oxidation reaction yields carbon-centered radicals mainly at C4 and C5, and these radicals undergo further reactions that yield different deoxyribose products. Under aerobic conditions, peroxyl radicals are formed and centered at C5′, and these are converted to an oxyl radical, which leads to β-cleavage and strand breakage followed by release of an altered sugar and an intact base. Subsequently, the lesion that is predominantly observed in DNA is a strand break that is mediated by iron and H_2O_2 [104, 107].

Due to its proximity near the internal membrane of the mitochondria, mtDNA is more exposed to ROS than nuclear DNA because, as previously described, ROS that produce the highest endogenous damage are generated in high concentrations by the respiratory chain. The attack mediated by ROS on mtDNA conduces two main mutagenic alterations: (a) formation of 8-OHdG because the oxidative modification of other bases is less frequent and (b) single- or double-stranded DNA breaks [106, 108]. An increasing number of experimental studies suggest that mtDNA mutations can be generated by replication of errors instead of cumulative oxidative damage and, thus, question the mitochondrial theory of aging [109].

4.4 Skin and Oxidative Stress

Skin cells are constantly exposed to various challenges such as oxidative stress that are associated with the formation of ROS from endogenous, as noted above, and exogenous sources such as ultraviolet radiation, chemical compounds, pollution, and inflammatory processes. Evidence suggests that $O_2^{\cdot-}$ and H_2O_2 are increased in aged skin and that aging is accompanied by an increase in lipoperoxides in keratinocytes, which is more marked in males and ovariectomized rats than in intact female rats and emphasizes a possible protective effect of estrogens from oxidative and inflammatory damage of the skin [44]. Constant exposure to ultraviolet A (UVA) radiation can generate ROS and causes the release of iron, which leads to oxidative damage in biomolecules. As a result of E2 loss, an increase in iron, which is generally released through desquamation occurs, and the skin becomes a main portal for the release of excess iron [110]. Furthermore, keratinocytes that are exposed to UVB radiation generate H_2O_2, which acts as an apoptotic mediator [111].

E2 deprivation has the following effects on skin cells: the capability of the stress response is reduced by the lack of estrogens, the oxidative alteration of collagen and its synthesis, insufficiency of the NO-dependent vasodilation mechanism, and glycoxidation, which causes OS, telomere shortening, and cellular senescence (Fig. 4.3).

Regarding the reduced capability of the stress response, some authors have shown that a significant decrease in mitochondrial membrane potential in ex vivo samples of human dermal fibroblasts from elderly donors occurs and is accompanied by a significant increase in ROS levels [112]. Ma et al. found that long-term exposure of cells to ROS initiates a vicious cycle that results in a reduced capability of the stress response, a reduction in ATP synthesis, and a further increase of ROS production in affected cells [113].

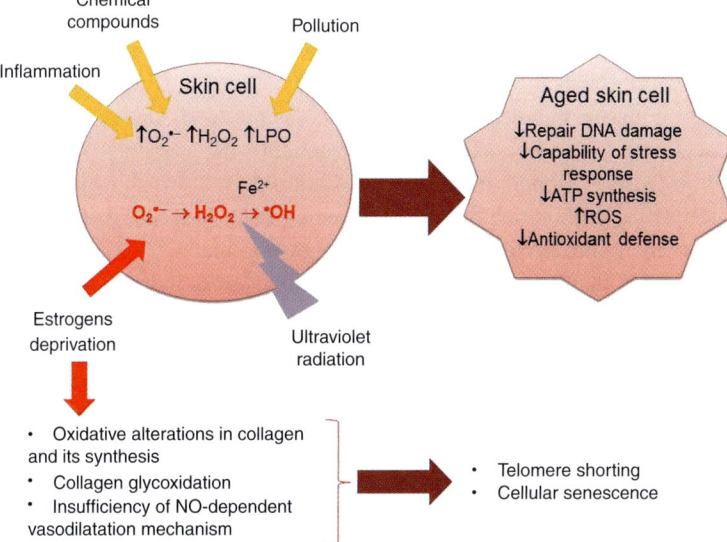

Fig. 4.3 Effect of oxidative stress and estrogens deprivation on skin cells. Prooxidant factors (*gold arrows*) induce that ROS increased and ultraviolet radiation causes iron release and H_2O_2 production, causing high oxidative stress. Estrogen deprivation (*red arrows*) causes high ROS levels in skin cells and some alterations in other skin cells mechanisms (see text). The final consequences of high oxidative stress in cells are some biochemical modifications that produce cellular senescence. $O_2^{\cdot-}$ superoxide anion, H_2O_2 hydrogen peroxide, $\cdot OH$ hydroxyl radical, *LPO* lipoperoxides, *ROS* reactive oxygen species, *NO* nitric oxide

Furthermore, as we age, human skin cells lose their ability to repair DNA damage; therefore, it is possible to say that the excess production of ROS and reduced antioxidant activity with advanced age significantly contributes to the clinical signs and chronological changes of aging [112].

Moreover, skin aging is characterized by a loss of collagen types I and III, among other matrix constituents, due to estrogen deficiency because this hormone enhances collagen synthesis, and estrogen and progesterone suppress collagenolysis by reducing matrix metalloproteinase (MMP) activity in fibroblasts, thereby maintaining skin thickness [114]. In postmenopausal women, reduced collagen levels in the dermis result from decreased procollagen synthesis and increased collagen degradation due to oxidative events. Some authors suggest that H_2O_2 increases the induction of MMP in keratinocytes and fibroblasts and demonstrate that E2 could interfere with the decrease in ROS-induced procollagen-I synthesis in human dermal fibroblasts, which counteracts the detrimental effects of OS in the dermal compartment during skin aging [27]. Additionally, in a study on SOD2-deficient mice, it was observed that the architecture of the collagen fibers was severely disturbed; they had thin and loosely packed collagen bundles, procollagen-I was reduced, and mitochondria from SOD2-deficient fibroblasts exhibited severe morphological damage [50], corroborating the oxidative modifications in collagen due to low antioxidant defense. Another factor related to oxidative damage in skin is the insufficiency of the NO-dependent vasodilation mechanism. In a study of women, a decrease-free NO• content in blood was observed that was possibly due to the decrease of NO• synthesis and the oxidative degradation of NO• in oxidative stress conditions. This finding led us to conclude that this insufficiency produces a disorder of subcutaneous vasodilatation that contributes to oxidative processes in the skin and its rapid aging [115].

Collagen is a long-lived protein that is susceptible to glycoxidation in diabetic and nondiabetic subjects, but glycoxidation is highest among diabetic subjects. It was reported that the collagen of diabetic subjects contained significantly increased quantities of FL and AGEs, which altered the characteristics of collagen during aging and resulted in diabetic complications. Data from this investigation showed that FL and AGE in skin correlated with functional abnormalities in other tissues such as the retina and kidney; thus, it is possible that glycoxidation may be implicated in the development of diabetic retinopathy and early nephropathy [116].

Investigations have revealed that human keratinocytes seem to have a greater antioxidant defense that counteracts the oxidative damage to which the skin is subjected. Conversely, mesenchymal stem cells from human skin do not have an efficient defense system because they are surrounded by a complex microenvironment that protects them from external insults. Therefore, they are less responsive to enhanced, prooxidant challenge [117].

The antioxidant effects of estrogens have also been proven in the skin. As noted above, estrogens function as antioxidants, due to their chemical structure, and as antioxidant-response inducers. In human Friedreich's ataxia skin fibroblasts, it was demonstrated that phenolic estrogens were able to prevent lipid peroxidation and $\Delta\Psi m$ collapse, maintain ATP at near control levels, increase oxidative phosphorylation, and maintain the activity of aconitase [118]. Additionally, it was shown that 17β-estradiol prevented H_2O_2-induced apoptosis in keratinocytes, suggesting that E2 may rescue these cells from oxidative stress-induced apoptosis by the action of the Bcl-2 protein (a protein that blocks apoptosis) [119].

Another antioxidant that is widely used for its effect on the skin is vitamin C, which is essential for collagen biosynthesis in connective tissues. Vitamin C serves as a cofactor for the prolysyl and lysyl hydroxylases, which are responsible for stabilizing and cross-linking collagen molecules, and it is capable of serving as an electron donor and thus helping to maintain the full activity of these hydroxylases. Additionally, ascorbate acts as an electron donor by keeping iron in its ferrous state by inhibiting the Fenton reaction and the reactions that cause skin aging, which were described previously [74, 120].

4.5 Menopause as Risk Factor for Oxidative Stress

It is known that OS increases with age [12], and menopause is considered the beginning of aging in women due to the decline in estrogen and the endocrinological changes that produce several symptoms, many of which have been reported as prooxidant factors.

Studies in animal models have demonstrated that E2 deprivation after ovariectomy alters the redox state of the animal by decreasing the release of NO$^\bullet$ and diminishing systemic vascular conductance. These studies also revealed an increase in $O_2^{\bullet-}$ production by NADPH oxidase in systemic and cerebral arteries because, as noted, E2 normally suppresses the $O_2^{\bullet-}$-generating activity of vascular NADPH oxidases. Furthermore, evidence suggests that levels of vascular ROS are lower in reproductive females than in ovariectomized females and male animals under healthy, hypertensive and atherosclerotic conditions [121, 122].

Studies in humans have investigated several different biomarkers and demonstrated an increase in OS in postmenopausal women. It has been reported that lipoperoxides, 4-hydroxynenal, and oxidized LDL levels are higher and GPx activity is lower in postmenopausal women compared with premenopausal women [123–125]. Likewise, we used an oxidative stress score that integrated oxidant and antioxidant markers to represent the dynamics of OS. This score has also shown that postmenopausal women have more OS than premenopausal women and that the degree of OS increases in postmenopausal women. Therefore, we suggest that the depletion of estrogen in postmenopausal women could cause OS as well as all of the abovementioned conditions and the known symptoms that also produce OS [125]. These results support the hypothesis that estradiol likely exerts its antioxidant action not only through its chemical structure but also through its influence on natural, cellular, antioxidant enzyme activity. Thus, it is likely that the action of estradiol can be mediated via intracellular signaling cascades and that it upregulates the expression of antioxidant and longevity-related genes [126].

Moreover, the relationship between OS and many symptoms of postmenopause that are considered prooxidant factors, such as somatic symptoms, insomnia, depression, and anxiety, and their effect on the quality of life have been reported.

Somatic symptoms such as hot flashes and insomnia have been shown to be directly associated with increased lipoperoxides levels [127, 128]. Additionally, a positive association between the total score of the Menopause Rating Scale, which is a test that assesses perimenopausal symptoms and is divided into three subscales (somatic, psychological, and urogenital), and lipoperoxides levels shows that more severe symptoms are a result of greater oxidative damage [125]. Additionally, it has been described that sleep provides an antioxidant function because it serves to restore the neurotransmitters that are necessary for brain neuronal synapses and thus neutralizes wear and repairs OS that are formed during wakefulness [129]. This result lead to the hypothesis that sleeps deprivation is associated with an accumulation of ROS.

Of the various functions of estrogens, one of their most important is their role in the functional integrity of the nervous system. In this sense, evidence links E2 to the development, maturation, differentiation, and function of brain cells. Furthermore, the presence of steroid hormone receptors in various brain regions has been demonstrated. In addition to the discovery that E2 is involved in stimulating cholinergic markers, E2 increases cerebral blood flow, which prevents neuronal atrophy and enhances sleep, memory, cognition, and other neurologic functions [63, 64]. Once E2 is secreted in erratic cycles, it generates a vicious cycle in which the depletion of E2 causes the abovementioned symptoms and OS increase the severity of those symptoms [130]. Anxiety, which is a common symptom that is reported by postmenopausal women, has not been studied in depth, but in a literature review, Bouayed et al. [131] note a link between oxidative stress and high-anxiety-related behavior. However, the analyzed studies do not explain the underlying mechanisms. A physiological depressive mood, which is another common symptom that is reported by postmenopausal women, has been shown by some researchers to be associated with OS and indicates a potential link between depression and cancer due to oxidative DNA damage via neutrophil activation [132–134].

Furthermore, in a study carried out by our research group, we observed that postmenopausal women who have severe symptoms and a low quality of life also have increased OS [135] because of an additive effect between estrogen deficiency and the severe symptoms that affect the quality of their lives. In fact, life events, such as a dysfunctional family and poor social support, were important modulators of postmenopausal symptoms, and their severity was correlated with each person's method of facing problems, which suggested that the vulnerability to stress contributed to the worsening of the postmenopausal symptoms [136, 137]. Therefore, if the severity of the symptoms is high, psychological stress is produced, and OS increases.

Finally, hormone therapy (HT) has shown positive effects on postmenopausal symptoms and on the prevention of some common diseases and degenerative changes that occur as women age. In this sense, our research group has found that HT has a powerful antioxidant effect, which is provided by E2 [135]. Therefore, estrogen therapy, when applied during the early postmenopausal stage, can be an alternative to counteract the OS that are associated with postmenopause. However, HT has negative effects over the short and long term; hence, the use of low-dose estrogen, which lacks side effects, and alternative therapies such as antioxidant vitamin supplementation, have been suggested to expand the therapeutic options to counteract OS and promote healthy aging.

Acknowledgments This work was supported by Dirección General de Asuntos del Personal Académico, Universidad Nacional Autónoma de México (DGAPA, UNAM), PAPIIT IN222213.

References

1. Hall G, Phillips TJ. Estrogen and skin: the effects of estrogen, menopause, and hormone replacement therapy on the skin. J Am Acad Dermatol. 2005;53:555–68.
2. Emmerson E, Hardman MJ. The role of estrogen deficiency in skin ageing and wound healing. Biogerontology. 2012;13(1):3–20.
3. Mofid A, Seyyed Alinaghi SA, Zandieh S, Yazdani T. Hirsutism. Int J Clin Pract. 2007;62:433–43.
4. Blume-Peytavi U, Atkin S, Gieler U, Grimalt R. Skin academy: hair, skin, hormones and menopause - current status/knowledge on the management of hair disorders in menopausal women. Eur J Dermatol. 2012;22:310–8.
5. Broekmans FJ, Soules MR, Fauser BC. Ovarian aging: mechanisms and clinical consequences. Endocr Rev. 2009;30:465–93.
6. Weiss G, Skurnick JH, Goldsmith LT, Santoro NF, Park SJ. Menopause and hypothalamic-pituitary sensitivity to estrogen. JAMA. 2004;292:2991–6.
7. Avis N, Brockwell S, Colvin A. A universal menopausal syndrome? Am J Med. 2005;118(12B):37S–46.
8. Troen BR. The biology of aging. Mt Sinai J Med. 2003;70:3–22.
9. Davidovic M, Milosevic DR. Are all dilemmas in gerontology being swept under the carpet of intra-individual variability? Med Hypotheses. 2006;66:432–6.
10. Goldsmith TC. Aging theories and the zero-sum game. Rejuvenation Res. 2014;17:1–2.
11. Tatone C, Amicarelli F, Carbone MC, Monteleone P, Caserta D, Marci R, et al. Cellular and molecular aspects of ovarian follicle ageing. Hum Reprod Update. 2008;14:131–42.
12. Mendoza-Núñez VM, Ruiz-Ramos M, Sánchez-Rodríguez MA, Retana-Ugalde R, Muñoz-Sánchez JL. Aging-related oxidative stress in healthy humans. Tohoku J Exp Med. 2007;231:261–8.
13. Moffatt O, Drury S, Tomlison M, Afnan M, Denny S. The apoptotic profile of human cumulus cells changes with patient age and after exposure to sperm but not in relation to oocyte maturity. Fertil Steril. 2002;77:1006–11.
14. Gold EB, Crawford SL, Avis NE, Crandall CJ, Matthews KA, Waetjen LE, et al. Factors related to age at natural menopause: longitudinal analyses from SWAN. Am J Epidemiol. 2013;178:70–83.
15. Shuster LT, Rhodes DJ, Gostout BS, Grossardt BR, Roccae WA. Premature menopause or early menopause: long-term health consequences. Maturitas. 2010;65:161–6.
16. Vajaranant TS, Pasquale LR. Estrogen deficiency accelerates aging of the optic nerve. Menopause. 2012;19:942–7.
17. Pansini F, Mollica G, Bergamini CM. Management of the menopausal disturbances and oxidative stress. Curr Pharm Des. 2005;11:2063–73.
18. Chen JT, Kotani K. An inverse relation between the simplified menopausal index and biological antioxidant potential. Climacteric. 2013;16:288–91.

19. Muchová J, Sustrová M, Garaiová I, Liptáková A, Blazıcek P, Kvasnicka P, et al. Influence of age on activities of antioxidant enzymes and lipid peroxidation products in erythrocytes and neutrophils of Down syndrome patients. Free Radic Biol Med. 2001;31:499–508.
20. de Haan JB, Cristiano F, Iannello R, Bladier C, Keiner MJ, Kola I. Elevation in the ratio of Cu/Zn-superoxide dismutase to glutathione peroxidase activity induces features of cellular senescence and this effect is mediated by hydrogen peroxide. Hum Mol Genet. 1996;5:283–92.
21. Esbensen AJ. Health conditions associated with aging and end of life of adults with Down syndrome. Int Rev Res Ment Retard. 2010;39(C):107–26.
22. Halliwell B. Biochemistry of oxidative stress. Biochem Soc Trans. 2007;35(part 5):1147–50.
23. Birben E, Sahiner UM, Sackesen C, Erzurum S, Kalayci O. Oxidative stress and antioxidant defense. World Allergy Organ J. 2012;5:9–19.
24. Gerschman R, Gilbert DL, Nye SW, Dwyer P, Fenn WO. Oxygen poisoning and X-irradiation: a mechanism in common. Science. 1954;119:623–6.
25. Harman D. Aging: a theory based on free radical and radiation chemistry. J Gerontol. 1956;11:298–300.
26. McCord JM, Fridovich I. Superoxide dismutase. An enzymic function for erythrocuprein (hemocuprein). J Biol Chem. 1969;244:6049–55.
27. Bottai G, Mancina R, Muratori M, Di Gennaro P, Lotti T. 17β-estradiol protects human skin fibroblasts and keratinocytes against oxidative damage. J Eur Acad Dermatol Venereol. 2012. doi:10.1111/j.1468-3083.2012.04697.
28. Babior BM. Phagocytes and oxidative stress. Am J Med. 2000;109:33–44.
29. Betteridge DJ. What is oxidative stress? Metabolism. 2000;49(2 Suppl 1):3–8.
30. Giles GI, Jacob C. Reactive sulfur species: an emerging concept in oxidative stress. Biol Chem. 2002;383:375–88.
31. Halliwell B, Gutteridge JMC, Cross CE. Free radicals, antioxidants, and human disease: where are we now? J Lab Clin Med. 1992;119:598–620.
32. Bunker VW. Free radicals, antioxidants and ageing. Med Lab Sci. 1992;49:299–312.
33. Guzik TJ, Harrison DG. Vascular NADPH oxidases as drug targets for novel antioxidant strategies. Drug Discov Today. 2006;11:524–33.
34. Mendoza-Núñez VM, Rosado-Pérez J, Santiago-Osorio E, Ortiz R, Sánchez-Rodríguez MA, Galván-Duarte RE. Aging linked to type 2 diabetes increases oxidative stress and chronic inflammation. Rejuvenation Res. 2011;14:25–31.
35. Bleier L, Dröse S. Superoxide generation by complex III: from mechanistic rationales to functional consequences. Biochim Biophys Acta. 2012. pii: S0005-2728(12)01102-4. doi: 10.1016/j.bbabio.2012.12.002.
36. Dröge W. Free radicals in the physiological control of cell function. Physiol Rev. 2002;82:47–95.
37. Kadenbach B, Ramzan R, Vogt S. High efficiency versus maximal performance – the cause of oxidative stress in eukaryotes: a hypothesis. Mitochondrion. 2012. doi:10.1016/j.mito.2012.11.005.
38. Miller DM, Buettner GR, Aust SD. Transition metals as catalysts of "autoxidation" reactions. Free Radic Biol Med. 1990;8:95–108.
39. Halliwell B. Free radicals and antioxidants: updating a personal view. Nutr Rev. 2012;70:257–65.
40. Lipinski B. Is it oxidative or free radical stress and why does it matter? Oxid Antioxid Med Sci. 2012;1:5–9.
41. Fukai T, Ushio-Fukai M. Superoxide dismutases: role in redox signaling, vascular function, and diseases. Antiox Redox Signal. 2011;15:1583–606.
42. Sosa V, Moliné T, Somoza R, Paciucci R, Kondoh H, LLeonart ME. Oxidative stress and cancer: an overview. Ageing Res Rev. 2013;12:376–90.
43. Gutteridge JM. Lipid peroxidation and antioxidants as biomarkers of tissue damage. Clin Chem. 1995;41:1819–28.
44. Tresguerres JA, Kireev R, Tresguerres AF, Borras C, Vara E, Ariznavarreta C. Molecular mechanisms involved in the hormonal prevention of aging in the rat. J Steroid Biochem Mol Biol. 2008;108:318–26.
45. Halliwell B, Hoult JR, Blake DR. Oxidants, inflammation, and anti-inflammatory drugs. FASEB J. 1988;2:2867–73.
46. Rusting LR. Why do we age? Sci Am. 1992;367(6):86–95.
47. Niki E, Noguchi N, Tsuchihashi H, Gotoh N. Interaction among vitamin C, vitamin E, and β-carotene. Am J Clin Nutr. 1995;62(6 Suppl):1322S–6.
48. Niki E. Assessment of antioxidant capability in vitro and in vivo. Free Radic Biol Med. 2010;49:503–15.
49. Liochev SI, Fridovich I. Mechanism of the peroxidase activity of Cu, Zn superoxide dismutase. Free Radic Biol Med. 2010;48:1565–9.
50. Treiber N, Maity P, Singh K, Ferchiu F, Wlaschek M, Scharffetter-Kochanek K. The role of manganese superoxide dismutase in skin aging. Dermatoendocrinol. 2012;4:232–5.
51. Kirkman HN, Rolfo M, Ferraris AM, Gaetani GF. Mechanisms of protection of catalase by NADPH. Kinetics and stoichiometry. J Biol Chem. 1999;274:13908–14.
52. Brigelius-Flohé R, Maiorino M. Glutathione peroxidases. Biochim Biophys Acta. 1830;2013:3289–303.
53. de Silva DM, Aust SD. Ferritin and ceruloplasmin in oxidative damage: review and recent finding. Can J Physiol Pharmacol. 1993;71:715–20.
54. Bourdon E, Blache D. The importance of proteins in defense against oxidation. Antioxid Redox Signal. 2001;3:293–311.
55. Roche M, Rondeau P, Singh NR, Tarnus E, Bourdon E. The antioxidant properties of serum albumin. FEBS Lett. 2008;582:1783–7.
56. Iwao Y, Ishima Y, Yamada J, Noguchi T, Kragh-Hansen U, Mera K, et al. Quantitative evaluation of

the role of cysteine and methionine residues in the antioxidant activity of human serum albumin using recombinant mutants. IUBMB Life. 2012;64:450–4.
57. Reif DW. Ferritin as a source of iron for oxidative damage. Free Radic Biol Med. 1992;12:417–27.
58. Galaris D, Pantopoulos K. Oxidative stress and iron homeostasis: mechanistic and health aspects. Crit Rev Clin Lab Sci. 2008;45:1–23.
59. Samokyszyn VM, Reif DW, Miller DM, Aust SD. Effects of ceruloplasmin on superoxide-dependent iron release from ferritin and lipid peroxidation. Free Radic Res Commun. 1991;12–13(Part 1):153–9.
60. Subbiah MT, Kessel B, Agrawal M, Rajan R, Abplanalp W, Rymaszewski Z. Antioxidant potential of specific estrogens on lipid peroxidation. J Clin Endocrinol Metab. 1993;77:1095–7.
61. Kumar S, Lata K, Mukhopadhyay S, Mukherjee TK. Role of estrogen receptors in pro-oxidative and anti-oxidative actions of estrogens: A perspective. Biochim Biophys Acta. 1800;2010:1127–35.
62. Tikkanen MJ, Vihma V, Hockerstedt A, Jauhiainen M, Helisten H, Kaamanen M. Lipophilic oestrogen derivatives contained in lipoprotein particles. Acta Physiol Scand. 2002;176:117–21.
63. Bhavnani BR. Estrogens and menopause: pharmacology of conjugated equine estrogens and their potential role in the prevention of neurodegenerative diseases such as Alzheimer's. J Steroid Biochem Mol Biol. 2003;85(2–5):473–82.
64. Markides C, Roy D, Liehr G. Concentration dependence of prooxidant and antioxidant properties of catecholestrogens. Arch Biochem Biophys. 1998;360:105–12.
65. Wassmann K, Wassmann S, Nickenig G. Progesterone antagonizes the vasoprotective effect of estrogen on antioxidant enzyme expression and function. Circ Res. 2005;97:1046–54.
66. Yager JD, Davidson NE. Estrogen carcinogenesis in breast cancer. N Engl J Med. 2006;354:270–82.
67. Bolton JL, Thatcher GR. Potential mechanisms of estrogen quinone carcinogenesis. Chem Res Toxicol. 2008;21:93–101.
68. Agte V, Tarwadi K, Mengale S, Finge A, Chiplonkar S. Vitamin profile of cooked foods: how healthy is the practice of ready-to-eat foods? Int J Food Sci Nutr. 2002;53:197–208.
69. Fairfield KM, Fletcher RH. Vitamins for chronic disease prevention in adults. JAMA. 2002;287:3116–26.
70. Faruqi R, de la Motte C, DiCorleto PE. Alpha-tocopherol inhibits agonist-induced monocytic cell adhesion to cultured human endothelial cells. J Clin Invest. 1994;94:592–600.
71. Devaraj S, Li D, Jialal I. The effects of alpha-tocopherol supplementation on monocyte function. Decreased lipid oxidation, interleukin 1 beta secretion, and monocyte adhesion to endothelium. J Clin Invest. 1996;98:756–63.
72. Lam YT, Stocker R, Dawes IW. The lipophilic antioxidants α-tocopherol and coenzyme Q_{10} reduce the replicative lifespan of *Saccharomyces cerevisiae*. Free Radic Biol Med. 2010;49:237–44.
73. Bowry VW, Ingold KU, Stocker R. Vitamin E in human low-density lipoprotein. When and how this antioxidant becomes a pro-oxidant. Biochem J. 1992;288:341–4.
74. Du J, Cullen JJ, Buettner GR. Ascorbic acid: chemistry, biology and the treatment of cancer. Biochim Biophys Acta. 1826;2012:443–57.
75. Pohanka M, Pejchal J, Snopkova S, Havlickova K, Karasova JZ, Bostik P, et al. Ascorbic acid: an old player with a broad impact on body physiology including oxidative stress suppression and immunomodulation: a review. Mini Rev Med Chem. 2012;12:35–43.
76. Schneider M, Niess AM, Rozario F, Angres C, Tschositsch K, Golly I, et al. Vitamin E supplementation does not increase the vitamin C radical concentration at rest and after exhaustive exercise in healthy male subjects. Eur J Nutr. 2003;42:195–200.
77. Traber MG, Stevens JF. Vitamins C and E: beneficial effects from a mechanistic perspective. Free Radic Biol Med. 2011;51:1000–13.
78. Ingold KU, Bowry VW, Stocker R, Walling C. Autoxidation of lipids and antioxidation by alpha-tocopherol and ubiquinol in homogeneous solution and in aqueous dispersions of lipids: unrecognized consequences of lipid particle size as exemplified by oxidation of human low density lipoprotein. Proc Natl Acad Sci U S A. 1993;90:45–9.
79. Sram RJ, Binkova B, Rossner Jr P. Vitamin C for DNA damage prevention. Mutat Res. 2012;733(1–2):39–49.
80. Childs A, Jacobs C, Kaminski T, Halliwell B, Leeuwenburgh C. Supplementation with vitamin C and N-acetyl-cysteine increases oxidative stress in humans after an acute muscle injury induced by eccentric exercise. Free Radic Biol Med. 2001;31:745–53.
81. Van Kuijk FJGM, Sevanian A, Handelman GJ, Dratz EA. A new role for phospholipase A2: protection of membrane from lipid peroxidation damage. Trends Biochem Sci. 1987;12:31–4.
82. Watson AD, Navab M, Hama SY, Sevanian A, Prescott SM, Stafforini DM, et al. Effect of platelet activating factor-acetylhydrolase on the formation and action of minimally oxidized low density lipoprotein. J Clin Invest. 1995;95:774–82.
83. Pacifici RE, Davies KJA. Protein, lipid and DNA repair systems in oxidative stress: the free-radical theory of aging revisited. Gerontology. 1991;37:166–80.
84. Fagbemi AF, Orelli B, Schärer OD. Regulation of endonuclease activity in human nucleotide excision repair. DNA Repair. 2011;10:722–9.
85. Bürkle A. DNA repair and PARP in aging. Free Radic Res. 2006;40:1295–302.
86. Dean RT, Fu SL, Stocker R, Davies MJ. Biochemistry and pathology of radical-mediated protein oxidation. Biochem J. 1997;324(Pt. 1):1–18.
87. Davies MJ. The oxidative environment and protein damage. Biochim Biophys Acta. 2005;1703:93–109.
88. Petropoulos I, Friguet B. Maintenance of proteins and aging: the role of oxidized protein repair. Free Radic Res. 2006;40:1269–76.

89. Dizdaroglu M, Jaruga P. Mechanisms of free radical-induced damage to DNA. Free Radic Res. 2012;46:382–419.
90. Niki E, Yoshida Y, Saito Y, Noguchi N. Lipid peroxidation: mechanisms, inhibition, and biological effects. Biochem Biophys Res Commun. 2005;338:668–76.
91. Yoshida Y, Umeno A, Shichiri M. Lipid peroxidation biomarkers for evaluating oxidative stress and assessing antioxidant capability in vivo. J Clin Biochem Nutr. 2013;52:9–16.
92. Niki E. Lipid peroxidation products as oxidative stress biomarkers. Biofactors. 2008;34:171–80.
93. Maccarrone M, Melino G, Finazzi-Agró A. Lipoxygenases and their involvement in programmed cell death. Cell Death Differ. 2001;8:776–84.
94. Stadtman ER. Protein oxidation and aging. Free Radic Res. 2006;40:1250–8.
95. Davies MJ. Protein and peptide alkoxyl radicals can give rise to C terminal decarboxylation and backbone cleavage. Arch Biochem Biophys. 1996;336:163–72.
96. Vilar-Rojas C, Guzmán-Grenfell AM, Hicks JJ. Participation of oxygen-free radicals in the oxidoreduction of proteins. Arch Med Res. 1996;27:1–6.
97. Ames BN. Prevention of mutation, cancer, and other age-associated diseases by optimizing micronutrient intake. J Nucleic Acids. 2010. doi:10.4061/2010/725071.
98. Sohal RS. Role of oxidative stress and protein oxidation in the aging process. Free Radic Biol Med. 2002;33:37–44.
99. Dyer DG, Blackledge JA, Thorpe SR, Baynes JW. Formation of pentosidine during nonenzymatic browning of proteins by glucose. Identification glucose other carbohydrates as possible precursors pentosidine in vivo. J Biol Chem. 1991;266:11654–60.
100. Dyer DG, Dunn JA, Thorpe SR, Bailie KE, Lyons TJ, McCance DR, et al. Accumulation of Maillard reaction products in skin collagen in diabetes and aging. J Clin Invest. 1993;91:2463–9.
101. Singh R, Barden A, Mori T, Beilin L. Advanced glycation end-products: a review. Diabetologia. 2001;44:129–46.
102. Nagai R, Unno Y, Hayashi MC, Masuda S, Hayase F, Kinae N, et al. Peroxynitrite induces formation of Nε(carboxymethyl)lisina by the cleavage of Amarodi product and generation of glucosone and glyoxal. Novel pathways for protein modification by peroxynitrite. Diabetes. 2002;51:2833–9.
103. Beckman KB, Ames BN. Oxidative decay of DNA. J Biol Chem. 1997;272:19633–6.
104. Aust AE, Eveleigh JF. Mechanisms of DNA oxidation. Proc Soc Exp Biol Med. 1999;222:246–52.
105. de Zwart LL, Meerman JHN, Commandeur JNM, Vermeulen NPE. Biomarkers of free radical damage applications in experimental animals and in humans. Free Radic Biol Med. 1999;26:202–6.
106. Gredilla R, Garm C, Stevnsner T. Nuclear and mitochondrial DNA repair in selected eukaryotic aging model systems. Oxid Med Cell Longev. 2012;2012:282438. doi:10.1155/2012/282438.
107. Floyd RA, Carney JM. Free radical damage to protein and DNA: mechanisms involved and relevant observations on brain undergoing oxidative stress. Ann Neurol. 1992;32(Suppl):S22–7.
108. Wiesner RJ, Zsurka G, Kunz WS. Mitochondrial DNA damage and the aging process – facts and imaginations. Free Radic Res. 2006;40:1284–94.
109. Lagouge M, Larsson NG. The role of mitochondrial DNA mutations and free radicals in disease and ageing. J Intern Med. 2013;273:529–43.
110. Pelle E, Jian J, Declercq L, Dong K, Yang Q, Pourzand C, Maes D, Pernodet N, Yarosh DB, Huang X. Protection against ultraviolet A-induced oxidative damage in normal human epidermal keratinocytes under post-menopausal conditions by an ultraviolet A-activated caged-iron chelator: a pilot study. Photodermatol Photoimmunol Photomed. 2011;27:231–5.
111. Peus D, Vasa RA, Beyerle A, Meves A, Krautmacher C, Pittelkow MR. UVB activates ERK1/2 and p38 signaling pathways via reactive oxygen species in cultured keratinocytes. J Invest Dermatol. 1999;112:751–6.
112. Poljsak B, Dahmane RG, Godic A. Intrinsic skin aging: the role of oxidative stress. Acta Dermatovenerol Alp Pannonica Adriat. 2012;21:33–6.
113. Ma YS, Wu SB, Lee WY, Cheng JS, Wei YH. Response to the increase of oxidative stress and mutation of mitochondrial DNA in aging. Biochim Biophys Acta. 2009;1790:1021–9.
114. Kanda N, Watanabe S. Regulatory roles of sex hormones in cutaneous biology and immunology. J Dermatol Sci. 2005;38:1–7.
115. Katsitadze A, Berianidze K, Kaladze K, McHedlishvili T, Sanikidze T. Nitric oxide dependent skin aging mechanism in postmenopausal women. Georgian Med News. 2012;208–209:66–71.
116. McCance DR, Dyer DG, Dunn JA, Bailie KE, Thorpe SR, Baynes JW, et al. Maillard reaction products and their relation to complications in insulin-dependent diabetes mellitus. J Clin Invest. 1993;91:2470–8.
117. Orciani M, Gorbi S, Benedetti M, Di Benedetto G, Mattioli-Belmonte M, Regoli F, et al. Oxidative stress defense in human-skin-derived mesenchymal stem cells versus human keratinocytes: different mechanisms of protection and cell selection. Free Radic Biol Med. 2010;49:830–8.
118. Richardson TE, Yu AE, Wen Y, Yang S-H, Simpkins JW. Estrogen prevents oxidative damage to the mitochondria in Friedreich's ataxia skin fibroblasts. PLoS One. 2012;7(4):e34600. doi:10.1371/journal.pone.0034600.
119. Kanda N, Watanabe S. 17β-estradiol inhibits oxidative stress-induced apoptosis in keratinocytes by promoting Bcl-2 expression. J Invest Dermatol. 2003;121:1500–9.
120. Traikovich SS. Use of topical ascorbic acid and its effects on photo damaged skin topography. Arch Otolaryngol Head Neck Surg. 1999;125:1091–8.

121. Hernandez I, Delgado JL, Diaz J, Quesada T, Teruel MJ, Llanos MC, et al. 17β-estradiol prevents oxidative stress and decrease blood pressure in ovariectomized rats. Am J Physiol Regul Integr Comp Physiol. 2000;279:R1599–605.
122. Miller AA, De Silva TM, Jackman KA, Sobey CG. Effect of gender and sex hormones on vascular oxidative stress. Clin Exp Pharmacol Physiol. 2007;34:1037–43.
123. Bednarek-Tupikowska G, Bohdanowicz-Pawlak A, Bidzińska B, Milewicz A, Antonowicz-Juchniewicz J, Andrzejak R. Serum lipid peroxide levels and erythrocyte glutathione peroxidase and superoxide dismutase activity in premenopausal and postmenopausal women. Gynecol Endocrinol. 2001;15:298–303.
124. Signorelli SS, Neri S, Sciacchitano S, Di Pino L, Costa MP, Marchese G, et al. Behaviour some indicators of oxidative stress in postmenopausal and fertile women. Maturitas. 2006;53:77–82.
125. Sánchez-Rodríguez MA, Zacarías-Flores M, Arronte-Rosales A, Correa-Muñoz E, Mendoza-Núñez VM. Menopause as risk factor for oxidative stress. Menopause. 2012;19:361–7.
126. Viña J, Borrás C, Gambini J, Sastre J, Pallardo FV. Why females live longer than males? Importance of the upregulation of longevity-associated genes by oestrogenic compounds. FEBS Lett. 2005;579:2541–5.
127. Leal M, Díaz J, Serrano E, Abellán J, Carbonell LF. Hormone replacement therapy for oxidative stress in postmenopausal women with hot flushes. Obstet Gynecol. 2000;95:804–9.
128. Hachul de Campos H, Brandao LC, Almeida VD, Grego BHC, Bittencourt LR, Tufik S, et al. Sleep disturbances, oxidative stress and cardiovascular risk parameters in postmenopausal women complaining of insomnia. Climacteric. 2006;9:312–9.
129. Tufik S, Andersen ML, Bittencourt RLA, De Mello MT. Paradoxical sleep deprivation: neurochemical, hormonal and behavioral alterations. Evidence from 30 years of research. An Acad Bras Cienc. 2009;81:521–38.
130. Cabrera T, Guevara-Pérez E, Cuza-Echevarría L, Domenech-García A, Urbizo-Cañón R. Estudio preliminar de indicadores del estrés oxidativo y los síntomas que aquejan con mayor frecuencia a las mujeres climatéricas. Rev Med Electrón. 2006;28(3). Available at: http://www.revmatanzas.sld.cu/revista medica/ano 2006/vol3 2006/tema08.htm.
131. Bouayed J, Rammal H, Soulimani R. Oxidative stress and anxiety. Oxid Med Cell Longev. 2009;2:63–7.
132. Tsuboi H, Shimoi K, Kinae N, Oguni I, Hori R, Kobayashi F. Depressive symptoms are independently correlated with lipid peroxidation in a female population. Comparison with vitamins and carotenoids. J Psychosom Res. 2004;56:53–8.
133. Irie M, Miyata M, Kasai H. Depression and possible cancer risk due to oxidative DNA damage. J Psychiatr Res. 2005;39:553–60.
134. Kodydková J, Vávrová L, Zeman M, Jirák R, Macášek J, Staňková B, et al. Antioxidative enzymes and increased oxidative stress in depressive women. Clin Biochem. 2009;42:1368–74.
135. Sánchez-Rodríguez MA, Zacarías-Flores M, Arronte-Rosales A, Mendoza-Núñez VM. Efecto de la terapia hormonal con estrógenos en el estrés oxidativo y la calidad de vida en mujeres posmenopáusicas. Ginecol Obstet Mex. 2013;81:11–22.
136. Igarashi M, Saito H, Morioka Y, Oiji A, Nadaoka T, Kashiwakura M. Stress vulnerability and climacteric symptoms: live events, coping behavior, and severity of symptoms. Gynecol Obstet Invest. 2000;49:170–7.
137. Binfa L, Castelo-Branco C, Blümel JE, Cancelo MJ, Bonilla H, Muñoz I, et al. Influence of psycho-social factors on climacteric symptoms. Maturitas. 2004; 48:425–31.

The Effect of Cytokines on Skin During Menopause

Marika Borg and Jean Calleja-Agius

Contents

5.1	Introduction	53
5.2	Tumor Necrosis Factor-Alpha (TNf-α)	54
5.3	Interleukin-1 (IL-1)	55
5.4	IL-6	57
5.5	IL-8	58
5.6	IL-10	58
5.7	IL-18	58
5.8	Interferons (IFNS)	59
5.8.1	IFN-α	59
5.8.2	IFN-β	59
5.8.3	IFN-γ	59
5.9	Cysteine-Rich Protein 61 (CRY61)	60
5.10	Transforming Growth Factor-β (TGF-β)	60
5.11	Skin Wrinkling	61
5.12	Hair Changes	62
5.13	Wound Healing	62
5.14	Photoaging	64
5.15	Summary	64
References		64

M. Borg
J. Calleja-Agius, MD, MRCOG, MRCPI, PhD (✉)
Department of Anatomy,
Faculty of Medicine and Surgery,
University of Malta, Msida MSD 2080, Malta
e-mail: marika.borg92@gmail.com;
jean.calleja-agius@um.edu.mt

5.1 Introduction

Cytokines are cell-signalling proteins that act as a communication link between cells. They play a crucial role in skin aging. Cytokines are produced in the skin by epithelial cells and keratinocytes, besides being synthesized by Langerhans cells as part of the immune system [1]. The concentration of cytokines in the human body is very low, usually in the nanomolar or femtomolar range, because cytokine receptors have a very high affinity to their ligand [1]. Cytokine concentration increases with infection and trauma. Cytokines may act simultaneously or in a consecutive manner. The receptors themselves or inhibitory cytokines bring the action of cytokines to an end. Various cytokines, especially the interleukins, have similarities in their amino acid sequence. This enables them to interact with the same cell receptor and thus to have pleiotropic and redundant effects [2].

Various cytokines are involved in the aging process of skin, including the interleukins, interferons, and tumor necrosis factor (TNF). Menopause brings with it a decrease in estrogen level and an imbalanced level of cytokines that bring about the menopausal complications including osteoporosis, cardiovascular disease, and skin aging [3–5].

Different epidermal and dermal cells produce a variety of cytokines as summarized in Table 5.1. A significant increase in the level of the proinflammatory cytokines IL-1, IL-6, and TNF-α has been reported in postmenopausal women [6, 7]. A low-grade chronic elevation of these cytokines

Table 5.1 Summary of the main cellular elements in the epidermis and dermis and the specific cytokines each cell type produces

Skin layer	Cellular element	Cytokines
Epidermis	Keratinocyte	TNF-α [1], IL-1α [34], IL-1ra [34], IL-6 [47], IL-8 [60], IL-10 [67]
	Langerhans cell	IL-8 [60], IL-18 [33]
	Melanocyte	IL-8 [60]
Dermis	Fibroblast	TNF-α [12], IL-6 [44], IL-8 [60], TGF-β [3], IFN-β [84]
	Macrophage	TNF-α [1], IL-10 [67], IL-18 [33]

IFN-β interferon-beta, *IL-1α* interleukin-1 alpha, *IL-1ra* interleukin-1 receptor antagonist, *TGF-β* transforming growth factor beta, *TNF-α* tumor necrosis factor alpha

drives the aging process [8]. Other changes in the immune system that follow hypoestrogenemia include a decrease in B- and CD4 T-lymphocytes, an increase in the response of cells to cytokines, and a decline in the natural killer cells' cytotoxic activity [6, 7].

Estrogen enhances the humoral immune response, while androgens and progesterone act as natural immunosuppressors. This difference between genders is partly responsible for the higher antibody titers and CD4+ve T cells and serum IgM in women and for the less vigorous immune response in males [9]. Changes in the sex hormone levels with menopause affect these immune mechanisms [7].

Immunosenescence is accompanied by changes in both the cellular and humoral immune responses to antigens. Fragile skin and reduced antibody production further reduce the immune response [10]. Sex hormones mediate the development of some diseases; women appear at a higher risk of developing infections and autoimmune diseases [7].

5.2 Tumor Necrosis Factor-Alpha (TNf-α)

Human TNF-α is a non-glycosylated protein that triggers inflammatory responses [11]. In the skin, TNF-α is synthesized by monocytes, macrophages, keratinocytes [1], and fibroblasts [12]. These cells produce membrane-bound TNF-α which is then converted to a soluble protein by TNF-α-converting enzyme. Both soluble and insoluble TNF-α are capable of forming non-covalently linked homotrimers that are biologically active [13].

Epidermal keratinocytes and dermal fibroblasts produce an increased amount of TNF-α on exposure to ultraviolet B (UVB) radiation which leads to increased inflammation [14]. Macrophages in old skin secrete only low levels of TNF-α compared to younger skin. In old skin less antigen-specific CD4+ T cells are recruited from the blood to skin areas where antigens enter because of defective activation of dermal blood vessels as a result of less TNF-α secretion [15]. As a consequence, old age brings with it decreased immunity [16] and increased skin infections [17]. This is reflected in decreased skin delayed-type hypersensitivity (DTH) responses when exposed to previously sensitized antigens [15].

Cutaneous macrophages have been studied in order to determine the reason for decreased TNF-α levels in old skin biopsies. Old cutaneous macrophages are inactivated, but not defective. This is because there is an increase in TNF-α secretion when Toll-like receptor (TLR) ligands are added [15]. CD4+Foxp3+ regulatory T cells inhibit TNF-α secretion from macrophages besides inhibiting macrophage activation [18]. These regulatory T cells occur in a high level in old people's skin [15, 19].

When intradermal injections of different recall antigens and organisms (*Candida albicans*, bacterium tuberculin purified protein derivative, and varicella zoster virus) are introduced into skin, there is a low DTH response in old skin [15]. Younger people are less susceptible to skin malignancy and infections, but the reaction of skin to antigens decreases with age [17]. This occurs because TNF-α aids leukocyte diapedesis from blood vessels into the skin dermis by increasing the expression of VCAM-1, ICAM-1, and E-selectin adhesion molecules on endothelial cells [15].

A defect with TLR4 expression and function of cutaneous macrophages has been detected in old skin [10, 20, 21], but this finding is not always present [22]. Secretion of TNF-α by macrophages may be low because of defective TLR1 and TLR2 function after ligands bind to the receptors [23]. This was noted when *C. albicans* was used as a recall antigen to infect skin [15]. The defect in these three different receptors seems to be reversible as skin monocytes and macrophages secrete a higher quantity of TNF-α when these receptors are stimulated in vitro [15]. However, the skin samples used by Agius et al. lacked the cytokine Interferon-gamma (IFN-γ) which is necessary for macrophages to become activated and reach their maximum functional capacity. This reason could contribute to the low number of T cells that moved to the antigen challenge site. Several cytokines are needed for macrophages to become activated besides signals from TLRs [15].

Various genes of macrophages including the major histocompatibility complex (MHC) class II genes need IFN-γ for their expression. Macrophage MHC class II present antigens to T cells [24]. This immune response does not take place in old people because antigen presentation does not occur, thus producing a block in the cascade [15]. Chronic nonspecific inflammatory responses are common in old age because there is decreased memory T cell immunosurveillance as a result of decreased macrophage activation. This can also predispose to malignancy and infection of aged skin, as well as to crystal arthritis, because debris is allowed to accumulate in blood vessels and skin tissue [15, 25].

The level of TNF-α in the circulation is higher after menopause [3, 26, 27], and this inhibits collagen synthesis while increasing collagenase synthesis [28].

TNF-α is involved in skin inflammatory responses. It modulates matrix metalloproteinase (MMP) gene expression and induces MMP-9 production. MMP-9 damages skin and inhibits its repair, thus causing the skin to age [29]. Persistent exposure of epidermal cells to TNF-α disturbs MMP-9 production and can damage the epidermis irreversibly [29]. MMP gene transcription is controlled by nuclear factor kappa B (NF-κB) [29] and activator protein-1(AP-1) [30], both of which are transcription factors. TNF-α increases MMP-9 production by increasing the binding activity of AP-1 and NF-κB to the MMP-9 DNA sequence [29].

The 3-deoxysappanchalcone decreases MMP-9 expression and inflammation [29]. 3-deoxysappanchalcone is a flavonoid that has antioxidant, anti-inflammatory, and antiallergic properties [31, 32]. It inhibits the expression and DNA binding activity of AP-1 proportionally to its concentration, hence decreasing MMP-9 protein expression [29]. Besides acting on AP-1, 3-deoxysappanchalcone directly inhibits NF-κB without affecting inhibitory kB (IκB) [29]. 3-deoxysappanchalcone inhibits MMP-9 expression at the mRNA and protein level in human keratinocytes. This is achieved by inhibiting the activation of AP-1 and NF-κB transcription factors. This is used by some pharmacological products that help skin renewal [29].

Epidermal TNF-α secretion increases after premalignant keratinocytes are irradiated with UVB. This leads to elimination of the G2/M checkpoint of the keratinocyte cell cycle and increases apoptosis while inhibiting DNA repair [13]. Since cells escape the checkpoint, they accumulate mutations and tumors develop. TNF-α regulates the atypical protein kinase C (aPKC) and activates protein kinase B (Akt). The aPKC-Akt axis reduces DNA repair. Treatment of keratinocytes with infliximab inhibits DNA repair despite enhancing the G2/M cell cycle checkpoint and apoptosis [13].

TNF-α increases cutaneous infections in old skin because of decreased skin immunity [16, 17]. It also inhibits collagen synthesis and increases collagen degradation hence producing skin aging [28, 29].

5.3 Interleukin-1 (IL-1)

IL-1 together with eight other cytokines belongs to the IL-1 structural family, also known as IL-F [33]. The outermost layer of the epidermis known as the stratum corneum contains active IL-1 [34]. IL-1α has both cytokine and transcription factor properties and it is located intracellularly. IL-1β is initially produced inactive until it is cleaved by cysteine protease caspase-1 [33]. IL-1β levels are raised in the inflammatory mechanisms of aging and atherosclerosis. They bring about elevated levels of amyloid A and C-reactive protein [33].

Keratinocytes produce both IL-1α and interleukin-1 receptor antagonist (IL-1ra). IL-1ra acts on several target cells by binding to common receptors by competitive inhibition [34]. This is however debatable as other investigators reported that IL-1ra binds to the IL-1 receptor type I only [33]. IL-1α release from keratinocytes is triggered by various stimuli including UVB radiation. It causes skin inflammation by activating different cytokines and adhesion molecules. IL-1α is inhibited by IL-1ra; the balance between these two cytokines maintains skin homeostasis [34].

The level of IL-1 in the stratum corneum in facial skin (exposed to UVB) does not change significantly with age, while IL-1α level is higher in aged skin samples taken from the inside of the upper arm (not exposed to UVB) compared with samples taken from younger skin. Conversely, the level of IL-1ra measured from skin biopsies taken from the inside of the upper arm was found to decrease with age [34]. However, an increase in the level of IL-1ra with aging has been observed in cultured human keratinocytes, while a decrease in level noted in photoaged cells [35]. No difference in the level of IL-1 cytokines present in the stratum corneum between males and females was observed [34].

IL-1 release form keratinocytes in the epidermis induces cortisol synthesis which controls wound healing [36]. Conversely, insulin-like growth factor-1 decreases the production of cortisol. The epidermis produces various enzymes necessary for de novo cortisol synthesis like steroid 11β-hydroxylase (CYP11B1) and 11β-hydroxysteroid dehydrogenase 2 (11βHSD2) that converts active cortisol into inactive cortisone and controls negative feedback responses. Glucocorticoids (GCs) inhibit the healing process of wounds and limit the degree of inflammation in acute wounds. CYP11B1 enzyme inhibitor (metyrapone) inhibits cortisol synthesis in skin keratinocytes while ACTH promotes synthesis [36].

Upon tissue injury, keratinocytes release preformed IL-1 [37]. IL-1 is the initial signal of tissue injury that has both autocrine and paracrine functions. It activates keratinocytes to migrate and proliferate while they secrete more proinflammatory molecules [38]. Cessation of inflammation and tissue healing is brought about by activated keratinocytes that transition into a differentiating phenotype [36]. This is facilitated by IL-10, IL-receptor antagonist, GCs, and transforming growth factor-β1 (TGF-β1) that reverse the activation of keratinocytes and bring about resolution [36]. Treatment of keratinocytes with GC inhibits the synthesis or signalling of several inflammatory cytokines including IL-1β, IL-4, IL-8, INF-γ, and TNF-α and growth factors like TGF-β, epidermal growth factor (EGF), and vascular endothelial growth factor (VEGF) that take part in the inflammatory part of wound healing [39]. IL-1, IL-6, and TNF-α act on the hypothalamic-pituitary-adrenal axis to increase cortisol synthesis [40].

IL-1β is a proinflammatory cytokine that increases the expression of CYP11B1 and hence the production of cortisol and activates the GR pathway involved in wound healing both in vivo and ex vivo. Epidermal cortisol synthesis may serve locally as a negative feedback to proinflammatory cytokines because when cortisol synthesis is inhibited, the production of IL-1β is increased. This regulatory mechanism prevents excessive inflammation form occurring during wound healing that may otherwise damage the tissue even more. When GC synthesis is inhibited, the wound closure process is faster in vivo [36].

The epidermis is unique in its properties and characteristics. Although it lacks its own vascular supply, it is the "first line of defense" that comes in contact with foreign antigens, pathogens, and commensals and is exposed to various forms of injury. Keratinocyte activation and timely regulated release of IL-1β together with other proinflammatory cytokines and growth factors are the main features that enable skin to function as an effective barrier [38].

In vitro studies showed that the production of both IL-1α and IL-1β increased in cocultured keratinocytes more than in monocultures. Keratinocytes by producing IL-1 actively stimulate fibroblasts to produce keratinocyte growth factor that stimulates the proliferation of keratinocytes. IL-1 does not have a direct effect on keratinocyte proliferation as was observed in monocultures. IL-1 thus regulates skin homeostasis through a double paracrine mechanism. This was also observed in blocking experiments; when IL-1α and IL-1β neutralizing antibodies together with IL-1 receptor antagonist were applied to cocultures, the proliferation of keratinocytes was reduced. This inhibition was reversible because when the antibodies were removed, keratinocyte proliferation rate was the same as in controls [41]. Various other cytokines and growth factors have been detected in keratinocytes and fibroblasts including IL-6, IL-8, TGF-α, TGF-β, granulocyte macrophage colony stimulating factor (GM-CSF), platelet-derived growth factor (PDGF), and nerve growth factor (NGF) [42].

Dermal fibroblasts in aged human skin produce a higher level of CCN1 than in younger skin. CCN1 upregulates the level of IL-1β, decreasing the skin collagen content in two ways: by increasing the amount of MMPs that degrade collagen and by downregulating the rate of collagen synthesis [43, 44]. IL-1β also downregulates TGF-β type II receptors impairing TGF-β signalling. This increases the risk of developing inflammatory and degenerative disease in osteoarthritis [43, 44].

5.4 IL-6

The postmenopausal drop in estrogen is accompanied by a rise in IL-6 level [3]. During infection or tissue injury, the level of IL-6 rises much more than the postmenopausal level [45].

IL-6 is both a pro- and anti-inflammatory cytokine. It achieves these opposite functions by working through different signalling mechanisms [46]. Human keratinocytes produces IL-6 upon induction by TGF-α [47]. The IL-6 produced stimulates keratinocyte proliferation [48]. However, other researchers did not observe a rise in keratinocyte proliferation upon IL-6 expression in transgenic mice [49]. The stratum corneum of transgenic mice became thicker after IL-6 expression, but epidermal proliferation was not increased, and there was no leukocyte infiltration. This suggested that although IL-6 is elevated in inflammatory conditions, it is does not have a direct proinflammatory activity on the skin [49]. IL-6 is also produced by dermal fibroblasts [44].

Besides TGF-α, IL-1, IL-4, TNF-α, and IFN-γ also induce the production of IL-6 in keratinocytes [50, 51]. CCN1 induces dermal fibroblasts to produce IL-6 through reactive oxygen species (ROS) and integrin pathways [44]. Ultraviolet radiation increases IL-6 production. IL-6 plays a role in skin aging, wrinkle formation [51], and tissue damage [44]. It is considered a health status marker in the elderly [52].

Chronic elevated levels of IL-6 together with IL-1β in aged skin contribute to sustained high levels of MMPs that degrade collagen, and thus these cytokines are negative regulators of collagen homeostasis. Furthermore, IL-6 decreases the rate of collagen synthesis [52].

In women aged between 25 and 82 years, there is no significant difference between 25-hydroxyvitamin D status (through UVB exposure) and IL-6 in women with regular versus not regular UVB exposure, unlike for serum TNF-α which had an inverse relationship with vitamin D level [53]. While most in vivo studies did not show that IL-6 serum levels are affected by vitamin D status [54], in vitro studies showed that 1,25-dihydoroxyvitamin D inhibits IL-6 production in different cells [55]. However, one study involving hemodialysis patients showed that a 6-month course treatment of both iv and oral 1,25-dihydroxyvitamin D significantly suppressed IL-6 concentrations [56]. Parathyroid hormone (PTH) induces IL-6 production by osteoblasts [57] although there is no significant relationship between circulating IL-6 and intact PTH ($p=0.8$) [53]. Vitamin D supplementation decreases the level of PTH and hence its indirect effect on IL-6 concentrations [53].

In a study involving 47 healthy postmenopausal women taking daily 1 g of calcium and 800 U cholecalciferol for 12 weeks, there was no change observed in serum IL-6 level. A significantly inverse correlation was found between IL-6 and osteoprotegerin ($p=0.004$). Furthermore, a significant correlation was obtained between insulin and IL-6 levels ($p=0.0005$) [58].

IL-6 plays a key role in bone resorption by activating osteoclasts. It is also involved in other diseases that occur more frequently in menopausal women like atherosclerosis, diabetes, and cardiovascular disease [3, 59].

A significant positive association was found between menopausal status and IL-6 ($R^2=0.0764$, $p=0.0246$) and between age and IL-6 ($R^2=0.09413$, $p=0.0116$) with analysis of potential covariates [53].

5.5 IL-8

IL-8, formerly known as neutrophil-activating peptide-I (NAP-I), serves to activate neutrophils and also as a chemoattractant. It is produced by fibroblasts, keratinocytes, melanocytes, endothelial cells, monocytes, and Langerhans cells [60]. Serum IL-8 level is significantly higher in menopausal women ($p=0.001$) compared to women in their reproductive age [61].

The expression of IL-8 is increased by IL-1 and TNF [62]. Besides being a neutrophil chemoattractant, IL-8 is also a T-cell chemoattractant. However it has no effect on monocytes and eosinophils. The action on neutrophils is brought about by increasing the expression of Mac-1 (a cell adhesion molecule) on neutrophils [1].

When IL-8 is injected into the dermis, it causes neutrophils to accumulate in the dermis surrounding the blood vessels [63]. Excess IL-8 is found in psoriatic skin and causes neutrophils to accumulate in the epidermis [64]. Excess IL-8 also plays a role in cutaneous T-cell lymphoma [65].

5.6 IL-10

IL-10, a potent anti-inflammatory cytokine [66], is known as cytokine synthesis inhibitory factor (CSIF) because it inhibits the production of several cytokines including IL-2, IL-3, TNF, and GM-CSF and also inhibits the proliferation of T lymphocytes [67–69]. It has an immunosuppressive role [67]. IL-10 is produced by keratinocytes, macrophages, and B lymphocytes [67]. UV light increases the production of IL-10 in human keratinocytes [1, 70].

The difference in circulating IL-10 levels is not significant between postmenopausal and fertile women [71]. Levels of 25-hydroxyvitamin D in healthy women showed no statistically significant relationship with circulating IL-10 measured using highly sensitive ELISA kits, suggesting that the body status of vitamin D does not affect the secretion of IL-10 into the systemic circulation in healthy individuals [53]. Furthermore, a positive relationship between 25-hydroxyvitamin D and IL-10 in the circulation was found in diseased individuals [72].

5.7 IL-18

IL-18 belongs to the IL-1 structural family and is similar in structure to IL-1β [33]. Previously, it was known as interferon-gamma-inducing factor (IGIF). IL-18 is produced by dendritic cells, macrophages, and epithelial cells [33]. IL-12 increases the expression of IL-18 receptors on natural killer cells, T lymphocytes, and thymocytes [73]. It functions as an immunoregulatory and proinflammatory cytokine and is involved in the aging process, atherosclerosis, and autoimmune diseases. The aging process might be slowed down by therapeutic strategies that reduce IL-18 [33]. IL-18 binding protein (IL-18BP) is an inhibitor of IL-18. When this inhibitor is overexpressed, mice deficient in apolipoprotein E do not develop atherosclerosis [33].

The circulating level of IL-18 is higher in postmenopausal women compared to fertile women [71]. IL-18 inactive precursor becomes active upon cleavage by cysteine protease caspase-1 [33]. This immunoregulatory cytokine has the ability to induce IFN-γ [74]. Research has shifted towards blocking IL-18 activity in autoimmune diseases as it inhibits the production of IFN-γ [33].

This proinflammatory cytokine enhances the production of cell adhesion molecules, nitric oxide, and chemokines [33]. It is also involved in type 2 T-helper cell (Th2) polarization. Both allergic and nonallergic skin inflammation are worsened with overexpression of IL-18 [75]. When combined with IL-12, IL-18 stops the production of immunoglobulin (Ig) E [33]. On the other hand, IL-18 prevents UV-induced immunosuppression and protects the skin from damage after exposure to UVB radiation by promoting DNA repair [76]. Unlike other proinflammatory cytokines, IL-18 does not produce fever [77] and prostaglandin E_2 [78].

The signalling cascade of IL-18 starts with IL-18 binding to IL-18 receptor α (IL-18Rα), which then recruits IL-18Rβ to bring the intracellular Toll domains in close proximity [33]. This complex recruits MyD88 protein that phosphorylates IL-1 receptor activating kinases (IRAKs). TNF factor is then phosphorylated followed by inhibitory κB kinases (IKK) α and β activation. IκB is then phosphorylated and NF-κB moves to the nucleus. Mitogen-activating protein (MAP) kinase p38 is also phosphorylated. IL-18BP located extracellularly can neutralize IL-18 and prevent it from binding to IL-18Rα. IL-18 bound to IL-18BP can form an inactive complex with IL-18Rβ, consuming IL-18Rβ chain to further decrease the chance of cell activation [33].

5.8 Interferons (IFNS)

IFNs are known for their antiproliferative activities, antiviral activities, and regulation of cell differentiation and proliferation [79]. Three major types of IFNs are recognized based on the type of receptors used in signalling: Type I includes IFN-α, IFN-β, and IFN-ω that bind to IFN-α receptor; type II is IFN-γ in humans and binds to interferon-gamma receptor (IFNGR) [80]. The class interferon type III which signals via IL10R2 and IFNLR1 is not universally accepted [81].

5.8.1 IFN-α

IFN-α is produced by leukocytes to take part in the innate immune response against viruses. When the skin is constantly exposed to IFN-α, the population doublings of dermal microvascular endothelial cells decrease and express a senescent phenotype [82].

CD1a+ (Langerhans) cells stimulate T-lymphocyte-dependent immune reactions to take place. These Langerhans cells decrease linearly with age, giving the skin decreased immunosurveillance. Studies where IFN-α cream was applied to preauricular skin biopsies showed that the biopsies taken from people whose ages varied between 57 and 75 years had a higher amount of cutaneous CD1a+ cells than before the cream was applied in comparison to younger people [83].

5.8.2 IFN-β

IFN-β is produced by fibroblasts. Like IFN-α, it is involved against viral infections in the innate immune response. Exposure of the skin to IFN-β causes dermal fibroblasts to senesce via a DNA damage signalling pathway [84]. Fibroblasts are the commonest cell type found in the dermis and produce mainly collagen types I and III [85].

5.8.3 IFN-γ

IFN-γ is produced by T-lymphocyte cells including those that reside in the skin which possess the cutaneous lymphocyte antigen (CLA). It forms part of the family of macrophage-activating factors [86]. The level of IFN-γ produced by peripheral blood mononuclear cells in healthy women decreases with age and is linked with the changes in circulating gonadal hormones [87] although there appears to be no change in the amount of IFN-γ-producing CLA+ T cells with old age [86]. There is a significant positive correlation between estrogen level and IFN-γ [87]. Other investigators reported that the decline in IFN-γ with age may also be due to the loss of lymphocyte functions as a result of aging such as cellular dysfunctions, impaired intracellular signalling, and weakened interaction between the receptors on T cells and antigen-presenting cells [7, 88].

IL-18 stimulates the production of IFN-γ though it does not achieve this on its own but requires IL-12. This is achieved via the transcription factor

T-bet [33]. IL-18BP promoter has two IFN-γ response elements that help regulate the level of IFN-γ produced [89]. When levels of IFN-γ are high, they stimulate IL-18BP to decrease the production of IFN-γ [33].

IFN-γ is considered to be the "signature" cytokine of natural killer cells and of CD4+ and CD8+ T cells [33]. IFN-γ is needed for the production of cytotoxic T cells and to induce type 1 T-helper (Th 1) cells and hence plays a role in graft versus host disease [33]. IFN-γ suppresses IgE synthesis and thus is involved in Th 2 polarization [33].

GCs produced in the epidermis suppress essentially all genes regulated by IFN-γ, such as STAT-1 and IFN-γ receptor [39]. Application of GCs to epidermal keratinocytes showed that IFN-γ-related genes were suppressed at 48 h and 72 h after GC treatment. This action is brought about through suppression of STAT-1 expression and preventing its activation [39]. Treating human keratinocytes with IFN-γ and GCs simultaneously blocks STAT-1 nuclear translocation and IFN-γ-mediated activation. This was even more enhanced when keratinocytes were pretreated with GCs for 4 h. Conversely, with IFN-γ pretreatment for two hours, translocation and activation occurred [39]. Both IFN-α and IFN-γ are able to modulate the growth of epidermal keratinocytes [90].

5.9 Cysteine-Rich Protein 61 (CRY61)

CRY61 forms part of the connective tissue growth factor, cysteine-rich protein, and nephroblastoma overexpressed gene (CCN) protein family that together with the other five matricellular protein members of this family, it interrelates with the extracellular matrix [44, 91]. CRY61 is also known as CCN1. Its function is to induce M1 macrophages to become activated and express a proinflammatory genetic profile. It also plays a role in Th 1 cell responses. CCN1 decreases the production of TGF-β, while it enhances the production of the cytokines TNF-α, IL-1α, IL-1β, IL-6, and IL-12b. Furthermore, it alters the mechanism of some cytokines, for example, it induces TNF-α to exhibit cytotoxic properties without inhibiting the activity of NF-κB [92]. This alteration in the genetic profile is brought about via either of two pathways: a delayed response achieved via CCN1-indcued TNF-α or through an immediate-early response that involves direct activation of CCN1 [92].

A high level of CCN1 in aged skin causes dermal fibroblasts to have an "age-associated secretory phenotype" [44]. Fibroblasts produce collagen that is the main component of the skin connective tissue. Fibroblasts also degrade collagen. The fibroblast phenotype in aged skin brings about abnormal homeostasis of type I collagen in the skin, where collagen production is low while degradation increased [93].

CCN1 interacts with integrins to increase the level of ROS [94] which in turn activates MAPK and NF-κB signalling pathways to increase the production of IL-1β and IL-6 [52]. IL-1β and IL-6 increase the production of MMPs in old dermal fibroblasts. These two cytokines further imbalance collagen homeostasis by lowering the rate of collagen production [43, 52]. TGF-β signalling is impaired in dermal fibroblasts of aged skin because IL-1β decreases the TGF-β type II receptors to have a negative effect on collagen homeostasis [93]. All these cause the skin connective tissue to age, and the skin loses its function and integrity [44].

5.10 Transforming Growth Factor-β (TGF-β)

TGF-β is a cytokine family that has many functions, for example, it suppresses inflammatory processes; regulates cell growth, differentiation, and proliferation; controls extracellular connective tissue synthesis; and plays a role in tissue repair and tissue recycling after injury [3, 95, 96]. It acts as an antagonist to proinflammatory cytokines [3]. Three isoforms of this cytokine family are found in mammals: TGF-β1, TGF-β2, and TGF-β3 [95]. They bind to either of the two cell-surface receptors – TGF-β type I receptor (TβRI) and TβRII – and the signal continues via the Sma and Mad (Smad) pathway to bring about their actions [97].

In the skin, TGF-β stimulates dermal fibroblasts to proliferate and increase the production and secretion of most ECM proteins including type I, III, and VII collagens [97] and fibronectin [98]. It also decreases the production of proteolytic enzymes including MMPs, collagenase, and stromelysin that break down the ECM proteins [99].

Estrogen increases the production of TGF-β in various tissue cells including fibroblasts, vascular smooth muscle, osteoclasts, and osteoblasts to inhibit bone resorption [3, 100]. Cutaneous wound biopsies taken from healthy postmenopausal women showed that they had a lower level of TGF-β in their wounds in comparison to younger women and this is associated with a slower rate of wound healing [95]. Application of topical estrogen after cutaneous injury in ovariectomized female rodents induces dermal fibroblasts to increase TGF-β1 secretion by stimulating the TGF-β/Smad pathway and this accelerates cutaneous wound healing [101].

Topical 17β-estradiol improves the symptoms of skin aging like loss of skin elasticity, thin dermal skin, and wrinkling [95]. This is achieved by increasing type I procollagen production which occurs to a bigger extent in the skin of aged females than in aged males [95]. Conversely, the effect of topical 17β-estradiol on MMPs and fibrillin-1 was not found to be significantly different between male and female skin although the investigators suggest that this could be due to the small number of volunteers that took part in the experiments [95]. When anti-TGFβ1 antibody was added together with 17β-estradiol to cultured fibroblasts, there was no increase in procollagen type I [95].

Studies suggest that 17β-estradiol application to aged skin stimulate the TGF-β/Smad pathway to increase fibrillin-1 and elastin production, two main fibers that give skin its elastic properties [95]. Aged skin has less elastin and increased elastic fiber breakdown than younger skin [102].

Although TGF-β inhibits epidermal keratinocyte growth [103], when 17β-estradiol is applied to old skin, there is increased proliferation of epidermal keratinocytes contributing to a thicker epidermis [95]. This might occur through activation of ERK or modulation of the level of estrogen receptors in the nucleus [104] instead of through the TGF-β/Smad pathway [95].

5.11 Skin Wrinkling

Skin aging is characterized by wrinkle formation that results from rapid loss of collagen which leads to decreased skin elasticity [105]. Climacteric skin aging is a separate entity from chronological aging and photoaging that contributes to cutaneous wrinkling [106]. The loss of collagen as a result of hypestrogenemia in the initial postmenopausal period occurs at a faster rate than that in later menopausal years, with about 30 % loss in the initial 5 years [107]. A study on 186 Korean females of ages varying between 20 and 89 showed that women with more than 10 years since the onset of menopause had significantly greater facial wrinkling than women with less than 5 years in their postmenopausal period, after controlling for sun exposure and age [106]. Korean women had 3.7 times greater risk to develop severe wrinkles than Korean men [108]. Conversely, men under the age of 50 had a significantly greater risk of wrinkling ($p<0.05$) than women of similar age [106]. Studies on white Caucasian individuals found out that females in their 60s had a 28-fold increased risk of developing wrinkles compared to women in their 40s, whereas men had only an 11.4-fold increased risk [109]. After the age of 50 years, facial wrinkles increase more rapidly with age in women than in men. This suggests that hypoestrogenism in postmenopausal women contributes more than chronological aging to the decline in skin collagen and wrinkling [106]. Collagen content decreases by 2.1 % every postmenopausal year [110].

HRT prevents wrinkle formation in postmenopausal women. HRT helps the skin to form more mature collagen fibers [111]. Estrogen enhances the production of hyaluronic acid and glycosaminoglycans which increase the water content of dermal collagen [112]. These two mechanisms serve as a protection against facial wrinkling [106].

Wrinkle formation starts with activation of receptors like interleukin-1 receptor, tumor necrosis factor receptor, epidermal growth factor receptor, platelet-derived growth factor receptor, and platelet-activating factor receptor, which lead to signal transduction which eventually activates AP-1 to stimulate the production of MMPs, which degrade collagen. C-jun transcription factor subunit is the limiting factor of AP-1 activity [105]. This subunit is found at a higher level in aged skin (80 years old) compared to younger skin (18–28 years old) [113]. C-jun is the common intermediate protein that takes part in all the five different signal transduction pathways involving all the mentioned receptors. Thus c-jun is the target for new drugs to prevent the wrinkle formation [105].

5.12 Hair Changes

Hair changes that may occur with menopause include a decrease in body hair and pubic hair and an increase in facial hair [114]. Scalp hair changes include fine-textured hair that inadequately covers the scalp and increased spaces between the hairs on the vertex in comparison to the occiput that is typical of female pattern hair loss (FPHL) [115]. Frontal fibrosing alopecia can also occur (see Chap. 9) [116]. Although hair density decreases with age, this is not related to menopausal status [115]. Estrogen regulates the growth of hair follicles and hair cycles [115]. Human hair follicles contain more estrogen receptor (ER)-β than ER-α [117]. Estradiol increases aromatase activity in scalp follicles of humans [116] to increase the production of estrogen from adrenal androgen [115]. Male and female frontotemporal hair follicles respond to 17β-estradiol differently. In the lower outer root sheath of male hair follicles, TGF-β2 immunoreactivity decreased, whereas it increased in follicles taken from females after 48 h from treatment with 17β-estradiol [118].

Estrogen modulates the production and activity of several cytokines, growth factors, and transcription factors that influence hair growth, but further research of the pathways involved is required [115]. On the other hand, the role of androgens on hair growth has been extensively studied as it has previously dominated the field of hair biology [115].

5.13 Wound Healing

Estrogen deprivation that occurs with menopause is a major risk factor for delayed and poor wound healing in humans, much more than chronological aging. A microarray study showed that only 3 % of genes differentially expressed between wounds in elderly and young men are age associated, while more than three-quarters of them are regulated by estrogen [119, 120]. Various comorbid conditions that might occur simultaneously in the elderly like diabetes mellitus, decreased innate immune defenses, vascular insufficiency, and local skin pressure further delay the healing process [96]. Chronic wounds are often difficult to treat. Acute wounds are usually repaired using paper strips rather than using sutures in the elderly because the skin is thin and sutures may tear the skin further [96].

The complex orchestrated process of inflammation and vascular and cellular proliferation, with remodelling that occurs in response to cutaneous injury in young skin, is not harmonically regulated in old skin. Aged skin is fragile and prone to trauma. Keratinocytes, fibroblasts, and endothelial cells involved in the healing process age, resulting in aberrant wound healing [120]. The innate inflammatory response that is initiated first in the healing process is disrupted in elderly skin. Wound healing in aged skin is characterized by an overproduction of MMPs and elastase [121–123] and underproduction of tissue inhibitors of metalloproteinases [124], as a result of prolonged recruitment of macrophages, delayed resolution, excess influx of neutrophils, and altered endothelial cell adhesion [125]. Wound healing of aged skin is also manifested by delayed angiogenesis [126], slow keratinocyte proliferation [127], decreased collagen deposition [128] and scar strength [129], and increased sensitivity to keratinocyte growth factor and epidermal growth factor [130]. On the other hand, the quality of the scar formed by matrix remodelling is improved [131].

While topical estrogen improves cutaneous wound healing in elderly people of both genders [131], HRT improves wound healing in postmenopausal women [101]. Estrogen therapy in elderly people improves wound healing by working on different cells in the dermis and epidermis including keratincoytes, fibroblasts, and inflammatory cells [120]. Estrogen treatment prevents excessive elastase production and neutrophil recruitment. Both collagen and fibronectin syntheses are increased [120]. Furthermore, HRT prevents the development of pressure ulcers and venous leg ulcers in postmenopausal women [132, 133]. HRT may also reduce the development of chronic wounds in elderly women as observed in a case-cohort retrospective study of elderly females above 65 years of age in the United Kingdom [96].

Accelerated cutaneous wound healing was observed with estrogen replacement in ovariectomized female mice and rats [134, 135]. The same was observed with dehydroepiandrosterone (DHEA) given systemically as it was locally converted to estrogen [136]. On the other hand, androgens are harmful to wound healing; testosterone delays repair [137] while blocking androgen receptors or castration improves wound healing in rodents [138, 139]. A randomized double-blind study showed that skin biopsies treated with estrogen before wounding healed more after 7 days than placebo patches and were stronger 80 days after wounding in both genders (mean age greater than 70 years). Biopsies also showed lower levels of elastase, neutrophils, and fibronectin degradation in both male and female upper arm skin wounded patches treated with estrogen compared to placebo skin areas [131].

Estrogen works at the cellular level by down-regulating L-selectins expressed by neutrophils. This avoids excess neutrophils and elastase from accumulating [131] besides helping the phagocytic activity of neutrophils [140]. Hypestrogenemia that occurs in menopausal women may result in hyperinflammation and a high proteolyitc environment that slow wound healing [96]. Estrogen reduces the expression of several proinflammatory cytokines, especially TNF-α, macrophage migration inhibitory factor (MIF), IL-1β, IL-6, and monocyte chemoattractant protein-1 (MCP-1) [141]. These cytokines cause inflammatory cells containing proteolytic enzymes to accumulate, further degrading the extracellular matrix. Overproduction of these cytokines may complicate the healing process by provoking immunosuppression [96].

Plasma MIF level correlates inversely with the level of systemic estrogen; the level is high in postmenopausal women and low after treatment with HRT [142, 143]. During hypestrogenemia, MIF causes excessive wound inflammation that leads to slow wound healing [144]. Low MIF levels following estrogen are very beneficial in wound healing [143, 145]. Being a keratinocyte mitogen [104], estrogen promotes migration and wound reepithelialization in ovariectomized mice [135]. In vitro studies showed that estrogen stimulates dermal fibroblasts to migrate both directly and indirectly [145, 146]. The indirect route is achieved via PDGF which stimulates macrophages. PDGF also stimulates wound contraction and angiogenesis [147]. After the basement membrane of capillaries is formed, endothelial cells take a capillary-like structure with the help of estradiol [148]. However, the role of estradiol in angiogenesis is debatable. Some studies reported decreased angiogenesis, while others showed no change after treatment with estrogen [149, 150].

Skin biopsies taken from wounds of healthy postmenopausal women contained a low level of TGF-β which was linked to a low wound healing rate [101]. TGF-β increases the synthesis of collagen and elastic fibers by fibroblasts and decreases the synthesis of MMPs [95].

Estrogen therapy, both alone and together with a progestin, helps to prevent wound formation by maintaining the skin thickness and collagen content to similar levels found in youthful skin. It also helps wound healing in postmenopausal females by preserving the extracellular matrix of the dermis [151].

5.14 Photoaging

Exposure to solar radiation brings about the loss of subcutaneous fat tissue which results in aging. When Li and associates investigated the expression of cytokine mRNA production by qRT-PCR and protein secretion by ELISA in cultured keratinocytes, fibroblasts, and other epidermal-dermal equivalents exposed to different doses of solar simulated radiation, it was observed that the secretion of TNF-α, IL-1α, IL-6, and IL-11 was induced. On the other hand, when sunscreen was used, it prevented the production of these cytokines [152].

The differentiation of facial human preadipocytes was studied using image analyses and the presence of adipocyte differentiation markers. When facial preadipocytes were exposed to conditioned medium from solar-irradiated equivalents, their differentiation was inhibited. Contrary, when solar-irradiated equivalents were first pretreated with sunscreen, the differentiation of preadipocytes into mature adipocytes was not inhibited. Using a variety of antibodies to TNF-α, IL-1α, IL-6, and IL-11 significantly reduced the inhibition on the differentiation of preadipocytes caused by solar simulator radiation [152].

5.15 Summary

Skin aging is one of the menopausal complications that concerns most women. It does not occur uniformly in all females but varies between individuals [114]. Three factors bring about aged skin: chronological aging [153], extrinsic skin aging [154], and hypoestrogenemia after menopause [155].

As seen, cytokines play a key role in the appearance of aged skin characteristics like easy bruising, dry skin, and delayed wound healing [114]. Cytokines are produced by a range of skin cells and cells of the immune system and have both overlapping and independent effects on skin aging and inflammation. Because of their overlapping roles, cytokines should be viewed as a network rather than individually [156]. Further research is necessary especially to identify the role of cytokines in the prevention and treatment of skin aging.

References

1. Feliciani C, Gupta AK, Saucier DN. Keratinocytes and cytokine/growth factors. Crit Rev Oral Biol Med. 1996;7(4):300–18.
2. Calleja-Agius J, Muttukrishna S, Jauniaux E. The role of tumor necrosis factor alpha (TNFα) in human female reproduction. Expert Rev Endocrinol Metab. 2009;4:273–82.
3. Pfeilschifter J, Koditz R, Pfohl M, Schatz H. Changes in proinflammatory cytokine activity after menopause. Endocr Rev. 2002;23:90–199.
4. Zupan J, Komadina R, Marc J. The relationship between osteoclastogenic and anti-osteoclastogenic pro-inflammatory cytokines differs in human osteoporotic and osteoarthritic bone tissues. J Biomed Sci. 2012;19:28.
5. Camilleri G, Borg M, Brincat S, Schembri-Wismayer P, Brincat M, Calleja-Agius J. The role of cytokines in cardiovascular disease in menopause. Climacteric. 2012;15(6):524–30.
6. Giglio T, Imro MA, Filaci G, Scudeletti M, Puppo F, De Cecco L, et al. Immune cell circulating subsets are affected by gonadal function. Life Sci. 1994;54(18):1305–12.
7. Gameiro CM, Romão F, Castelo-Branco C. Menopause and aging: changes in the immune system–a review. Maturitas. 2010;67:316–20.
8. Franceschi C, Capri M, Monti D, Giunta S, Olivieri F, Sevini F, et al. Inflammaging and anti-inflammaging: a systemic perspective on aging and longevity emerged from studies in humans. Mech Ageing Dev. 2007;128:92–105.
9. Goldsby AR, Kindt JT, Osborne AB. Kuby immunology. 4th ed. New York: W.H. Freeman and Company; 2000.
10. Krabbe KS, Pedersen M, Brunsgaard H. Inflammatory mediators in the elderly. Exp Gerontol. 2004;39(5):687–99.
11. Dada LA, Sznajder JI. Mitochondrial Ca2+ and ROS take center stage to orchestrate TNF-α–mediated inflammatory responses. J Clin Invest. 2011;121(5):1683–5.
12. Bashir MM, Sharma MR, Werth VP. TNF-alpha production in the skin. Arch Dermatol Res. 2009;301(1):87–91.
13. Faurschou A. Role of tumor necrosis factor-α in the regulation of keratinocyte cell cycle and DNA repair after ultraviolet-B radiation. Dan Med Bull. 2010;57(10):B4179.
14. Bashir MM, Sharma MR, Werth VP. UVB and proinflammatory cytokines synergistically activate TNF-alpha production in keratinocytes

15. Agius E, Lacy KE, Vukmanovic-Stejic M, Jagger AL, Papageorgiou AP, Hall S, et al. Decreased TNF-α synthesis by macrophages restricts cutaneous immunosurveillance by memory CD4+ T cells during aging. Exp Med. 2009;206(9):1929–40.
16. Yoshikawa TT. Epidemiology and unique aspects of aging and infectious diseases. Clin Infect Dis. 2000;30:931–3.
17. Laube S. Skin infections and aging. Aging Res Rev. 2004;3:69–89.
18. Tiemessen MM, Jagger AL, Evans HG, van Herwijnen MJ, John S, Taams LS. CD4+CD25+ Foxp3+ regulatory T cells induce alternative activation of human monocytes/macrophages. Proc Natl Acad Sci U S A. 2007;104(49):19446–51.
19. Vukmanovic-Stejic M, Zhang Y, Cook JE, Fletcher JM, McQuaid A, Masters JE, et al. Human CD4+ CD25hi Foxp3+ regulatory T cells are derived by rapid turnover of memory populations in vivo. J Clin Invest. 2006;116:2423–33.
20. Renshaw M, Rockwell J, Engleman C, Gewirtz A, Katz J, Sambhara S. Cutting edge: impaired Toll-like receptor expression and function in aging. J Immunol. 2002;169:4697–701.
21. van den Biggelaar AH, Huizinga TW, de Craen AJ, Gussekloo J, Heijmans BT, Frölich M, et al. Impaired innate immunity predicts frailty in old age. The Leiden 85-plus study. Exp Gerontol. 2004;39:1407–14.
22. van Duin D, Shaw AC. Toll-like receptors in older adults. J Am Geriatr Soc. 2007;55:1438–44.
23. van Duin D, Mohanty S, Thomas V, Ginter S, Montgomery RR, Fikrig E, et al. Age-associated defect in human TLR-1/2 function. J Immunol. 2007;178:970–5.
24. Cullell-Young M, Barrachina M, López-López C, et al. From transcription to cell surface expression, the induction of MHC class II I-A alpha by interferon-gamma in macrophages is regulated at different levels. Immunogenetics. 2001;53:136–44.
25. Richards A, Kavanagh D, Atkinson JP. Inherited complement regulatory protein deficiency predisposes to human disease in acute injury and chronic inflammatory states the examples of vascular damage in atypical hemolytic uremic syndrome and debris accumulation in age-related macular degeneration. Adv Immunol. 2007;96:141–77.
26. Pacifici R, Brown C, Puscheck E, Friedrich E, Slatopolsky E, Maggio D, et al. Effect of surgical menopause and estrogen replacement on cytokine release from human blood mononuclear cells. Proc Natl Acad Sci U S A. 1991;88:5134–8.
27. Deswal A, Petersen NJ, Feldman AM, Young JB, White BG, Mann DL. Cytokines and cytokine receptors in advanced heart failure: an analysis of the cytokine database from the Vesnarinone Trial (VEST). Circulation. 2001;103:2055–9.
28. Chou DH, Lee W, McCulloch CA. TNF-alpha inactivation of collagen receptors: implications for fibroblast function and fibrosis. J Immunol. 1996;156(11):4354–62.
29. Youn UJ, Nam KW, Kim HS, Choi G, Jeong WS, Lee MY, et al. 3-Deoxysappanchalcone inhibits tumor necrosis factor-α-induced matrix metalloproteinase-9 expression in human keratinocytes through activated protein-1 inhibition and nuclear factor-kappa B DNA binding activity. Biol Pharm Bull. 2011;34(6):890–3.
30. Crawford HC, Matrisian LM. Mechanisms controlling the transcription of matrix metalloproteinase genes in normal and neoplastic cells. Enzyme Protein. 1996;49(1–3):20–37.
31. Ban HS, Suzuki K, Lim SS, Jung SH, Lee S, Ji J, et al. Inhibition of lipopolysaccharide-induced expression of inducible nitric oxide synthase and tumor necrosis factor-alpha by 2′-hydroxychalcone derivatives in RAW 264.7 cells. Biochem Pharmacol. 2004;67(8):1549–57.
32. Yodsaoue O, Cheenpracha S, Karalai C, Ponglimanont C, Tewtrakul S. Anti-allergic activity of principles from the roots and heartwood of Caesalpinia sappan on antigen-induced beta-hexosaminidase release. Phytother Res. 2009;23(7):1028–31.
33. Dinarello CA. Interleukin 1 and interleukin 18 as mediators of inflammation and the aging process. Am J Clin Nutr. 2006;83:S2447–55.
34. Hirao T, Aoki H, Yoshida T, Sato Y, Kamoda H. Elevation of Interleukin 1 receptor antagonist in the stratum corneum of sun-exposed and ultraviolet B-irradiated human skin. J Invest Dermatol. 1996;106(5):1102–7.
35. Garmyn M, Yaar M, Boileau N, Backendorf C, Gilchrest BA. Effect of aging and habitual sun exposure on the genetic response of cultured human keratinocytes to solar-simulated irradiation. J Invest Dermatol. 1992;99(6):743–8.
36. Vukelic S, Stojadinovic O, Pastar I, Rabach M, Krzyzanowska A, Lebrun E, et al. Cortisol synthesis in epidermis is induced by IL-1 and tissue injury. J Biol Chem. 2011;286(12):10265–75.
37. Kupper TS. The activated keratinocyte: a model for inducible cytokine production by non-bone marrow-derived cells in cutaneous inflammatory and immune responses. J Invest Dermatol. 1990;94(6 Suppl):146S–50.
38. Freedberg IM, Tomic-Canic M, Komine M, Blumenberg M. Keratins and the keratinocyte activation cycle. J Invest Dermatol. 2001;116(5):633–40.
39. Stojadinovic O, Lee B, Vouthounis C, Vukelic S, Pastar I, Blumenberg M, et al. Novel genomic effects of glucocorticoids in epidermal keratinocytes: inhibition of apoptosis, interferon-gamma pathway, and wound healing along with promotion of terminal differentiation. J Biol Chem. 2007;282(6):4021–34.
40. Rhen T, Cidlowski JA. Anti-inflammatory action of glucocorticoids – new mechanisms for old drugs. N Engl J Med. 2005;353(16):1711–23.

(continued from previous page)
through enhanced gene transcription. J Invest Dermatol. 2009;129(4):994–1001.

41. Maas-Szabowski N, Shimotoyodome A, Fusenig NE. Keratinocyte growth regulation in fibroblast cocultures via a double paracrine mechanism. J Cell Sci. 1999;112(Pt 12):1843–53.
42. Kupper TS, Groves RW. The interleukin-1 axis in cutaneous inflammation. J Invest Dermatol. 1995;105:62S–6.
43. Bauge C, Legendre F, Leclercq S, Elissalde JM, Pujol JP, Galera P, et al. Interleukin-1 beta impairment of transforming growth factor beta1 signaling by down-regulation of transforming growth factor beta receptor type II and upregulation of Smad7 in human articular chondrocytes. Arthritis Rheum. 2007;56:3020–32.
44. Quan T, Qin Z, Robichaud P, Voorhees JJ, Fisher GJ. CCN1 contributes to skin connective tissue aging by inducing age-associated secretory phenotype in human skin dermal fibroblasts. J Cell Commun Signal. 2011;5(3):201–7.
45. Cohen MC, Cohen S. Cytokine function: a study in biologic diversity. Am J Clin Pathol. 1996;105:589–98.
46. Rose-John S. IL-6 Trans-Signaling via the Soluble IL-6 Receptor: importance for the pro-inflammatory activities of IL-6. Int J Biol Sci. 2012;8(9):1237–47.
47. Aragane Y, Yamada H, Schwarz A, Poppelmann B, Luger TA, Tezuka T, et al. Transforming growth factor-alpha induces interleukin-6 in the human keratinocyte cell line HaCaT mainly by transcription activation. J Invest Dermatol. 1996;106(6):1192–7.
48. Grossman RM, Krueger J, Yourish D, Granelli-Piperno A, Murphy DP, May LT, et al. Interleukin 6 is expressed in high levels in psoriatic skin and stimulates proliferation of cultured human keratinocytes. Proc Natl Acad Sci U S A. 1989;86(16):6367–7631.
49. Turksen K, Kupper T, Degenstein L, Williams I, Fuchs E. Interleukin 6: insights to its function in skin by overexpression in transgenic mice. Proc Natl Acad Sci U S A. 1992;89(11):5068–72.
50. Maas-Szabowski N, Fusenig NE. Interleukin-1 induced growth factor expression in postmitotic and resting fibroblasts. J Invest Dermatol. 1996;107:849–55.
51. Omoigui S. The Interleukin-6 inflammation pathway from cholesterol to aging – Role of statins, bisphosphonates and plant polyphenols in aging and age-related diseases. Immun Ageing. 2007;4:1.
52. Maggio M, Guralnik JM, Longo DL, Ferrucci L. Interleukin-6 in aging and chronic disease: a magnificent pathway. J Gerontol A Biol Sci Med Sci. 2006;61:575–84.
53. Peterson CA, Heffernan ME. Serum tumor necrosis factor-alpha concentrations are negatively correlated with serum 25(OH)D concentrations in healthy women. J Inflamm. 2008;5:10.
54. Gannage-Yared MH, Azoury M, Mansour I, Baddoura R, Halaby G, Naaman R. Effects of a short-term calcium and vitamin D treatment on serum cytokines, bone markers, insulin and lipid concentrations in healthy post-menopausal women. J Endocrinol Invest. 2003;26:748–53.
55. Evans KN, Nguyen L, Chan J, Innes BA, Bulmer JN, Kilby MD, et al. Effects of 25-hydroxyvitamin D3 and 1,25-dihydroxyvitamin D3 on cytokine production by human decidual cells. Biol Reprod. 2006;75:816–22.
56. Turk S, Akbulut M, Yildiz A, Gurbilek M, Gonen S, Tombul Z, Yeksan M. Comparative effect of oral pulse and intravenous calcitriol treatment in hemodialysis patients: the effect on serum IL-1 and IL-6 levels and bone mineral density. Nephron. 2002;90:188–94.
57. Greenfield EM, Shaw SM, Gornik SA, Banks MA. Adenyl cyclise and interleukin-6 are downstream effectors of parathyroid hormone resulting in stimulation of bone resorption. J Clin Invest. 1995;96:1238–44.
58. Gannagé-Yared MH, Azoury M, Mansour I, Baddoura R, Halaby G, Naaman R. Effects of a short-term calcium and vitamin D treatment on serum cytokines, bone markers, insulin and lipid concentrations in healthy post-menopausal women. J Endocrinol Invest. 2003;26(8):748–53.
59. Tonet AC, Nóbrega OT. Immunosenescence: the association between leukocytes, cytokines and chronic diseases. Rev Bras Geriatr Gerontol. 2008;11(2):259–73.
60. Yoshimura T, Matsushima K, Tanaka S, Robinson EA, Appella E, Oppenheim JJ, et al. Purification of a human monocyte-derived neutrophil chemotactic factor that shows sequence homology with other host defence cytokines. Proc Natl Head Sci U S A. 1987;84:9233–9.
61. Tani A, Yasui T, Matsui S, Kato T, Kunimi K, Tsuchiya N, et al. Different circulating levels of monocyte chemoattractant protein-1 and interleukin-8 during the menopausal transition. Cytokine. 2013;62(1):86–90.
62. Kristensen MS, Paludan K, Larsen CG, Zachariae OC, Deleuran BW, Jensen PKA, et al. Quantitative determination of IL-1a-induced IL-8 mRNA levels in cultured human keratinocytes, dermal fibroblasts, endothelial cells and monocytes. J Invest Dermatol. 1991;97:506–10.
63. Leonard EJ, Yoshimura T, Tanaka S, Raffeld M. Neutrophil recruitment by intradermally injected neutrophil attractant/activation protein-1. J Invest Dermatol. 1991;96(5):690–4.
64. Schroder JM, Christofer E. Identification of C5a des arg and an anionic neutrophil-activating peptide (ANAP) in psoriatic scales. J Invest Dermatol. 1986;87:53–8.
65. Wismer JM, McKenzie RC, Sauder DN. Interleukin-8 immunoreactivity in epidermis of cutaneous T-cell lymphoma patients. Lymphokine Cytokine Res. 1994;13:21–7.
66. Bortesi L, Rossato M, Schuster F, Raven N, Stadlmann J, Avesani L, et al. Viral and murine interleukin-10 are correctly processed and retain

their biological activity when produced in tobacco. BMC Biotechnol. 2009;9:22.
67. MacNeil IA, Suda T, Moore KW, Momann TR, Zlotnik A. IL-10, a novel growth factor for mature and immature T-cells. Immunology. 1990;145: 4167–73.
68. Fiorentino DF, Zlotnik A, Viera P. IL-10 acts on the antigen presenting cell to inhibit cytokine production byTHl cells. J Immunol. 1991;146:3444–51.
69. Taga K, Tosato G. IL-10 inhibits human T-cell proliferation and IL-2 production. J Immunol. 1992;148: 1143–8.
70. Enk CD, Sredni D, Blauvelt A, Katz SI. Induction of IL-10 gene expression in human keratinocytes by UVB exposure in vivo and in vitro. Immunology. 1995;154:4851–6.
71. Cioffi M, Esposito K, Vietri MT, Gazzerro P, D'Auria A, Ardovino I, et al. Cytokine pattern in postmenopause. Maturitas. 2002;41(3):187–92.
72. Schleithoff SS, Zittermann A, Tenderich G, Berthold HK, Stehle P, Koerfer R. Vitamin D supplementation improves cytokine profiles in patients with congestive heart failure: a doubleblind, randomized, placebo-controlled trial. Am J Clin Nutr. 2006;83: 754–9.
73. Neumann D, Martin MU. Interleukin-12 upregulates the IL-18Rb chain in BALB/c thymocytes. J Interferon Cytokine Res. 2001;21:635–42.
74. Nakamura K, Okamura H, Wada M, Nagata K, Tamura T. Endotoxininduced serum factor that stimulates gamma interferon production. Infect Immun. 1989;57:590–5.
75. Kawase Y, Hoshino T, Yokota K, Kuzuhara A, Kirii Y, Nishiwaki E, et al. Exacerbated and prolonged allergic and non-allergic inflammatory cutaneous reaction in mice with targeted interleukin-18 expression in the skin. J Invest Dermatol. 2003;121: 502–9.
76. Schwarz A, Maeda A, Ständer S, van Steeg H, Schwarz T. IL-18 reduces ultraviolet radiation-induced DNA damage and thereby affects photoimmunosuppression. J Immunol. 2006;176(5):2896–901.
77. Li S, Goorha S, Ballou LR, Blatteis CM. Intracerebroventricular interleukin-6, macrophage inflammatory protein-1 beta and IL-18: pyrogenic and PGE(2)-mediated? Brain Res. 2003;992:76–84.
78. Lee JK, Kim SH, Lewis EC, Azam T, Reznikov LL, Dinarello CA. Differences in signalling pathways by IL-1beta and IL-18. Proc Natl Acad Sci U S A. 2004; 101:8815–20.
79. Pestka S. Identification of functional type I and type II interferon receptors. Hokkaido Igaky Zasshi. 1994;69(6):1301–19.
80. Liu YJ. IPC: professional type 1 interferon-producing cells and plasmacytoid dendritic cell precursors. Annu Rev Immunol. 2005;23:275–306.
81. Uzé G, Monneron D. IL-28 and IL-29: newcomers to the interferon family. Biochimie. 2007;89(6–7): 729–34.
82. Pammer J, Reinisch C, Birner P, Pogoda K, Sturzl M, Tschachler E. Interferon-alpha prevents apoptosis of endothelial cells after short-term exposure but induces replicative senescence after continuous stimulation. Lab Invest. 2006;86:997–1007.
83. Ghersetich I, Lotti T. Alpha-interferon cream restores decreased levels of Langerhans/indeterminate (CD1a+) cells in aged and PUVA-treated skin. Skin Pharmacol. 1994;7:118–20.
84. Moiseeva O, Mallette FA, Mukhopadhyay UK, Moores A, Ferbeyre G. DNA damage signaling and p53-dependent senescence after prolonged beta-interferon stimulation. Mol Biol Cell. 2006;17(4): 1583–92.
85. Brincat M, Studd J. Skin and the menopause. In: Studd J, Whitehead MI, editors. The menopause. London: Blackwell Scientific Publications; 1988. p. 85–101.
86. Neuber K, Schmidt S, Mensch A. Telomere length measurement and determination of immunosenescence-related markers (CD28, CD45RO, CD45RA, interferon-γ and interleukin-4) in skin-homing T cells expressing the cutaneous lymphocyte antigen: indication of a non-ageing T-cell subset. Immunology. 2003;109:24–31.
87. Priyanka HP, Sharma U, Gopinath S, Sharma V, Hima L, Thyaga Rajan S. Menstrual cycle and reproductive aging alters immune reactivity, NGF expression, antioxidant enzyme activities, and intracellular signaling pathways in the peripheral blood mononuclear cells of healthy women. Brain Behav Immun. 2013;32:131–43.
88. Larbi A, Franceschi C, Mazzatti D, Solana R, Wikby A, Pawelec G. Aging of the immune system as a prognostic factor for human longevity. Physiology. 2008;23:64–74.
89. Hurgin V, Novick D, Rubinstein M. The promoter of IL-18 binding protein: activation by an IFN-gamma-induced complex of IFN regulatory factor 1 and CCAAT/enhancer binding protein beta. Proc Natl Acad Sci U S A. 2002;99:16957–62.
90. Nickoloff BJ, Basham TY, Merigorn TC. Antiproliferative effects of recombinant alpha and gamma interferons on cultured human keratinocytes. Lab Invest. 1984;51:697–73.
91. Chen CC, Lau LF. Functions and mechanisms of action of CCN matricellular proteins. Int J Biochem Cell Biol. 2009;41:771–83.
92. Bai T, Chen C, Lau LF. Matricellular protein CCN1 activates a proinflammatory genetic program in murine macrophages. J Immunol. 2010;184:3223–32.
93. Quan T, He T, Shao Y, Lin L, Kang S, Voorhees JJ, et al. Elevated cysteine-rich 61 mediates aberrant collagen homeostasis in chronologically aged and photoaged human skin. Am J Pathol. 2006;169: 482–90.
94. Jun JI, Lau LF. The matricellular protein CCN1 induces fibroblast senescence and restricts fibrosis in cutaneous wound healing. Nat Cell Biol. 2010;12: 676–85.

95. Son ED, Lee JY, Lee S, Kim MS, Lee BG, Chang IS, et al. Topical application of 17beta-estradiol increases extracellular matrix protein synthesis by stimulating tgf-Beta signalling in aged human skin in vivo. J Invest Dermatol. 2005;124(6):1149–61.
96. Katz H, Prystowsky J. Menopause and the skin. In: Lobo RA, Kelsey J, Marcus R, editors. Menopause: biology and pathobiology. Amsterdam: Elsevier B.V; 2007. p. 243–4.
97. Massague J. TGF-beta signal transduction. Annu Rev Biochem. 1998;67:753–91.
98. Hocevar BA, Brown TL, Howe PH. TGF-beta induces fibronectin synthesis through a c-Jun N-terminal kinase-dependent, Smad4-independent pathway. EMBO J. 1999;18(5):1345–56.
99. Hall MC, Young DA, Waters JG, Rowan AD, Chantry A, Edwards DR, et al. The comparative role of activator protein 1 and Smad factors in the regulation of Timp-1 and MMP-1 gene expression by transforming growth factor-beta 1. J Biol Chem. 2003;278:10304–13.
100. Oursler MJ, Cortese C, Keeting P, Anderson MA, Bonde SK, Riggs BL, et al. Modulation of transforming growth factor-beta production in normal human osteoblast-like cells by 17 beta-estradiol and parathyroid hormone. Endocrinology. 1991;129: 3313–20.
101. Ashcroft GS, Dodsworth J, van Boxtel E, Tarnuzzer RW, Horan MA, Schultz GS, et al. Estrogen accelerates cutaneous wound healing associated with an increase in TGF-beta1 levels. Nat Med. 1997;3: 1209–15.
102. Braverman IM, Fonferko E. Studies in cutaneous aging: I. The elastic fiber network. J Invest Dermatol. 1982;78:434–43.
103. Massague J. How cells read TGF-beta signals. Nat Rev Mol Cell Biol. 2000;1:169–78.
104. Verdier-Sevrain S, Yaar M, Cantatore J, Traish A, Gilchrest BA. Estradiol induces proliferation of keratinocytes via a receptor mediated mechanism. FASEB J. 2004;18(11):1252–4.
105. Chauhan P, Shakya M. Modeling signaling pathways leading to wrinkle formation: identification of the skin aging target. Indian J Dermatol Venereol Leprol. 2009;75:463–8.
106. Youn CS, Kwon OS, Won CH, Hwang EJ, Park BJ, Eun HC, et al. Effect of pregnancy and menopause on facial wrinkling in women. Acta Derm Venereol. 2003;83:419–24.
107. Brincat M, Kabalan S, Studd JW, Moniz CF, de Trafford J, Montgomery J. A study of the decrease of skin collagen content, skin thickness, and bone mass in the postmenopausal woman. Obstet Gynecol. 1987;70:840–5.
108. Chung JH, Lee SH, Youn CS, Park BJ, Kim KH, Park KC. Cutaneous photodamage in Koreans: influence of sex, sun exposure, smoking, and skin color. Arch Dermatol. 2001;137:1043–51.
109. Ernster VL, Grady D, Miike R, Black D, Selby J, Kerlikowske K. Facial wrinkling in men and women by smoking status. Am J Public Health. 1995;85: 78–82.
110. Brincat M, Moniz CF, Kabalan S, Versi E, O'Dowd T, Magos AL, et al. Decline in skin collagen content and metacarpal index after the menopause and its prevention with sex hormone replacement. Br J Obstet Gynaecol. 1987;94:126–9.
111. Holland EF, Studd JW, Mansell JP, Leather AT, Bailey AJ. Changes in collagen composition and cross-links in bone and skin of osteoporotic postmenopausal women treated with percutaneous estradiol implants. Obstet Gynecol. 1994;83:180–3.
112. Vogel H. Age dependence of mechanical properties of human skin. Part II: hysteresis, relaxation, creep, and repeated strain experiments. Bioeng Skin. 1987;3:141–76.
113. Fisher GJ, Kang S, Varani J, Bata-Csorgo Z, Wan Y, Datta S, et al. Mechanism of photoageing and chronological skin ageing. Arch Dermatol. 2002;138: 1462–70.
114. Calleja-Agius J, Muscat-Baron Y, Brincat MP. Skin ageing. Menopause Int. 2007;13(2):60–4.
115. Mirmirani P. Hormonal changes in menopause: do they contribute to a 'midlife hair crisis' in women? Br J Dermatol. 2011;165 Suppl 3:7–11.
116. Hoffmann R, Niiyama S, Huth A, Kissling S, Happle R. 17alphaestradiol induces aromatase activity in intact human anagen hair follicles ex vivo. Exp Dermatol. 2002;11:376–80.
117. Thornton MJ, Taylor AH, Mulligan K, Al-Azzawi F, Lyon CC, O'Driscoll J, et al. Estrogen receptor beta is the predominant estrogen receptor in human scalp skin. Exp Dermatol. 2003;12:181–90.
118. Conrad F, Ohnemus U, Bodo E, Biro T, Tychsen B, Gerstmayer B, et al. Substantial sex-dependent differences in the response of human scalp hair follicles to estrogen stimulation in vitro advocate gender-tailored management of female versus male pattern balding. J Investig Dermatol Symp Proc. 2005;10: 243–6.
119. Hardman MJ, Ashcroft GS. Estrogen, not intrinsic aging, is the major regulator of delayed human wound healing in the elderly. Genome Biol. 2008; 9(5):R80.
120. Emmerson E, Hardman MJ. The role of estrogen deficiency in skin ageing and wound healing. Biogerontology. 2012;13(1):3–20.
121. Ashcroft GS, Horan MA, Herrick SE, Tarnuzzer RW, Schultz GS, Ferguson MW. Age-related differences in the temporal and spatial regulation of matrix metalloproteinases (mmps) in normal skin and acute cutaneous wounds of healthy humans. Cell Tissue Res. 1997;290(3):581–91.
122. Ashcroft GS, Kielty CM, Horan MA, Ferguson MW. Age-related changes in the temporal and spatial distributions of fibrillin and elastin mRNAs and proteins in acute cutaneous wounds of healthy humans. J Pathol. 1997;183(1):80–9.
123. Herrick S, Ashcroft G, Ireland G, Horan M, McCollum C, Ferguson M. Up-regulation of elastase

in acute wounds of healthy aged humans and chronic venous leg ulcers are associated with matrix degradation. Lab Invest. 1997;77(3):281–8.
124. Ashcroft GS, Herrick SE, Tarnuzzer RW, Horan MA, Schultz GS, Ferguson MW. Human ageing impairs injury induced in vivo expression of tissue inhibitor of matrix metalloproteinases (timp)-1 and -2 proteins and mrna. J Pathol. 1997;183(2):169–76.
125. Ashcroft GS, Horan MA, Ferguson MW. Aging alters the inflammatory and endothelial cell adhesion molecule profiles during human cutaneous wound healing. Lab Invest. 1998;78(1):47–58.
126. Ashcroft GS, Horan MA, Ferguson MW. Aging is associated with reduced deposition of specific extracellular matrix components, an upregulation of angiogenesis, and an altered inflammatory response in a murine incisional wound healing model. J Invest Dermatol. 1997;108(4):430–7.
127. Stanulis-Praeger BM, Gilchrest BA. Growth factor responsiveness declines during adulthood for human skin derived cells. Mech Ageing Dev. 1986;35(2):185–98.
128. Lenhardt R, Hopf HW, Marker E, Akca O, Kurz A, Scheuenstuhl H, et al. Perioperative collagen deposition in elderly and young men and women. Arch Surg. 2000;135(1):71–4.
129. Lindstedt E, Sandblom P. Wound healing in man: tensile strength of healing wounds in some patient groups. Ann Surg. 1975;181(6):842–6.
130. Gilchrest BA, Szabo G, Flynn E, Goldwyn RM. Chronologic and actinically induced aging in human facial skin. J Invest Dermatol. 1983;80(Suppl):81s–5s.
131. Ashcroft GS, Greenwell-Wild T, Horan MA, Wahl SM, Ferguson MW. Topical estrogen accelerates cutaneous wound healing in aged humans associated with an altered inflammatory response. Am J Pathol. 1999;155(4):1137–46.
132. Berard A, Kahn SR, Abenhaim L. Is hormone replacement therapy protective for venous ulcer of the lower limbs? Pharmacoepidemiol Drug Saf. 2001;10(3):245–51.
133. Margolis DJ, Knauss J, Bilker W. Hormone replacement therapy and prevention of pressure ulcers and venous leg ulcers. Lancet. 2002;359(9307):675–7.
134. Hardman MJ, Emmerson E, Campbell L, Ashcroft GS. Selective estrogen receptor modulators accelerate cutaneous wound healing in ovariectomized female mice. Endocrinology. 2008;149(2):551–7.
135. Emmerson E, Campbell L, Ashcroft GS, Hardman MJ. The phytestrogen genistein promotes wound healing by multiple independent mechanisms. Mol Cell Endocrinol. 2010;321(2):184–93.
136. Mills SJ, Ashworth JJ, Gilliver SC, Hardman MJ, Ashcroft GS. The sex steroid precursor dhea accelerates cutaneous wound healing via the estrogen receptors. J Invest Dermatol. 2005;125(5):1053–62.
137. Gilliver SC, Ruckshanthi JP, Hardman MJ, Zeef LA, Ashcroft GS. 5alpha- dihydrotestosterone (DHT) retards wound closure by inhibiting re-epithelialization. J Pathol. 2009;217(1):73–82.
138. Gilliver SC, Wu F, Ashcroft GS. Regulatory roles of androgens in cutaneous wound healing. Thromb Haemost. 2003;90(6):978–85.
139. Gilliver SC, Ashworth JJ, Mills SJ, Hardman MJ, Ashcroft GS. Androgens modulate the inflammatory response during acute wound healing. J Cell Sci. 2006;119(Pt 4):722–32.
140. Magnusson U, Einarsson S. Effects of exogenous estradiol on the number and functional capacity of circulating mononuclear and polymorphonuclear leukocytes in the sow. Vet Immunol Immunopathol. 1990;25(3):235–47.
141. Kovacs EJ, Faunce DE, Ramer-Quinn DS, Mott FJ, Dy PW, Frazier-Jessen MR. Estrogen regulation of je/mcp-1 mrna expression in fibroblasts. J Leukoc Biol. 1996;59(4):562–8.
142. Aloisi AM, Pari G, Ceccarelli I, Vecchi I, Ietta F, Lodi L, et al. Gender-related effects of chronic non-malignant pain and opioid therapy on plasma levels of macrophage migration inhibitory factor (mif). Pain. 2005;115(1–2):142–51.
143. Hardman MJ, Waite A, Zeef L, Burow M, Nakayama T, Ashcroft GS. Macrophage migration inhibitory factor: a central regulator of wound healing. Am J Pathol. 2005;167(6):1561–74.
144. Ashcroft GS, Mills SJ, Lei K, Gibbons L, Jeong MJ, Taniguchi M, et al. Estrogen modulates cutaneous wound healing by downregulating macrophage migration inhibitory factor. J Clin Invest. 2003;111(9):1309–18.
145. Emmerson E, Campbell L, Ashcroft GS, Hardman MJ. Unique and synergistic roles for 17beta-estradiol and macrophage migration inhibitory factor during cutaneous wound closure are cell type specific. Endocrinology. 2009;150(6):2749–57.
146. Campbell L, Emmerson E, Davies F, Gilliver SC, Krust A, Chambon P, et al. Estrogen promotes cutaneous wound healing via estrogen receptor beta independent of it's anti-inflammatory activities. J Exp Med. 2010;207(9):1825–33.
147. Battegay EJ, Rupp J, Iruela-Arispe L, Sage EH, Pech M. Pdgf-bb modulates endothelial proliferation and angiogenesis in vitro via pdgf beta-receptors. J Cell Biol. 1994;125(4):917–28.
148. Morales DE, McGowan KA, Grant DS, Maheshwari S, Bhartiya D, Cid MC, et al. Estrogen promotes angiogenic activity in human umbilical vein endothelial cells in vitro and in a murine model. Circulation. 1995;91(3):755–63.
149. Nyman S. Studies on the influence of estradiol and progesterone on granulation tissue. J Periodontal Res. 1971;Suppl 7:1–24.
150. Lundgren D. Influence of estrogen and progesterone on exudation, inflammatory cell migration and granulation tissue formation in preformed cavities. Scand J Plast Reconstr Surg. 1973;7(1):10–4.
151. Brincat MP, Muscat-Baron YM, Galea R. Estrogens and the skin. Climacteric. 2005;8(2):110–23. Review.

152. Li WH, Pappas A, Zhang L, Ruvolo E, Cavender D. IL-11, IL-1α, IL-6, and TNF-α are induced by solar radiation in vitro and may be involved in facial subcutaneous fat loss in vivo. J Dermatol Sci. 2013;71(1):58–66.
153. Sugimoto M, Yamashita R, Ueda M. Telomere length of the skin in association with chronological aging and photoaging. J Dermatol Sci. 2006;43(1):43–7.
154. Baumann L. Skin ageing and its treatment. J Pathol. 2007;211:241–51.
155. Raine-Fenning N, Brincat M, Muscat-Baron Y. Skin aging and menopause implications for treatment. Am J Clin Dermatol. 2003;4(6):371–8.
156. Townsend MJ, McKenzie AN. Unravelling the net? Cytokines and diseases. J Cell Sci. 2000;113 (Pt 20):3549–50.

The Role of Estrogen Deficiency in Skin Aging and Wound Healing

6

Charis R. Saville and Matthew J. Hardman

Contents

6.1	Skin Structure and Function	71
6.2	Skin Aging	72
6.3	Intrinsic Aging	72
6.4	Extrinsic Aging	73
6.5	Mechanisms of Aging	73
6.6	Estrogen Synthesis	74
6.7	Estrogen Receptors	74
6.8	Menopause and Skin Changes	75
6.9	Murine Studies	76
6.10	Aging Delays Wound Healing	77
6.10.1	Inflammation	77
6.10.2	Re-epithelialisation	77
6.10.3	Matrix Deposition	78
6.10.4	Angiogenesis	78
6.11	Estrogen Effects on Wound Healing	78
6.12	Inflammation	79
6.13	Re-epithelialisation	79
6.14	Matrix Deposition and Angiogenesis	79
6.15	ERS and Wound Healing	80
6.16	SERMs and Future Therapies	80
6.17	Summary	80
References		81

C.R. Saville, BSc, PhD • M.J. Hardman, PhD (✉)
The Healing Foundation Centre,
Faculty of Life Sciences, University of Manchester,
Oxford Road, Manchester M13 9PT, UK
e-mail: Charis.Saville@manchester.ac.uk;
matthew.j.hardman@manchester.ac.uk

6.1 Skin Structure and Function

Human skin is a complex, multilayered tissue that forms the largest organ of the body. Its primary function is to provide an essential barrier to the external environment, protecting against mechanical stresses and chemical or pathogenic incursion. Other functions are diverse and include sensory perception, prevention of fluid loss, maintenance of body temperature and biosynthesis [1]. Structurally the skin can be divided into three principle layers, an outermost epidermis, underlying dermis and innermost hypodermis [2]. The avascular epidermis is composed mainly of keratinocytes originating from a pool of progenitor cells in the basal layer of the epidermis and the bulge region of the hair follicle [3, 4]. These progenitor cells give rise to daughter cells that transit through the suprabasal layers of the epidermis undergoing a tightly regulated programmed terminal differentiation, regulated at least in part by an epidermal calcium gradient [5]. The ultimate aim of terminal differentiation is the synthesis of components of the outermost epidermal layer, the stratum corneum, which imparts the majority of epidermal barrier function (reviewed in [6]) [7]. These include filaggrin, loricrin, SPRR and LCE proteins, which become cross-linked to form the impermeable cornified envelope, and lipid bodies, which are extruded to form the stratum corneum lipid lamellae. Non-keratinocyte epidermal cell types include melanocytes, which synthesise melanin for UV protection; Langerhans cells, which are responsible for antigen presentation and protection from pathogens; and Merkel cells, which complex with nerve fibres acting as touch receptors [8, 9].

The underlying dermis is connected to the epidermis by a basement membrane termed the dermal epidermal junction (DEJ). This region has a complex structure of anchoring proteins including collagen VII, laminins and fibrillin-1 [10, 11]. The dermis is highly vascularised and relatively acellular, instead composed of a structurally diverse extracellular matrix (ECM) comprised of fibrillar collagens, elastic fibres and proteoglycans. These ECM proteins are responsible for much of the strength and structure of the skin providing a physical scaffold. The fibrillar collagens are mechanically very strong, resisting tensile forces. This tensile strength is complemented by the elastic fibres, which only comprise around 2 % of the dermal ECM but confer passive recoil in this dynamic tissue [12]. The elastic fibres are complex macromolecules comprising an elastin-rich core surrounded by fibrillin-rich microfibrils [13]. In the human skin they assemble into a characteristic arrangement with thick elastin-rich fibres running parallel in the deeper dermis and branching into perpendicular fibrillin-rich fibres towards the DEJ [14]. The dermis also contains a diverse range of proteoglycans, which primarily maintain skin hydration and resist compressive forces via hydrophilic GAG chains [15].

6.2 Skin Aging

A combination of intrinsic and extrinsic factors contributes to altered homeostasis in aged skin resulting in dramatic changes that manifest as wrinkling, sagging, fragility, atrophy and increased laxity. These changes have a significant impact on skin structure (Fig. 6.1) and function, rendering skin both more susceptible to injury and less able to repair once injured. Indeed, advanced age is a primary risk factor for developing chronic, non-healing skin wounds.

6.3 Intrinsic Aging

Intrinsic aging, mainly genetically programmed, presents clinically as uniform pigmentation, loss of elasticity and reduced appendage density (hair follicles, sweat and sebaceous glands; [16]). Intrinsically aged skin is characterised by fine wrinkles, a flattened DEJ and a thinning of both the dermis and epidermis. Intrinsic aging is reported to result in an overall loss of around 1 % of total collagen per adult year [17], while elastic fibres are gradually lost from the papillary dermis

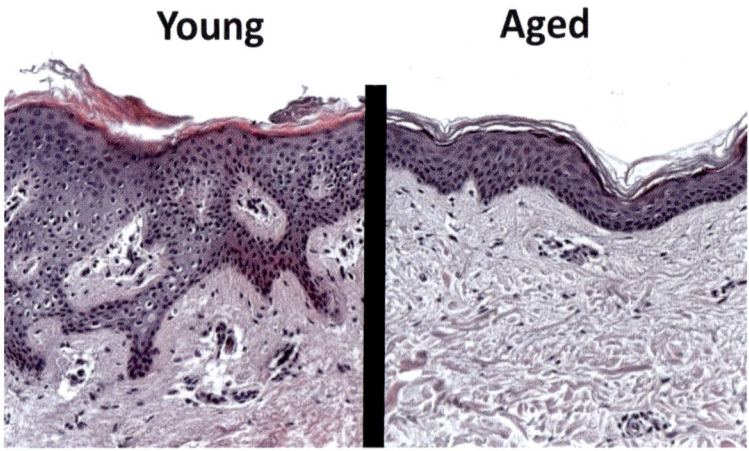

Fig. 6.1 Human skin is structurally altered with age. *Left* inner arm skin from a young subject with abundant rete ridges. *Right* inner arm skin from an aged subject lacks rete ridges with a thinner epidermis. In addition, dermal cellularity is reduced with less dermal extracellular matrix

[18]. Reduction in total proteoglycans, which have important roles in binding water, leads to the increasingly dry skin associated with age [19, 20]. Dermal fibroblasts are reduced in number [17, 21] and functionally altered producing more matrix metalloproteinases (MMPs) and less extracellular matrix proteins [21, 22]. Mast cells are generally reported to be reduced in aged tissue [17]. However, Gunin et al. 2011 [23] report increased mast cells in aged skin which they suggest to be an important driver of tissue damage in aging. Mechanically the skin becomes stiffer and more fragile with a loss of resilience [24] making aged skin more susceptible to damage. Intriguingly, skin components are not equally affected by skin aging. Hair follicles, for example, age relatively slowly and continue to function even at advanced age [25].

6.4 Extrinsic Aging

While all tissues undergo intrinsic aging, the skin is also uniquely subject to extrinsic aging resulting from extensive exposure to environmental factors. The effects of extrinsic aging are particularly evident on the face, chest, hands and arms, which are subject to a high degree of UV exposure over a lifetime. Extrinsically aged skin is characterised by deeper wrinkles, a leathery appearance, irregular pigmentation and extensive loss of elasticity [26, 27]. At the cellular level the effects of extrinsic aging are extensive. Confusingly the epidermis of extrinsically aged skin is reported to be thickened due to hyperplasia or thinned as a result of tissue atrophy dependent on the level and duration of UV damage [28]. However, it is the changes in the dermal components of photo-aged skin which have the most profound impact on appearance. Fibrillar collagens (type I and III) are dramatically reduced and become more fragmented [29, 30], directly leading to reduced tissue tensile strength. Collagen VII anchoring fibrils are specifically lost from the DEJ along with both fibrillin 1 and fibulin 5 [31]. Severe photo-aging causes extensive profound remodelling of the elastic fibres. In young skin elastic fibres are highly ordered in structure; thick elastin-rich fibres in the deeper dermis that run parallel to the DEJ branch into perpendicular fibrillin-rich fibres in the papillary dermis. In severely photo-damaged skin, this structure is lost completely, and elastic fibre production is pathologically increased, resulting in abundant randomly orientated elastic material [31]. In contrast to intrinsically aged skin, proteoglycans are also increased and abnormally distributed as a result of extrinsic aging co-localising with the elastic fibre material [32].

6.5 Mechanisms of Aging

With the exception of severe photo damage, aged skin is characterised by a cumulative loss of components and function. Numerous theories have been proposed to drive aging (reviewed in [33]). These range from the idea that aging is due to wear and tear and an accumulation of damage with the passage of time to more specific concepts of preprogrammed life span defined by specific age-related genes. Of direct relevance to the role of hormones in the skin is the endocrine theory of aging, which places the HPA (hypothalamic pituitary axis) as a "master regulator", signalling the termination and onset of life stages. In reality it is probably a complex accumulation of multiple different factors (i.e. aspects of each theory) that defines skin aging and in turn drives age-associated pathologies.

Aged cells are both slower to divide and compromised in their repair mechanisms. Aged fibroblasts in culture, for example display a threefold reduction in population doubling time [34], with older cells reported to have an increased G0/G1 phase proportion due to repression of cell cycle progression genes [35]. Accumulation of DNA damage is particularly detrimental to the numerous stem cell populations that reside in the skin. Accumulated damage severely impairs the function of aged stem cells ultimately leading to loss of tissue homeostasis [36]. In aged dermis, fibroblasts are reduced in both number and capacity to synthesise ECM proteins [17] contributing to age-associated atrophy. MMP overexpression is accompanied by reduced expression of the TIMP family of MMP inhibitors [37, 38].

One of the key contributors to the aging phenotype is the generation of reactive oxygen species (ROS). These highly reactive molecules cause damage to DNA, proteins and lipids via breaks, cross-links and degradation. Intriguingly, active ROS generation is emerging as an essential early signal in wound repair [39]. Mechanistically, ROS acts via AP-1 to upregulate MMP transcription and also directly activates MMPs [40–42], ultimately contributing to overall degradation of the ECM. Once activated these degradative mechanisms are maintained by a positive-feedback loop whereby MMPs are upregulated by fragmented ECM components [43].

Another central contributor to organismal aging is cellular senescence. First observed in 1961, Hayflick and Moorhead [44] reported the phenomenon of replicative growth arrest in cultured human fibroblasts. Subsequent studies revealed that the number of cell divisions at which this limit was reached is inversely proportional to the age of the donor [45], now known to be a consequence of progressive telomere shortening [46]. Telomeres form a cap of repeated DNA sequence at the ends of chromosomes; during cell division these become progressively shorter until cells can no longer divide. Senescent cells, which were originally thought quiescent, have more recently emerged as an active driver of tissue aging, secreting a number of proteases and cytokines, termed senescence-associated phenotype (SASP), which damage surrounding tissue [47]. In addition to the overexpression of proteases [37], there is also a reduction in the expression of TIMPs [38] to inhibit the actions of MMPs.

6.6 Estrogen Synthesis

All estrogens are derived from the precursor cholesterol via multiple biosynthetic steps. While the majority of circulating estrogens are gonadally derived, estrogens can also be synthesised peripherally in nonreproductive tissues such as the liver, heart, bone and skin. Specifically, the skin contains all the components required for local estrogen synthesis, including 17β-hydroxysteroid dehydrogenase (17β-HSD), 3β-hydroxysteroid dehydrogenase (3β-HSD), aromatase and 5α-reductase [48–51]. Indeed, peripheral synthesis is thought to provide the majority of estrogens post menopause, functioning as paracrine and/or intracrine factors to maintain important tissue-specific functions [52, 53]. Prior to menopause 17β-estradiol (E_2) is the main gonadally derived circulating hormone. Following menopause estrone (E) plays an important role, with high levels reportedly synthesised in adipose tissue from the adrenally derived precursor DHEA [54, 55]. Estrogen can also be locally regulated by interconversion between E, E2 and E3 forms or by estrogen-sulfotransferase-mediated conversion to inactive forms [56]. Thus, at any one time the local levels of active estrogens depend on finely balanced biosynthetic, metabolic and deactivation pathways. It remains unclear exactly how menopause influences peripheral estrogen synthesis. Our data from both murine models and humans suggest that estrogen deficiency leads to widespread downregulation of peripheral hormone synthetic enzymes [57, 58]. The one exception is the enzyme aromatase, which is increased in subcutaneous adipose tissue with advancing age [59].

Aromatase, a key player in peripheral hormone synthesis, is widely expressed across many tissues [60]. Its regulation is particularly complex, with the human aromatase gene containing ten validated tissue-specific promoters [61]. In the skin, as in the bone, aromatase expression is driven by the glucocorticoid responsive distal promoter I.4 [61]. It is likely that skin injury and/or disease will alter aromatase promoter usage, as is the case in breast cancer where promoter usage switches to the cAMP responsive promoter [62]. Aromatase activity can also be regulated at the level of posttranslational modification, most notably phosphorylation [63]. Skin-derived fibroblasts and adipocytes display high aromatase activity [64, 65] as do human osteoblasts [66].

6.7 Estrogen Receptors

Estrogen signals via two distinct nuclear hormone receptors, estrogen receptor alpha (ERα) and estrogen receptor beta (ERβ) encoded by separate genes (ESR1 and ESR2), located on different chromosomes. ER expression is widespread throughout the body; in some organs both receptors are expressed at similar levels, whereas in others one receptor is more highly expressed. For example, a large body of literature documents a predominance of ERα in reproductive tissues [67]. In the skin both receptors are widely expressed; however, distribution varies depending on cell type and source. Both receptors are reported in human dermal fibroblasts [68] and sebaceous glands [69]. ERβ appears to be the dominant receptor in human eccrine and apocrine glands [70] and hair follicles, being expressed in dermal papilla cells, the outer root sheath and the bulge [69]. Keratinocyte expression is more contentious. Both receptors have been reported in neonatal foreskin-derived keratinocytes with estradiol specifically upregulating ERα [71]; however, ERβ was reportedly highly expressed in human scalp skin with no ERα expression [72]. More recently still Inoue et al. [73] report significantly reduced ERβ expression in the skin of subjects over 70. By contrast, both receptors have been reported in the upper inner arm epidermis of both young and old female subjects [74]. The receptors function as homo- or heterodimers, and in this context ERβ's function in heterodimers has been suggested to dampen ERα-mediated gene expression [75, 76]. In addition, insulinlike growth factor-1 (IGF-1) has been shown to signal through ERs in various tissues [77].

6.8 Menopause and Skin Changes

Post menopause, there is a rapid decline in the macroscopic and histological appearance of the skin with an increase in wrinkling, sagging and dryness [78, 79] (Fig. 6.2). The use of hormone replacement therapy (HRT) can prevent many of these changes, increasing extracellular matrix components, skin hydration and elasticity and reducing wrinkles [80–82]. One area that remains contentious in skin biology, as in other tissues, is the extent to which estrogen replacement can

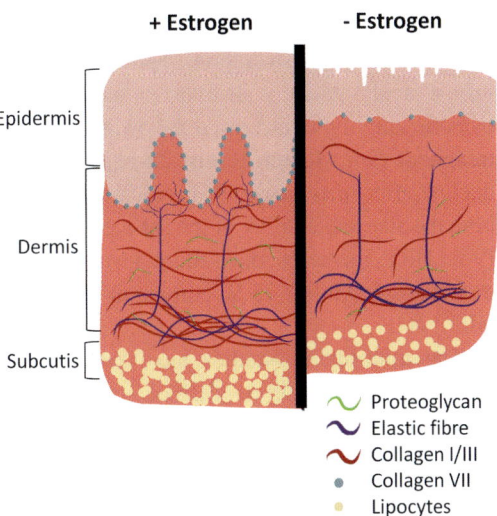

Fig. 6.2 Estrogen deficiency accelerates skin aging. *Right* postmenopausal estrogen deficiency leads to profound structural changes in the skin, including epidermal atrophy and wrinkling, reduced dermal elastic fibres and collagen. Collectively these changes lead to altered skin function and increased susceptibility to damage

reverse detrimental changes that have already occurred and whether estrogen is beneficial in skin that is decades post menopause rather than in the perimenopause period.

Extensive clinical studies over recent decades have assessed the beneficial effects of HRT post menopause. The epidermis is considerably thinner post menopause [83], while HRT orally administered for 3 months or 6 months increases epidermal thickness [81, 84, 85]. Mechanistically, estrogen has been shown to directly influence keratinocyte proliferation over a far shorter period [86] and to prevent H_2O_2-induced apoptosis at least in vitro [87]. A large study of nearly 4,000 women found postmenopausal skin to be significantly dryer, with estrogen use functionally reversing this [78, 88]. Here HRT has been shown to significantly increase the ability of the stratum corneum to hold water [89]. More specifically, epidermal sphingolipids have been shown to be altered only in aged female skin [90], an effect that can be reversed by HRT [91, 92]. Postmenopausal changes in skin hydration are, in part, also due to changes in the dermal polysaccharides and changes in sebum levels. Here Danforth et al. [93] demonstrate that the high estrogen levels in pregnancy are linked to increased dermal hydration. Moreover, hyaluronic acid, which is known to have a high osmotic activity, is increased following estrogen treatment [94]. Sebum levels are also found to decline after menopause [95] with a decrease in both the size and activity of the sebaceous glands [96]. HRT increases the sebum level of postmenopausal skin by 35 % compared to without HRT [91].

The majority of studies have assessed the effect of menopause on dermal structure and function. The dermal extracellular matrix provides skin with many of its mechanical properties, such as resilience and tensile strength. Type I collagen is the major component of adult dermis providing tensile strength. Loss of collagen is one of the major changes implicated in the development of skin wrinkles [78, 97, 98]. Following menopause, dermal collagen content has been reported to fall by 2–5 % per year [80, 99, 100], leading to reduced dermal thickness and density. This decrease in dermal composition correlated only to postmenopausal years and not to chronological age. Affinito et al. [100] reported a decline in both collagen I and III and a specific change in the ratio of these collagen types. Brincat et al. [80] quantified the rapid loss of collagen in the initial postmenopausal period accompanied by a 1.1 % reduction in dermal thickness per year. The beneficial effects of estrogen on dermal collagen have been reported across a number of studies and trials. Topically applied estrogen increases type I and III collagen expression [101–103]. In a double-blind randomised trial, Maheux et al. [104] reported up to 30 % increase in postmenopausal skin dermal thickness following estrogen treatment. Estrogen appears to act by preferentially inducing new expression of type III collagen in aged skin, presumably invoking a "developmental"-type programme of expression [101, 105].

The skin tensile strength provided by fibrillar collagens is complemented by the elastic fibre network which endows skin with resilience, allowing it to return to a resting state following deformation. Skin resilience also negatively correlates with postmenopausal years. Using a suction device Sumino et al. [106] were able to quantify a 0.55 % decline in skin elasticity per postmenopausal year. The same study also reported a 5.2 % increase in skin forearm elasticity following 12 months of HRT. These observations are in line with previous studies that reported beneficial effects of HR on the extensibility and elasticity of forearm skin [82] and facial skin [107]. These changes in gross mechanical properties following estrogen treatment correlate with specific beneficial changes at the histological level. Punnonen et al. [108] report that topical estrogen treatment modifies the elastic fibre network, increasing elastic fibre number and improving orientation. In addition, estradiol increases cutaneous expression of tropoelastin and fibrillin proteins, key modulators of elastic fibre assembly and function [102]. By contrast, Bolognia et al. [109] report that women entering early menopause show premature degradation of elastic fibres with signs of splitting and fragmentation.

6.9 Murine Studies

Murine models provide an opportunity to mechanistically address hormonal aspects of skin aging. The ovariectomised (OVX) mouse is widely used as a model of the human menopausal state; surgical removal of the ovaries leads to a rapid decline in circulating sex steroid hormones that mimics the menopause. OVX mice are widely used to model a range of human age-associated pathologies, including osteoporosis, neurodegeneration and cardiac dysfunction, as well as perimenopausal symptoms, such as depression and hot flushes [110–112]. It is therefore surprising that comparatively little skin research has been carried out with this model. OVX is known to enhance the sensitivity of rat skin to UV-induced photo-aging, measured as wrinkling, a loss of elasticity and damage to elastic fibres [113]. This is supported by a mouse study where effects on skin extensibility and elastic recoil were measured. Here ovariectomy significantly increased recoil time in

UV-exposed skin associated with elevated tissue elastase activity [114]. Very recently Fang et al. [115] have combined cryo-sectioning with AFM to reveal nanoscale changes in morphology of dermal collagen fibrils in ovine OVX samples. Other studies have explored the role of estrogen in protecting from ROS [116] and cellular senescence [117]. There are suggestions from the literature that estrogen may act as a direct antioxidant as well as induce antioxidant enzymes. Direct functional evidence was provided by Baeza et al. [118] who showed that OVX rats had increased levels of oxidised glutathione, lipid peroxidation and mitochondrial DNA damage all of which could be reversed by estrogen replacement. More recently Bottai et al. [119] report that 17β-estradiol protects both human skin fibroblasts and keratinocytes against oxidative damage.

The second major advantage of mice is their genetic tractability, crucial in the context of unravelling estrogen signalling. Mice have been generated lacking one or both of the ERs [120–125], or aromatase (ArKO), which disrupts estrogen biosynthesis [126], or more complex Cre/LoxP conditional ER nulls [121, 127, 128] and point mutants [129–131]. Phenotypic analysis of these mice had provided, and continues to provide, insight into ER-mediated physiological roles across a range of tissues (reviewed in [132]). Relevant here ER null mice display a number of skin phenotypes. First to be reported were effects on hair follicles. Moverare et al. [133] identified a role for ERα, but not ERβ, in regulating hair cycling. In a subsequent study Ohnemus et al. [134] demonstrated that ERβ does play a role, regulating catagen induction. In the same studies ERα was suggested to be important for estrogen's effects on epidermal thickness. Markiewicz et al. [135] have recently reported increased skin collagen content in ERα null mice with decreased collagen content in ERβ nulls. Meanwhile Cho et al. [136] report a key role for ERβ in mediating UV-induced photoimmune modulation. Clearly ERs play an important role in skin homeostasis, often with directly opposite effects, supporting "ying-yang" ER interactions [75, 76].

6.10 Aging Delays Wound Healing

Under normal circumstances the skin has evolved a highly coordinated response to injury, whereby numerous cell types are sequentially activated to orchestrate rapid tissue repair (reviewed in [137]). However, with increasing age the skin not only becomes more fragile and susceptible to damage but also less able to effectively heal following injury. Indeed, numerous studies have revealed significant cellular changes in age-associated delayed healing: altered haemostasis [138, 139], reduced re-epithelialisation [140, 141], an excessive inflammatory response [142, 143] and upregulated protease activity associated with reduced matrix deposition [144]. Collectively, these age-associated changes lead to delayed acute wound healing in the elderly that predisposes to the development of chronic wounds [145]. Moreover, Wicke et al. [146] report a clinically measurable delay in chronic wound closure in those over 60 years of age versus younger patients.

6.10.1 Inflammation

The inflammatory response is delayed in elderly humans, and the overall number of inflammatory cells recruited to sites of injury is increased [142, 144, 147]. Despite these higher numbers aged macrophages are less active, with altered expression and function of TLRs [148], decreased cytokine and growth factor production [149] and reduced phagocytic activity compared to macrophages from younger counterparts [150]. Functional significance has been demonstrated in adoptive transfer experiments where macrophages from young mice are able to promote healing in aged mice [151]. Aged neutrophils are also functionally altered with reduced chemotaxis and phagocytosis [152].

6.10.2 Re-epithelialisation

Multiple studies have reported delayed re-epithelisation in aged mice and humans [140,

144, 147]. This observed delay is likely multifactorial. Key cytokines and growth factors required to stimulate keratinocyte migration and proliferation, such as PDGF, EGF and KGF, are reduced with age [153, 154]. Keratinocytes from aged donors are also intrinsically altered with reduced hypoxia-induced migration [155]. Additionally, aged keratinocytes fail to induce MMPs and other proteases required to successfully migrate through the wound granulation tissue [155]. Finally, we have recently shown that the wound-induced switch to weak keratinocyte adhesion fails in chronic wounds from aged patients [156].

6.10.3 Matrix Deposition

Fibroblasts are essential for effective repair, depositing and remodelling ECM and mediating wound contraction. Aged fibroblasts display reduced collagen synthesis [157] and impaired migration [158]. The general consensus is that aged fibroblasts are more prone to senescence with decreased proliferation with a reduced ability to respond to growth factors [159–161]. This is supported by studies indicating dysfunction in fibroblasts isolated from chronic wounds [162–164]. Intriguingly, other studies report no change in fibroblast responsiveness with age [165].

6.10.4 Angiogenesis

The literature on age-associated changes in new blood vessel formation following wounding is also conflicting. Ashcroft et al. [144] and Swift et al. [147] report increased and decreased angiogenesis, respectively, in aged mice. While this may in part reflect the different wound models used (incisional versus excisional), subsequent in vitro studies have shown that reduced angiogenic growth factors are responsible for an age-associated reduction in angiogenesis [166]. Specifically FGF2 and VEGF are decreased in the wounds of aged mice [147].

6.11 Estrogen Effects on Wound Healing

Post menopause, there is a rapid decline in wound healing ability. Studies have linked a range of menopause-associated hormones to this altered healing including progesterone [167], DHEA [168] and testosterone/DHT [169, 170]. The majority of research has, however, focussed on estrogen's role in healing (Fig. 6.3). Studies by Ashcroft and colleagues were first to show that HRT treatment could protect against delayed healing in postmenopausal women [171]. In a

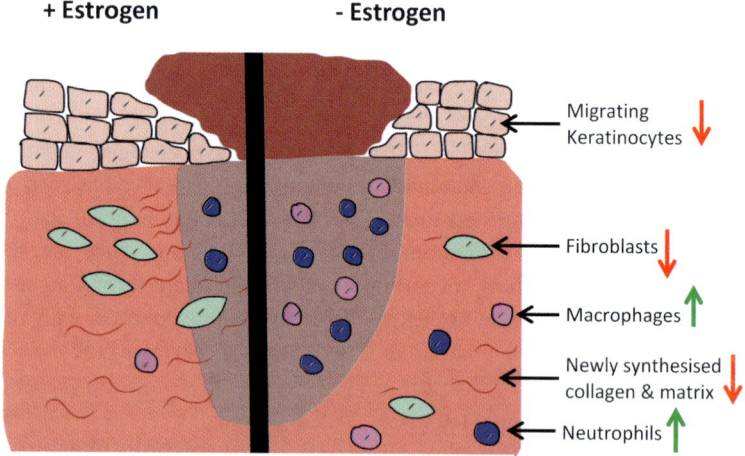

Fig. 6.3 Estrogen deficiency has a profound effect on skin wound healing. *Right* postmenopausal reduced estrogen leads to an inappropriately excessive but ineffective inflammatory response and retarded re-epithelialisation. Suppressed fibroblast function, decreased collagen synthesis and increased MMPs lead to a reduction in extracellular matrix

subsequent study topical estrogen was shown to accelerate acute wound repair in healthy elderly men and women [172]. Shortly after came the key observation that HRT was protective against developing chronic wounds, both pressure sores (age-adjusted relative risk 0.68) and venous ulcers (age-adjusted relative risk 0.65) [173, 174]. More recently we have used microarray profiling to demonstrate that the vast majority (78 %) of genes differentially expressed in wounds from elderly versus young men were estrogen-regulated [58]. Thus, estrogen is clearly clinically and physiologically important for effective skin repair.

Subsequent studies focusing on estrogen's mechanism of action have largely employed ovariectomised (OVX) rodents. OVX mice and rats display a pronounced delay in healing with altered re-epithelialisation, inflammation, ECM deposition and protease levels. Short-term estrogen replacement reverses these effects promoting keratinocyte migration, increasing matrix deposition and dampening inflammation [58, 171, 175].

6.12 Inflammation

In vitro studies have functionally linked estrogen to a range of inflammatory cells, including neutrophils, macrophages and mast, dendritic and Langerhans cells [176, 177]. In acute healing estrogen acts to dampen the inflammatory response and in human studies prevents excessive neutrophil recruitment via downregulation of L-selectin, inhibiting homing to the wound site [172]. The subsequent dampening of wound neutrophil-derived elastase levels prevents excessive degradation of ECM proteins. Estrogen also appears essential for the switch from classical (TH1; CA) to alternative (TH2: AA) macrophage polarisation. Wounds from OVX rodents contain highly CA polarised macrophages [167, 178], while estrogen treatment shifts to AA polarisation, in line with a pro-healing role [58, 167]. Estrogen is also potently anti-inflammatory in other tissues, such as the brain, where it protects against neurodegeneration [179]. Estrogen specifically dampens the expression of numerous proinflammatory cytokines, including TNF-α, MCP-1, Il-1β, Il-6 and macrophage migration inhibitory factor (MIF) [92, 180, 181]. MIF is particularly interesting and expressed by a range of wound cell types. *MIF* null mice are entirely resistant to the detrimental effects of OVX, implying that MIF acts as a key downstream mediator of both the detrimental effects of estrogen deficiency and the beneficial effects of estrogen replacement on skin wound healing [57, 175, 182]. Of clinical relevance, human plasma MIF levels increase post menopause and fall following HRT [57].

6.13 Re-epithelialisation

A failure of re-epithelialisation is a key aspect of both age-associated delayed acute healing and chronic wounds. Estrogen is a keratinocyte mitogen [71] directly promoting in vitro scratch wound closure in both mouse and human cells [128, 175] and in vivo re-epithelisation in murine acute wounds [183, 184]. In humans the delayed re-epithelisation associated with the postmenopausal state can be entirely reversed following 3 months of HRT [171] or short-term topical estrogen treatment [172].

6.14 Matrix Deposition and Angiogenesis

Wound collagen deposition and subsequent remodelling are delayed post menopause and promoted by HRT or topical estrogen treatment [171, 172]. Indeed in vivo estrogen promotes fibroblast proliferation and migration, with increased collagen deposition conferring increased wound strength. Estrogen directly promotes fibroblast migration demonstrated via in vitro cell assays [128, 175, 185–187] and indirectly via macrophage-produced platelet-derived growth factor (PDGF). Estrogen-driven PDGF production has a significant effect on angiogenesis, with estrogen demonstrated to be proangiogenic both in vitro and in vivo [188].

6.15 ERS and Wound Healing

Estrogen signals via two nuclear hormone receptors: ERα predominates in reproductive tissues and is strongly associated with cancer [189], while ERβ is more widely expressed in peripheral tissues [190, 191]. Estrogen's pleiotropic role in healing is supported by widespread cellular ER expression in wound tissue and skin from a range of body sites in both mouse and human [72, 128, 192–195]. Indeed, very recently we have employed the ERE-luciferase reporter mouse [196] to directly assess ER-mediated signalling following in vivo wounding [197]. Shortly after injury ER-mediated signalling is robustly upregulated in the skin immediately adjacent to the wound. Subsequent immunohistochemical analysis revealed the signal to be predominantly localised to wound edge keratinocytes and inflammatory cells.

Crucially, in OVX mice ER-specific agonists confer entirely different effects. Treatment with the ERβ-specific agonist DPN promotes wound healing as effectively as estrogen treatment, while the ERα-specific agonist PPT has no effect. These agonist treatment effects are confirmed by estrogen replacement studies in OVX ER null mice, where ERβ null mice display a pronounced delay in healing [128]. Thus signalling through ERβ is beneficial and ERα detrimental to repair. Taking these observations further, epidermal-specific (K14-cre mediated) ER null mice were shown to phenocopy global ER nulls, and the ERβ agonist DPN was shown to directly promote keratinocyte migration in vitro, suggesting a key role for epidermal ERβ [128]. These studies are entirely consistent with clinical reports that polymorphisms in the human ERβ gene are significantly associated with venous ulceration in the Caucasian population [74, 198]. However, an alternative picture emerges for a skin flap necrosis model where the beneficial effects of 17β-estradiol on outcome are reportedly mediated via ERα [199]. The discrepancy between the two models may be explained by the observation that ERα, not ERβ, is important for controlling wound inflammation in response to IGF1 [200].

6.16 SERMs and Future Therapies

Pharmacological modulators of ERs have been developed. These include specific agonists that are experimentally invaluable and the more clinically relevant mixed agonist/antagonists, termed selective estrogen receptor modulators (SERMs). Here the SERMs tamoxifen, raloxifene and genistein have been shown to promote skin healing [183, 184]. Raloxifene acts as an antagonist in breast tissue and an agonist in bone tissue [201]. It has been shown to have a positive effect on wound healing [184]; this could be in part due to its ability to stimulate collagen synthesis in cultured fibroblasts [202] and also reduce inflammation in the wound [184]. As well as the improvement in wound healing, raloxifene is also shown to improve skin elasticity in humans following 12 months of treatment [203]. Tamoxifen was also shown to have a similar effect on wound healing reducing inflammation and restoring wound healing time in the OVX mouse to that of the intact control and estrogen treated [184]. Tamoxifen has also been studied in the formation of keloid scars in burn patients where it appears to improve scarring, decreasing collagen synthesis via reduction of TGF-β signalling and reducing fibroblast proliferation [204]. In the context of skin aging, the ERβ-selective ligand, WAY-200070, has been suggested to dampen inflammation and MMP expression in UV-damaged skin [205]. The phytoestrogen genistein has also been reported to improve gross skin changes in OVX rats [206]. In summary SERMs, which are used clinically in tissues such as bone, clearly influence physiology of postmenopausal skin; however, the mechanisms remain to be fully elucidated.

6.17 Summary

The skin undergoes widespread functional deterioration with age and following menopause. It is now widely accepted that the age-associated reduction in circulating hormones, particularly estrogen, directly accelerates skin aging, a major clinical consequence being delayed repair leading to an increased incidence of chronic wounds.

Numerous studies have shown that estrogen replacement (in the form of HRT) can protect against, and possibly even reverse, skin aging, promoting repair. While macroscopic and ultrastructural aspects of these hormone-mediated effects on skin have been documented, much remains unknown. Recent studies revealing differential roles for the two estrogen receptors in skin biology and pathology have opened exciting new avenues for therapeutic intervention.

References

1. Chuong CM, Nickoloff BJ, Elias PM, Goldsmith LA, Macher E, Maderson PA, Sundberg JP, et al. What is the 'true' function of skin? Exp Dermatol. 2002;11(2):159–87.
2. Casey G. Physiology of the skin. Nurs Stand. 2002; 16(34):47–51; quiz 53, 55.
3. Lai-Cheong JM, McGrath JA. Structure and function of skin, hair and nails. Medicine. 2009;37(5):223–6.
4. Cotsarelis G. Epithelial stem cells: a folliculocentric view. J Invest Dermatol. 2006;126(7):1459–68.
5. Eckert RL, Rorke EA. Molecular biology of keratinocyte differentiation. Environ Health Perspect. 1989;80:109–16.
6. Elias PM, Feingold KR. Lipids and the epidermal water barrier: metabolism, regulation, and pathophysiology. Semin Dermatol. 1992;11(2):176–82.
7. Winsor T, Burch GE. Differential roles of layers of human epigastric skin on diffusion rate of water. Arch Intern Med. 1944;74:428–36.
8. Maricich SM, Wellnitz SA, Nelson AM, Lesniak DR, Gerling GJ, Lumpkin EA, et al. Merkel cells are essential for light-touch responses. Science. 2009; 324(5934):1580–2.
9. Holikova Z, Hercogová J, Pizák J, Smetana Jr K. Dendritic cells and their role in skin-induced immune responses. J Eur Acad Dermatol Venereol. 2001;15(2):116–20.
10. Steplewski A, Kasinskas A, Fertala A. Remodeling of the dermal-epidermal junction in bilayered skin constructs after silencing the expression of the p.R2622Q and p.G2623C collagen VII mutants. Connect Tissue Res. 2012;53(5):379–89.
11. Burgeson RE, Christiano AM. The dermal-epidermal junction. Curr Opin Cell Biol. 1997;9(5):651–8.
12. Makrantonaki E, Zouboulis CC. The skin as a mirror of the aging process in the human organism – state of the art and results of the aging research in the German National Genome Research Network 2 (NGFN-2). Exp Gerontol. 2007;42(9):879–86.
13. Kielty CM, Sherratt MJ, Shuttleworth CA. Elastic fibers. J Cell Sci. 2002;115(Pt 14):2817–28.
14. Braverman IM, Fonferko E. Studies in cutaneous aging: I. The elastic fiber network. J Invest Dermatol. 1982;78(5):434–43.
15. Frantz C, Stewart KM, Weaver VM. The extracellular matrix at a glance. J Cell Sci. 2010;123(Pt 24): 4195–200.
16. Kohl E, Steinbauer J, Landthaler M, Szeimies RM. Skin aging. J Eur Acad Dermatol Venereol. 2011;25(8):873–84.
17. Fenske NA, Lober CW. Structural and functional changes of normal aging skin. J Am Acad Dermatol. 1986;15(4 Pt 1):571–85.
18. Francis C, Robert L. Elastin and elastic fibers in normal and pathologic skin. Int J Dermatol. 1984;23: 166–79.
19. Ghersetich I, Lotti T, Campanile G, Grappone C, Dini G. Hyaluronic acid in cutaneous intrinsic aging. Int J Dermatol. 1994;33(2):119–22.
20. Naylor EC, Watson RE, Sherratt MJ. Molecular aspects of skin aging. Maturitas. 2011;69(3): 249–56.
21. Langton AK, Sherratt MJ, Griffiths CE, Watson RE. A new wrinkle on old skin: the role of elastic fibers in skin aging. Int J Cosmet Sci. 2010;32(5): 330–39.
22. Varani J, Warner RL, Gharaee-Kermani M, Phan SH, Kang S, Chung JH, et al. Vitamin A antagonizes decreased cell growth and elevated collagen-degrading matrix metalloproteinases and stimulates collagen accumulation in naturally aged human skin. J Invest Dermatol. 2000;114(3):480–6.
23. Gunin AG, Kornilova NK, Vasilieva OV, Petrov VV. Age-related changes in proliferation, the numbers of mast cells, eosinophils, and cd45-positive cells in human dermis. J Gerontol A Biol Sci Med Sci. 2011;66(4):385–92.
24. Gilchrest BA. Age-associated changes in the skin. J Am Geriatr Soc. 1982;30(2):139–43.
25. Tobin DJ, Paus R. Graying: gerontobiology of the hair follicle pigmentary unit. Exp Gerontol. 2001; 36(1):29–54.
26. Kligman LH, Kligman AM. The nature of photoaging: its prevention and repair. Photodermatol. 1986; 3(4):215–27.
27. Jenkins G. Molecular mechanisms of skin aging. Mech Aging Dev. 2002;123(7):801–10.
28. Gilchrest BA, Yaar M. Aging and photoageing of the skin: observations at the cellular and molecular level. Br J Dermatol. 1992;127 Suppl 41: 25–30.
29. El-Domyati M, Attia S, Saleh F, Brown D, Birk DE, Gasparro F, et al. Intrinsic aging vs. photoaging: a comparative histopathological, immunohistochemical, and ultrastructural study of skin. Exp Dermatol. 2002;11(5):398–405.
30. Talwar HS, Griffiths CE, Fisher GJ, Hamilton TA, Voorhees JJ. Reduced type I and type III procollagens in photodamaged adult human skin. J Invest Dermatol. 1995;105(2):285–90.

31. Watson RE, Kielty CM, Griffiths CE, Craven NM, Shuttleworth CA. Fibrillin-rich microfibrils are reduced in photoaged skin. Distribution at the dermal-epidermal junction. J Invest Dermatol. 1999;112(5):782–7.
32. Bernstein EF, Underhill CB, Hahn PJ, Brown DB, Uitto J. Chronic sun exposure alters both the content and distribution of dermal glycosaminoglycans. Br J Dermatol. 1996;135(2):255–62.
33. Weinert BT, Timiras PS. Invited review: theories of aging. J Appl Physiol. 2003;95:1706–16.
34. Yoon IK, Kim HK, Kim YK, Song IH, Kim W, Kim S, et al. Exploration of replicative senescence-associated genes in human dermal fibroblasts by cDNA microarray technology. Exp Gerontol. 2004;39(9):1369–78.
35. Yaar M, Eller MS, Gilchrest BA. Fifty years of skin aging. J Investig Dermatol Symp Proc. 2002;7(1):51–8.
36. Rossi DJ, Bryder D, Seita J, Nussenzweig A, Hoeijmakers J, Weissman IL. Deficiencies in DNA damage repair limit the function of haematopoietic stem cells with age. Nature. 2007;447(7145):725–9.
37. Zeng G, Millis AJ. Differential regulation of collagenase and stromelysin mRNA in late passage cultures of human fibroblasts. Exp Cell Res. 1996;222(1):150–6.
38. Khorramizadeh MR, Tredget EE, Telasky C, Shen Q, Ghahary A. Aging differentially modulates the expression of collagen and collagenase in dermal fibroblasts. Mol Cell Biochem. 1999;194(1–2):99–108.
39. Love NR, Chen Y, Ishibashi S, Kritsiligkou P, Lea R, Koh Y, et al. Amputation-induced reactive oxygen species are required for successful Xenopus tadpole tail regeneration. Nat Cell Biol. 2013;15(2):222–8.
40. Haorah J, Ramirez SH, Schall K, Smith D, Pandya R, Persidsky Y. Oxidative stress activates protein tyrosine kinase and matrix metalloproteinases leading to blood-brain barrier dysfunction. J Neurochem. 2007;101(2):566–76.
41. Sardy M. Role of matrix metalloproteinases in skin aging. Connect Tissue Res. 2009;50(2):132–8.
42. Pimienta G, Pascual J. Canonical and alternative MAPK signaling. Cell Cycle. 2007;6(21):2628–32.
43. Booms P, Pregla R, Ney A, Barthel F, Reinhardt DP, Pletschacher A, et al. RGD-containing fibrillin-1 fragments upregulate matrix metalloproteinase expression in cell culture: a potential factor in the pathogenesis of the Marfan syndrome. Hum Genet. 2005;116(1–2):51–61.
44. Hayflick L, Moorhead PS. The serial cultivation of human diploid cell strains. Exp Cell Res. 1961;25:585–621.
45. Schneider EL, Mitsui Y. The relationship between in vitro cellular aging and in vivo human age. Proc Natl Acad Sci U S A. 1976;73(10):3584–8.
46. Olovnikov AM. Telomeres, telomerase, and aging: origin of the theory. Exp Gerontol. 1996;31(4):443–8.
47. Campisi J. Aging, cellular senescence, and cancer. Annu Rev Physiol. 2012;75:685–705.
48. Hughes SV, Robinson E, Bland R, Lewis HM, Stewart PM, Hewison M. 1,25-dihydroxyvitamin D3 regulates estrogen metabolism in cultured keratinocytes. Endocrinology. 1997;138(9):3711–8.
49. Sawaya ME, Penneys NS. Immunohistochemical distribution of aromatase and 3B-hydroxysteroid dehydrogenase in human hair follicle and sebaceous gland. J Cutan Pathol. 1992;19(4):309–14.
50. Thiboutot D, Martin P, Volikos L, Gilliland K. Oxidative activity of the type 2 isozyme of 17beta-hydroxysteroid dehydrogenase (17beta-HSD) predominates in human sebaceous glands. J Invest Dermatol. 1998;111(3):390–5.
51. Thiboutot D, Bayne E, Thorne J, Gilliland K, Flanagan J, Shao Q, et al. Immunolocalization of 5alpha-reductase isozymes in acne lesions and normal skin. Arch Dermatol. 2000;136(9):1125–9.
52. Labrie F, Luu-The V, Lin SX, Simard J, Labrie C. Role of 17 beta-hydroxysteroid dehydrogenases in sex steroid formation in peripheral intracrine tissues. Trends Endocrinol Metab. 2000;11(10):421–7.
53. Inoue T, Miki Y, Abe K, Hatori M, Hosaka M, Kariya Y, et al. Sex steroid synthesis in human skin in situ: the roles of aromatase and steroidogenic acute regulatory protein in the homeostasis of human skin. Mol Cell Endocrinol. 2012;362(1–2):19–28.
54. Cauley JA, Gutai JP, Glynn NW, Paternostro-Bayles M, Cottington E, Kuller LH. Serum estrone concentrations and coronary artery disease in postmenopausal women. Arterioscler Thromb. 1994;14(1):14–8.
55. Tapiero H, Ba GN, Tew KD. Estrogens and environmental estrogens. Biomed Pharmacother. 2002;56(1):36–44.
56. Kotov A, Falany JL, Wang J, Falany CN. Regulation of estrogen activity by sulfation in human Ishikawa endometrial adenocarcinoma cells. J Steroid Biochem Mol Biol. 1999;68(3–4):137–44.
57. Hardman MJ, Waite A, Zeef L, Burow M, Nakayama T, Ashcroft GS. Macrophage migration inhibitory factor: a central regulator of wound healing. Am J Pathol. 2005;167(6):1561–74.
58. Hardman MJ, Ashcroft GS. Estrogen, not intrinsic aging, is the major regulator of delayed human wound healing in the elderly. Genome Biol. 2008;9(5):R80.
59. Misso ML, Jang C, Adams J, Tran J, Murata Y, Bell R, et al. Adipose aromatase gene expression is greater in older women and is unaffected by postmenopausal estrogen therapy. Menopause. 2005;12(2):210–5.
60. Santen RJ, Brodie H, Simpson ER, Siiteri PK, Brodie A. History of aromatase: saga of an important biological mediator and therapeutic target. Endocr Rev. 2009;30(4):343–75.
61. Simpson ER, Zhao Y, Agarwal VR, Michael MD, Bulun SE, Hinshelwood MM, et al. Aromatase expression in health and disease. Recent Prog Horm Res. 1997;52:185–213; discussion 213–4.

62. Harada N, Utsumi T, Takagi Y. Tissue-specific expression of the human aromatase cytochrome P-450 gene by alternative use of multiple exons 1 and promoters, and switching of tissue-specific exons 1 in carcinogenesis. Proc Natl Acad Sci U S A. 1993;90(23):11312–6.
63. Charlier TD, Harada N, Balthazart J, Cornil CA. Human and quail aromatase activity is rapidly and reversibly inhibited by phosphorylating conditions. Endocrinology. 2011;152(11):4199–210.
64. Cleland WH, Mendelson CR, Simpson ER. Aromatase activity of membrane fractions of human adipose tissue stromal cells and adipocytes. Endocrinology. 1983;113(6):2155–60.
65. Berkovitz GD, Fujimoto M, Brown TR, Brodie AM, Migeon CJ. Aromatase activity in cultured human genital skin fibroblasts. J Clin Endocrinol Metab. 1984;59(4):665–71.
66. Watanabe M, Noda M, Nakajin S. Aromatase expression in a human osteoblastic cell line increases in response to prostaglandin E(2) in a dexamethasone-dependent fashion. Steroids. 2007;72(9–10):686–92.
67. Hewitt SC, Korach KS. Oestrogen receptor knockout mice: roles for oestrogen receptors alpha and beta in reproductive tissues. Reproduction. 2003;125(2):143–9.
68. Haczynski J, Tarkowski R, Jarzabek K, Wolczynski S, Magoffin DA, Czarnocki KJ, et al. Differential effects of estradiol, raloxifene and tamoxifen on estrogen receptor expression in cultured human skin fibroblasts. Int J Mol Med. 2004;13(6):903–8.
69. Thornton MJ, Taylor AH, Mulligan K, Al-Azzawi F, Lyon CC, O'Driscoll J. The distribution of estrogen receptor beta is distinct to that of estrogen receptor alpha and the androgen receptor in human skin and the pilosebaceous unit. J Investig Dermatol Symp Proc. 2003;8(1):100–3.
70. Beier K, Ginez I, Schaller H. Localization of steroid hormone receptors in the apocrine sweat glands of the human axilla. Histochem Cell Biol. 2005;123(1):61–5.
71. Verdier-Sevrain S, Yaar M, Cantatore J, Traish A, Gilchrest BA. Estradiol induces proliferation of keratinocytes via a receptor mediated mechanism. FASEB J. 2004;18(11):1252–4.
72. Thornton MJ, Taylor AH, Mulligan K, Al-Azzawi F, Lyon CC, O'Driscoll J, et al. Oestrogen receptor beta is the predominant oestrogen receptor in human scalp skin. Exp Dermatol. 2003;12(2):181–90.
73. Inoue T, Miki Y, Abe K, Hatori M, Hosaka M, Kariya Y, et al. The role of estrogen-metabolizing enzymes and estrogen receptors in human epidermis. Mol Cell Endocrinol. 2011;344(1–2):35–40.
74. Ashworth JJ, Smyth JV, Pendleton N, Horan M, Payton A, Worthington J, et al. The dinucleotide (CA) repeat polymorphism of estrogen receptor beta but not the dinucleotide (TA) repeat polymorphism of estrogen receptor alpha is associated with venous ulceration. J Steroid Biochem Mol Biol. 2005;97(3):266–70.
75. Liu Y, Gao H, Marstrand TT, Ström A, Valen E, Sandelin A, et al. The genome landscape of ERalpha- and ERbeta-binding DNA regions. Proc Natl Acad Sci U S A. 2008;105(7):2604–9.
76. Charn TH, Liu ET, Chang EC, Lee YK, Katzenellenbogen JA, Katzenellenbogen BS. Genome-wide dynamics of chromatin binding of estrogen receptors alpha and beta: mutual restriction and competitive site selection. Mol Endocrinol. 2010;24(1):47–59.
77. Klotz DM, Hewitt SC, Ciana P, Raviscioni M, Lindzey JK, Foley J, et al. Requirement of estrogen receptor-alpha in insulin-like growth factor-1 (IGF-1)-induced uterine responses and in vivo evidence for IGF-1/estrogen receptor cross-talk. J Biol Chem. 2002;277(10):8531–7.
78. Verdier-Sevrain S, Bonte F, Gilchrest B. Biology of estrogens in skin: implications for skin aging. Exp Dermatol. 2006;15(2):83–94.
79. Brincat MP. Hormone replacement therapy and the skin. Maturitas. 2000;35(2):107–17.
80. Brincat M, Versi E, Moniz CF, Magos A, de Trafford J, Studd JW. Skin collagen changes in postmenopausal women receiving different regimens of estrogen therapy. Obstet Gynecol. 1987;70(1):123–7.
81. Hall G, Phillips TJ. Estrogen and skin: the effects of estrogen, menopause, and hormone replacement therapy on the skin. J Am Acad Dermatol. 2005;53(4):555–68; quiz 569–72.
82. Pierard GE, Letawe C, Dowlati A, Piérard-Franchimont C. Effect of hormone replacement therapy for menopause on the mechanical properties of skin. J Am Geriatr Soc. 1995;43(6):662–5.
83. Sauerbronn AV, Fonseca AM, Bagnoli VR, Saldiva PH, Pinotti JA. The effects of systemic hormonal replacement therapy on the skin of postmenopausal women. Int J Gynaecol Obstet. 2000;68(1):35–41.
84. Rauramo L, Punnonen R. Effect of oral estrogen treatment with estriol succinate on the skin of castrated women. Z Haut Geschlechtskr. 1969;44(13):463–70.
85. Punnonen R. Effect of castration and peroral estrogen therapy on the skin. Acta Obstet Gynecol Scand Suppl. 1972;21:3–44.
86. Kanda N, Watanabe S. 17beta-estradiol stimulates the growth of human keratinocytes by inducing cyclin D2 expression. J Invest Dermatol. 2004;123(2):319–28.
87. Kanda N, Watanabe S. 17beta-estradiol inhibits oxidative stress-induced apoptosis in keratinocytes by promoting Bcl-2 expression. J Invest Dermatol. 2003;121(6):1500–9.
88. Dunn LB, Damesyn M, Moore AA, Reuben DB, Greendale GA. Does estrogen prevent skin aging? Results from the First National Health and Nutrition Examination Survey (NHANES I). Arch Dermatol. 1997;133(3):339–42.
89. Pierard-Franchimont C, Letawe C, Goffin V, Piérard GE. Skin water-holding capacity and transdermal

estrogen therapy for menopause: a pilot study. Maturitas. 1995;22(2):151–4.
90. Denda M, Koyama J, Hori J, Horii I, Takahashi M, Hara M, Tagami H. Age- and sex-dependent change in stratum corneum sphingolipids. Arch Dermatol Res. 1993;285(7):415–7.
91. Callens A, Vaillant L, Lecomte P, Berson M, Gall Y, Lorette G. Does hormonal skin aging exist? A study of the influence of different hormone therapy regimens on the skin of postmenopausal women using non-invasive measurement techniques. Dermatology. 1996;193(4):289–94.
92. Sator PG, Schmidt JB, Sator MO, Huber JC, Hönigsmann H. The influence of hormone replacement therapy on skin aging: a pilot study. Maturitas. 2001;39(1):43–55.
93. Danforth DN, Veis A, Breen M, Weinstein HG, Buckingham JC, Manalo P. The effect of pregnancy and labor on the human cervix: changes in collagen, glycoproteins, and glycosaminoglycans. Am J Obstet Gynecol. 1974;120(5):641–51.
94. Grosman N, Hvidberg E, Schou J. The effect of oestrogenic treatment on the acid mucopolysaccharide pattern in skin of mice. Acta Pharmacol Toxicol (Copenh). 1971;30(5):458–64.
95. Pochi PE, Strauss JS, Downing DT. Age-related changes in sebaceous gland activity. J Invest Dermatol. 1979;73(1):108–11.
96. Zouboulis CC, Boschnakow A. Chronological aging and photoaging of the human sebaceous gland. Clin Exp Dermatol. 2001;26(7):600–7.
97. Contet-Audonneau JL, Jeanmaire C, Pauly G. A histological study of human wrinkle structures: comparison between sun-exposed areas of the face, with or without wrinkles, and sun-protected areas. Br J Dermatol. 1999;140(6):1038–47.
98. Bosset S, Barré P, Chalon A, Kurfurst R, Bonté F, André P, et al. Skin aging: clinical and histopathologic study of permanent and reducible wrinkles. Eur J Dermatol. 2002;12(3):247–52.
99. Brincat M, Moniz CJ, Studd JW, Darby A, Magos A, Emburey G, et al. Long-term effects of the menopause and sex hormones on skin thickness. Br J Obstet Gynaecol. 1985;92(3):256–9.
100. Affinito P, Palomba S, Sorrentino C, Di Carlo C, Bifulco G, Arienzo MP, et al. Effects of postmenopausal hypoestrogenism on skin collagen. Maturitas. 1999;33(3):239–47.
101. Schmidt R, Fazekas F, Reinhart B, Kapeller P, Fazekas G, Offenbacher H, et al. Estrogen replacement therapy in older women: a neuropsychological and brain MRI study. J Am Geriatr Soc. 1996;44(11):1307–13.
102. Son ED, Lee JY, Lee S, Kim MS, Lee BG, Chang IS, et al. Topical application of 17beta-estradiol increases extracellular matrix protein synthesis by stimulating tgf-Beta signaling in aged human skin in vivo. J Invest Dermatol. 2005;124(6):1149–61.
103. Varila E, Rantala I, Oikarinen A, Risteli J, Reunala T, Oksanen H, et al. The effect of topical oestradiol on skin collagen of postmenopausal women. Br J Obstet Gynaecol. 1995;102(12):985–9.
104. Maheux R, Naud F, Rioux M, Grenier R, Lemay A, Guy J, et al. A randomized, double-blind, placebo-controlled study on the effect of conjugated estrogens on skin thickness. Am J Obstet Gynecol. 1994;170(2):642–9.
105. Savvas M, Bishop J, Laurent G, Watson N, Studd J. Type III collagen content in the skin of postmenopausal women receiving oestradiol and testosterone implants. Br J Obstet Gynaecol. 1993;100(2):154–6.
106. Sumino H, Ichikawa S, Abe M, Endo Y, Ishikawa O, Kurabayashi M. Effects of aging, menopause, and hormone replacement therapy on forearm skin elasticity in women. J Am Geriatr Soc. 2004;52(6):945–9.
107. Henry F, Piérard-Franchimont C, Cauwenbergh G, Piérard GE. Age-related changes in facial skin contours and rheology. J Am Geriatr Soc. 1997;45(2):220–2.
108. Punnonen R, Vaajalahti P, Teisala K. Local oestriol treatment improves the structure of elastic fibers in the skin of postmenopausal women. Ann Chir Gynaecol Suppl. 1987;202:39–41.
109. Bolognia JL, Braverman IM, Rousseau ME, Sarrel PM. Skin changes in menopause. Maturitas. 1989;11(4):295–304.
110. Edwards MW, Bain SD, Bailey MC, Lantry MM, Howard GA. 17 beta estradiol stimulation of endosteal bone formation in the ovariectomized mouse: an animal model for the evaluation of bone-targeted estrogens. Bone. 1992;13(1):29–34.
111. Bekku N, Yoshimura H. Animal model of menopausal depressive-like state in female mice: prolongation of immobility time in the forced swimming test following ovariectomy. Psychopharmacology (Berl). 2005;183(3):300–7.
112. Kai M, Tominaga K, Okimoto K, Yamauchi A, Kai H, Kataoka Y. Ovariectomy aggravates nifedipine-induced flushing of tail skin in mice. Eur J Pharmacol. 2003;481(1):79–82.
113. Tsukahara K, Moriwaki S, Ohuchi A, Fujimura T, Takema Y. Ovariectomy accelerates photoaging of rat skin. Photochem Photobiol. 2001;73(5):525–31.
114. Tsukahara K, Nakagawa H, Moriwaki S, Kakuo S, Ohuchi A, Takema Y, et al. Ovariectomy is sufficient to accelerate spontaneous skin aging and to stimulate ultraviolet irradiation-induced photoaging of murine skin. Br J Dermatol. 2004;151(5):984–94.
115. Fang M, Liroff KG, Turner AS, Les CM, Orr BG, Holl MM. Estrogen depletion results in nanoscale morphology changes in dermal collagen. J Invest Dermatol. 2012;132(7):1791–7.
116. Borras C, Gambini J, Gómez-Cabrera MC, Sastre J, Pallardó FV, Mann GE, et al. 17beta-oestradiol up-regulates longevity-related, antioxidant enzyme expression via the ERK1 and ERK2[MAPK]/NFkappaB cascade. Aging Cell. 2005;4(3):113–8.

117. Imanishi T, Hano T, Nishio I. Estrogen reduces endothelial progenitor cell senescence through augmentation of telomerase activity. J Hypertens. 2005;23(9):1699–706.
118. Baeza I, Fdez-Tresguerres J, Ariznavarreta C, De la Fuente M. Effects of growth hormone, melatonin, oestrogens and phytoestrogens on the oxidized glutathione (GSSG)/reduced glutathione (GSH) ratio and lipid peroxidation in aged ovariectomized rats. Biogerontology. 2010;11(6):687–701.
119. Bottai G, Mancina R, Muratori M, Di Gennaro P, Lotti T. 17beta-estradiol protects human skin fibroblasts and keratinocytes against oxidative damage. J Eur Acad Dermatol Venereol. 2013;27(10):1236–43.
120. Cicatiello L, Cobellis G, Addeo R, Papa M, Altucci L, Sica V, et al. In vivo functional analysis of the mouse estrogen receptor gene promoter: a transgenic mouse model to study tissue-specific and developmental regulation of estrogen receptor gene transcription. Mol Endocrinol. 1995;9(8):1077–90.
121. Dupont S, Krust A, Gansmuller A, Dierich A, Chambon P, Mark M. Effect of single and compound knockouts of estrogen receptors alpha (ERalpha) and beta (ERbeta) on mouse reproductive phenotypes. Development. 2000;127(19):4277–91.
122. Korach KS. Insights from the study of animals lacking functional estrogen receptor. Science. 1994;266(5190):1524–7.
123. Krege JH, Hodgin JB, Couse JF, Enmark E, Warner M, Mahler JF, et al. Generation and reproductive phenotypes of mice lacking estrogen receptor beta. Proc Natl Acad Sci U S A. 1998;95(26):15677–82.
124. Lubahn DB, Moyer JS, Golding TS, Couse JF, Korach KS, Smithies O. Alteration of reproductive function but not prenatal sexual development after insertional disruption of the mouse estrogen receptor gene. Proc Natl Acad Sci U S A. 1993;90(23):11162–6.
125. Shughrue PJ, Askew GR, Dellovade TL, Merchenthaler I. Estrogen-binding sites and their functional capacity in estrogen receptor double knockout mouse brain. Endocrinology. 2002;143(5):1643–50.
126. Fisher CR, Graves KH, Parlow AF, Simpson ER. Characterization of mice deficient in aromatase (ArKO) because of targeted disruption of the cyp19 gene. Proc Natl Acad Sci U S A. 1998;95(12):6965–70.
127. Antal MC, Krust A, Chambon P, Mark M. Sterility and absence of histopathological defects in nonreproductive organs of a mouse ERbeta-null mutant. Proc Natl Acad Sci U S A. 2008;105(7):2433–8.
128. Campbell L, Emmerson E, Davies F, Gilliver SC, Krust A, Chambon P, et al. Estrogen promotes cutaneous wound healing via estrogen receptor beta independent of its antiinflammatory activities. J Exp Med. 2010;207(9):1825–33.
129. Jakacka M, Ito M, Weiss J, Chien PY, Gehm BD, Jameson JL. Estrogen receptor binding to DNA is not required for its activity through the nonclassical AP1 pathway. J Biol Chem. 2001;276(17):13615–21.
130. Swope DL, Castranio T, Harrell JC, Mishina Y, Korach KS. AF-2 knock-in mutation of estrogen receptor alpha: Cre-loxP excision of a PGK-neo cassette from the 3′ UTR. Genesis. 2002;32(2):99 101.
131. Jakacka M, Ito M, Martinson F, Ishikawa T, Lee EJ, Jameson JL. An estrogen receptor (ER)alpha deoxyribonucleic acid-binding domain knock-in mutation provides evidence for nonclassical ER pathway signaling in vivo. Mol Endocrinol. 2002;16(10):2188–201.
132. Couse JF, Korach KS. Estrogen receptor null mice: what have we learned and where will they lead us? Endocr Rev. 1999;20(3):358–417.
133. Moverare S, Lindberg MK, Faergemann J, Gustafsson JA, Ohlsson C. Estrogen receptor alpha, but not estrogen receptor beta, is involved in the regulation of the hair follicle cycling as well as the thickness of epidermis in male mice. J Invest Dermatol. 2002;119(5):1053–8.
134. Ohnemus U, Uenalan M, Conrad F, Handjiski B, Mecklenburg L, Nakamura M, et al. Hair cycle control by estrogens: catagen induction via estrogen receptor (ER)-alpha is checked by ER beta signaling. Endocrinology. 2005;146(3):1214–25.
135. Markiewicz M, Znoyko S, Stawski L, Ghatnekar A, Gilkeson G, Trojanowska M. A role for estrogen receptor-alpha and estrogen receptor-beta in collagen biosynthesis in mouse skin. J Invest Dermatol. 2013;133(1):120–7.
136. Cho JL, Allanson M, Domanski D, Arun SJ, Reeve VE. Estrogen receptor-beta signaling protects epidermal cytokine expression and immune function from UVB-induced impairment in mice. Photochem Photobiol Sci. 2008;7(1):120–5.
137. Shaw TJ, Martin P. Wound repair at a glance. J Cell Sci. 2009;122(Pt 18):3209–13.
138. Boldt J, Hüttner I, Suttner S, Kumle B, Piper SN, Berchthold G. Changes of haemostasis in patients undergoing major abdominal surgery – is there a difference between elderly and younger patients? Br J Anaesth. 2001;87(3):435–40.
139. Pleym H, Wahba A, Videm V, Asberg A, Lydersen S, Bjella L, et al. Increased fibrinolysis and platelet activation in elderly patients undergoing coronary bypass surgery. Anesth Analg. 2006;102(3):660–7.
140. Holt DR, Kirk SJ, Regan MC, Hurson M, Lindblad WJ, Barbul A. Effect of age on wound healing in healthy human beings. Surgery. 1992;112(2):293–7; discussion 297–8.
141. Usui ML, Mansbridge JN, Carter WG, Fujita M, Olerud JE. Keratinocyte migration, proliferation, and differentiation in chronic ulcers from patients with diabetes and normal wounds. J Histochem Cytochem. 2008;56(7):687–96.
142. Ashcroft GS, Horan MA, Ferguson MW. Aging alters the inflammatory and endothelial cell adhesion molecule profiles during human cutaneous wound healing. Lab Invest. 1998;78(1):47–58.

143. Ashcroft GS, Jeong MJ, Ashworth JJ, Hardman M, Jin W, Moutsopoulos N, et al. Tumor necrosis factor-alpha (TNF-alpha) is a therapeutic target for impaired cutaneous wound healing. Wound Repair Regen. 2012;20(1):38–49.
144. Ashcroft GS, Horan MA, Ferguson MW. Aging is associated with reduced deposition of specific extracellular matrix components, an upregulation of angiogenesis, and an altered inflammatory response in a murine incisional wound healing model. J Invest Dermatol. 1997;108(4):430–7.
145. Mustoe T. Understanding chronic wounds: a unifying hypothesis on their pathogenesis and implications for therapy. Am J Surg. 2004;187(5A):65S–70.
146. Wicke C, Bachinger A, Coerper S, Beckert S, Witte MB, Königsrainer A. Aging influences wound healing in patients with chronic lower extremity wounds treated in a specialized Wound Care Center. Wound Repair Regen. 2009;17(1):25–33.
147. Swift ME, Kleinman HK, DiPietro LA. Impaired wound repair and delayed angiogenesis in aged mice. Lab Invest. 1999;79(12):1479–87.
148. van Duin D, Mohanty S, Thomas V, Ginter S, Montgomery RR, Fikrig E, et al. Age-associated defect in human TLR-1/2 function. J Immunol. 2007;178(2):970–5.
149. Agius E, Lacy KE, Vukmanovic-Stejic M, Jagger AL, Papageorgiou AP, Hall S, et al. Decreased TNF-alpha synthesis by macrophages restricts cutaneous immunosurveillance by memory CD4+ T cells during aging. J Exp Med. 2009;206(9):1929–40.
150. Swift ME, Burns AL, Gray KL, DiPietro LA. Age-related alterations in the inflammatory response to dermal injury. J Invest Dermatol. 2001;117(5):1027–35.
151. Danon D, Kowatch MA, Roth GS. Promotion of wound repair in old mice by local injection of macrophages. Proc Natl Acad Sci U S A. 1989;86(6):2018–20.
152. Butcher SK, Chahal H, Nayak L, Sinclair A, Henriquez NV, Sapey E, et al. Senescence in innate immune responses: reduced neutrophil phagocytic capacity and CD16 expression in elderly humans. J Leukoc Biol. 2001;70(6):881–6.
153. Gilchrest BA. In vitro assessment of keratinocyte aging. J Invest Dermatol. 1983;81(1 Suppl):184s–9.
154. Ross C, Alston M, Bickenbach JR, Aykin-Burns N. Oxygen tension changes the rate of migration of human skin keratinocytes in an age-related manner. Exp Dermatol. 2011;20(1):58–63.
155. Xia YP, Zhao Y, Tyrone JW, Chen A, Mustoe TA. Differential activation of migration by hypoxia in keratinocytes isolated from donors of increasing age: implication for chronic wounds in the elderly. J Invest Dermatol. 2001;116(1):50–6.
156. Thomason HA, Cooper NH, Ansell DM, Chiu M, Merrit AJ, Hardman MJ, et al. Direct evidence that PKCalpha positively regulates wound re-epithelialization: correlation with changes in desmosomal adhesiveness. J Pathol. 2012;227(3):346–56.
157. Varani J, Dame MK, Rittie L, Fligiel SE, Kang S, Fisher GJ, et al. Decreased collagen production in chronologically aged skin: roles of age-dependent alteration in fibroblast function and defective mechanical stimulation. Am J Pathol. 2006;168(6):1861–8.
158. Kondo H, Yonezawa Y. Changes in the migratory ability of human lung and skin fibroblasts during in vitro aging and in vivo cellular senescence. Mech Aging Dev. 1992;63(3):223–33.
159. Plisko A, Gilchrest BA. Growth factor responsiveness of cultured human fibroblasts declines with age. J Gerontol. 1983;38(5):513–8.
160. Bruce SA, Deamond SF. Longitudinal study of in vivo wound repair and in vitro cellular senescence of dermal fibroblasts. Exp Gerontol. 1991;26(1):17–27.
161. Bruce SA. Ultrastructure of dermal fibroblasts during development and aging: relationship to in vitro senescence of dermal fibroblasts. Exp Gerontol. 1991;26(1):3–16.
162. Stanley AC, Park HY, Phillips TJ, Russakovsky V, Menzoian JO. Reduced growth of dermal fibroblasts from chronic venous ulcers can be stimulated with growth factors. J Vasc Surg. 1997;26(6):994–9; discussion 999–1001.
163. Cook H, Davies KJ, Harding KG, Thomas DW. Defective extracellular matrix reorganization by chronic wound fibroblasts is associated with alterations in TIMP-1, TIMP-2, and MMP-2 activity. J Invest Dermatol. 2000;115(2):225–33.
164. Wall IB, Moseley R, Baird DM, Kipling D, Giles P, Laffafian I, et al. Fibroblast dysfunction is a key factor in the non-healing of chronic venous leg ulcers. J Invest Dermatol. 2008;128(10):2526–40.
165. Freedland M, Karmiol S, Rodriguez J, Normolle D, Smith Jr D, Garner W. Fibroblast responses to cytokines are maintained during aging. Ann Plast Surg. 1995;35(3):290–6.
166. Arthur WT, Vernon RB, Sage EH, Reed MJ. Growth factors reverse the impaired sprouting of microvessels from aged mice. Microvasc Res. 1998;55(3):260–70.
167. Routley CE, Ashcroft GS. Effect of estrogen and progesterone on macrophage activation during wound healing. Wound Repair Regen. 2009;17(1):42–50.
168. Mills SJ, Ashworth JJ, Gilliver SC, Hardman MJ, Ashcroft GS. The sex steroid precursor DHEA accelerates cutaneous wound healing via the estrogen receptors. J Invest Dermatol. 2005;125(5):1053–62.
169. Gilliver SC, Ruckshanthi JP, Hardman MJ, Zeef LA, Ashcroft GS. 5alpha-dihydrotestosterone (DHT) retards wound closure by inhibiting re-epithelialization. J Pathol. 2009;217(1):73–82.
170. Ashcroft GS, Mills SJ. Androgen receptor-mediated inhibition of cutaneous wound healing. J Clin Invest. 2002;110(5):615–24.
171. Ashcroft GS, Dodsworth J, van Boxtel E, Tarnuzzer RW, Horan MA, Schultz GS, et al. Estrogen accelerates

cutaneous wound healing associated with an increase in TGF-beta1 levels. Nat Med. 1997;3(11):1209–15.
172. Ashcroft GS, Greenwell-Wild T, Horan MA, Wahl SM, Ferguson MW. Topical estrogen accelerates cutaneous wound healing in aged humans associated with an altered inflammatory response. Am J Pathol. 1999;155(4):1137–46.
173. Margolis DJ, Knauss J, Bilker W. Hormone replacement therapy and prevention of pressure ulcers and venous leg ulcers. Lancet. 2002;359(9307):675–7.
174. Berard A, Kahn SR, Abenhaim L. Is hormone replacement therapy protective for venous ulcer of the lower limbs? Pharmacoepidemiol Drug Saf. 2001;10(3):245–51.
175. Emmerson E, Campbell L, Ashcroft GS, Hardman MJ. Unique and synergistic roles for 17beta-estradiol and macrophage migration inhibitory factor during cutaneous wound closure are cell type specific. Endocrinology. 2009;150(6):2749–57.
176. Seillet C, Rouquié N, Foulon E, Douin-Echinard V, Krust A, Chambon P, et al. Estradiol promotes functional responses in inflammatory and steady-state dendritic cells through differential requirement for activation function-1 of estrogen receptor alpha. J Immunol. 2013;190(11):5459–70.
177. Hunt JS, Miller L, Roby KF, Huang J, Platt JS, DeBrot BL. Female steroid hormones regulate production of pro-inflammatory molecules in uterine leukocytes. J Reprod Immunol. 1997;35(2):87–99.
178. Campbell L, Saville CR, Murray PJ, Cruickshank SM, Hardman MJ. Local arginase 1 activity is required for cutaneous wound healing. J Invest Dermatol. 2013;133(10):2461–70.
179. Vegeto E, Belcredito S, Etteri S, Ghisletti S, Brusadelli A, Meda C, et al. Estrogen receptor-alpha mediates the brain antiinflammatory activity of estradiol. Proc Natl Acad Sci U S A. 2003;100(16):9614–9.
180. Pfeilschifter J, Köditz R, Pfohl M, Schatz H. Changes in proinflammatory cytokine activity after menopause. Endocr Rev. 2002;23(1):90–119.
181. Zhang B, Subramanian S, Dziennis S, Jia J, Uchida M, Akiyoshi K, et al. Estradiol and G1 reduce infarct size and improve immunosuppression after experimental stroke. J Immunol. 2010;184(8):4087–94.
182. Ashcroft GS, Mills SJ, Lei K, Gibbons L, Jeong MJ, Taniguchi M, et al. Estrogen modulates cutaneous wound healing by downregulating macrophage migration inhibitory factor. J Clin Invest. 2003;111(9):1309–18.
183. Emmerson E, Campbell L, Ashcroft GS, Hardman MJ. The phytoestrogen genistein promotes wound healing by multiple independent mechanisms. Mol Cell Endocrinol. 2010;321(2):184–93.
184. Hardman MJ, Emmerson E, Campbell L, Ashcroft GS. Selective estrogen receptor modulators accelerate cutaneous wound healing in ovariectomized female mice. Endocrinology. 2008;149(2):551–7.
185. Stevenson S, Taylor AH, Meskiri A, Sharpe DT, Thornton MJ. Differing responses of human follicular and nonfollicular scalp cells in an in vitro wound healing assay: effects of estrogen on vascular endothelial growth factor secretion. Wound Repair Regen. 2008;16(2):243–53.
186. Stevenson S, Nelson LD, Sharpe DT, Thornton MJ. 17beta-estradiol regulates the secretion of TGF-beta by cultured human dermal fibroblasts. J Biomater Sci Polym Ed. 2008;19(8):1097–109.
187. Stevenson S, Sharpe DT, Thornton MJ. Effects of oestrogen agonists on human dermal fibroblasts in an in vitro wounding assay. Exp Dermatol. 2009;18(11):988–90.
188. Morales DE, McGowan KA, Grant DS, Maheshwari S, Bhartiya D, Cid MC, et al. Estrogen promotes angiogenic activity in human umbilical vein endothelial cells in vitro and in a murine model. Circulation. 1995;91(3):755–63.
189. Ali S, Coombes RC. Estrogen receptor alpha in human breast cancer: occurrence and significance. J Mammary Gland Biol Neoplasia. 2000;5(3):271–81.
190. Kuiper GG, Carlsson B, Grandien K, Enmark E, Häggblad J, Nilsson S, et al. Comparison of the ligand binding specificity and transcript tissue distribution of estrogen receptors alpha and beta. Endocrinology. 1997;138(3):863–70.
191. Couse JF, Lindzey J, Grandien K, Gustafsson JA, Korach KS. Tissue distribution and quantitative analysis of estrogen receptor-alpha (ERalpha) and estrogen receptor-beta (ERbeta) messenger ribonucleic acid in the wild-type and ERalpha-knockout mouse. Endocrinology. 1997;138(11):4613–21.
192. Miller JG, Gee J, Price A, Garbe C, Wagner M, Mac NS. Investigation of oestrogen receptors, sex steroids and soluble adhesion molecules in the progression of malignant melanoma. Melanoma Res. 1997;7(3):197–208.
193. Reed CA, Berndtson AK, Nephew KP. Dose-dependent effects of 4-hydroxytamoxifen, the active metabolite of tamoxifen, on estrogen receptor-alpha expression in the rat uterus. Anticancer Drugs. 2005;16(5):559–67.
194. Mosselman S, Polman J, Dijkema R. ER beta: identification and characterization of a novel human estrogen receptor. FEBS Lett. 1996;392(1):49–53.
195. Cho LC, Hsu YH. Expression of androgen, estrogen and progesterone receptors in mucinous carcinoma of the breast. Kaohsiung J Med Sci. 2008;24(5):227–32.
196. Ciana P, Di Luccio G, Belcredito S, Pollio G, Vegeto E, Tatangelo L, et al. Engineering of a mouse for the in vivo profiling of estrogen receptor activity. Mol Endocrinol. 2001;15(7):1104–13.
197. Emmerson E, Rando G, Meda C, Campbell L, Maggi A, Hardman MJ. Estrogen receptor-mediated signalling in female mice is locally activated in response to wounding. Mol Cell Endocrinol. 2013;375(1–2):149–56.
198. Ashworth JJ, Smyth JV, Pendleton N, Horan M, Payton A, Worthington J, et al. Polymorphisms

spanning the ON exon and promoter of the estrogen receptor-beta (ERbeta) gene ESR2 are associated with venous ulceration. Clin Genet. 2008;73(1): 55–61.
199. Toutain CE, Filipe C, Billon A, Fontaine C, Brouchet L, Guéry JC, et al. Estrogen receptor alpha expression in both endothelium and hematopoietic cells is required for the accelerative effect of estradiol on reendothelialization. Arterioscler Thromb Vasc Biol. 2009;29(10):1543–50.
200. Emmerson E, Campbell L, Davies FC, Ross NL, Ashcroft GS, Krust A, et al. Insulin-like growth factor-1 promotes wound healing in estrogen-deprived mice: new insights into cutaneous IGF-1R/ERalpha cross talk. J Invest Dermatol. 2012;132(12):2838–48.
201. Shu YY, Maibach HI. Estrogen and skin: therapeutic options. Am J Clin Dermatol. 2011;12(5):297–311.
202. Surazynski A, Jarzabek K, Haczynski J, Laudanski P, Palka J, Wolczynski S. Differential effects of estradiol and raloxifene on collagen biosynthesis in cultured human skin fibroblasts. Int J Mol Med. 2003;12(5):803–9.
203. Sumino H, Ichikawa S, Kasama S, Takahashi T, Kumakura H, Takayama Y, et al. Effects of raloxifene and hormone replacement therapy on forearm skin elasticity in postmenopausal women. Maturitas. 2009;62(1):53–7.
204. Mousavi SR, Raaiszadeh M, Aminseresht M, Behjoo S. Evaluating tamoxifen effect in the prevention of hypertrophic scars following surgical incisions. Dermatol Surg. 2010;36(5):665–9.
205. Chang KC, Wang Y, Oh IG, Jenkins S, Freedman LP, Thompson CC, et al. Estrogen receptor beta is a novel therapeutic target for photoaging. Mol Pharmacol. 2010;77(5):744–50.
206. Polito F, Marini H, Bitto A, Irrera N, Vaccaro M, Adamo EB, et al. Genistein aglycone, a soy-derived isoflavone, improves skin changes induced by ovariectomy in rats. Br J Pharmacol. 2012;165(4): 994–1005.

Skin and Effect of Hormones and Menopause

Miranda A. Farage, Kenneth W. Miller, Ghebre E. Tzeghai, Enzo Berardesca, and Howard I. Maibach

Contents

7.1	Introduction	89
7.2	Sex Hormones and the Skin	90
7.3	Estrogen, Skin, and Aging	90
7.3.1	Skin Thickness	91
7.3.2	Skin Moisture	91
7.3.3	Skin Elasticity	92
7.3.4	Sebum Production	92
7.3.5	Wound Healing	92
7.3.6	Skin Cellular Immunity	92
7.3.7	Hair Growth	93
7.3.8	Vulvar Skin Changes	93
7.4	Estrogen and Skin Diseases	93
7.5	Photoaging and Sex Hormones	94
References		94

M.A. Farage, MSc, PhD (✉)
Clinical Innovative Sciences,
The Procter and Gamble Company,
6110 Center Hill Avenue, Cincinnati,
OH 45224, USA
e-mail: farage.m@pg.com

K.W. Miller, PhD
Global Product Stewardship,
The Procter & Gamble Company,
Cincinnati, OH, USA
e-mail: miller.kw.1@pg.com

G.E. Tzeghai, PhD
Quantitative Sciences and Innovation,
Corporate R&D, The Procter & Gamble Co,
Mason, OH, USA
e-mail: Tzeghai.ge@pg.com

7.1 Introduction

Gender-based differences, which occur mainly due to the discrepancy in the sex hormones between men and women, are seen in histology/pathology, immunology, and specific disease conditions of various physiological systems, including the skin, as well as overall quality of life (QoL). Estrogen and other gonadal steroid hormones are powerful biological influences on the skin as well as the central nervous system (CNS).

In the brain, estrogen stimulates growth and repair of neurons and also overall brain function [1]. Menopause, the permanent cessation of menstruation, results in dramatic decrease in the circulating estrogen levels [2]. This depletion of estrogen would potentially deteriorate mental health and function in older women [3]. These effects of chronological estrogen decline on mental health of women are discussed in detail in a subsequent chapter of this book.

The skin is the largest organ in the body and its primary function is protection of the body

E. Berardesca, MD
Clinical Dermatology,
San Gallicano Dermatological Institute,
Rome, Italy
e-mail: berardesca@berardesca.it

H.I. Maibach, MD
Department of Dermatology,
University of California, School of Medicine,
San Francisco, CA, USA
e-mail: maibachh@derm.ucsf.edu

against the external environment. In addition to protecting the body against pathogens, the other functions include insulation, temperature regulation, sensation, production of vitamin D folates, and protection against excessive water loss. Gender differences in basic skin structure not only help us to understand the histological and physiological alterations that occur in dermatologic skin conditions but also explains the pathogenesis of several skin diseases (such as atopic dermatitis). Similarly, gender differences in the immune system justify the variability in the pathogenesis of diseases with cutaneous manifestations and the process of wound healing. Lastly, differences in response to skin conditions, partly influenced by societal expectations and responses to ideals of attractiveness, can significantly alter the QoL among individuals coping with similar severities of identical dermatologic conditions.

Table 7.1 Localization of receptor activity in the skin[a]

Skin structure	Sex steroid receptors			
	AR	PR	ER-α	ER-β
Epidermal keratinocytes	+	+	+	
Melanocytes	+		+	+
Hair follicles				
Follicular keratinocytes	+		+	
Root sheath			+	
Matrix epithelium	+		+	
Dermal papilla cells	+	+	+	
Sebaceous glands	+	+	+	+
Sweat glands	+			
Eccrine			+	+
Apocrine	+		+	
Dermal fibroblasts	+		+	+
Endothelial cells	+		+	

Abbreviations: *AR* androgen receptor, *ER-α* estrogen receptor-alpha, *ER-β* estrogen receptor-beta, *PR* progesterone receptor
+ shows that the receptor is present
[a]Adapted from [5, 7]

7.2 Sex Hormones and the Skin

Molecular studies suggest that sex steroid hormones, estrogen, progesterone, and androgen play an important role in the gender-based pathophysiological differences observed in skin structure, function, and pathology [4]. These sex steroids not only include circulating hormones but also androgens and estrogens synthesized locally in the skin. The expression of sex steroid receptors in the skin varies by cell type and by sex. Nuclear androgen (AR), progesterone (PR), and estrogen (ER) receptors that prevail in the skin facilitate hormone-driven interactions [5]. Testosterone and dihydrotestosterone (DHT) act through AR, which are present in epidermal and follicular keratinocytes, sebocytes, sweat glands, dermal papilla cells, dermal fibroblasts, endothelial cells, and genital melanocytes [6]. Both PR and ER-β are observed in fibroblasts, keratinocytes, and macrophages, whereas ER-α are seen only in fibroblasts and keratinocytes [7]. Also, women have more ERs than men. Estrogens play an important role in promoting skin elasticity and structural integrity of the skin as well as the water-binding capacity of the stratum corneum. Estrogen effects in the skin and hair are mainly mediated by ER-β [8]. In postmenopausal women, estradiol upregulates the expression of ER-β in dermal fibroblasts. Sebocytes, sweat glands, and dermal papilla hair cells express enzymes that convert adrenal prohormones into testosterone and DHT [9]. Sebocytes play a key role in maintaining androgen homeostasis. Also, the sebaceous glands, the outer and inner root sheath cells of anagen terminal hair follicles, and dermal papilla cells express aromatase enzyme that converts testosterone and androstenedione into estrogens [10]. Aromatase expression is much higher in scalp hair follicles of women than men, and it is rarely expressed in telogen hair follicles [11]. The presence of receptor activity in the skin is shown in Table 7.1.

7.3 Estrogen, Skin, and Aging

Intrinsic factors such as chronologic aging and hormonal levels as well as extrinsic factors such as sunlight exposure and smoking levels influence skin biology and skin aging [12]. The normal process of aging of the skin comprises of gradual thinning, atrophy, dryness, skin fragility, and wrinkling. Exposed photoaged skin shows more pronounced signs of aging as compared to the sun-protected sites. With progressing age, the growth rate of hair and nail also slows down. The nail surface becomes rigid and lusterless and the plate thins, whereas the hair loses pigment and the density of hair follicles decrease. Vellus hairs in the ears, nose, and eyebrows of men and hair on the upper lip and chin of women convert to more obvious terminal hairs.

7.3.1 Skin Thickness

The human male skin is thicker and drier than the female skin from the age of 5 through 90. In men, linear decline in skin thickness is observed from age 20 onwards. However, in women, skin thickness remains constant until menopause and thereafter declines drastically. The decrease in thickness of the epidermis is on average about 6.4 % per decade, whereas dermal thickness decreases by up to 20 %. Thinning of aging skin is mainly due to reduction of dermal thickness [13].

Collagen, elastin, and hyaluronic acid are the major extracellular components of the dermis. Collagen provides the required tensile strength. Type I (80 %) and type III (15 %) are most prevalent in the human skin among over 14 types of collagen. Collagen fibers become sparse, thicker, and increasingly disorganized with age thereby disrupting the tension on dermal fibroblasts. In addition, elastin turnover also declines with age. Thus, the skin becomes less elastic, less extensible under force, and more vulnerable to injury by shear forces. In women, collagen content declines at an average of 2.1 % per year for the first 15 postmenopausal years [14]. Women receiving hormone replacement therapy (HRT) showed no such reduction in skin thickness [15]. Also, oral, topical, or subcutaneous estrogen supplementation has also shown to increase collagen content [14].

Dehydroepiandrosterone (DHEA) regulates the turnover of extracellular matrix protein by promoting procollagen synthesis by decreasing the synthesis of collagenase and matrix metalloproteases and limiting collagen degradation by increasing the production of tissue inhibitor of matrix metalloproteinase. DHEA, the primary source of sex steroid production in the skin, declines tangibly with age, resulting in lower procollagen synthesis and higher collagen degradation. Baulieu et al. showed that oral DHEA treatment in men and women aged 60–79 improved epidermal thickness and skin hydration, increased sebum production, and reduced facial pigmentation, with effects being more dramatic in women over 70 than in men [16].

Though the interplay between estrogens and androgens is not clearly understood, androgens are known to affect epidermal hyperplasia in humans, which may partly contribute to greater skin thickness in men and in women with excess of androgen [7].

7.3.2 Skin Moisture

Another important sign of aging skin is dryness. The water-holding capacity of both the epidermis and the dermis is affected by age with no significant gender-related difference [17]. The water content of the stratum corneum, which is related to skin barrier function and the composition and organization of stratum corneum lipids, is much lower in aged skin [18]. Aging fibroblasts produce lower levels of glycosaminoglycans and hyaluronic acid, thereby reducing the water-holding capacity of the dermis [19]. Schmidt et al. showed that topical estradiol 0.01 % and estriol 0.3 % improved skin moisture in perimenopausal or postmenopausal women [20]. Also, a large population-based cohort study demonstrated that postmenopausal women taking HRT were less likely to experience dry skin as compared to those not taking HRT [21]. Estrogen is known to increase acid mucopolysaccharides and hyaluronic acid in the dermis which leads to increase in dermal water content [22]. Also, the higher levels of sebum in postmenopausal women receiving HRT suggest that estrogen may prevent the decrease in glandular secretion otherwise seen in aging skin [23]. Estrogen therapy also leads to increased water-holding capacity of the stratum corneum and a decrease in the rate of water accumulation in postmenopausal women, thereby improving the ability of the stratum corneum to prevent water loss [24, 25]. Estrogen enhancement of skin barrier function potentially aids in maintaining homeostasis [26].

7.3.3 Skin Elasticity

Loss of skin elasticity, epidermal thickness, and elastic degradation results in skin wrinkling. The study by Henry et al. demonstrated that facial skin wrinkling is characterized by an increase in extensibility and decrease in elasticity [27]. Topical application of estrogen results in significant decrease in fine wrinkles and wrinkle depth [20, 21]. The observed improvement in skin wrinkles by estrogen is due to its ability to increase the proportion of type III collagen. The application of estriol ointments to the skin of postmenopausal women also leads to histologic changes of the skin in some individuals. These changes include thickening of the elastic fibers in the papillary dermis. The elastic fibers were also noted to be in better orientation and slightly increased in number. Estrogen causes an increase in the hyaluronic acid in the dermis which improves the water-holding capacity. Thus, HRT seems to improve skin wrinkling in postmenopausal women. However, Castelo-Branco et al. pointed out this improvement is seen only in nonsmoking women and not in smokers. This is possibly due to the side effects of tobacco use, which include a destruction of the ground substance, decreased blood flow in the skin, and direct toxic effects of tobacco [28].

7.3.4 Sebum Production

Sebum levels stay consistent in men after puberty until age 80, whereas in women, a gradual decrease in sebum secretion is observed from menopause through the 70s. Estrogen deprivation also affects sebum production, causing skin dryness [23, 29]. HRT showed a 35 % increase in sebum levels in postmenopausal women [30]. Estrogen appears to increase sebum production primarily by regulating the expression of insulin-like growth factor (IGF)-1 receptors and increasing the production of IGF-1 from fibroblasts. Increased IGF-1, in turn, induces lipogenesis in human sebocytes via the phosphatidylinositol 3 kinase-stimulated pathway, leading to increased sebum production in the skin [31].

7.3.5 Wound Healing

Aged skin is more vulnerable to shear forces due to increased fragility caused by the flattening of the dermoepidermal junctions [32]. In the aged, wound healing is slower to start and slower to proceed. Epidermal turnover slows by 30–50 % between the third and eighth decades and the tensile strength also decreased after age 70 [33]. In general, men show slower wound healing than women at all ages. Wound healing is influenced by the balance of circulating estrogens and androgens and gender differences in the response to the hormones. Keratinocytes on wound edge, infiltrating inflammatory cells, and dermal fibroblasts express AR. Androgens increase local inflammation and promote excessive proteolysis, which depress wound healing [34]. Androgens delay regression of inflammatory response as well as matrix degradation. Induction of tissue inhibitors of metalloproteinases (TIMP-1 and TIMP-2) that promote wound healing is defective in elderly people [35]. DHT also inhibits wound closure by affecting the migration of epidermal keratinocytes [35]. Estrogens are very critical to the process of wound healing; estrogen inhibits inflammation and promotes deposition of matrix components [36]. Estrogen's mitogenic effect on keratinocytes increases re-epitheliazation of wounds [37]. In postmenopausal women with impaired wound healing, estrogen treatment accelerates re-epithelization and local collagen deposition. Estrogen also regulates the expression of macrophage inhibitory factor (MIF), a proinflammatory cytokine involved in hormonal regulation of wound healing [38].

7.3.6 Skin Cellular Immunity

Estrogen receptors are present on nearly every type of cell in the immune system including β cells, CD4+T cells, CD8 +T cells, dendritic cells, macrophages, mast cells, neutrophils, and thymocytes [39]. Estrogen exposure activates ER at the cell membrane to modulate signal transduction cascades [40]. Estrogen produces thymic atrophy and decreases the number and function of thymocytes which in turn downregulates T-cell mediated immune function [41]. Estrogens enhance humoral immunity by stimulating CD4+TH2 cells and β cells. Systemic lupus erythematosus (SLE), an autoimmune disease with a female-to-male ratio of 3:1 before puberty, 10–15:1 during the reproductive years, and 8:1 after menopause, has higher prevalence in menopausal women taking estrogen supplement [42]. Scleroderma and rheumatoid arthritis (RA) are some of the other autoimmune diseases which seem to be affected by sex hormones. It is increasingly evident that women have to cope with the immune-inducing effects of increased estrogen levels during reproductive years and after menopause, increased autoreactive monocyte survival as a result of decreased activation of the Fas/Fas ligand system due to decrease in estrogen levels [13].

7.3.7 Hair Growth

Remarkable gender differences are observed in hair growth, since both androgens and estrogens affect hair follicle stimulation [43]. Androgenic effects on hair follicles are mediated by DHT, produced by 5α-reductase from testosterone. DHT interacts with AR on dermal papilla cells, which causes release of growth factors that act on other cells in the hair follicle. In androgen-dependent areas such as the male beard and pubic hair, androgens promote enlargement of hair follicles, whereas they also cause miniaturization of scalp follicles, leading to male pattern baldness [44]. Female pattern hair loss (FPHL), usually involving the frontal and parietal scalp areas and independent of androgen levels, begins after age 30 and is more prevalent after menopause. Women's frontal and occipital hair follicles have less than one-third 5α-reductase and 40 % lower AR levels compared to men [45]. Scalp hair follicles express six times more aromatase activity in women than in men, leading to formation of estrogen from testosterone which probably acts as a protective factor [46]. Hair loss (alopecia) and hirsutism are two major changes seen during menopause. The most common form of alopecia in elderly women [47] is FPHL. The amount of body hair in women keeps increasing until menopause, after which it begins to decrease. In contrast, facial hair increases even after menopause [48].

7.3.8 Vulvar Skin Changes

Unlike the bulk of cutaneous epithelium, the vulvar area derives from three different embryonic layers. The cutaneous epithelia of the mons pubis, labia, and clitoris, which originate from the embryonic ectoderm, exhibit keratinized, stratified structure. The nonkeratinized mucosa of the vulvar vestibule originates from the embryonic ectoderm. The vagina, derived from the embryonic mesoderm, is mainly responsive to estrogen cycling. Hormonal changes at menopause perturb morphological and physiological changes of the vulva and vagina. After menopause, the vaginal epithelium and the labia atrophies, cervicovaginal secretions reduce, vaginal pH rises, atrophic vaginitis becomes more common, collagen and water content decrease, pubic hair becomes sparse and gray, and the labia majora loses subcutaneous fat. The thinned and dry tissue is more susceptible to irritation and infection [49].

7.4 Estrogen and Skin Diseases

It is a well-established fact that estrogen signaling depends principally on the balanced expression of ER-α and ER-β, and the disturbance of this fine balance leads to neoplasm in estrogen target sites such as breast and ovaries. Similarly, multiple studies have shown that estrogens may influence the growth of malignant melanoma (MM) [50]. The occurrence of MM is rare in women before puberty, rises throughout reproductive years, and then decreases during menopausal years [51]. Pregnancy, oral contraceptives (OCs), and HRT seem to cause changes in pigmentation and proliferation of melanocytes. However, several recent epidemiological studies demonstrate that neither the use of OCs or HRT nor pregnancy seems to influence the prognosis of MM in women [50]. Interestingly, recent immunohistochemical and molecular analyses have shown that ER-β expression is higher in atypical melanocyte lesions and reduced with increasing Breslow depth in MMs, suggesting a role for the loss of ER-β in MM progression [52]. However, overall the evidence of the role of estrogen in melanoma remains in most part inconclusive.

7.5 Photoaging and Sex Hormones

Skin is in direct contact with the environment, including ultraviolet (UV) irradiation from the sun. Sun-induced aging, similar to chronological aging, is a cumulative process. But unlike chronological aging of the skin affected by the age-dependent changes in the hormonal levels, photoaging depends primarily on the degree of sun exposure and skin pigmentation [53]. Individuals with higher exposure to the sun and light pigmentation experience higher degree of photoaging. The emerging information over the last decade affirms that chronological hormonal aging and photoaging share fundamental molecular pathways [54]. Also, the effects of chronological aging are more pronounced in skin areas exposed to the sun, mainly due to combined effect of both photoaging and chronological aging [55]. Oral or topical estrogen therapy have shown to reduce the symptoms of dry skin, wrinkling, and reduced elasticity of skin damaged by the sun irradiations [56].

References

1. McEwen BS, Alves SE. Estrogen actions in the central nervous system. Endocr Rev. 1999;20(3):279–307.
2. Burger HG, Dudley EC, Robertson DM, Dennerstein L. Hormonal changes in the menopause transition. Recent Prog Horm Res. 2002;57:257–75.
3. Birge SJ. HRT and cognition: what the evidence shows. OBG Manag. 2000;42:40–59.
4. Kanda N, Watanabe S. Regulatory roles of sex hormones in cutaneous biology and immunology. J Dermatol Sci. 2005;38(1):1–7.
5. Pelletier G, Ren L. Localization of sex steroid receptors in human skin. Histol Histopathol. 2004;19(2):629–36.
6. Zouboulis CC, Degitz K. Androgen action on human skin – from basic research to clinical significance. Exp Dermatol. 2004;13(4):5–10.
7. Farage MA, Miller KW, Zouboulis CC, Piérard GE, Maibach HI. Gender differences in skin aging and the changing profile of the sex hormones with age. J Steroids Horm Sci. 2012;3:109.doi:10.4172/2157-7536.1000109.
8. Haczynski J, Tarkowski R, Jarzabek K, Slomczynska M, Wolczynski S, Magoffin DA, et al. Human cultured skin fibroblasts express estrogen receptor alpha and beta. Int J Mol Med. 2002;10(2):149–53.
9. Zouboulis CC, Chen WC, Thornton MJ, Qin K, Rosenfield R. Sexual hormones in human skin. Horm Metab Res. 2007;39(2):85–95.
10. Fritsch M, Orfanos CE, Zouboulis CC. Sebocytes are the key regulators of androgen homeostasis in human skin. J Invest Dermatol. 2001;116(5):793–800.
11. Sawaya ME, Price VH. Different levels of 5alpha-reductase type I and II, aromatase, and androgen receptor in hair follicles of women and men with androgenetic alopecia. J Invest Dermatol. 1997;109(3):296–300.
12. Quatresooz P, Piérard-Franchimont C, Gaspard U, Piérard GE. Skin climacteric aging and hormone replacement therapy. J Cosmet Dermatol. 2006;5(1):3–8.
13. Dao HJ, Kazin RA. Gender differences in skin: a review of the literature. Gend Med. 2007;4(4):308–28.
14. Brincat M, Versi E, Moniz CF, Magos A, de Trafford J, Studd JW. Skin collagen changes in postmenopausal women receiving different regimens of estrogen therapy. Obstet Gynecol. 1987;70(1):123–7.
15. Chen L, Dyson M, Rymer J, Bolton PA, Young SR. The use of high-frequency diagnostic ultrasound to investigate the effect of hormone replacement therapy on skin thickness. Skin Res Technol. 2001;7(2):95–7.
16. Baulieu EE, Thomas G, Legrain S, Lahlou N, Roger M, Debuire B, et al. Dehydroepiandrosterone (DHEA), DHEA sulfate, and aging: contribution of the DHEAge Study to a sociobiomedical issue. Proc Natl Acad Sci U S A. 2000;97(8):4279–84.
17. Jemec GB, Serup J. Scaling, dry skin and gender. A bioengineering study of dry skin. Acta Derm Venereol Suppl (Stockh). 1992;177:26–8.
18. Jackson SM, Williams ML, Feingold KR, Elias PM. Pathobiology of the stratum corneum. West J Med. 1993;158(3):279–85.
19. Südel KM, Venzke K, Mielke H, Breitenbach U, Mundt C, Jaspers S, et al. Novel aspects of intrinsic and extrinsic aging of human skin: beneficial effects of soy extract. Photochem Photobiol. 2005;81(3):581–7.
20. Schmidt JB, Binder M, Demschik G, Bieglmayer C, Reiner A. Treatment of skin aging with topical estrogens. Int J Dermatol. 1996;35(9):669–74.
21. Dunn LB, Damesyn M, Moore AA, Reuben DB, Greendale GA. Does estrogen prevent skin aging? Results from the First National Health and Nutrition Examination Survey (NHANES I). Arch Dermatol. 1997;133(3):339–42.

22. Grosman N. Study on the hyaluronic acid-protein complex, the molecular size of hyaluronic acid and the exchangeability of chloride in skin of mice before and after oestrogen treatment. Acta Pharmacol Toxicol (Copenh). 1973;33(3):201–8.
23. Pochi PE, Strauss JS, Downing DT. Age-related changes in sebaceous gland activity. J Invest Dermatol. 1979;73(1):108–11.
24. Paquet F, Piérard-Franchimont C, Fumal I, Goffin V, Paye M, Piérard GE. Sensitive skin at menopause; dew point and electrometric properties of the stratum corneum. Maturitas. 1998;28(3):221–7.
25. Piérard-Franchimont C, Letawe C, Goffin V, Piérard GE. Skin water-holding capacity and transdermal estrogen therapy for menopause: a pilot study. Maturitas. 1995;22(2):151–4.
26. Shah MG, Maibach HI. Estrogen and skin. An overview. Am J Clin Dermatol. 2001;2(3):143–50.
27. Henry F, Piérard-Franchimont C, Cauwenbergh G, Piérard GE. Age-related changes in facial skin contours and rheology. J Am Geriatr Soc. 1997;45(2):220–2.
28. Castelo-Branco C, Figueras F, Martínez de Osaba MJ, Vanrell JA. Facial wrinkling in postmenopausal women. Effects of smoking status and hormone replacement therapy. Maturitas. 1998;29(1):75–86.
29. Piérard-Franchimont C, Piérard GE. Postmenopausal aging of the sebaceous follicle: a comparison between women receiving hormone replacement therapy or not. Dermatology. 2002;204(1):17–22.
30. Shu YY, Maibach HI. Estrogen and skin: therapeutic options. Am J Clin Dermatol. 2011;12(5):297–311.
31. Makrantonaki E, Vogel K, Fimmel S, Oeff M, Seltmann H, Zouboulis CC. Interplay of IGF-I and 17beta-estradiol at age-specific levels in human sebocytes and fibroblasts in vitro. Exp Gerontol. 2008;43(10):939–46.
32. Grove GL. Physiologic changes in older skin. Clin Geriatr Med. 1989;5(1):115–25.
33. Holt DR, Kirk SJ, Regan MC, Hurson M, Lindblad WJ, Barbul A. Effect of age on wound healing in healthy human beings. Surgery. 1992;112(2):293–7; discussion 297–8.
34. Gilliver SC, Ashworth JJ, Ashcroft GS. The hormonal regulation of cutaneous wound healing. Clin Dermatol. 2007;25(1):56–62.
35. Gilliver SC, Ruckshanthi JPD, Atkinson SJ, Ashcroft GS. Androgens influence expression of matrix proteins and proteolytic factors during cutaneous wound healing. Lab Invest. 2007;87(9):871–81.
36. Ashcroft GS, Greenwell-Wild T, Horan MA, Wahl SM, Ferguson MW. Topical estrogen accelerates cutaneous wound healing in aged humans associated with an altered inflammatory response. Am J Pathol. 1999;155(4):1137–46.
37. Ashcroft GS, Dodsworth J, van Boxtel E, Tarnuzzer RW, Horan MA, Schultz GS, et al. Estrogen accelerates cutaneous wound healing associated with an increase in TGF-beta1 levels. Nat Med. 1997;3(11):1209–15.
38. Hardman MJ, Waite A, Zeef L, Burow M, Nakayama T, Ashcroft GS. Macrophage migration inhibitory factor: a central regulator of wound healing. Am J Pathol. 2005;167(6):1561–74.
39. Farage MA, Miller KW, Berardesca E, Maibach H. Sex hormones, the skin and the immune system: interactions and implication for skin testing. Treat Strateg Dermatol. 2011;1(1):62–70.
40. Ackerman LS. Sex hormones and the genesis of autoimmunity. Arch Dermatol. 2006;142(3):371–6.
41. Straub RH. The complex role of estrogens in inflammation. Endocr Rev. 2007;28(5):521–74.
42. Lahita RG. The role of sex hormones in systemic lupus erythematosus. Curr Opin Rheumatol. 1999;11(5):352–6.
43. Paus R, Cotsarelis G. The biology of hair follicles. N Engl J Med. 1999;341(7):491–7.
44. Rebora A. Pathogenesis of androgenetic alopecia. J Am Acad Dermatol. 2004;50(5):777–9.
45. Price VH. Androgenetic alopecia in women. J Investig Dermatol Symp Proc. 2003;8(1):24–7.
46. Hoffmann R, Niiyama S, Huth A, Kissling S, Happle R. 17alpha-estradiol induces aromatase activity in intact human anagen hair follicles ex vivo. Exp Dermatol. 2002;11(4):376–80.
47. Dinh QQ, Sinclair R. Female pattern hair loss: current treatment concepts. Clin Interv Aging. 2007;2(2):189–99.
48. Rittmaster RS. Hirsutism. Lancet. 1997;349(9046):191–5.
49. Farage MA, Miller KW, Elsner P, Maibach HI. Intrinsic and extrinsic factors in skin ageing: a review. Int J Cosmet Sci. 2008;30(2):87–95.
50. Gupta A, Driscoll MS. Do hormones influence melanoma? Facts and controversies. Clin Dermatol. 2010;28(3):287–92.
51. Strouse JJ, Fears TR, Tucker MA, Wayne AS. Pediatric melanoma: risk factor and survival analysis of the surveillance, epidemiology and end results database. J Clin Oncol. 2005;23(21):4735–41.
52. de Giorgi V, Gori A, Grazzini M, Rossari S, Scarfì F, Corciova S, et al. Estrogens, estrogen receptors and melanoma. Expert Rev Anticancer Ther. 2011;11(5):739–47.
53. Fisher GJ, Kang S, Varani J, Bata-Csorgo Z, Wan Y, Datta S, et al. Mechanisms of photoaging and chronological skin aging. Arch Dermatol. 2002;138(11):1462–70.
54. Lavker RM. Cutaneous aging: chronologic versus photoaging. In: Gilchrest B, editor. Photodamage. Cambridge: Blackwell Science; 1995. p. 123–35.
55. Yaar M, Gilchrest BA. Aging of skin. In: Freedberg IM, Eisen AZ, Wolff K, Austen KF, Goldsmith LA, Katz SI, editors. Fitpatrick's dermatology in general medicine. New York: McGraw-Hill; 2003. p. 1386–98.
56. Sauerbronn AV, Fonseca AM, Bagnoli VR, Saldiva PH, Pinotti JA. The effects of systemic hormonal replacement therapy on the skin of postmenopausal women. Int J Gynaecol Obstet. 2000;68(1):35–41.

Effects of Hormone Replacement Therapy on Skin Viscoelasticity During Climacteric Aging

Gérald E. Piérard, Trinh Hermanns-Lê, Sébastien Piérard, and Claudine Piérard-Franchimont

Contents

8.1	Climacteric Aging	98
8.2	Oral and Transdermal Hormone Replacement Therapy	98
8.3	Skin Viscoelasticity Assessment	99
8.4	Variables Influencing Tensile Characteristics of Skin	99
8.5	Experimental Test Procedure	100
8.6	Observational Study on Skin Viscoelasticity During WCA	101
8.7	Summary	101
	References	102

G.E. Piérard, MD, PhD (✉) • T. Hermanns-Lê, MD, PhD • C. Piérard-Franchimont, MD, PhD
Department of Dermatopathology,
University Hospital of Liège,
Boulevard de l'Hôpital, Liège 4000, Belgium
e-mail: gerald.pierard@ulg.ac.be;
trinh.hermanns@chu.ulg.be;
claudine.franchimont@ulg.ac.be

S. Piérard, MD, PhD
Telecommunications and Imaging Laboratory,
Montefiore Institute, Intelsig, University of Liège,
Liège, Belgium
e-mail: sebastien.pierard@ulg.ac.be

From an engineering viewpoint, the skin and subcutaneous tissues correspond to a complex integrated and heterogeneous load-transmitting structure. However, it is almost impossible to ascribe a given aspect of the skin tensile strength (STS) to a specific component of the skin. However, in a biomechanical perspective, the skin is featured as a four-layer organ comprising: (1) the stratum corneum, (2) the combination of the interwoven stratum Malpighi and papillary dermis, (3) the reticular dermis and (4) the hypodermis and other subcutaneous structures.

Over most of the body surface, the major part of STS is supported by the reticular dermis and hypodermis, with a discrete contribution from the epidermis and papillary dermis. For each layer, both its thickness and intimate structure play prominent functional roles. In addition, there are intimate connections between the papillary dermis and epidermis, as well as between the viscoelastic function of the dermis and hypodermis. It is virtually impossible to isolate the dermal properties from those of its neighbouring structures when mechanical tests are performed in vivo. Inevitably, the performed procedures involve, in part, the epidermal layers and the subcutaneous functions. Clearly, the relative involvement of the different tissue layers depends on the size of the tested site. The scope of these tests must be born in mind when interpreting their results.

8.1 Climacteric Aging

Human aging is a physiologic process corresponding to a progressive failure in homeostatic capacity of the body systems. Such a process ultimately increases the skin vulnerability to a number of environmental threats and to certain disorders. Aging progresses differently among subjects sharing similar life duration. In addition, senescence is heterogenous among organs and their constitutive tissues, cells, subcellular organelles and molecular components [1]. Each human organ develops and ultimately fails at its own rate. Any stage of this process is referred to as its own biologic age [2]. Such a systematic aging process occurs everywhere in the body from 30 to 45 years of age. Further regional variability of skin aging is expressed over the body. At any time in adult life, any given body site shows peculiar manifestations of aging. In addition, scrutinizing skin aging reveals a patchwork of aging severity at different tissue levels (epidermis, dermis, hypodermis, hair follicle) and further at the cellular level (keratinocyte, melanocyte, fibroblast, dermal dendrocyte, endothelial cell, etc.).

Woman aging represents a multifaceted darling topic for laypeople, the media and the medical community as well. Any new purported treatment in this domain is avidly watched by anti-aging worshippers. Targeting early signs of wear and tear is indeed common in Western countries. However, from time out of mind, only few novel corrective treatments fulfilled the appealing promises. Beyond new management advances in this field, the forefront in the scientific knowledge of skin aging relies on an increased understanding of the relationships between cell biology, global skin physiology and any perceptible improvement in the ultimate clinical appearance.

The skin represents a hormone-dependent organ [3–5]. Quite distinctly, skin manifestations of some endocrinopathies possibly mimic or interfere with skin aging [3, 4]. Thus, a few direct consequences of endocrine gland aging interfere with skin senescence. They are mostly related to the decline in the activity of the pituitary gland, adrenal glands, ovaries and testes.

Menopause is defined by the initial 12-month amenorrhea following the ultimate menstruations. It results from a permanent collapse in ovarian estrogen production and release, while serum levels of the follicular stimulating hormone (FSH) are pushed up [5]. Some younger women under cancer chemotherapy suffer from treatment-induced amenorrhea. Yet, this condition is not a reliable model for the regular menopausal condition, as the ovarian function occasionally remains intact and possibly resumes despite initial anovulation and amenorrhea [6].

Women climacteric aging (WCA) represents a specific time- and gender-linked part of the global aging progress [7]. It affects all women during perimenopause. Skin alterations during WCA lead to a decline in a number of physiologic functions of any of its components. In particular, the dermal connective tissue is subjected to a progressive atrophy mainly characterized by a global decline in (a) the cohesion between collagen fibrils forming bundles and (b) the amount in non-fibrillar components of the extracellular matrix (ECM). As a result, skin atrophic withering and wrinkling are commonly initiated during WCA. Post-menopausal aging (PMA) is perceived as a late critical WCA phase. Severe cutaneous PMA aspects were occasionally identified in some women. The most prominent signs were featured by progressive epidermal atrophy with xerosis, skin looseness, withering and wrinkling, as well as by altered sebum production and increased hair loss. Many other tissues and organs are commonly altered during the WCA period [8, 9].

8.2 Oral and Transdermal Hormone Replacement Therapy

Oral hormone replacement therapy (HRT) using estrogens or a combination estrogen-progesterone derivative is expected to prevent, at least in part, some adverse effects caused by the decline in estrogens. Thus, HRT has long been used for controlling a series of undesirable WCA ailments and PMA disorders. The high steroid doses administered in oral HRT were shown to be responsible for a boosted release of liver proteins including C-reactive protein (CRP), insulinlike growth factor (IGF)-1, various clotting factors and the sex hormone-binding globulin (SHBG) [10].

Some concerns arose, particularly in the United States, regarding adverse events associated with oral HRT [11]. In particular, a conjugated equine estrogen and medroxyprogesterone acetate combination was reported to be responsible for a discrete risk increase in breast cancer and thrombotic events in menopausal women [12, 13]. However, subsequent guidelines supported the continued use of estrogens at lower doses to alleviate WCA symptomatology [14]. More recently, it was recognized that oral HRT exerted beneficial effects particularly in the absence of any body overweight [5]. In these women, oral HRT reduced the severity of osteoporosis, the risk of bone fractures and the perception of vasomotor instability [8, 15–17]. It remains that HRT effects were unfrequently investigated on the skin despite the frequent skin ailments during PMA [18–20]. Of note, HRT efficacy was not similar in all treated women. Groups of good and poor skin responders to oral HRT were apparently distinguished [21].

HRT has advanced in sophistication by replacing oral estrogen administration while keeping the safety and efficacy in life quality. For that purpose, transdermal delivery of native estradiol is used [22]. Transdermal estrogen therapy (TET) for menopausal women transfers bioactive sex steroid estradiol directly into the skin microcirculation where its delivery represents a close simulation of natural hormonal secretion [22]. In such a WCA management, there is no involvement of a first-pass hepatic transformation or deactivation.

8.3 Skin Viscoelasticity Assessment

The global aging process is associated with obvious changes in skin viscoelasticity. However, the distinct influence of sex hormone deficiency during perimenopause has not been fully explored so far in relation with functional skin changes [23–26]. Normal skin is anisotropic both in its structure and viscoelasticity [27, 28]. In addition, each skin viscoelastic parameter is time-dependent and likely related to the thickness of the involved tissues. Globally, data vary with the body site, the subject's age and gender as well as the duration and repetition of the mechanical test procedure. They are further influenced by the impact of various specific environmental conditions [27].

In recent decades, various instrumentations were used for in vivo skin viscoelasticity assessments [26, 29]. The diverse procedures determining STS included uniaxial and biaxial stretchings, torsion, elevation, indentation, suction and ballistometry tests, as well as measurements of ultrasound shear wave velocity [27]. Objective noninvasive assessments of the skin tensile strength are expected to document the functional impact of both PMA and HRT effects on the dermal ECM. The time-honoured suction method measures the skin deformation caused by any pressure reduction exerted over a circumscribed skin area [28–31]. Skin deformation depends on the suction force, its time of application and the surface area of the stressed skin [28, 29, 31]. It is regarded as a convenient in vivo expression of the overall skin viscoelasticity.

8.4 Variables Influencing Tensile Characteristics of Skin

Skin viscoelasticity is commonly complex to assess and interpret. Such a difficulty is linked to the heterogenous structure of cutaneous tissues. Their physiologic functions depend on two major aspects. First, the intrinsic mechanical response of each structural component is variable within the wide range of different force intensities. Second, the mutual interdependence of the skin components prevents the allocation of any given mechanical response to a specific structure or tissue. In some instances, the comparative inter- and intraobserver observations of subjective clinical STS assessment are not reliable. By contrast, measuring STS objectively is more reliable. However, the biomechanical field occasionally remains confusing because it is influenced by a diversity of factors including body posture, age

[32, 33], cumulative ultraviolet light exposures and gender influences [34].

To add complications, STS is a time-dependent macrocharacteristic during a measurement procedure. Under mechanical stress a time-rate dependence prevails with a rapid elastic extension taking place initially to give way to a second viscoelastic phase exhibiting much lower extension rate. If the load is stabilized for a period of time, further creep or viscous extension gradually takes place [31]. A similar phenomenon occurs when a series of stresses are successively applied and released. Because of the aforementioned considerations, the time-dependent STS depends to some extent on the rate of load application. Its duration and any previous stress history correspond to skin preconditioning at the test site. Unfortunately, a large portion of the literature reporting careful and well-meant work is of questionable value in this time factor.

The skin is globally under the influence of sustained and variable anisotropic stresses. This was initially explored by Dupuytren [35], Malgaigne [36] and Langer [37]. The relaxed skin tension lines correspond to the orientation of the long and straight furrows produced by pinching the skin in a relaxed position. All observations dismiss any doubts as to the presence of intrinsic mechanical tensions in the skin and about the variability in their orientations. They are obviously influenced by the amount of subcutaneous fat and by joint mobility. Relaxed skin tension lines are usually oriented in concordance with joint motion. Their presence apparently depends on subtle tridimensional conformational characteristics in the network of connective tissue fibres. For instance, parallelism between such lines and the main orientation of primary lines seen at the skin surface is present at specific sites on the human body. The skin response to extrinsic stretching forces seems to correlate well with the orientation of the furrows, revealing a close relationship between skin topography and the three-dimensional fibrous structure of the superficial dermis. The forces generated in the dermis influence the skin surface topography so that stretching the skin alters its surface geometric configuration, the fine lines of the skin surface serving as a reservoir facilitating deformation. Marked differences in STS appear when measurements are taken from different surface sizes on a given test area and for different force intensities [38]. The relevance of some measurement designs and their interpretations are occasionally doubtful.

It is noteworthy that the environmental conditions at the time of assessments particularly influence the physical attributes of the stratum corneum which in turn marginally affects the overall STS. Hence, controlling the ambient temperature and relative humidity (i.e. the dew point) is of importance when the tensile functions of the stratum corneum are specifically explored [39, 40]. Similarly, the presence of residual topical products at the skin surface clearly alters the results.

8.5 Experimental Test Procedure

A group of 200 healthy Caucasian women without any past medical history requiring long-standing treatments were enrolled [41]. Eligible participants had a body mass index (weight: height^2) ranging from 19 to 23 corresponding to a normal range for nonobese women in Western Europe. The women were assigned to three age distinct groups corresponding to 50 nonmenopausal women aged 29–50 years (40±4), 75 menopausal women aged 48–61 years (54±3) out of HRT and 75 menopausal women aged 48–58 years (53±2) under oral HRT. The measuring device was a Cutometer® MPA 580 (C+K electronic, Cologne, Germany) equipped with a 4-mm hollow probe. The hand-held probe was maintained onto the skin under controlled pressure. An outer concentric 55-mm diameter guard ring was affixed to the skin by a double-side adhesive film [28, 31, 41]. Adhesive tapes (acrylate or silicone type) were further placed in a crosswise pattern between the outer guard ring and the probe.

A progressive suction modality was applied with a stress-versus-strain recording. It corresponded to a single cycle comprising a two-step procedure involving the successive application of increasing and decreasing suction forces at a constant pace. Under such a procedure, the skin deformation was always more prominent under the decreasing suction than in the increasing phase at the same force [28, 31, 41]. Measurements were performed as single time assessments on the mid part of the inner aspect of both forearms. At each evaluation time, the maximum vertical skin deformation (MD, Uf) corresponding to the skin stiffness was measured following application of a progressive suction force at a 25 mbar/s rate for 20 s. This procedure was followed by a similar linear decrease in suction during a 20-s relaxation period. At the issue of the test, the strain values never returned immediately to the baseline value, and the intercept of the curve on the strain axis defined the residual deformation (RD, Ua). This parameter typically shows an initial limitation phase in elastic recovery. The biologic elasticity (BE) expressed in per cent was defined as $10^2(MD-RD)MD^{-1}$. The stress-versus-strain curve during the increasing suction phase was never superposed to the relaxation curve. The area delimited by these two curves corresponded to the hysteresis loop [24, 26, 28–31, 41].

8.6 Observational Study on Skin Viscoelasticity During WCA

Women sex hormones exert a variety of biologic effects on the skin [4, 5, 44–47]. In WCA, the administration of estrogens alone or in combination with progesterone derivatives prevents or reverses some aspects of skin xerosis, increases the dermal versican-hyaluronic acid load and abates the occurrence of withered skin atrophy and wrinkling associated with WCA. Estrogens are expected to stimulate keratinocyte renewal and to downregulate apoptosis, thus preventing epidermal atrophy. The combination of estrogens and progesterone is expected to reduce collagenolysis through the inhibition of matrix metalloproteinases (MMP) activity, thereby contributing to the upholding of the skin thickness. Furthermore, these hormones possibly enhance collagen synthesis [9]. In addition, estrogens are expected to contribute to hold the global skin moisture by increasing the hyaluronic acid and versican amounts in the dermis. Progesterone is involved in sustained sebum excretion.

Both the climacteric and andropause negatively affect the skin. HRT during the climacteric period is expected to limit some of these changes [48–50]. However, there is a limitation because there seems to exist good and poor responders to the treatments [21]. Smoking habit possibly limits the HRT result [51].

In experimental and routine clinical measurements, various distinct soft tissues such as the skin, adipose tissue and skeletal muscle contribute to the overall mechanical behaviour. Unfortunately, the relative effects of different soft tissues on the measured response remain unsettled. Mechanical properties of skin have been investigated using negative pressure loading in a number of recent studies [42, 52, 53].

The human skin mostly corresponds to a heterogeneous material composed of collagen and elastic fibres. Skin ECM is modelled as a fibril-reinforced tissue [54]. The measured skin responses under negative pressure were globally distinct among the presently identified three age groups of women [41]. The non-menopausal women had MD values lower than both the other groups of menopausal women with and without HRT [41]. No significant differences were yielded in MD values between menopausal women receiving HRT and those who were not. In untreated menopausal women, BE values were significantly decreased, and hysteresis was increased compared to the younger group. A significant hysteresis increase and a trend in BE reduction were disclosed in HRT-treated women.

8.7 Summary

The influence of woman sex hormones on mechanical properties of the skin seems obvious. Some previous assessments in young women suggested an increased dermal hydration during the premenstrual phase [55]. This review focused on the variations in skin biomechanics during climacteric modulated or not by HRT. At present, the effect of TET on these properties is not clearly established by large-scale studies.

References

1. Piérard GE. Aging across the life span: time to think again. J Cosmet Dermatol. 2004;3:50–3.
2. Braverman ER. Ageprint for anti-ageing medicine. J Eur Anti-Ageing Med. 2005;1:7–8.
3. Kanda N, Watanabe S. Regulatory roles of sex hormones in cutaneous biology and immunology. J Dermatol Sci. 2005;38:1–7.
4. Quatresooz P, Piérard-Franchimont C, Kharfi M, Al Rustom K, Chian CA, Garcia R, et al. Skin in maturity. The endocrine and neuroendocrine pathways. Int J Cosmet Sci. 2007;29:1–6.
5. Farage M, Miller KW, Zouboulis CC, Maibach H. Gender differences in skin aging and the changing profile of the sex hormones with age. Steroid Hormon Sci. 2012;3:1000109.
6. Murthy V, Chamberlain RS. Menopausal symptoms in young survivors of breast cancer: a growing problem without an ideal solution. Cancer Control. 2012;19:317–29.
7. Piérard GE. The quandary of climacteric skin ageing. Dermatology. 1996;193:273–4.
8. Li C, Samsioe G, Borgfeldt C, Lidfeldt J, Agardh CD, Nerbrand C. Menopause-related symptoms: what are the background factors? A prospective population-based cohort study of Swedish women (The Women's Health in Lund Area Study). Am J Obstet Gynecol. 2003;189:1646–53.
9. Calleja-Agius J, Brincat M. The effect of menopause on the skin and other connective tissues. Gynecol Endocrinol. 2012;28:273–7.
10. Shifren JL. Androgens, estrogens, and metabolic syndrome at midlife. Menopause. 2009;16:226–8.
11. Rossouw JE, Anderson GL, Prentice RL, LaCroix AZ, Kooperberg C, Stefanick ML, et al. Risks and benefits of estrogen plus progestin in healthy postmenopausal women: principal results from the Women's Health Initiative randomized controlled trial. JAMA. 2002;288:321–33.
12. Chlebowski RT, Hendrix SL, Langer RD, Stefanick ML, Gass M, Lane D, et al. Influence of estrogen plus progestin on breast cancer and mammography in healthy postmenopausal women: the Women's Health Initiative Randomized Trial. JAMA. 2003;289:3243–53.
13. Wassertheil-Smoller S, Hendrix SL, Limacher M, Heiss G, Kooperberg C, Baird A, et al. Effect of estrogen plus progestin on stroke in postmenopausal women: the Women's Health Initiative Randomized Trial. JAMA. 2003;289:2673–84.
14. Seifert-Klauss V, Kingwell E, Hitchcock CL, et al. Estrogen and progestogen use in peri- and postmenopausal women. March 2007 position statement of the North American Menopause Society. Menopause. 2007;14:168–82.
15. Marjoribanks J, Farquhar C, Roberts H, Lethaby A. Long term hormone therapy for perimenopausal and postmenopausal women. Cochrane Database Syst Rev. 2012;(7):CD004143.
16. Eriksen EF. Hormone replacement therapy or SERMS in the long term treatment of osteoporosis. Minerva Ginecol. 2012;64:207–21.
17. Patrelli TS, Gizzo S, Franchi L, Berretta R, Pedrazzi G, Volpi L, et al. A prospective, case-control study on the lipid profile and the cardiovascular risk of menopausal women on oestrogen plus progestogen therapy in a northern Italy province. Arch Gynecol Obstet. 2013;288:91–7.
18. Piérard-Franchimont C, Piérard GE. Post-menopausal aging of the sebaceous follicle. A comparison between women receiving hormone replacement therapy or not. Dermatology. 2002;204:17–22.
19. Thirion L, Piérard-Franchimont C, Arrese JE, Quatresooz P, Gaspard U, Piérard GE. The skin and menopause. Rev Med Liege. 2006;61:159–62.
20. Quatresooz P, Piérard GE. Downgrading skin climacteric aging by hormone replacement therapy. Expert Rev Dermatol. 2007;2:373–6.
21. Piérard-Franchimont C, Cornil F, Dehavay J, Deleixhe-Mauhin F, Letot B, Piérard GE. Climacteric skin ageing of the face. A prospective longitudinal intent-to-treat trial on the effect of oral hormone replacement therapy. Maturitas. 1999;32:87–93.
22. Buster JE. Transdermal menopausal hormone therapy: delivery through skin changes the rules. Expert Opin Pharmacother. 2010;11:1489–99.
23. Piérard GE, Letawe C, Dowlati A, Piérard-Franchimont C. Effect of hormone replacement therapy for menopause on the mechanical properties of skin. J Am Geriatr Soc. 1995;43:662–5.
24. Piérard GE, Henry F, Piérard-Franchimont C. Comparative effect of short-term topical tretinoin and glycolic acid on mechanical properties of photodamaged facial skin in HRT-treated menopausal women. Maturitas. 1996;23:273–7.
25. Ryu HS, Joo YH, Kim SO, Park KC, Youn SW. Influence of age and regional differences on skin elasticity as measured by the Cutometer. Skin Res Technol. 2008;14:354–8.
26. Krueger N, Luebberding S, Oltmer M, Streker M, Kerscher M. Age-related changes in skin mechanical properties: a quantitative evaluation of 120 female subjects. Skin Res Technol. 2011;17:141–8.
27. Piérard GE. EEMCO guidance to the in vivo assessment of tensile functional properties of the skin. Part 1: relevance to the structures and ageing of the skin and subcutaneous tissues. Skin Pharmacol Phys. 1999;12:352–62.
28. Piérard GE, Hermanns-Lê T, Piérard-Franchimont C. Scleroderma: skin stiffness, assessment using the stress-strain relationship under progressive suction. Expert Opin Med Diag. 2013;7:119–25.
29. Rodriguez L, EEMCO Group. EEMCO guidance to the in vivo assessment of tensile functional properties of the skin. Part 2: instrumentation and test modes. Skin Pharmacol Appl Skin Physiol. 2001;14:52–67.
30. Diridollou S, Black D, Lagarde JM, Gall Y, Berson M, Vabre V, et al. Sex- and site-dependent variations in

the thickness and mechanical properties of human skin in vivo. Int J Cosmet Sci. 2000;22:421–5.
31. Piérard GE, Piérard S, Delvenne P, Piérard-Franchimont C. In vivo evaluation of the skin tensile strength by the suction method. Pilot study coping with hysteresis and creep extension. Int Scholarly Res Network Dermatol. 2013;2013:841217.
32. Malm M, Samman M, Serup J. In vivo skin elasticity of 22 anatomical sites. The vertical gradient of skin extensibility and implications in gravitational aging. Skin Res Technol. 1995;1:61–7.
33. Piérard GE, Henry F, Castelli D, Ries G. Ageing and rheological properties of facial skin in women. Gerontology. 1998;44:159–61.
34. Berardesca E, Gabba P, Farinelli N, Borroni G, Rabbiosi G. Skin extensibility time in women. Changes in relation to sex hormones. Acta Derm Venereol. 1989;69:431–3.
35. Dupuytren G. Traité théorique et pratique des blessures par armes de guerre. Bruxelles: Librairie Dumont; 1835. p. 1–66.
36. Malgaigne JF. Traité d'anatomie chirurgical et de chirurgie expérimentale. Paris: Librairie Baillère; 1838.
37. Langer K. Zur Anatomie und Physiologie der Haut. III- Uber die Elasticität der Cutis. Sitzungsber Math CI Kaiserlich Acad Wiss. 1862;45:156.
38. Piérard GE, Nikkels-Tassoudji N, Piérard-Franchimont C. Influence of the test area on the mechanical properties of skin. Dermatology. 1995;191:9–15.
39. Piérard-Franchimont C, Letawe C, Goffin V, Piérard GE. Skin water-holding capacity and transdermal estrogen therapy for menopause. A pilot study. Maturitas. 1995;22:151–4.
40. Paquet F, Piérard-Franchimont C, Fumal I, Goffin V, Paye M, Piérard GE. Sensitive skin at menopause: dew point and electrometric properties of the stratum corneum. Maturitas. 1998;28:221–7.
41. Piérard GE, Hermanns-Lê T, Paquet P, Piérard-Franchimont C. Skin viscoelasticity during hormone replacement therapy for climacteric ageing. Int J Cosmet Sci. 2014;36(1):88–92.
42. Diridollou S, Patat F, Gens F, et al. In vivo model of the mechanical properties of the human skin under suction. Skin Res Technol. 2000;6:214–21.
43. Piérard GE, Piérard-Franchimont C, Vanderplaetsen S, Franchimont N, Gaspard U, Malaise M. Relationships between bone mass density and tensile strength of the skin in women. Eur J Clin Invest. 2001;31:731–5.
44. Piérard GE, Vanderplaetsen S, Piérard-Franchimont C. Comparative effect of hormone replacement therapy on bone mass density and skin tensile properties. Maturitas. 2001;40:221–7.
45. Thurston RC, Santoro N, Matthews KA. Adiposity and hot flashes in midlife women: a modifying role of age. J Clin Endocrinol Metab. 2011;96:e1588–95.
46. Wend K, Wend P, Krum SA. Tissue-specific effects of loss of estrogen during menopause and aging. Front Endocrinol. 2012;3:19.
47. Farage M, Miller KW, Zouboulis CC, Maibach H. Gender differences in skin aging and the changing profile of the sex hormones with age. J Steroid Hormonal Sci. 2012;2:1000109.
48. Quatresooz P, Piérard-Franchimont C, Gaspard U, Piérard GE. Skin climacteric aging and hormone replacement therapy. J Cosmet Dermatol. 2006;5:3–8.
49. Sator PG, Sator MO, Schmidt JB, Nahavandi H, Radakovic S, Huber JC, et al. A prospective, randomized, double-blind, placebo-controlled study on the influence of a hormone replacement therapy on skin aging in postmenopausal women. Climacteric. 2007;10:320–34.
50. Verdier-Sévrain S. Effect of estrogens on skin aging and the potential role of selective estrogen receptor modulators. Climacteric. 2007;10:289–97.
51. Castelo-Branco C, Figueras F, Martinez de Osaba MJ, Vanrell JA. Facial wrinkling in postmenopausal women effects of smoking status and hormone replacement therapy. Maturitas. 1998;20:75–86.
52. Hendriks FM, Brokken D, Oomens CW, Bader DL, Baaijens FP. The relative contributions of different skin layers to the mechanical behavior of human skin in vivo using suction experiments. Med Eng Phys. 2006;28:259–66.
53. Deallau A, Josse G, Lagarde JM, Zahouani H, Bergheau JM. A non-linear elastic behavior to identify the mechanical parameters of human skin in vivo. Skin Res Technol. 2008;14:152–64.
54. Goh KL, Meakin JR, Aspden RM, Hukins DW. Stress transfer in collagen fibrils reinforcing connective tissues: effects of collagen fibril slenderness and relative stiffness. J Theor Biol. 2007;245:305–11.
55. Berardesca E, Gabba P, Farinelli N, Borroni G, Rabbiosi G. Skin extensibility time in women. Changes in relation to sex hormones. Acta Dermatol Venereol. 1989;69:431–3.

Frontal Fibrosing Alopecia

Alexandra Katsarou-Katsari
and Konstantina M. Papagiannaki

Contents

9.1 Introduction 105
9.2 Clinical Features, Etiology, and Epidemiology 105
9.3 Diagnosis 106
9.4 Differential Diagnosis 107
9.5 Treatment 107
References 108

9.1 Introduction

Frontal fibrosing alopecia (FFA) is a form of cicatricial hair loss characterized by progressive recession of the frontotemporal hairline and affects mainly postmenopausal women [1, 2]. However, in the last few years, there have been multiple case reports of FFA in premenopausal women [3–7], and a few cases in men have also been reported [8, 9]. FFA is considered a clinical variant of lichen planopilaris (LPP) that primarily involves the scalp hair over the frontal hairline. It was first described by Kossard in 1994 [4]; its origin remains unknown, but the prevalence of the disease appears to be increasing in recent years [10, 11].

9.2 Clinical Features, Etiology, and Epidemiology

FFA is a clinically distinctive condition characterized by perifollicular erythema, follicular hyperkeratosis, and scarring affecting the frontotemporal hairline. Eyebrow loss is frequently recorded (50–83 % of cases) [1, 4, 6, 7], but body hair loss elsewhere has been less commonly reported (0–77 %) [1, 6, 12, 13].

The origin is unknown, but in analogy with other lichen-like dermatoses, a lymphocyte T-mediated autoimmune reaction appears to play a predominant role in its genesis [14, 15]. Most cases of FFA reported are in postmenopausal women, but there are few reports of its occurrence

A. Katsarou-Katsari, MD, PhD (✉)
Department of Dermatology,
University Clinic, "A.Syggros" Hospital,
National Kapodistian University of Athens,
5, I. Dragoumi Street, Athens 16121, Greece
e-mail: alkats.duoa@yahoo.gr

K.M. Papagiannaki, MD
Dermatology Department,
Sismanoglio General Hospital, Athens, Greece
e-mail: nantiapapagianaki@yahoo.gr

in premenopausal women showing that FFA is not a disease that is exclusively postmenopausal. However, hormonal changes following menopause possibly play a role in the etiology of the disease. Moreover, response to treatment with finasteride suggests that androgens may be responsible in the pathogenesis of the disease [7, 16]. The fact that FFA is becoming increasingly common may also suggest that environmental factors could be involved in etiology [7].

Eyebrow involvement in FFA is common (73 %) [6, 7], whereas eyelash involvement is rare (3 %) [3]. Body hair loss is not uncommon in FFA, a finding that is likely unreported. Alopecia of the upper limbs in FFA is indeed common and histopathologically shows features of lichen planopilaris and scarring, similar to findings in the scalp and eyebrows [13].

9.3 Diagnosis

Histologically, FFA is characterized by a variably dense lymphocytic infiltrate around the infundibulum, isthmus, and bulge regions of the affected hair follicles. Inflammation results in loss of sebaceous glands, permanent destruction of the follicle, and replacement with fibrotic scar tissue. The histological findings seen in FFA are indistinguishable from those in lichen planopilaris and the other lymphocyte-mediated cicatricial alopecia [4].

Most studies utilize a numerical clinical score, the Lichen Planopilaris Activity Index (LPPAI), to assess the treatment efficacy in patients with FFA. The LPPAI has been validated to correlate with clinical responses in LPP and ranges from 0 (no evidence of clinical active disease) to 10 (most severe activity). The index comprises eight subjective and objective surrogate markers of disease activity: pruritus, pain, burning, erythema, perifollicular erythema, perifollicular scale, anagen pull test, and spreading. The index was created by weighing its criteria according to reproducibility and objectivity. Therefore, surrogate markers were measured with the following scale: 0 no spreading, 1 indeterminate, and 2 spreading. LPPAI values are calculated using the following equation [17]:

$$LPPAI = (itch + pain + burning)/3 + (scalp\,erythema + perifollicular\,erythema + perifollicular\,scale)/3 + 2.5(pull\,test) + 1.5(spreading/2)$$

Having been described recently little is known about the natural history of frontal fibrosing alopecia. Frontal recession may progress as far as the mid-scalp and occasionally beyond. Continuance of recession is not inevitable, and in most women it appears that the disease eventually stabilizes. However, the degree to which it progresses before stabilization in an individual patient cannot be predicted. Recent studies report an average rate of 0.9 mm as far as the frontotemporal recession is concerned [15]. It is not possible to restart hair growth where hair follicles have been destroyed, and the aim of treatment must be to arrest the progression of the disease. In view of the slow and variable course of the disease, this is difficult to assess although measuring the distance between the glabella and the frontal hairline may be a simple procedure to monitor the progression of the disease [7].

FFA is currently considered a variant of LPP, but it would also appear that lichen planus associated with FFA is more common than believed. To date there are several cases reported with FFA in combination with lichen planus lesions. A single case is reported in the English-speaking literature in which Faulkner et al. presented a case of FFA associated with cutaneous lichen planus affecting the wrists and feet in a premenopausal woman [5]. Samrao et al. included in their study three patients with FFA, LPP, and lesions of either cutaneous or mucous membrane LP [4]. This supports the hypothesis that FFA is a variant of lichen planopilaris.

Autoimmune associations occur more frequently than expected in FFA. The study of MacDonald et al. included 18 out of 60 (30 %) patients with FFA and associated autoimmune diseases [1]. This percentage is higher than the percentage reported for FFA (16.5 %) by Tan et al. [7] and significantly higher than the levels of thyroid dysfunction expected in general female population (3–10 %) [18, 19]. Miteva et al. reported a case of FFA occurring on the scalp vitiligo [20], and Trueb et al. reported a case of FFA and Sjögren syndrome [21].

9.4 Differential Diagnosis

Differential diagnoses include lichen androgenetic alopecia (AGA), alopecia areata, chronic cutaneous lupus, familial high frontal hairline, and traction alopecia. AGA usually spares the frontal hairline, and it is not associated with scarring, perifollicular erythema, or loss of eyebrows. The histopathologic findings reveal miniaturization of follicles and nonspecific superficial perivascular inflammation [22]. The sudden onset of progressive hair loss in the scalp margin and eyebrows may lead to a wrong diagnosis of alopecia areata (AA). The lack of scarring changes and the clinical presentation of AA are important features to take in consideration. Chronic cutaneous lupus may result in broken hairs, patchy frontal alopecia, and scarring. In these cases, the scalp often shows gross scarring and hyperkeratinization with mottled hyperpigmentation and hypopigmentation. Biopsy specimens with positive immunofluorescence from areas of alopecia in chronic cutaneous lupus erythematosus are important to rule out this condition. A familial high frontal hairline may be present in some women. It usually has an early age of onset and is not associated with scarring and loss of eyebrows, and there is no evidence of perifollicular erythema [10]. Prolonged tension on the hair root from certain hairstyles leads to traction alopecia (TA), which can over time result in irreversible scarring alopecia. This condition is frequently observed among some groups (e.g., African American women) as a result of cultural hair care practices [23]. TA may produce hair loss localized to the frontal hairline associated with a ragged border and broken hairs of uneven lengths. Biopsy specimens show no significant lymphocytic inflammation, contrasting with FFA. Dermoscopy can be very useful in the diagnosis of the disease. Dermoscopy shows absence of follicular openings, perifollicular scale, and a variable degree of perifollicular erythema [24].

9.5 Treatment

Treatments that have been used for FFA include topical and systemic steroids, topical retinoids, oral isotretinoin, topical minoxidil, hydroxychloroquine, and finasteride. In most cases the disease is stabilized with time, and it is not possible to determine whether the disease stabilization is the result of the treatment or a part of the natural history of the disease. Local treatment is generally used in conjunction with systemic therapy or to patients who respond well to systemic treatment as a maintenance therapy. Fernandes et al. conducted a study that included 11 patients with FFA treated with different drugs depending on the stage of the disease. No significant improvement was observed in the majority of cases, except in one patient with a rapidly and recent (less than a year) regressing disease who received intralesional corticosteroids on the frontal hairline and oral hydroxychloroquine 400 mg per day for 12 months. In this case the initial biopsy specimen revealed a predominance of inflammatory changes. After a mean follow-up of 30 months, progression of the condition stopped in ten patients (90.9 %) [14]. This study suggests that early anti-inflammatory therapy could have some benefits in the recession of the disease in accordance with the study of Moreno-Raminez et al. [6].

The study of Samrao et al. included 36 adults with FFA, treated with hydroxychloroquine, doxycycline, and mycophenolate mofetil. Hydroxychloroquine and mycophenolate were initiated in patients with FFA when biopsy specimen showed a moderate to dense inflammatory infiltrate. Doxycycline was given when the infiltrate was sparse. The study revealed that hydroxychloroquine is significantly effective in reducing signs and symptoms of FFA after both 6 and 12 months of treatment. The lack of a significant reduction in signs and symptoms between 6 and 12 months indicates that the maximal benefits of hydroxychloroquine are evident within the first 6 months of use [3]. This study is in accordance with the study conducted by Chiang et al. which demonstrated response to treatment with hydroxychloroquine in 40 patients with LPP, including 11 patients with FFA. The data showed a statistically significant reduction in LPPAI at 6 months with continued reduction in LPPAI scores at 12 months [17].

Racz et al. conducted a literature search in order to find all primary studies on the treatment of FFA and LPP trying to determine the effectiveness of available options for FFA and LPP and to identify promising treatment options for future studies. According to their study, there is currently no effective treatment of FFA. Comparing all the systemic treatments, oral 5-alpha-reductase inhibitors, which were provided more often, seem to be the most effective treatment resulting in good clinical response in 45 % of the patients, possibly affecting the accompanying androgenic alopecia. Hydroxychloroquine resulted in good clinical response in 30 % of the 29 treated patients. Topical corticosteroids are ineffective in FFA, and the remaining treatments were all reported in less than ten patients. There is still an argument whether cyclosporine A could be a good candidate for future studies on the treatment of FFA. Ladizinsky et al. performed a retrospective review of 19 patients with FFA seen at Duke University. A number of treatments, including topical and intralesional steroids, antibiotics, and immunomodulators, were used with disappointing results in most patients. Moreover, stabilization of hair loss was seen in 7 of 10 (70 %) patients treated with dutasteride (2 in combination with doxycycline and 1 in combination with topical tacrolimus and topical class I steroid), in 1 of 3 (33 %) patients treated with finasteride, in 2 of 4 (50 %) patients on hydroxychloroquine, in 1 of 3 (33 %) on methotrexate, and in 1 of 2 on minocycline (in combination with topical tacrolimus). However, the majority of patients on dutasteride experienced disease stabilization, but no therapy was associated with significant hair regrowth [11]. MacDonald et al. conducted a review of 60 patients with FFA treated with several different modalities, none consistently effective. According to their study, potent topical corticosteroids and calcineurin inhibitors reduced inflammation but without clear benefit in slowing the alopecia. The most frequently used systemic medication, hydroxychloroquine, was without consistent benefit, and the number of patients treated with other modalities (tetracycline, intralesional triamcinolone, and UVB) precludes any conclusion regarding efficacy [1]. At the end, another study conducted by Tan et al. is in agreement with previous reports showing that it is not clear whether treatment with topical and systemic steroids, topical retinoids, oral isotretinoin, topical minoxidil, hydroxychloroquine and finasteride stops the progression of the disease or the stabilization of FFA is part of the natural history of the disease [7].

Effective management of FFA would best be established by multicenter randomized controlled trials. However, foreseeable difficulties would be assessment of disease activity and progression, and a prolonged time frame for observation would be required. Until then, management of this fascinating disorder will remain unsatisfactory.

References

1. MacDonald A, Clark C, Holmes S. Frontal fibrosing alopecia: a review of 60 cases. J Am Acad Dermatol. 2012;67:955–61.
2. Donati A, Molina L, Doche I, Valente NS, Romiti R. Facial papules in frontal fibrosing alopecia. Arch Dermatol. 2011;147:1425–7.
3. Kossard S, Lee MS, Wilkinson B. Postmenopausal frontal fibrosing alopecia: a frontal variant of lichen planopilaris. J Am Acad Dermatol. 1997;36:59–66.
4. Samrao A, Chew A-L, Price V. Frontal fibrosing alopecia: a clinical review of 36 patients. Br J Dermatol. 2010;163:1296–300.
5. Faulkner CF, Wilson NJ, Jones SK. Frontal fibrosing alopecia associated with cutaneous lichen planus in

premenopausal woman. Australas J Dermatol. 2002;43:65–7.
6. Moreno-Raminez D, Camacho MF. Frontal fibrosing alopecia: a survey in 16 patients. J Eur Acad Dermatol Venereol. 2005;19:700–5.
7. Tan KT, Messenger AG. Frontal fibrosing alopecia: clinical presentations and prognosis. Br J Dermatol. 2009;160:75–9.
8. Kossard S, Shiell RC. Frontal fibrosing alopecia developing after hair transplantation for androgenetic alopecia. Int J Dermatol. 2005;44:321–3.
9. Stockmeier M, Kunte C, Sander CA, Wolff H. Frontale fiebrosierende Alopezie Kossard bei einem Mann. Hautarzt. 2002;53:409–11.
10. Kossard S. Postmenopausal fibrosing alopecia. Arch Dermatol. 1994;130:770–4.
11. Ladinsky B, Bazakas A, Selim A. Frontal fibrosing alopecia: a retrospective review of 19 patients seen at Duke University. J Am Acad Dermatol. 2012;68(5):749–55.
12. Camacho Martinez F, Garcia-Hernandez MJ, Majuecos BJ. Post menopausal frontal fibrosing alopecia. Br J Dermatol. 1999;140:1181–2.
13. Chew AL, Bashir SJ, Wain EM, Fenton DA, Stefanato CM. Expanding the spectrum of frontal fibrosing alopecia: a unifying concept. J Am Acad Dermatol. 2010;63:653–60.
14. Conde Fernandes I, Selores M, Machado S. Frontal fibrosing alopecia: a review of eleven patients. Eur J Dermatol. 2011;21(5):750–2.
15. Vaisse V, Matard B, Assouly P, Jouannique C, Reygagne P. Postmenopausal frontal alopecia: 20 cases. Ann Dermatol Venereol. 2003;130:607–10.
16. Tosti A, Piraccini BM, Iorizzo M, Misciali C. Frontal fibrosing alopecia in postmenopausal women. J Am Acad Dermatol. 2005;52:55–60.
17. Chiang C, Sah D, Cho B, Ochoa BE, Price VH. Hydroxychloroquine and lichen planopilaris: efficacy and introduction of lichen planopilaris activity index scoring system. J Am Acad Dermatol. 2010;62:387–92.
18. Empson M, Flood V, Ma G, Eastman CJ, Mitchell P. Prevalence of thyroid disease in an older Australian population. Int Med J. 2007;37:448–55.
19. Leese GP, Flynn RV, Jung RT, Macdonald TM, Murphy MJ, Morris AD. Increasing prevalence and incidence of thyroid disease in Tayside, Scotland: the thyroid epidemiology audit and research study. Clin Endocrinol. 2008;68:311–6.
20. Miteva M, Aber C, Torres F, Tosti A. Frontal fibrosing alopecia occurring on a scalp vitiligo: report of four cases. Br J Dermatol. 2011;165:445–7.
21. Sato M, Saga K, Takahashi H. Postmenopausal frontal fibrosing alopecia a Japanese woman with Sjogren's syndrome. J Dermatol. 2008;35:729–31.
22. Whiting DA. Diagnostic and predictive value of horizontal sections of scalp biopsy specimens in male pattern androgenic alopecia. J Am Acad Dermatol. 1993;28:755–63.
23. Wright DR, Gathers R, Kapke A, Johnson D, Joseph CL. Hair care practices and their association with scalp and hair disorders in African American girls. J Am Acad Dermatol. 2011;64:253–62.
24. Rubegni P, Mandato F, Fimiani M. Frontal fibrosing alopecia: role of dermoscopy in differential diagnosis. Case Rep Dermatol. 2010;2:40–5.

Female-Specific Pruritus from Childhood to Postmenopause: Clinical Features, Hormonal Factors, and Treatment Considerations

10

Lauren P. Rimoin, Gil Yosipovitch, and Marilynne McKay

Contents

10.1	**Introduction**	111
10.2	**Prepubertal Vulvar Pruritus**	112
10.2.1	Atopic and Irritant Dermatitis	113
10.2.2	Psoriasis	113
10.2.3	Lichen Sclerosus	113
10.2.4	Infectious Vulvovaginitis	114
10.3	**Reproductive-Age Vulvar Pruritus**	114
10.3.1	Vulvovaginal Candidiasis	115
10.3.2	Allergic and Irritant Contact Dermatitis	115
10.3.3	Lichen Simplex Chronicus and Neuropathic Itch	116
10.3.4	Psoriasis	116
10.4	**Pruritus in Pregnancy**	117
10.4.1	Polymorphic Eruption of Pregnancy	118
10.4.2	Pemphigoid Gestationis	119
10.4.3	Intrahepatic Cholestasis of Pregnancy (ICP)	120
10.4.4	Atopic Eruption of Pregnancy	120
10.5	**Postmenopausal Vulvar Pruritus**	121
10.5.1	Atrophic Vulvovaginitis	121
10.5.2	Lichen Sclerosus	121
10.5.3	Irritant Contact Dermatitis	122
10.5.4	Squamous Cell Carcinoma	122
10.6	**Summary**	123
	References	123

L.P. Rimoin, MD (✉)
Department of Dermatology,
Emory University, Atlanta, GA, USA
e-mail: lrimoin@gmail.com

G. Yosipovitch, MD
Department of Dermatology, Temple University,
3322 North Broad Street Medical Office
Building – Suite 212, Philadelphia, PA 19140, USA
e-mail: gyosipov@wakehealth.edu

10.1 Introduction

New light has been shed on the pathophysiology of pruritus and the various etiologies underlying itch in recent literature, and an increasing number of reports are describing the pruritic dermatoses specific to women. As a result, pruritic conditions in women are being more widely studied, as are the underlying mechanisms that cause female itch. It is important to distinguish between genders when considering the basic pathophysiology and manifestations of these dermatoses. On an anatomical level, the vulva has distinct epithelial characteristics in its different regions that are important to a number of disease processes (Table 10.1). In addition, women have unique temporal hormonal shifts that lead to cyclical changes across the age spectrum in the skin's basic composition.

It appears that female-specific temporal shifts in the expression of hormones and receptors modulate cyclical changes in the skin's basic composition. For example, it has been noted that keratinocytes have estrogen receptors that respond to rising and falling levels of estrogen. Through these receptors, estrogen can directly generate changes in skin hydration, collagen content, and in the concentration of glycosaminoglycans that form the skin barrier and, as a result,

M. McKay, MD
Department of Dermatology, Emory University
School of Medicine, Atlanta, GA, USA
e-mail: mmckayatl@comcast.net

affect the sensation of itch [1]. Downstream effects include changes in vulvovaginal pH and varying microflora compositions [1]. Alterations in pH may be an important factor in the aggravation of itch since increasing pH is known to activate the PAR2 receptor, a well-known itch mediator. Given the extensive alteration of hormones throughout a female lifetime, there exists a diversity of skin pathologies and phenotypes that tend to fall into hormonal-dependent groupings (prepubertal, reproductive age, postmenopausal).

These conditions are known to cause significant discomfort, significantly impacting the quality of women's lives. However, little effort has been placed on studying female-specific itch to date. This is particularly true in the case of vulvar dermatoses, which are often under-recognized and undertreated. Herein, we will examine the causes, manifestations, and management options of vulvar itch in women from childhood to postmenopause (Fig. 10.1).

Table 10.1 Vulvar structures, epithelial patterns, and associated diseases

Vulvar skin type	Epithelial characteristics	Associated diseases
Labia majora and outer minora	Keratinized stratified squamous epithelium	Psoriasis
	Eccrine, apocrine, and sebaceous glands	Lichen sclerosus
		Allergic and irritant dermatitis
		Atopic eczema
Inner labia minora	Nonkeratinized stratified squamous epithelium	Lichen planus
	No adnexal structures	
Vaginal vestibule	Mucosa	Lichen planus
		Vulvovaginal candidiasis
	No adnexal structures	Atrophic vulvovaginitis

10.2 Prepubertal Vulvar Pruritus

From birth to menarche, the vulvar and vaginal epithelium are characterized by low estrogen levels, a high vulvovaginal pH, and a lack of genital lactobacillus colonization. The main pruritic dermatoses in this age range are atopic and irritant dermatitis, psoriasis, and lichen sclerosus. Of note, streptococcal infection of the vulva occurs *exclusively* in prepubertal girls. Finally, poor hygiene, foreign bodies, and sexual abuse should also be considered as causes of vulvar pruritus in this age group.

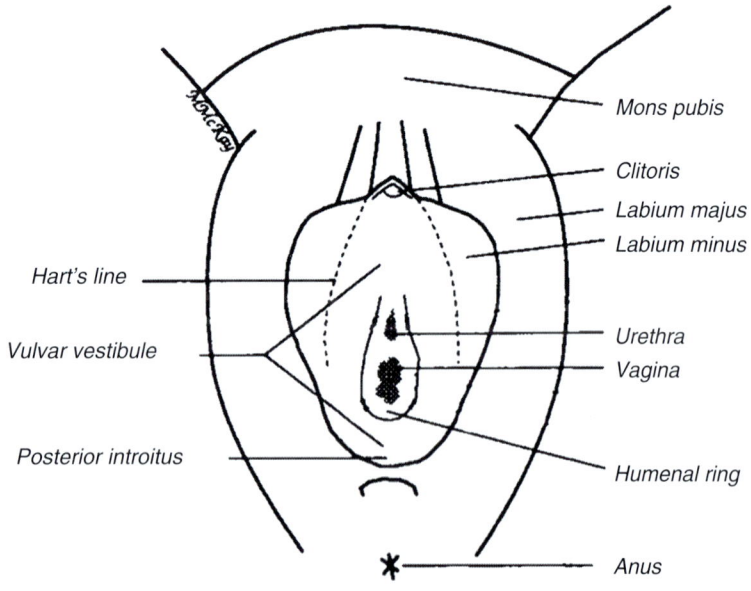

Fig. 10.1 Vulvar anatomy showing Hart's line, the demarcation between keratinized (lateral to Hart's line) and nonkeratinized epithelium (Figure courtesy of Marilynne McKay, MD)

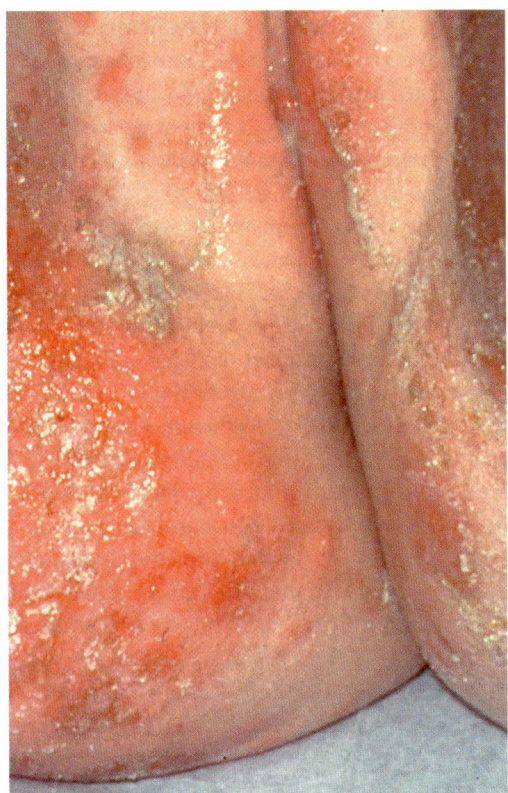

Fig. 10.2 Secondarily infected dermatitis in an atopic child with intense vulvar itching. Staphylococcus and streptococcus were both present (Photograph courtesy of Marilynne McKay, MD)

10.2.1 Atopic and Irritant Dermatitis (Fig. 10.2)

Atopic and irritant dermatitis are the most common causes of prepubertal vulvar itch, and they often occur together [2]. These conditions manifest as fluctuating, poorly defined erythematous patches and plaques involving the vulvar area that are exacerbated by excessive washing and overuse of antifungal creams [3]. The labia majora may have scale and slight rugosity, while the labia minora can present with desquamation and redness [3]. The pruritus is often so intense that scratching is difficult to control. As such, disturbances in sleep and parental embarrassment are not uncommon.

While superinfection by *Staphylococcus aureus* may occur, it rarely yields positive cultures [3]. Management of atopic and irritant dermatitis focuses on the reduction of irritant exposures (commonly urine, feces, soaps, and bubble baths), as well as application of low-dose topical steroids [2]. Secondary skin infections can be treated with topical antimicrobials such as mupirocin 2 % ointment, although more severe cases may require oral antibiotics.

10.2.2 Psoriasis

Vulvar psoriasis more commonly affects children than adults [2]. These lesions first present as a persistent diaper rash in babies. As children age, the lesions become pruritic, well demarcated, symmetric red plaques without scale in the vulvar and perianal regions [3]. When psoriasis is limited to the vulva, diagnosis may be difficult. In such cases, the presence of other manifestations of psoriasis such as nail pitting, history of cradle cap, and scalp/postauricular rashes can help confirm the etiology [3]. Vulvar psoriasis is managed with high-potency topical steroids or topical tacrolimus.

10.2.3 Lichen Sclerosus (Fig. 10.3)

Lichen sclerosus (LS) affects approximately 1 in 900 girls in the United States, with 7–15 % of all cases found in the prepubertal age group [4]. This chronic, autoimmune, mucocutaneous inflammatory dermatosis of unknown etiology classically presents as a white plaque with secondary atrophy and subcutaneous hemorrhage of the vulvar and perianal skin [2] in a figure of eight configuration. Extragenital lesions include pale "confetti" spots, which can occasionally be seen on the inner wrists or elsewhere on the body; these macules are often asymptomatic. The vulvar rash is characterized by severe pruritus, which may lead to subsequent soreness, dysuria, and chronic constipation [3]. The presence of petechiae and purpura can trigger inappropriate investigations into sexual abuse in this age group [2]. LS typically first presents between the ages

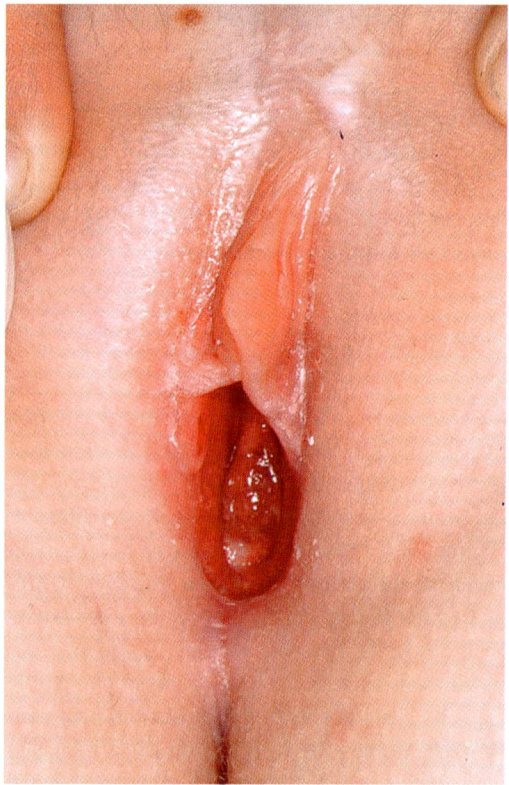

Fig. 10.3 Lichen sclerosus in a 7-year old. Note pale appearance of the inner labia majora with early resorption of the labia minora. Early involvement of the clitoral hood is typical and the perineal body shows early atrophic changes. The vagina is easily visualized due to loss of vulvar architecture (Figure courtesy of Marilynne McKay, MD)

of 4 and 5 years old, but diagnosis often lags for at least 1 year after onset of symptoms [4]. Complications include loss of genital architecture secondary to scarring and subsequent effacement of the labia minora and clitoris [5]. While some pediatric LS resolves with puberty, other cases may silently progress into adulthood. Long-standing LS is associated with a less than 5 % chance of squamous cell carcinoma later in life [6–8]. Treatment of LS includes high-potency topical steroids and topical calcineurin inhibitors with frequent follow-up [5].

10.2.4 Infectious Vulvovaginitis

Infectious vulvovaginitis in the female prepubertal age group typically occurs secondary to group A beta-hemolytic streptococcal infection [9]. Streptococcal bacterial infections of the vulva may present in acute or subacute forms. In the more severe, acute form, patients present with erythematous, painful, edematous plaques with discharge. Alternatively, they may present with subacute inflammation, manifested as pruritic erythematous patches and plaques in the vulvar and perianal regions. Streptococcal infections are diagnosed via culture and sensitivity of vaginal swabs. Treatment includes oral antibiotics such as penicillin, amoxicillin, or cephalexin (if penicillin allergic). Although streptococcus accounts for most cases of infectious vulvovaginitis in these prepubertal girls, more rare infections include staphylococcus, haemophilus, and shigella [2]. Beyond bacterial infections, pinworm is a common etiology of vulvar and perianal pruritus and may be associated with an eczematous rash. Mebendazole is the treatment of choice for pinworm [3]. Although tinea infections can occasionally be seen in girls, vulvovaginal candidiasis does not occur before menarche in immunocompetent patients.

10.3 Reproductive-Age Vulvar Pruritus

With the onset of menstruation, baseline estrogen levels rise and cyclic hormonal changes are triggered, creating a new cutaneous environment. At puberty, estrogen begins to act on maturing keratinocytes, causing vulvovaginal pH to decrease from an average of 7 in prepubertal girls to an average of 4 in adult females [10]. During this hormonal transition, the vulvar epithelium becomes rich in glycogen, and lactobacilli begin to colonize the vulvovaginal area. After menarche, monthly variations in vaginal physiology and pH significantly alter the cutaneous environment. In the first 2 weeks of the menstrual cycle, estrogen levels rise, and vulvovaginal epithelial cells proliferate. In the second 2 weeks, progesterone reigns as the primary hormonal player, and as a result, these keratinocytes desquamate [11]. Cyclical hormonal changes also modulate the bacterial flora composition of the vulvovaginal region. Finally, hormonal pH changes associated with the menstrual cycle have a direct relationship with itch stimulation, as increasing pH is known to activate a well-known itch mediator, the PAR2 receptor [12].

Common causes of vulvar pruritus in reproductive-age, nonpregnant women include vulvovaginal candidiasis, allergic and irritant dermatitis, lichen simplex chronicus, psoriasis, and to a lesser extent lichen sclerosus. Other, less common, causes are lichen planus, vaginal infections, herpes vulvovaginitis, and seborrheic dermatitis.

10.3.1 Vulvovaginal Candidiasis

Most reproductive-age women experience at least one episode of vulvovaginal candidiasis (VVC) in their lifetime, and approximately half of these women endure multiple episodes [13]. Estrogen mediates the colonization of the vulvovaginal region with yeast. Because of this hormonal control, vulvovaginal candidiasis occurs almost exclusively in the reproductive years. Since estrogen levels are highest in the premenstrual period, candidal infections occur more commonly during the second half of the menstrual cycle [13]. Among women of different age groups, vulvovaginal candidal colonization has been estimated to have a prevalence of 11–22 % [14–16]. Certain conditions and medications may increase estrogen levels and lead to more frequent colonization as well as infections. These include pregnancy, antibiotic use, the use of hormonal birth control methods, hormone replacement therapy, and tamoxifen [2, 13–16]. Changes in immune regulation can also cause yeast infections, including diabetes, HIV, thyroid disease, lupus, corticosteroid use, and inheritance of a polymorphism associated with low production of mannose-binding lectin [13].

The typical presentation of VVC includes itching and burning of the vulva, with or without white discharge and vulvovaginal redness. Some patients also experience dysuria and dyspareunia. It should be noted that VVC is largely overdiagnosed in women with vulvar itch; self-diagnosis is poor, particularly in cases of recurrent vulvovaginal symptoms [13]. Diagnosis is usually made by wet prep to visualize fungal elements. However, when wet prep is indeterminate, culture or PCR may be used along with a normal vaginal pH to rule out bacterial vaginosis, atrophic vaginitis, and trichomoniasis [13]. Treatment involves topical or systemic antifungal azoles, with expected resolution of symptoms in 2–3 days [13]. Older proven therapies include topical treatment with Silvadine 1 %.

Recurrent VVC is defined as the occurrence of at least four episodes within 1 year or at least three episodes in 1 year not associated with antibiotic use [2]. These women are usually otherwise healthy and develop a hypersensitivity-like reaction to *Candida*. Recurrent vulvovaginal candidiasis (RVVC) may require a long-term treatment regimen of a weekly or biweekly suppressive azole antifungal [18].

Most VVC cases are associated with *Candida albicans*, although other species such as *C. glabrata, C. tropicalis,* and *C. parapsilosis* should be considered in relatively treatment-resistant cases. In such circumstances, fungal culture, rather than wet mount alone, is necessary for diagnosis [17].

10.3.2 Allergic and Irritant Contact Dermatitis (Fig. 10.4)

Approximately 50 % of chronic vulvovaginal pruritus cases are due to allergic and irritant contact dermatitis [13]. These dermatoses present in a nonspecific fashion, with sudden or gradual onset of itching, burning, and erythema of the vulvovaginal region. The common offending agents in allergic and irritant dermatitis are displayed in Table 10.2.

In acute irritant contact dermatitis, redness can be localized to the area of contact (if in solid or cream form) or may be diffuse (if in water soluble or liquid form). Subacute and chronic cases are characterized by erythema, swelling, and lichenification of the affected area. While vesicles and bullae occur with irritant dermatitis on other parts of the body; they are uncommon on the vulva [13]. New popular types of cosmetic hair removal may make the skin more sensitive to a host of irritants that were previously unknown.

Allergic contact dermatitis of the vulva has a similar presentation to irritant contact dermatitis, but may be delayed or intermittent in nature. Continuous exposure to an allergen triggers an itch-scratch cycle that leads to the development of the typical thickened plaques of lichen simplex chronicus. Medical history is the key to accurate diagnosis. While patch testing is not routinely performed, it can be helpful in certain cases. Allergic contact dermatoses are treated by removing the offending agent, avoiding overwashing, and applying topical steroids.

10.3.3 Lichen Simplex Chronicus and Neuropathic Itch
(Fig. 10.5)

Lichen simplex chronicus (LSC) occurs as a result of chronic rubbing and scratching of the skin. On the vulva, the skin becomes thickened, lichenified, and often hyperpigmented. Various etiologies of LSC exist; the condition can occur secondary to pruritic conditions such as LS or allergic contact dermatitis (ACD). Alternatively, it may be part of a systemic neuropathy or, in some cases, is a primary psychogenic process [13]. When LSC is suspected in the vulvar area, it is important to rule out neuropathic itch associated with sacral spinal compression: a lumbar X-ray may be helpful in identifying possible involvement of the dorsal root ganglia [19]. Other types of neuropathic itch include postherpetic neuralgia and diabetic neuropathy. To successfully treat neuropathic itch and LSC, patients must break the cycle of itching and scratching. This may be accomplished with behavior modification, anti-itch medications, anticonvulsants such as gabapentin and pregabalin [20], and topical steroids.

10.3.4 Psoriasis (Fig. 10.6)

Women who suffer from psoriasis often complain of vulvar itch. In rare cases, the vulva may exclusively be affected [21]. The vulva is relatively more hydrated than exposed skin, and as a result, psoriatic plaques in the vulvar region lack

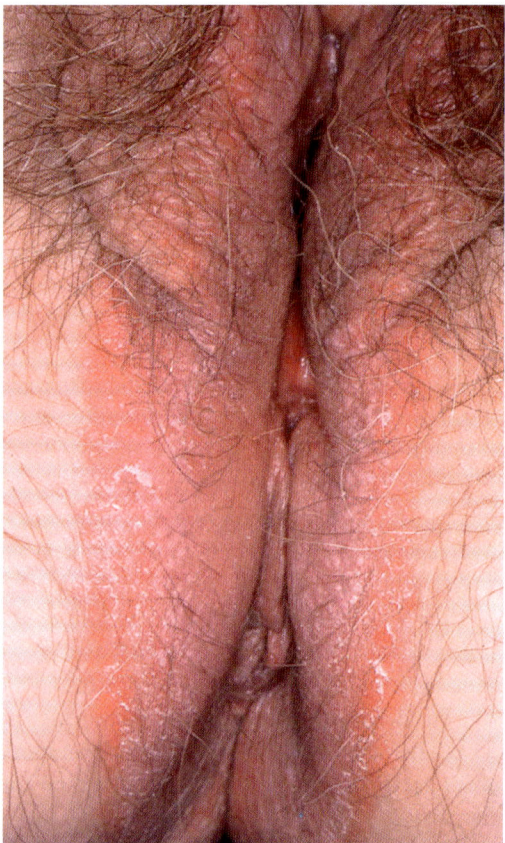

Fig. 10.4 Chronic contact dermatitis due to neomycin ointment. Note that the rash extends into the gluteal cleft and perineal area where the patient applied the medication (Figure courtesy of Marilynne McKay, MD)

Table 10.2 Common offending agents in allergic and irritant contact dermatitis of the female genital area [2, 13]

Allergic contact dermatitis	Neomycin
	Clobetasol
	Benzocaine
	Lanolin
	Dyes (clothing and black hair dye)
	Thiuram (in rubber condoms)
	Sanitary pads
	Perfumes
	Sodium metabisulfite (in topical antifungal creams)
Irritant contact dermatitis	Antifungal or menstrual-related topical creams and liquids
	Harsh soaps and antiseptics
	Urine
	Douches
	Lubricants and spermicides
	Tampons and sanitary pads
	Synthetic underwear

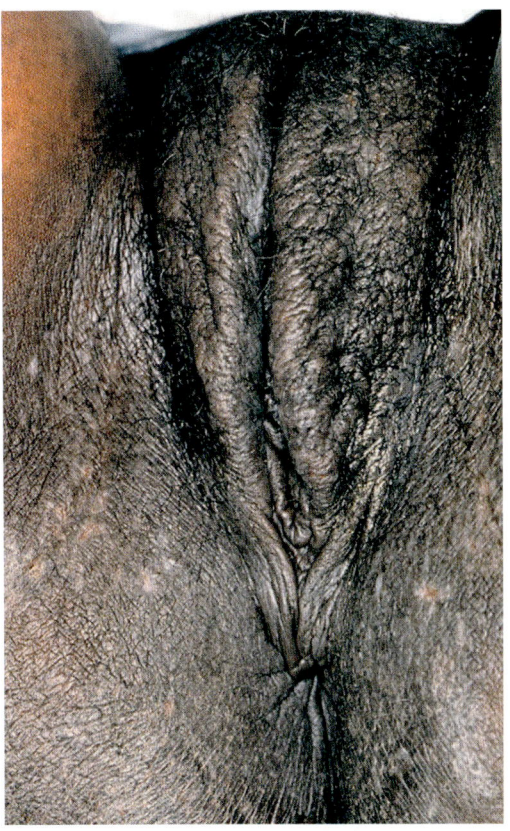

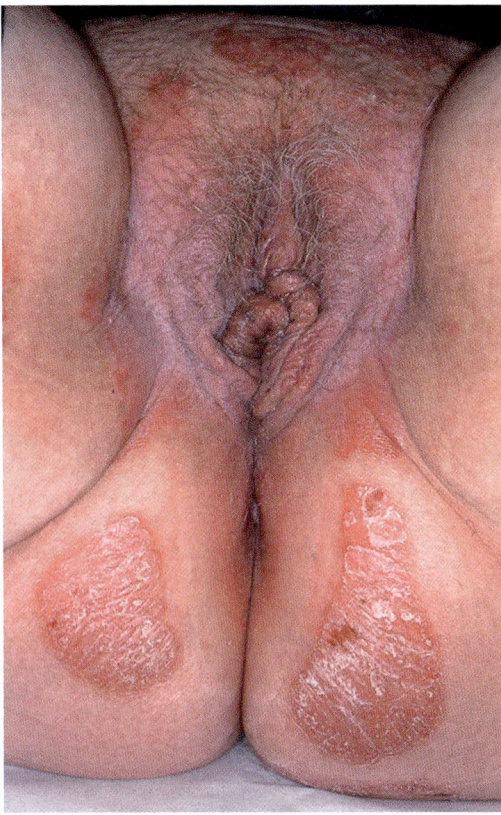

Fig. 10.5 Lichen simplex chronicus (*LSC*) due to chronic rubbing and scratching of pruritic skin. The surface shows thickening with increased skin markings and hairs have been broken due to trauma. Hyperpigmentation is a common finding in black patients with LSC (Figure courtesy of Marilynne McKay, MD)

Fig. 10.6 Psoriasis on the vulva can be intensely red. This patient has typical dry scaly psoriatic plaques on the buttocks, but the vulva appears white due to maceration, retention of moisture in the thickened stratum corneum (Figure courtesy of Marilynne McKay, MD)

scale and maceration is common [13]. Psoriasis affects keratinized skin; as such, affected areas in the vulvovaginal area include the labia majora and mons pubis while the vestibule and vagina are spared. Lesions on the labia majora tend to be well defined, symmetric, salmon pink to beefy red plaques, whereas intertriginous areas tend to appear glossy, smooth, and red. Vulvar itching may occur in the absence of visible vulvar lesions in psoriatic patients. Because of this, diagnosis of vulvar psoriasis can be difficult. In such cases, personal or family history of psoriasis and visualization of psoriatic lesions elsewhere on the body are important [2]. Treatment of vulvar psoriasis includes moderate- to high-potency topical steroids and topical calcineurin inhibitors.

10.4 Pruritus in Pregnancy

Pregnancy is the most well-studied stage of the female lifespan with regard to pruritic skin conditions. While the classic dermatoses of pregnancy are universally recognized by dermatologists, there is less familiarity with the pregnancy-associated physiologic changes in normal skin, as well as alterations of preexisting or acquired skin disease including other dermatoses. In this section, we will focus on the four specific dermatoses of pregnancy: pemphigoid gestationis, polymorphic eruption of pregnancy, intrahepatic cholestasis of pregnancy, and atopic eruption of pregnancy (specific features of these conditions can also be found in Table 10.3). While this section will not focus on meralgia paresthetica, it should be highlighted as a common source of

Table 10.3 Pregnancy-related skin diseases associated with itch [23, 26]

Condition	Presentation	Pathophysiology	Diagnosis	Treatment
Polymorphic eruption of pregnancy	Polymorphous eruption	Unknown	Negative immune studies	Topical or oral corticosteroids
	Urticarial papules within striae distensae	Thought to be due to abdominal distension, hormonal, and immunological factors	Typical histology with spongiosis and superficial perivascular infiltrate	Antihistamines
	Papules and plaques spread to buttocks and thighs			
	Spares periumbilical region			
Pemphigoid gestationis	Pruritic urticarial and bullous eruption	Autoimmune	Direct IF of perilesional skin	Topical or oral corticosteroids
	Pre-bullous stage with urticarial papules	IgG antibodies bind BP-180 in hemidesmosomes of DEJ	Linear C3 deposition along DEJ on IF	
	Bullous stage with tense bullae			
Intrahepatic cholestasis of pregnancy	Exclusively secondary changes caused by scratching	Defect in excretion of bile salts	Rise in serum bile acids level >11 micromol/l	Ursodeoxycholic acid (15 mg/kg/day or 1 g/day qday or BID-TID)
	Pruritus begins on palms/soles and then generalizes	Elevated bile acids in serum cause pruritus	LFTs may be normal	
	Excoriations and prurigo nodules on extensor surfaces			
Atopic eruption of pregnancy	Widespread eczematous eruption	Immunologic changes of pregnancy trigger underlying atopic reaction	Elevated IgE	Topical or oral corticosteroids
	Excoriated papules and nodules			Antihistamines

pruritus that occurs secondary to neuropathy of the lateral femoral cutaneous nerve by a growing abdomen [22]. This condition typically presents with itch over the lateral and anterolateral thigh [22]. Finally, Table 10.4 provides a list of acceptable and contraindicated antihistamines in the treatment of itchy dermatoses of pregnancy.

10.4.1 Polymorphic Eruption of Pregnancy

Polymorphic eruption of pregnancy, also known as pruritic urticarial papules and plaques of pregnancy (PUPPP), toxic erythema of pregnancy, and late-onset prurigo of pregnancy, is a self-limited, pruritic inflammatory condition that usually occurs in late pregnancy or postpartum. This condition is associated with increasing maternal weight and a history of multiple pregnancies. The pathophysiology of this condition is unknown, but some theories suggest that the lesions are triggered by distention and overstretching of the skin, which is why it occurs in first pregnancies and pregnancies in which a mother carries more than one fetus. Early lesions usually present as pruritic papules that coalesce into plaques; eventually, they may become vesicular, targetoid, and eczematous. These papules and plaques typically first present in the striae distensae of the abdomen and later spread to the buttocks and proximal thighs. The rash characteristically spares the umbilical region, unlike other dermatoses of pregnancy. This is particularly helpful in distinguishing polymorphic eruption of pregnancy from pemphigus gestationis, which can otherwise look very similar. Diagnosis hinges on clinical picture and history, and the rash generally resolves within 6 weeks of delivery without insult to the mother or fetus. Recurrence in subsequent pregnancies is rare with the exception of multiple gestational pregnancies. Treatment is focused on symptom control with topical corticosteroids with or without antihistamines.

Table 10.4 Acceptable and contraindicated antipruritic medications in pregnancy [27]

Acceptable antipruritic medications during pregnancy (classes A and B)	Contraindicated antipruritic medications during pregnancy (classes C, D and X)
Chlorpheniramine	Hydroxyzine
First-generation antihistamine	First-generation antihistamine
FDA pregnancy class B	FDA pregnancy class C
Drug of choice, preferred over second-generation antihistamines for embryonic, fetal, and perinatal periods	May be associated with increased risk of congenital malformations
Moderately safe in lactation period	May induce infant withdrawal in lactation period
Diphenhydramine	Fexofenadine
First-generation antihistamine	Second-generation antihistamine
FDA pregnancy class B	FDA pregnancy class C
Second line of the first-generation antihistamines for embryonic period	Adverse fetal effects in animals
May cause uterine contractions with third trimester exposure	Moderately safe in lactation period
Moderately safe in lactation period	
Loratadine	Doxepin
Second-generation antihistamine	Tricyclic antidepressant
FDA pregnancy class B	FDA pregnancy class B topically
First line of the second-generation antihistamines for embryonic, fetal, perinatal periods	FDA pregnancy class C orally
Safest in lactation period	May cause hypotonia, emesis, weak suck with third trimester exposure
	May cause dangerous respiratory depression in lactation period
Cetirizine	
Second-generation antihistamine	
FDA pregnancy class B	
Second line of the second-generation antihistamines for embryonic, fetal, perinatal periods	
Moderately safe in lactation period	

10.4.2 Pemphigoid Gestationis

Pemphigoid gestationis, also known as herpes gestationis, is a rare bullous autoimmune disease similar to bullous pemphigoid but limited to pregnancy. This condition tends to occur late in pregnancy, usually in the third trimester or immediately postpartum. In fact, 75 % of patients flare at delivery [23]. Patients present with intensely pruritic erythematous urticarial papules and plaques that progress to vesicles and bullae on the abdomen. It should be noted that pruritus may precede skin changes. These lesions classically involve the umbilical region but can spread to all skin surfaces (although bullae rarely appear in the mucous membranes). Diagnosis can be difficult in the early, pre-bullous stage, because it often mimics the presentation of polymorphic eruption of pregnancy clinically, with the exception of umbilical involvement [23].

The underlying pathophysiology of pemphigoid gestationis features circulating IgG antibodies that bind to bullous pemphigoid antigen 2 (BP-180) in the hemidesmosomes of the DEJ, with subsequent damage to the membrane and tense bullae production [23]. Diagnosis is made with histopathology and direct immunofluorescence of perilesional skin. The condition is self-limited and tends to resolve within weeks to months of delivery. Pemphigoid gestationis has been associated with a higher risk of premature and small-for-gestational-age babies due to chronic placental insufficiency, although there is no impact on fetal or maternal mortality [23]. Affected women may experience recurrent flares with menstruation and oral contraceptive use. Patients with mild disease can be treated with mid-potency topical corticosteroids and oral antihistamines. If these are ineffective, more severe cases may require systemic corticosteroids (prednisone 0.5–1 mg/kg/day).

10.4.3 Intrahepatic Cholestasis of Pregnancy (ICP)

Intrahepatic cholestasis of pregnancy is an intensely pruritic condition of late pregnancy triggered by cholestasis. This condition is seen more commonly in South American populations, as well as in multiple gestation pregnancies. Unlike other dermatoses of pregnancy, this disease is not associated with any primary skin lesions; instead, patients present with secondary lesions such as excoriations and prurigo nodules from chronic scratching and rubbing. These secondary changes tend to appear on the extensor surfaces of the arms and legs, although patients will usually describe a sudden-onset pruritus that starts in the palmoplantar regions and quickly becomes generalized to the entire body. Jaundice only occurs in approximately 10 % of cases [23].

Intrahepatic cholestasis of pregnancy is characterized by ineffective excretion of bile salts with a subsequent build up of serum bile acid levels. While this condition is relatively harmless to mothers, there is an increased risk of prematurity, fetal distress, and stillbirths; as such, prompt diagnosis and treatment is necessary. Interestingly, a new association has been found between ICP and highly elevated levels of serum autotaxin [24], an enzyme that converts lysophosphatidylcholine into lysophosphatidic acid (LPA) as the active compound. LPA is a very potent signaling lipid that can activate nerve cells to transmit itch [25].

The diagnosis of intrahepatic cholestasis of pregnancy should be made by clinical history and evidence of serum bile acid levels over 11.0 µmol/L. Other liver function tests may not be helpful; transaminases may be normal or elevated, and hyperbilirubinemia only occurs in approximately 10–20 % of patients. This condition is treated with ursodeoxycholic acid (UDCA), which reduces serum bile acid levels to reduce maternal pruritus and fetal prognosis. Given the serious consequences ICP may have on the fetus, close follow-up with early delivery after complete lung maturity is recommended. Recurrence may occur in subsequent pregnancies or with oral contraceptive use.

10.4.4 Atopic Eruption of Pregnancy

Atopic eruption of pregnancy is the most common pruritic dermatosis of pregnancy, as well as the newest classified condition. The new umbrella condition encompasses pruritic conditions previously known as atopic dermatitis, prurigo of pregnancy, and pruritic folliculitis of pregnancy. Atopic eruption of pregnancy is a benign pruritic disorder that serves as a diagnosis of exclusion in patients with atopy; it accounts for half of patients with a pregnancy-related dermatosis and tends to recur in subsequent pregnancies. Only 20 % of cases have a preexisting atopic dermatitis, while 80 % are experiencing eczematous changes for the first time (or have a distant childhood eczema history) [23]. Unlike other dermatoses of pregnancy, atopic eruption tends to occur early, typically in the first or second trimester. Most patients present with widespread pruritic, eczematous lesions generalized to the face, neck, and flexural surfaces of the extremities. A third of patients will alternatively present with papular lesions disseminated on the trunk and limbs, usually with prurigo nodules on the extremities.

Pathophysiology is felt to be secondary to a normal reduction in maternal cell-mediated immune function, tipping the Th1 to Th2 ratio towards a more Th2-dominant atopic state.

Diagnosis is made by clinical presentation. Elevated IgE levels can be seen in approximately 50–70 % of patients [23]. Both maternal and fetal prognosis is good. Treatment with topical corticosteroids is usually effective, although systemic corticosteroids, antihistamines, and UVB phototherapy may be required in severe cases.

10.5 Postmenopausal Vulvar Pruritus

Menopause is characterized by a drop in systemic estrogen and a rising vaginal pH, which essentially returns the vulva to a premenarcheal stage. However, changes in epidermal thickness, skin moisture, collagen content, wound healing, capillary strength, and vulvovaginal microflora distinguish the two phases from each other pathophysiologically. Common causes of vulvar itch in the postmenopausal age group are atrophic vulvovaginitis, lichen sclerosus, squamous cell carcinoma of the vulva, and irritant dermatitis.

10.5.1 Atrophic Vulvovaginitis

Most postmenopausal women are affected by atrophic vulvovaginitis, a condition that tends to worsen with time [28]. Although most women experience mild genital changes, up to half of patients complain of at least one debilitating symptom such as vulvovaginal itching, dryness, dyspareunia abnormal discharge, and recurrent urinary tract infections [28]. The postmenopausal vulva is characterized by thin, atrophic tissue that is easily irritated and susceptible to secondary infection [29]. Atrophic vulvovaginitis presents with pale, thin vulvovaginal epithelium lacking rugae; occasionally, petechiae may be present [29, 30]. Diagnosis is often made by clinical appearance alone, although a swab or biopsy may be indicated to rule out other diagnoses. The treatment of atrophic vulvovaginitis hinges on topical estrogen therapy (rings, creams, or pessaries), which reverses atrophy to premenopausal levels within 1–2 weeks [29]. Other therapies include systemic low-dose estradiol therapy, with the understanding that long-term hormone replacement therapy may increase breast cancer risk [30]. Superinfections should be treated and bland soaps and lubricants should be adopted to prevent further irritation.

10.5.2 Lichen Sclerosus
(Figs. 10.7 and 10.8)

Adult LS is a remitting and relapsing mucocutaneous disease that presents with intense vulvar itch and scarring. This condition affects all ages

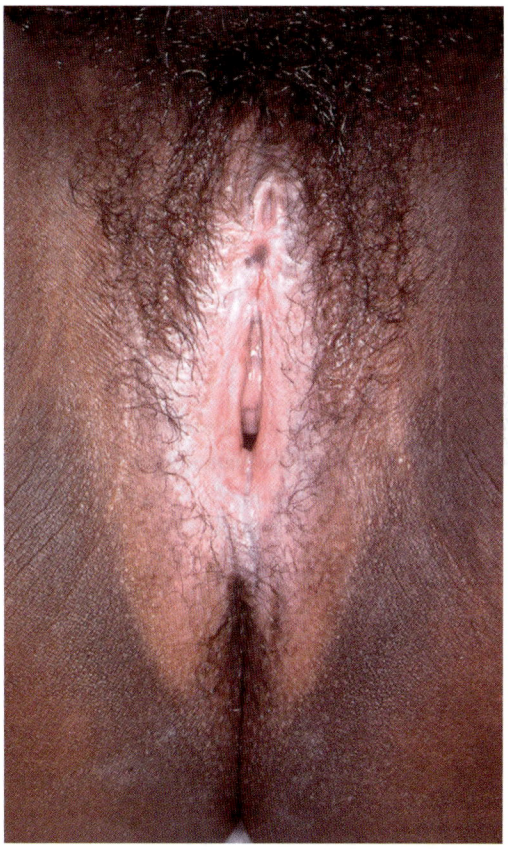

Fig. 10.7 Lichen sclerosus often forms a "figure of eight" pattern of vulvar and perianal involvement. The black patient was refereed for a "pigmented lesion," but this is merely bleeding under atrophic skin

are at increased risk for vulvar carcinoma. LS is treated with high-potency topical steroids to manage symptoms and prevent scarring, which should theoretically reduce the risk of cancer. Biopsies should be performed of thickened areas, as older patients may not be aware of asymptomatic changes. Patients with LS should be closely followed. Counseling is also recommended, as the disease can be quite disfiguring and emotionally challenging.

10.5.3 Irritant Contact Dermatitis

Irritant dermatitis occurs frequently in the postmenopausal group secondary to increased sensitivity of atrophic skin, especially with fecal and/or urinary incontinence. On the other hand, allergic contact dermatitis is much less common in this age group. While postmenopausal pH is already high, urinary incontinence causes an even more potent alkaline environment, which leads to activation of the PAR2 receptor with subsequent increased itching [12]. Irritant contact dermatitis presents as redness in the area of contact with or without edema, scaling, and erosions [30]. Secondary LSC can also occur in the setting of chronic scratching. To treat irritant contact dermatitis, offending agents must be identified and avoided, and protective barrier ointments may be used to protect the skin from irritants. Additionally, low- to medium-potency topical steroids may be used short term, and superinfections should be treated appropriately [30].

10.5.4 Squamous Cell Carcinoma (Fig. 10.9)

Squamous cell carcinoma (SCC) should always be considered as a potential diagnosis in postmenopausal women presenting with vulvar symptoms. Examination may reveal bleeding, nonhealing ulcers, persistent plaques, lumps, or pain and pruritus that does not respond to treatment [30]. Any suspicion of SCC should prompt immediate lesional biopsy.

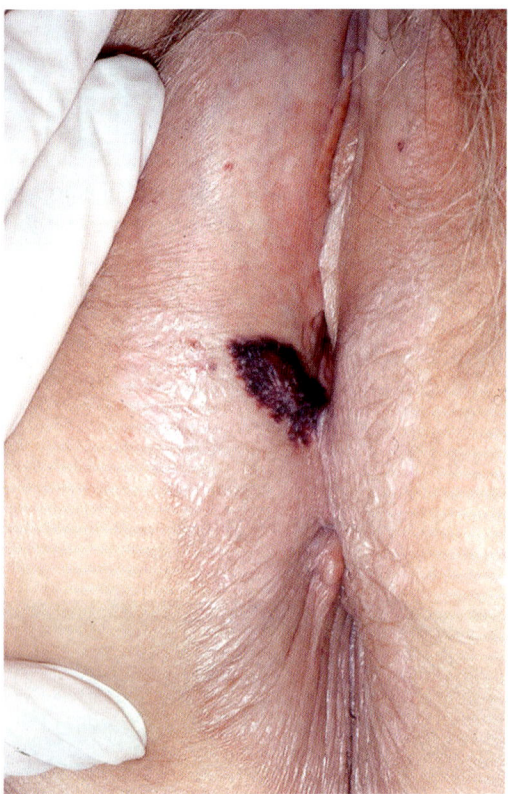

Fig. 10.8 This figure clearly shows marked sclerotic loss of vulvar architecture with narrowing of the introitus consistent with lichen sclerosus as well as purpura (Figure courtesy of Marilynne McKay, MD)

and races, but occurs with a bimodal peak in prepubertal and peri-/postmenopausal Caucasian women [13]. LS tends to occur more frequently in the setting of autoimmune disorders compared to controls [31]. LS presents as white, polygonal, atrophic papules, and plaques on the vulvar and perineal regions. The classic "figure of eight" sclerotic lesion occurs in advanced disease; it involves the introitus and anus and spares the vaginal mucosa. Vulvar architecture is often altered or lost, with flattening of the folds of the labia majora and minora and fibrotic binding of the clitoral hood. Scratching can induce secondary changes such as petechiae, purpura, and fissures. Approximately 11 % of patients with LS experience extragenital lesions on the neck, shoulders, inner thigh, and beneath the breast [13]. Patients with this condition

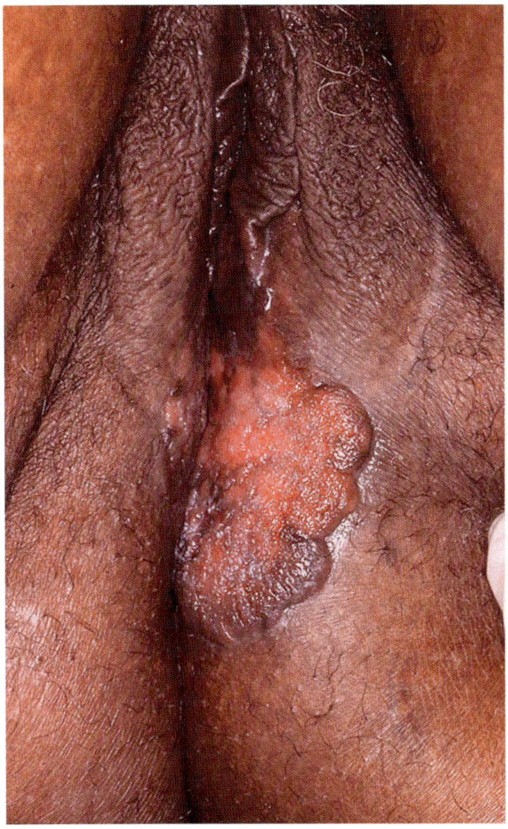

Fig. 10.9 A plaque of squamous cell carcinoma (vulvar intraepithelial neoplasia, *VIN*) in an elderly patient (Figure courtesy of Marilynne McKay, MD)

10.6 Summary

Pruritic conditions in women highly impact quality of life and early diagnosis and treatment can greatly improve morbidity. However, vulvar dermatoses are still underdiagnosed and undertreated.

Acknowledgments The authors would like to thank Dr. Marilynne McKay for providing important editorial suggestions and high-quality clinical photographs.

References

1. Raine-Fenning NJ, Brincat MP, Muscat-Baron Y. Skin aging and menopaus : implications for treatment. Am J Clin Dermatol. 2003;4(6):371–8.
2. Welsh B, Howard A, Cook K. Vulval itch. Aust Fam Physician. 2004;33(7):505–10.
3. Fischer GO. Vulval disease in pre-pubertal girls. Aust J Dermatol. 2001;42(4):225–34; quiz, 235–6.
4. Poindexter G, Morrell DS. Anogenital pruritus: lichen sclerosus in children. Pediatr Ann. 2007;36(12):785–91.
5. Neill SM, Lewis FM, Tatnall FM, Cox NH. British Association of Dermatologists' guidelines for the management of lichen sclerosus 2010. Br J Dermatol. 2010;163(4):672–82.
6. Pugliese JM, Morey AF, Peterson AC. Lichen sclerosus: review of the literature and current recommendations for management. J Urol. 2007;178(6):2268–76.
7. Hart WR, Norris HJ, Helwig EB. Relation of lichen sclerosus et atrophicus of the vulva to development of carcinoma. Obstet Gynecol. 1975;45(4):369–77.
8. Wallace HJ. Lichen sclerosus et atrophicus. Trans St Johns Hosp Dermatol Soc. 1971;57(1):9–30.
9. Olson D, Edmonson MB. Outcomes in children treated for perineal group A beta-hemolytic streptococcal dermatitis. Pediatr Infect Dis J. 2011;30(11):933–6.
10. Brabin L, Roberts SA, Fairbrother E, Mandal D, Higgins SP, Chandiok S, et al. Factors affecting vaginal pH levels among female adolescents attending genitourinary medicine clinics. Sex Transm Infect. 2005;81(6):483–7.
11. Keane FE, Ison CA, Taylor-Robinson D. A longitudinal study of the vaginal flora over a menstrual cycle. Int J STD AIDS. 1997;8(8):489–94.
12. Lee SE, Jeong SK, Lee SH. Protease and protease-activated receptor-2 signaling in the pathogenesis of atopic dermatitis. Yonsei Med J. 2010;51(6):808–22.
13. Farage MA, Miller KW, Ledger WJ. Determining the cause of vulvovaginal symptoms. Obstet Gynecol Surv. 2008;63(7):445–64.
14. Xu J, Schwartz K, Bartoces M, Monsur J, Severson RK, Sobel JD. Effect of antibiotics on vulvovaginal candidiasis: a MetroNet study. J Am Board Fam Med. 2008;21(4):261–8.
15. Ahmad A, Khan AU. Prevalence of Candida species and potential risk factors for vulvovaginal candidiasis in Aligarh, India. Eur J Obstet Gynecol Reprod Biol. 2009;144(1):68–71.
16. Pirotta MV, Garland SM. Genital Candida species detected in samples from women in Melbourne, Australia, before and after treatment with antibiotics. J Clin Microbiol. 2006;44(9):3213–7.
17. Rodriguez MI, Leclair CM. Benign vulvar dermatoses. Obstet Gynecol Surv. 2012;67(1):55–63.
18. Fidel Jr PL, Sobel JD. Immunopathogenesis of recurrent vulvovaginal candidiasis. Clin Microbiol Rev. 1996;9(3):335–48.
19. Cohen AD, Vander T, Medvendovsky E, Biton A, Naimer S, Shalev R, et al. Neuropathic scrotal pruritus: anogenital pruritus is a symptom of lumbosacral radiculopathy. J Am Acad Dermatol. 2005;52(1):61–6.
20. Edwards L. New concepts in vulvodynia. Am J Obstet Gynecol. 2003;189(3 Suppl):S24–30.
21. Meeuwis KAP, Van de Kerkhof PCM, Massuger LFAG, De Hullu JA, Van Rossum MM. Patients' experience of psoriasis in the genital area. Dermatology (Basel). 2012;224(3):271–6.

22. Van Slobbe AM, Bohnen AM, Bernsen RMD, Koes BW, Bierma-Zeinstra SMA. Incidence rates and determinants in meralgia paresthetica in general practice. J Neurol. 2004;251(3):294–7.
23. Ambros-Rudolph CM, Müllegger RR, Vaughan-Jones SA, Kerl H, Black MM. The specific dermatoses of pregnancy revisited and reclassified: results of a retrospective two-center study on 505 pregnant patients. J Am Acad Dermatol. 2006;54(3): 395–404.
24. Kremer AE, Martens JJWW, Kulik W, Ruëff F, Kuiper EMM, Van Buuren HR, et al. Lysophosphatidic acid is a potential mediator of cholestatic pruritus. Gastroenterology. 2010;139(3): 1008–18. 1018.e1.
25. Oude Elferink RPJ, Kremer AE, Martens JJWW, Beuers UH. The molecular mechanism of cholestatic pruritus. Dig Dis. 2011;29(1):66–71.
26. Ambros-Rudolph CM. Dermatoses of pregnancy – clues to diagnosis, fetal risk and therapy. Ann Dermatol. 2011;23(3):265–75.
27. Murase JE, Heller MM, Butler DC. Safety of dermatologic medications in pregnancy and lactation: part I. Pregnancy. J Am Acad Dermatol. 2014;70(3):401. e1–14.
28. Stika CS. Atrophic vaginitis. Dermatol Ther. 2010;23(5):514–22.
29. Wines N, Willsteed E. Menopause and the skin. Australas J Dermatol. 2001;42(3):149–8; quiz 159.
30. Kingston A. Vulval disease in the postmenopausal patient: a guide to current management. Menopause Int. 2010;16(3):117–20.
31. Cooper SM, Ali I, Baldo M, Wojnarowska F. The association of lichen sclerosus and erosive lichen planus of the vulva with autoimmune disease: a case-control study. Arch Dermatol. 2008;144(11):1432–5.

Gender Differences in Production and Circulating Levels of Sex Hormones and Their Impact on Aging Skin

11

Miranda A. Farage, Kenneth W. Miller, Christos C. Zouboulis, Gérald E. Piérard, and Howard I. Maibach

Contents

11.1	Introduction	125
11.2	Sources of the Sex Steroids	126
11.3	**Age-Related Changes in the Sex Steroids**	126
11.3.1	Changes in Prohormone and Androgen Production	126
11.3.2	Changes in Estrogen Production	131
11.3.3	Intracrine Production of the Sex Steroids	132
11.3.4	Sex Steroid Receptor Localization in the Skin	133
11.4	**Effects of Sex Hormones on the Structure, Characteristics, and Physiology of Aging Skin**	133
11.4.1	Skin Structure and Thickness	136
11.4.2	Wrinkles	137
11.4.3	Skin Barrier Function	138
11.4.4	Skin Moisture and Water-Holding Capacity	138
11.4.5	Sweating and Thermoregulation	139
11.4.6	Sebum Production	139
11.4.7	Hair Growth	140
11.4.8	Wound Healing	141
11.5	**Summary**	142
References		143

M.A. Farage, MSc, PhD (✉)
Clinical Innovative Sciences,
The Procter and Gamble Company,
6110 Center Hill Avenue,
Cincinnati, OH 45224, USA
e-mail: farage.m@pg.com

K.W. Miller, PhD
Global Product Stewardship,
The Procter & Gamble Company,
Cincinnati, OH USA
e-mail: miller.kw.1@pg.com

C.C. Zouboulis, MD
Departments of Dermatology, Venereology,
Allergology and Immunology, Dessau Medical Center, Dessau, Saxony-Anhalt, Germany
e-mail: christos.zouboulis@gmx.de

G.E. Piérard, MD, PhD
Department of Dermatopathology,
University Hospital of Liege, Liege, Belgium
e-mail: gerald.pierard@ulg.ac.be

H.I. Maibach, MD
Department of Dermatology,
University of California, School of Medicine,
San Francisco, CA, USA
e-mail: MaibachH@derm.ucsf.edu

11.1 Introduction

Endocrine function changes with age. Three endocrine systems affect skin aging: the hypothalamic-pituitary-gonadal axis, which affects gonadal production of the sex steroids; the adrenals, which produce the sex hormone precursor dehydroepiandrosterone (DHEA); and the growth hormone (GH)/insulin-like growth factor I (IGF-I) axis, which affects GH production and IGF-I release by

---

A version of this chapter appeared as an open-access article by Farage et al., *Journal of Steroids Hormonal Science* 2012, 3:2, (OMICS Publishing Group, www.omicsonline.org) http://dx.doi.org/10.4172/2157-7536.1000109 and is reproduced under the terms of the Creative Commons Attribution License.

systemic organs such as the liver. Changes in gonadal, adrenal, and peripheral production of the sex hormones impacts skin physiology [1]. This review focuses on gonadal, adrenal, and intracrine sources of the sex hormones and the impact of age-related changes in these hormones on the skin.

11.2 Sources of the Sex Steroids

Sex steroids are produced by the gonads, the adrenals, and by peripheral tissues. The ovaries are a primary source of estradiol in younger women and the testes a primary source of testosterone in younger men. Estrogens and androgens produced by the gonads enter the circulation for transport to distant target sites. The adrenals secrete inactive prohormones, DHEA and androstenedione, that serve as precursors of androgens and estrogens produced in peripheral tissues.

DHEA and its sulfate form, DHEAS (interconvertible by extra-adrenal sulfotransferase and sulfatase activity), are the most abundant sex steroids in plasma. Plasma DHEAS levels in adult men and women are 100–500 times higher than those of testosterone and 1,000–10,000 times higher than those of estradiol (Table 11.1). Circulating DHEA and DHEAS form a reservoir of prohormones for peripheral conversion to active androgens (testosterone and 5α-dihydrotestosterone (DHT)) and estrogens (estradiol, E2, and estrone, E1) (Fig. 11.1). The hydroxysteroid dehydrogenases transform DHEA into androstenediol and androstenedione, precursors of testosterone. Tissue aromatization of androstenedione and testosterone gives rise to estrone and estradiol, respectively. Only testosterone and its highly potent metabolite, dihydrotestosterone, have direct receptor-mediated androgenic activity [17]. Estradiol, which exerts its effects through interaction with nuclear and membrane-bound receptors, is the more potent estrogen.

The action of sex steroids on target tissue depends both on circulating levels and on local formation within the tissue itself (Fig. 11.2). Androgens and estrogens produced within tissues can act on neighboring cells (paracrine activity) or within the same cells (intracrine activity). Sex steroids produced in peripheral tissues (such as adipose tissue) also enter the circulation, and this source becomes especially significant as gonadal production declines with age. In postmenopausal women, for example, peripherally synthesized estrone is the primary source of estrogen. In men aged 60–75, adrenal DHEA contributes about 40 % to the total pool of androgens [18]. In older men and women, comparable amounts of sex steroids are synthesized outside the gonads [8, 18]: using circulating DHT metabolites as a measure, it is estimated that postmenopausal women synthesize almost half as much androgen as men of similar age, the excess in men being attributable to testicular origin [13].

11.3 Age-Related Changes in the Sex Steroids

Overall trends in circulating levels of sex hormones in aging men and women are summarized in Table 11.2. Factors affecting circulating levels of prohormones, androgens, and estrogens in each sex are described below.

11.3.1 Changes in Prohormone and Androgen Production

Production of DHEA and DHEAS begins during adrenarche. Serum concentrations of DHEAS reach their peak (in the order of 10^{-8} and 10^{-6} M, respectively) between the ages of 20 and 30 years [8]. Then DHEAS concentrations decline with age, being reduced to 20 % of peak levels by age 70 and 5 % of peak levels by age 90 [4, 6, 19–21]. Because DHEAS and DHEA serve as sex steroid precursors in peripheral tissue, this decline in circulating levels is thought to contribute to some of the degenerative changes seen with aging.

Gender differences exist in serum concentrations of these hormones (see Table 11.1). Circulating levels of DHEAS in adult women are consistently lower than those in men at all ages [20, 22, 23]. The decline in these prohormones is clinically important in both sexes, but especially so in women. In men, gonadal androgen production

Table 11.1 Serum concentrations of the sex hormones by age and gender

Hormone or binding protein	Younger adults				Older adults			
	Men	Reference	Women (premenopause)	Reference	Men	Reference	Women (postmenopause)	Reference
DHEAS	≈12 µmol/L Age 20 years	Labrie et al. [2]	≈6 µmol/L Age 20 years	Labrie et al. [2]	≈3 µmol/L Age 60 years	Labrie et al. [2]	≈1.5 µmol/L Age 60 years	Labrie et al. [2]
	8.5 µmol/L	Ravaglia et al. [3]	7.7 µmol/L	Ravaglia et al. [3]	1.5 µmol/L	Ravaglia et al. [3]	1.0 µmol/L	Ravaglia et al. [3]
	(3110 ng/mL) Age <40 years		(2,824 ng/mL) Age <40 years		(551 ng/mL) Age 90–99		(364 ng/mL) Age 90–99	Age 90–99
	7.0±4.0 µmol/L (2,600±1,500 ng/mL) Ages 40–70	Feldman et al. [4]	3.64 µmol/L (95 % CI 1.6–1.72)	Feldman et al. [4]	4.3±2.7 µmol/L (1,600±1,000 ng/mL)	Kaaks et al. [5]	1.9 nmol/L (95 % CI 0.8–4.4)	Burger et al. [6]
					Ages 46–80		Median age, 54	
DHEA	20–25 nmol/L Ages 20–30	Burger [7]	20–27 nmol/L	Burger [7]	4–6 nmol/L Ages 50–80	Labrie et al. [8]	6–7 nmol/L	Labrie et al. [8]
Total testosterone	13–40 nmol/L Age 30	Harman et al. [9]	0.6–2.5 nmol/L (0.2–0.7 ng/mL) Age unspecified	Harman et al. [9]	6–26 nmol/L Age 80	Harman et al. [9]	0.56±0.26 nmol/L Ages 50–89	Laughlin et al. [10]
	18.0±6.1 nmol/L (5.2±1.8 ng/mL) Ages 40–70	Feldman et al. [4]	1.66 nmol/L (95 % CI 1.6–1.72) Age <50	Feldman et al. [4]	15.7±5.6 nmol/L (4.5±1.6 ng/mL) Ages 46–80	Feldman et al. [4]	1.4 nmol/L (95 % CI 0.6–2.4) Median age, 54	Burger et al. [6]
	22±7 nmol/L	Gapstur et al. [11]	1.2±0.7 nmol/L	Sinha-Hikim et al. [12]	15.8±0.17 nmol/L (4.57±0.05 ng/mL) Ages 69–80	Labrie et al. [13]	0.5±0.01 nmol/L (0.14±0.004 ng/mL) Ages 55–65	Labrie et al. [13]
Free testosterone	0.097±0.039 ng/mL (0.34±0.14 nmol/L) Ages 40–70	Feldman et al. [4]	12.8±5.5 pmol/L	Sinha-Hikim et al. [12]	0.075±0.032 ng/mL (0.26±0.11 nmol/L) Ages 46–80	Feldman et al. [4]	0.14±0.07 nmol/L Ages 50–89	Laughlin et al. [10]
DHT	0.91±0.58 nmol/L (0.26±0.17 ng/mL) Ages 40–70	Feldman et al. [4]	0.43 nmol/L (0.12 ng/mL) Ages 30–49	Secreto et al. [14]	1.19±0.70 nmol/L (0.35±0.20 ng/mL)	Feldman et al. [4]	0.22±0.11 nmol/L (62.4±32 pg/mL) Age ≤69	Secreto et al. [15]

(continued)

Table 11.1 (continued)

Hormone or binding protein	Younger adults						Older adults					
	Men	Reference	Women (premenopause)	Reference			Men	Reference	Women (postmenopause)	Reference		
SHBG	32±16 nmol/L Ages 40–70	Feldman et al. [4]	53.1 nmol/L (95 % CI 50.7–50.5) Age <50	Kaaks et al. [5]			32±16 nmol/L Ages 46–80	Feldman et al. [4]	50.5 nmol/L (95 % CI 21.0–99.8) Median age, 54	Burger et al. [6]		
Estradiol	84.0±22.4 pmol/L Ages 24–31	Vermeulen et al. [16]	381 pmol/L (95 % CI 356–407.6)	Kaaks et al. [5]			88.1±24.6 pmol/L Ages 70–79	Vermeulen et al. [16]	18±9 pmol/L Ages 50–89	Laughlin et al. [10]		
	81.5±23.1 pmol/L Ages 37–46	Vermeulen et al. [16]					79.0±1.1 pmol/L (21.5±0.3 pg/mL) Ages 69–80	Labrie et al. [13]	15.4±0.7 pmol/L (4.2±0.2 pg/mL) Ages 55–65	Labrie et al. [13]		
Estrone	156±75 pmol/L Ages 40–70	Feldman et al. [4]	409.9 pmol/L (95 % CI 383.4–436.4)	Kaaks et al. [5]			124±78 pmol/L Ages 46–80	Feldman et al. [4]	70±34 pmol/L Ages 50–89	Labrie et al. [13]		
							139±2 pmol/L Ages 69–80	Labrie et al. [13]	65.9±1.8 pmol/L Ages 55–65	Labrie et al. [13]		

11 Gender Differences in Production and Circulating Levels of Sex Hormones

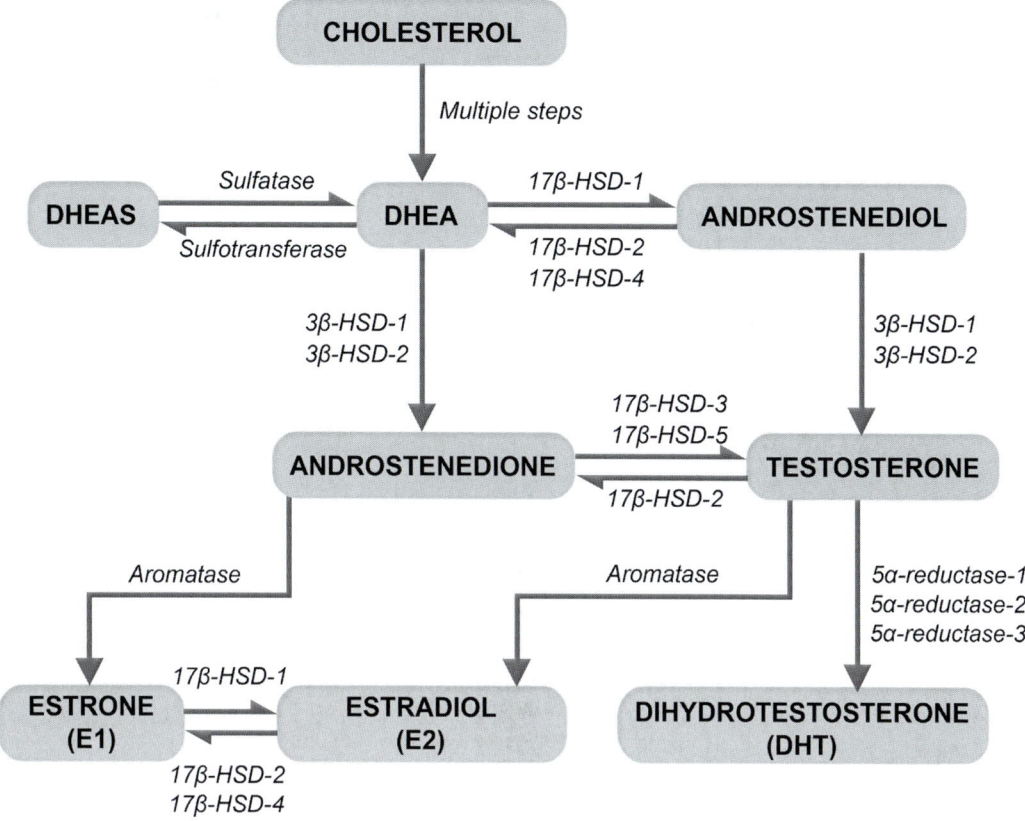

Fig. 11.1 Production of sex steroids from the adrenal precursors, dehydroepiandrosterone (*DHEA*) and its sulfate form (*DHEAS*). DHEA, an inactive prohormone, is produced by the adrenal glands from cholesterol. DHEA and DHEAS are interconvertible by the actions of sulfatases and sulfotransferases. In peripheral tissues, the hydroxysteroid dehydrogenases (*HSD*) convert DHEA to androstenedione and androstenediol, precursors of testosterone. The action of 5α-reductases converts testosterone to its potent metabolite, dihydrotestosterone (*DHT*). Aromatases produce estrogens by converting testosterone to estradiol and androstenedione to estrone

declines slowly, such that peripheral production of contributes some 40 % to the total androgen pool in men by age 65 [18]. By contrast, in postmenopausal women, DHEA is the exclusive source of sex steroids for all tissues except the uterus [18]. Nevertheless, large variability exists in the circulating levels of DHEA among women: an almost eightfold difference between high and low levels has been found [24], with the low end being barely detectable. This wide range could help explain why some older women experience fewer signs of hormone deficiency after menopause, while others experience significant signs and symptoms [24].

About 30–50 % of total androgens in adult men [25] and about 50–100 % in adult women, depending on age, are derived from DHEA and DHEAS [26]. In women, androstenedione levels decline with age up to menopause, remain fairly stable in the early years after menopause [10, 27], and then decline by about 20 % by 30 years after menopause [10]. Early studies suggested that the postmenopausal ovary was a source of androgens [26], but this is controversial. Recent studies indicate that expression of steroidogenic enzymes by the postmenopausal ovary is limited [28, 29], and that, absent the adrenal production, postmenopausal women have no detectable circulating androgens [30].

Testosterone and its highly potent metabolite, dihydrotestosterone (DHT), exert receptor-mediated activity. About 1–2 % of circulating testosterone is free, 32 % loosely bound to albumin,

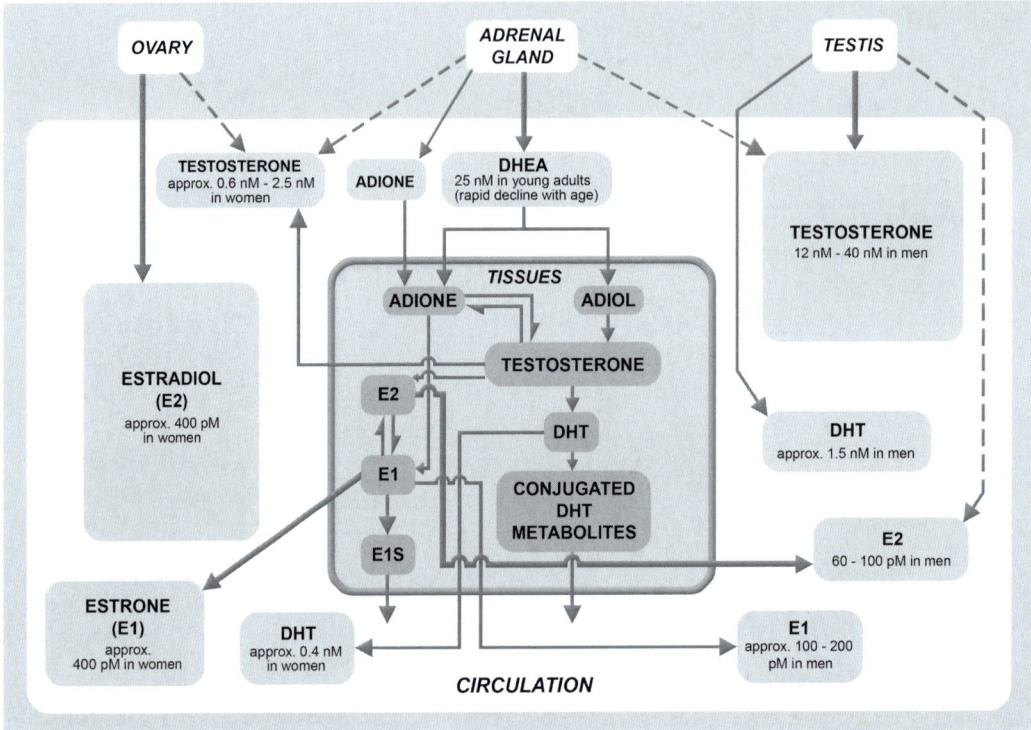

Fig. 11.2 Sources of the sex steroids in young men and women. Sex hormones are produced by the gonads, the adrenals, and by peripheral tissues. The ovary, adrenal gland, and testis are shown at the top of the chart. The *white box* in the central field denotes the circulatory compartment. The left side of the circulatory compartment below the ovary shows circulating levels of the sex hormones in young women; the right side of the circulatory compartment, below the testis, shows circulating levels of sex hormones in young men. The *gray box with a bold border* below the adrenal gland denotes the peripheral tissue compartment and illustrates peripheral conversion of the adrenal prohormone, DHEA, to sex hormones. *Bold arrows* denote primary sources of the sex hormones. The ovaries and testes are primary sources of circulating estradiol and testosterone in young women and men, respectively. The peripheral tissues (mainly adipose tissue) are a primary source of circulating estradiol in men and of estrone in both sexes. *DHEA* dehydroepiandrosterone, *ADIONE* androstenedione, *ADIOL* androstenediol, *DHT* dihydrotestosterone, *E2* estradiol, *E1* estrone

Table 11.2 Trends in circulating levels of sex steroids in aging men and women

Prohormone or hormone	Change with advancing age	
	Men	Women
DHEAS	Substantial decrease	Substantial decrease
DHEA	Decrease	Decrease
Testosterone	Decrease	Decrease
DHT	No significant change	No significant change
Estradiol	No significant change	Substantial decrease
Estrone	No significant change	Decrease

and 66 % bound to sex hormone-binding globulin (SHBG). Free and albumin-bound testosterones are bioavailable to tissues.

In younger men, the testicular Leydig cells produce 95 % of testosterone and a smaller amount of DHT (see Fig. 11.2). In premenopausal women, 25 % of circulating testosterone comes from the adrenals, 25 % from the ovaries [31], and the rest from peripheral conversion of androstenedione in adipose tissue [32].

In healthy men, total testosterone and free testosterone decline slowly with age [4, 33, 34]. The decline in total testosterone is modest, but comparatively greater for free testosterone due to the concurrent age-related rise in SHBG [35]. Data from a large, population-based cohort of men aged 40–70 at baseline who were followed for 7–10 years (the Massachusetts Male Aging Study) showed that total testosterone declined by age cross-sectionally (between subjects) at 0.8 %/year, free and albumin-bound testosterone declined at about 2 %/year, and SHBG concentrations rose about 1.6 %/year. Longitudinally (within subjects), total testosterone declined 1.6 %/year, bioavailable testosterone declined by 2–3 %/year, and SHBG levels rose at 1.3 %/year [4].

The age-related decline in testosterone in men is due to reductions in the number of productive Leydig cells as well as to changes in the response to leutinizing hormone (LH) and human chorionic gonadotropin (hCG). Moreover, obesity is associated with lower total and free testosterone and SHBG; a change in BMI from nonobese (<25 kg/m^2) to obese (≥30 kg/m^2) is equivalent to a 15-year fall in testosterone levels [35]. It has been postulated that age primarily affects testicular function, whereas obesity impairs hypothalamic and pituitary function. In addition, the circadian rhythm, with higher testosterone levels in the morning than in the evening, is lost in older men [36].

In women, testosterone levels decline between the ages of 20 and 50 [37]. However, the menopausal transition itself does not appear to affect testosterone levels significantly. A prospective study in 172 women failed to show a change in total testosterone in the time span from 5 years before to 7 years after the final menstrual period [6]. Other studies found a slight decrease in levels of bioavailable testosterone in the early years after menopause [10, 27], followed by a rise to premenopausal levels in the second decade following the menopausal transition [10]. Hence, declines during the decades preceding menopause have the most significant impact on testosterone levels in older women. These observations may reflect the relative importance of adrenal and peripheral sources of androgens in women.

11.3.2 Changes in Estrogen Production

In women of reproductive age, the ovaries are the principal source of estradiol. Menopause occurs when senescence of the ovarian follicles reduces the gonadal production of estradiol to miniscule levels (see Table 11.1). During this transition, circulating levels of estradiol decline from over 300 pmol/L to about 20 pmol/L [27, 38].

Estrone, a weaker estrogen produced from androstenedione in peripheral tissues, is the predominant form of estrogen in postmenopausal women (see Fig. 11.2). Estrone is also the principal source of postmenopausal estradiol, although only 5 % of estrone is thus converted [39]. Adipose tissue is a major site of peripheral estrone synthesis; hence, estrogen levels are higher in postmenopausal women with a high body mass index.

In men, 80 % of plasma estradiol is produced by peripheral aromatization of testosterone, which occurs principally in fat tissue [40]; the testes produce only 20 % of plasma estradiol [41, 42]. In younger men, 20 μg/day of estradiol derives from peripheral conversion of plasma testosterone, 5 μg/day from androstenedione, and 5–10 μg/day from the testicular Leydig cells [16]. As in women, plasma estrone derives principally from tissue aromatization of androstenedione, with 20 % secreted directly by the adrenals. The mean plasma estradiol concentration in men is 2–3 ng/dL (about 80 pmol/L), and the mean concentration of estrone is 3–6 ng/dL (about 100–200 pmol/L) (see Table 11.1) [43].

In men, plasma estradiol levels do not decrease significantly with age [19, 33, 44] (see Tables 11.1 and 11.2), although some investigators have reported declines [45, 46]. It has been postulated that plasma estradiol levels remain relatively unchanged despite declines in testosterone because of a rise in aromatase activity coincident with the age-associated increase in body fat mass [47, 48]. Consequently, plasma estradiol levels in older men are significantly higher than in postmenopausal women (see Table 11.1).

11.3.3 Intracrine Production of the Sex Steroids

The skin is affected not only by the action of circulating sex steroids but also by locally synthesized androgens and estrogens. Local production depends on the expression of androgen- and estrogen-synthesizing enzymes in individual skin structures and cell types (Table 11.3). Moreover, the expression of sex steroid receptors in the skin varies by cell type and by sex. Cytochrome p450c17, an enzyme necessary for the synthesis of DHEA and androstenedione from cholesterol, is not expressed to a great extent in androgen target cells, such as sebocytes; however, sebocytes, sweat glands, and dermal papilla hair cells do express enzymes that convert these adrenal prohormones into biologically active testosterone and DHT [49, 50]. Indeed, human sebocytes selectively use DHEA to produce active androgens [51]. A newly identified pathway in human sebocytes synthesizes DHT from DHEA without requiring testosterone as an intermediate. The sebaceous glands, the outer and inner root sheath cells of anagen terminal hair follicles, and dermal papilla cells express aromatases that convert testosterone and androstenedione into estrogens (see Table 11.3) [52, 53].

As in other steroidogenic organs, six enzyme systems are involved in the activation and deactivation of androgens in the skin: steroid sulfatase, 3β-hydroxysteroid dehydrogenase Δ^{5-4} isomerase (3β-HSD), 17β-hydroxysteroid dehydrogenase (17β-HSD), steroid 5α-reductase, 3α-hydroxysteroid dehydrogenase (3α-HSD), and aromatase [54]. The pilosebaceous unit and the sweat glands contribute to local synthesis of androgens and estrogens. Steroid sulfatase hydrolyses DHEAS to DHEA [55] (possibly in the sebocytes or in the dermal papillae of terminal hair follicles, which show enzymatic activity).

Within the pilosebaceous unit, testosterone is both produced from adrenal precursors as well as inactivated; this maintains androgen homeostasis [51, 52]. In sebocytes, the 1- isotype of 3β-HSD converts DHEA to androstenedione, and the 3- and 5- isotypes of 17β-HSD convert androstenedione to testosterone. Conversely, the 2- isotype (present in the root sheath cells of hair follicles) and the 4- isotype (in epidermal keratinocytes)

Table 11.3 Localization of sex steroidogenic enzymes and androgen and estrogen receptor activity in the skin

Skin structure	Enzyme activity				Sex steroid receptors		
	17β-HSD	3β-HSD	5α-Reductase	Aromatase	AR	ERβ	ERα
Epidermal keratinocytes	+ (4- isotype)		+ (1- isotype)		+	+	
Melanocytes					+	+	+
Hair follicles			+ (1- isotype) (2- isotype in beard)				
Follicular keratinocytes					+	+	
Root sheath	+ (2-isotype)			+		+	
Matrix epithelium					+	+	
Dermal papilla cells				+	+	+	
Sebaceous glands	+ (3- and 5- isotypes)	+ (1- isotype)	+ (1- isotype)	+	+	+	+
Sweat glands			+ (1- isotype)		+		
Eccrine						+	
Apocrine			+		+	+	
Dermal fibroblasts					+	+	+
Endothelial cells					+	+	

HSD hydroxysteroid dehydrogenase, *AR* androgen receptor, *Erβ* estrogen receptor-beta, *Erα* estrogen receptor-alpha deactivate testosterone in the reverse direction and play a protective role against androgen excess [54]. Keratinocytes also are responsible for androgen degradation [52].

Sebocytes are likely the major site of 5α-reductase activity in the skin. The type 1 isotype of 5α-reductase, expressed in sebaceous glands and sweat glands (with lesser activity in epidermal cells and hair follicles) [56], converts testosterone to the highly potent androgen, DHT. The type 2 isotype is active in beard hair follicles. A newly detected type 3 isotype, sensitive to finasteride (a 5α-reductase inhibitor), is strongly expressed in sebaceous gland cells [57]. Two isozymes of 3α-HSD deactivate DHT by conversion to 3α-androstanediol.

Aromatases in the sebaceous glands, the outer and inner root hair cells of anagen hair follicles, and dermal papillae cells [52, 53] convert androstenedione and testosterone to estrogens. Aromatase expression is much higher in scalp hair follicles of women than of men, and the enzyme is rarely expressed in telogen hair follicles [58].

11.3.4 Sex Steroid Receptor Localization in the Skin

Androgens (specifically testosterone and 5α-dihydrotestosterone (DHT)) and estrogens (specifically estradiol) mediate their skin effects by activating specific cellular receptors. Testosterone and DHT act through a single nuclear androgen receptor (AR), and their activity on the skin depends on receptor distribution. AR is present in epidermal and follicular keratinocytes, sebocytes, sweat glands, dermal papilla cells, dermal fibroblasts, endothelial cells, and genital melanocytes [59, 60].

Two distinct intracellular estrogen receptors, ERα and ERβ, belong to a superfamily of nuclear hormone receptors. Cell membrane-bound estrogen receptors also exist that activate signaling cascades via second messengers. ERβ is the predominant receptor in adult human scalp skin, strongly expressed in the stratum basale and stratum spinosum of the epidermis [59, 61]. ERα and ERβ are expressed in the sebaceous gland [59] and in primary cultures of dermal fibroblasts [62, 63].

Studies suggest that ERβ is the mediator of estrogen effects on skin and hair. ERβ is strongly expressed in anagen hair follicles of the human scalp, where it is localized to nuclei of the outer root sheath, epithelial matrix, and dermal papilla cells [59]. ERβ is also highly expressed in the epidermis, sebaceous glands, blood vessels, and dermal fibroblasts (see Table 11.3).

The apocrine gland develops from the hair follicle. ERβ but not ERα is expressed in the secretory epithelium of the apocrine gland [59] as well as in the eccrine gland. Estrogen receptor also is expressed in normal melanocytes [64] and in nevi of pregnant and nonpregnant women [65].

11.4 Effects of Sex Hormones on the Structure, Characteristics, and Physiology of Aging Skin

Clinically obvious signs of skin aging are wrinkling, pigmentary changes, loss of skin elasticity, and sagging. Skin exposed to UV damage has coarser and deeper wrinkles; a roughened, leathery surface; mottled pigmentation; and a more pronounced loss of elasticity. Intrinsically aged skin, which reflects purely chronological changes, has a dry, smoother texture, with fine wrinkles and an unblemished surface; loss of elasticity is less severe than in skin exposed to UV light. Aging skin is also thinner and more vulnerable to damage.

In addition to changes in structure, the growth rate of the hair and nails slows with age, the nail plate thins, and its surface becomes ridged and lusterless. The hair loses pigment and the density of hair follicles on the scalp decreases, independent of androgenetic alopecia (genetically driven patterns of balding). Vellus hairs in the ears, nose, and eyebrows of men and hair on the upper lip and chin of women convert to more obvious terminal hairs.

The influence of the sex steroids on these changes and the resulting gender differences in aging skin aging are summarized in Table 11.4 and reviewed below.

Table 11.4 Age-related changes in skin structure and physiology affected by the sex steroids in men and women

Parameter	Change	Gender differences	Impact of sex hormones
Wrinkles	Develop and become more pronounced with age	No established gender differences	Wrinkling may be related to reduced stimulation of collagen and glycosaminoglycan synthesis by estrogen
Skin thickness	Becomes thinner with age in both sexes (atrophy) Epidermal thickness decreases 6.4 % per decade [67] Dermal thickness decreases 20 % by old age [68]	Skin of adult men is thicker than that of women [66] Skin thickness decreases faster in older women than in older men [67]	Much of the decrease in skin thickness is thought to result from collagen changes in the dermis (see below)
Collagen (dermis)	Fibers more disorganized; balance between synthesis and degradation shifts toward greater degradation [69] Collagen matrix degrades and fibroblasts collapse [74, 75]	See above	Androgens promote thicker skin and higher collagen production in murine models [70, 71] DHEA declines result in lower procollagen synthesis and more collagen degradation [72, 73] DHEA is the principal source of estrogen synthesis in postmenopausal women. Estrogen supplementation in postmenopausal women increases skin collagen content [76, 77]
Elastin (dermis)	Fibers degrade; skin less elastic	Alterations more pronounced in older women [68] In the first 5 years following menopause, facial skin elasticity declines 1.5 %/year [78, 79]	Women who received HRT in the first 5 years following menopause exhibited no significant change in skin elasticity [78, 79]
Skin barrier function	Baseline barrier function (as measured by TEWL) unchanged [80, 81] Once compromised, barrier integrity takes longer to be restored [81, 86, 87]	No established gender differences [82]	Androgens reduce skin barrier function and estrogens increase it [83–85]
Skin moisture and water-holding capacity	Reduced water content of stratum corneum [88] Reduced water-holding capacity of the dermis due to declines in glycosaminoglycans and hyaluronic acid [93]	No established gender differences	Estrogens increase skin moisture and water-holding capacity [89] by increasing levels of hyaluronic acids [90, 91] and glycosaminoglycans [92]

Table 11.4 (continued)

Parameter	Change	Gender differences	Impact of sex hormones
Sweating and thermoregulation	Impaired with advancing age [94–96]	Men sweat to a greater degree than women in similar situations [97, 98]	Sweat glands express 5α-reductase (which converts androgens to DHT) and the androgen receptor through which DHT exerts its action
		Elevated temperature thresholds for sweating and reduced sweat response more pronounced in older women than in men [96]	
Sebum production	Gradual decrease in women	In men, sebum levels change minimally from puberty until about age 80	Sebocytes regulate the effect of androgens in the skin
			DHEA enhances sebum production in both sexes [99], but not through direct action on sebocytes [100]
			Testosterone promotes DHT synthesis in sebocytes and stimulates sebum production [101]
			In older women, estrogen supplementation suppresses sebum production; progesterone overcomes this effect [102]
		In women, sebum secretion decreases gradually from menopause through age 80, after which no appreciable change occurs [104]	Sebum production is affected by the interplay of growth factors (IGF-1), estrogen, progesterone, and androgens (DHEA) [100, 103]
Hair growth	Androgenetic alopecia usually begins around age 30 in genetically susceptible men and women	Male-pattern baldness is more common and severe and can start as early as late adolescence	Both androgens and estrogens affect hair growth. DHT acts on hair follicles to release growth factors in androgen-dependent areas (beard, axilla, pubis) [105]
		Female-pattern baldness is less common and usually milder	In male androgenetic alopecia, DHT causes susceptible scalp follicles to miniaturize; the number of follicles in anagen phase decreases
			In women, scalp hair follicles have lower 5α-reductase levels, lower AR levels, and higher aromatase activity, limiting the impact of DHT
			Estrogens act on hair follicles through ERβ, which is present at sites of hair renewal in follicles of women but not of men

(continued)

Table 11.4 (continued)

Parameter	Change	Gender differences	Impact of sex hormones
Wound healing	Skin is more susceptible to mechanical damage [106] and wound healing declines [107]	Men display lower rates of wound healing at all ages	Androgens depress wound healing by increasing inflammation, proteolysis, and matrix degradation [108]
			Estrogens promote wound healing by inhibiting inflammation and promoting keratinocyte mitogenesis, deposition of matrix components, and angiogenesis [109]
			Subcutaneous DHEA restores wound healing rates in ovariectomized mice and promoted wound healing in aged mice, likely through local conversion to estrogen [110]

11.4.1 Skin Structure and Thickness

Human male skin is thicker and drier than female skin throughout the life span (from ages 5 to 90 years) [66, 111]. In part, this is because androgens stimulate epidermal hyperplasia in adult human skin [83]. Although the skin thins with age in both sexes, in men, skin thickness decreases linearly beginning at age 20, whereas in women, it remains relatively constant until about age 50 and then decreases [112]. Epidermal thickness decreases about 6.4 % per decade on average, but faster in postmenopausal women than in men [67]. Dermal thickness decreases by up to 20 % in both genders [68], although in sun-protected sites, significant dermal thinning occurs only after the eighth decade [113].

The decline in dermal thickness accounts for most of the measurable thinning of aging skin. The major extracellular components of the dermis (collagen, elastin, and hyaluronic acid) are affected by age. Collagen fibers become disorganized, especially in photoaged skin, as the matrix metalloproteinases, which degrade collagen, are upregulated by UV exposure [69]. When the balance between collagen synthesis and degradation is disturbed, the collagen fibers fragment, disrupting the tension on dermal fibroblasts that exists in a healthy collagen matrix and causing fibroblasts to collapse [74, 75].

Elastin calcifies and degrades with age and its turnover declines [114]. These changes make the skin less elastic, less extensible under force, and more vulnerable to injury by shear forces. These properties erode more dramatically in women than in men [68].

DHEA plays a role in maintaining skin structure. It regulates the synthesis and degradation of extracellular matrix protein; it promotes procollagen synthesis; and it limits collagen degradation by decreasing the synthesis of collagenase and matrix metalloproteases and increasing the production of tissue inhibitors of matrix metalloproteinase [72, 73]. Consequently, the substantial decline in DHEA with age reduces procollagen synthesis and elevates collagen degradation.

Oral DHEA treatment in men and women aged 60–79 for 1 year improved epidermal thickness and skin hydration, increased sebum production, and reduced facial pigmentation, with effects being more dramatic in women over 70 than in men [99]. DHEA is the primary source of sex steroid production in skin: because older women have lower circulating levels of DHEA than older men, they may have benefited to a relatively greater degree from DHEA supplementation.

Most studies on the effects of estrogen on aging skin have examined the uses of systemic or topical estrogens in postmenopausal women. Estrogen slows or reverses these manifestations of skin aging, maintaining skin thickness, collagen content, and hydration.

Estrogens affect skin thickness and elasticity primarily through their impact on constituents of the dermis. Hormone replacement therapy maintains or improves skin thickness following menopause, largely by affecting dermal thickness. For example, nuns treated with oral conjugated estrogens for 1 year experienced a significant increase in dermal and overall skin thickness compared to placebo-treated controls [115]. Other studies found that postmenopausal women receiving HRT achieved skin thickness levels comparable to those of premenopausal women [116].

Collagen reduction is a major factor responsible for skin atrophy. The declines in the quality of collagen and elastin with age are more pronounced in aging women, probably due to estrogen deficiency. After a slight delay following the onset of menopause [76], total collagen content declines an average of 2.1 %/year in the first 15 postmenopausal years [76, 117]. Clinical studies have demonstrated beneficial effects of oral, topical, and subcutaneous estrogen treatment on collagen content (reviewed in [118–120]). The benefits of HRT or estrogen supplementation on collagen content are proportional to baseline levels at the time of treatment [76, 117].

Estrogen also benefits skin elasticity. In the first 5 years following menopause, facial skin distensibility increases 1.1 %/year and elasticity decreases by 1.5 %/year [78, 79, 121]. Women who received HRT during this time period experienced no significant changes in skin elasticity. Studies of oral, transdermal, and topical estrogen treatment also showed benefits [79, 102, 122, 123], although topical estrogen treatment seems to be effective only in sun-protected skin [124]. The extent to which the effect is due to improvements in elastin fiber quality is unclear.

Androgens also affect skin thickness, but the interplay between estrogens and androgens is incompletely defined. Androgens affect epidermal hyperplasia in humans, which may partly contribute in part to greater skin thickness in men [83]. Moreover, women with androgen excess who are hirsute display greatly increased skin thickness and skin collagen content [125].

Animal studies implicate androgens as important modulators of skin collagen content. In wild-type mice, skin collagen content is greater in maturing males than females, depending on the stage of development [71]. The skin of male and female mice with an X-linked mutation that eliminates a functional androgen receptor exhibited significantly decreased levels of collagen, implicating a role for the androgen receptor in modulating skin collagen content. In other studies, treatment of murine skin with DHT and DHEA increased dermal thickness by 22 and 19 %, respectively [70]. DHT administration to cultures of vulvar skin fibroblasts from healthy women resulted in significant increases in collagen production, whereas DHT treatment produced no change in cultures of perineal fibroblasts from a male patient with androgen insensitivity syndrome [126].

Although studies on the impact of these sex hormones have focused principally on the role of estrogens in aging female skin and the role androgens in male skin, the concentration profiles of both androgens and estrogens must contribute to differential skin thinning and changes in skin tone in aging men and women. Because women have thinner skin and lower skin collagen content to begin with, age-related thinning may be apparent earlier in this sex. Interestingly, skin thickness decreases linearly with age in men but accelerates in women after age 50 [112]. It may be pertinent that in men, androgen levels decline slowly with age while estradiol levels remain constant and comparable to those of premenopausal women, whereas in women, both androgen and estrogen concentrations decrease with age, with a precipitous drop in estradiol levels following menopause. These profiles could explain why skin thinning is more gradual and less pronounced in men and more dramatic in postmenopausal women.

11.4.2 Wrinkles

Wrinkling is related to loss of connective tissue and elasticity. Studies on wrinkling have focused on the potential benefits of estrogen supplementation in women. A large epidemiologic study in 3,875 postmenopausal women (NHANES I) found the odds of wrinkling to be substantially lower in estrogen users after adjusting for age, body mass index, and sunlight exposure [127]. Clinical trials of estrogen supplementation have given divergent results, some showing improvements in fine wrinkling and wrinkle depth with topical estrogen treatment [128, 129] and others showing effects on thickness but not on hydration or wrinkling [130]. The effects of estrogen on collagen and glycosaminoglycan content of the skin may account for the impact of estrogen on wrinkles.

11.4.3 Skin Barrier Function

The stratum corneum barrier depends on the composition and arrangement of intercellular lipids. Total lipid content declines by as much as 65 % with age, depleting levels of some ceramides, triglycerides, and sterol esters [131]. However, measurements of transepidermal water loss (TEWL) revealed no age-related differences in baseline skin barrier function, although lipid content declined [80, 81]. Nevertheless, when barrier integrity is compromised, recovery is slower in aged skin [81, 86, 87].

No gender differences in epidermal barrier function have been established [82]. However, the research suggests that androgens have a negative impact on skin barrier function, whereas estrogens help restore it. For example, measurements of skin barrier function in a hypogonadal man who received intermittent testosterone supplementation showed that barrier recovery rates were highest when serum testosterone levels were at a nadir and lowest when serum testosterone was at its peak [83]. Studies of the recovery of skin barrier function after tape stripping in castrated mice showed that recovery was delayed by systemic testosterone replacement [83]. Topical application of testosterone and androsterone delayed barrier recovery after tape stripping in hairless mice, a delay that was overcome by co-application of estradiol [84]. Moreover, male fetal mice develop barrier function more slowly than female littermates. Estrogen administration to pregnant mothers accelerated fetal barrier development; conversely, DHT administration delayed fetal skin barrier development, an effect that was reversed by treating with a testosterone receptor antagonist [85].

In aging men, testosterone levels decline while estradiol levels remain fairly constant, whereas in women, androgens decline slowly and estrogens decline dramatically following menopause. Consequently, gender differences in the balance of androgens and estrogens with age might be expected to affect skin barrier function; however, to our knowledge, systematic comparisons of this parameter in age-matched men and women have not been published.

11.4.4 Skin Moisture and Water-Holding Capacity

The water-holding capacity of both the epidermis and the dermis is affected by age. The water content of the stratum corneum is lower in aged skin [88]. Water content of the stratum corneum is related to skin barrier function and to the composition and organization of stratum corneum lipids. The water-holding capacity of the dermis also declines because aging fibroblasts produce lower levels of glycosaminoglycans and hyaluronic acid [93].

Estrogens affect skin dryness and water-holding capacity. Dry skin is very common among older women. A large epidemiologic study in 3,875 postmenopausal women found that women not on HRT were significantly more likely to experience dry skin compared to women taking estrogen [127]. In a pilot study of transdermal estrogen, the water-holding capacity of the stratum corneum increased at the treatment site [89]. In mice, estrogen treatment increased hyaluronic acid levels of aged skin [90, 132] and induced dermal glycosaminoglycans markedly within 2 weeks of therapy [92]. No gender-related differences in skin water-holding capacity have been found [133].

11.4.5 Sweating and Thermoregulation

Eccrine and apocrine glands located in the dermis produce sweat. Eccrine glands are distributed over the body, whereas apocrine glands are located in the axillar, areola, perineal, and perianal areas. Sweat glands express 5α-reductase (which converts testosterone to DHT) and express the AR through which DHT acts.

Men sweat more than women do in similar situations (approximately 800 mL/h for men vs. 450 mL/h for women during exercise). When corrected for body surface area, the sweat rate in men is still 30–40 % higher [97, 98]. Androgens initiate the differentiation of sweat glands during puberty, but may not be required to maintain function, because androgen treatment does not increase sweat rate in women and androgen antagonists do not diminish sweat rates in men. However, possibly the apocrine rather than eccrine sweat glands remain an androgen target, as type 1 5α-reductase predominates in apocrine glands of patients with excessive sweat odor, irrespective of sex [134].

Sweating and thermoregulation are impaired with age [94]. The number of eccrine glands diminishes and the output of both the eccrine and apocrine glands is reduced. Men over 60 or 70 display lower sweat rates and higher core temperatures in response to exercise than young men or boys [95, 96], and the temperature threshold to induce sweating is 0.5 °C higher in aged men [96]. The elevated temperature threshold for sweating and reduced sweat response was even more pronounced in aged women [96]. However, a small study comparing 8 women aged 50–62 with eight young women aged 20–30 found that in a hot-dry environment, the older women's whole body and local sweat rates were significantly lower than those of younger women, but in a warm-humid environment, there was no age-related difference [135].

11.4.6 Sebum Production

Most sebaceous glands are connected to hair follicles. Their concentration is greatest on the scalp, forehead, cheeks, and chin. Beginning at puberty, androgens act in conjunction with ligands of the peroxisome-proliferator-activated receptor (PPAR) to stimulate the proliferation and differentiation of the sebaceous gland and the production of sebum. The degree of proliferation depends on the anatomical location; the effect is greatest on facial sebocytes [136]. A Korean study of 30 men and women found a strong positive correlation between the male sex, pore size, and sebum excretion [137]. DHT is thought to stimulate sebaceous gland activity, especially in acne [138].

In men, sebum levels change minimally after puberty until about age 80, whereas in women, a gradual decrease in sebum secretion occurs from menopause through the seventh decade, after which no appreciable change occurs [104].

As noted earlier, sebocytes play a critical role in modulating androgen levels in the skin [52]. Due to the decline of their activity in aged individuals, sebaceous glands become hypertrophic to compensate this dysfunction (sebaceous gland hypertrophy) [139]. In human sebocytes, testosterone is converted to DHT, which stimulates sebum production. Cofactors such as linoleic acid, a ligand of the PPAR, exert synergistic effects [101]. By contrast, estrogen replacement in older women suppresses sebum production, although the addition of progesterone overcomes this effect [102].

In vitro, the treatment of sebocytes with a mixture of growth factors (IGF-1), estrogen, progesterone, and androgens (DHEA), at quantities that approximate the circulating levels at different ages, mimics the reduction of sebum production seen with age in vivo [100, 103]. Although oral supplementation for 1 year with the sex steroid precursor DHEA enhanced sebum production in both sexes [99], direct DHEA treatment of human sebocytes in vitro at age-specific levels has no effect on their activity [100]. Taken together, these observations indicate that changes in sebum production with age require the conversion of DHEA to sex hormones and are modulated by the interplay of both the sex hormone and the growth hormone signaling pathways.

11.4.7 Hair Growth

A hair follicle consists of epithelial components (inner and outer root sheath and hair shaft) and mesenchymal components (the dermal papillae and connective tissue sheath). The hair growth cycle involves anagen (growing), catagen (transitional), and telogen (resting) phases. The bulge region of the outer root sheath contains stem cells for hair follicle keratinocytes that regenerate the follicle during each anagen phase of the hair cycle; the dermal papilla cells provide the signal that initiates anagen and instructs the follicular stem cells to divide [140]. The hair growth cycle is not synchronized: each hair strand is in its own phase of development.

Both androgens and estrogens affect hair growth, and the interplay of their signaling pathways is relevant to gender differences in hair follicle stimulation. DHT, produced by the action of 5α-reductase on testosterone, mediates androgenic effects on hair follicles. DHT interacts with the AR on dermal papilla cells [56, 141], causing the release of growth factors that then act on other cells in the hair follicle [105]. The response to androgens at different body areas is genetically determined; single polymorphisms in AR are associated with hirsutism in women and androgenetic alopecia in men. In androgen-dependent areas (male beard, axillary and pubic hair), androgens promote enlargement of hair follicles; however, in scalp follicles of susceptible men, they cause the follicles to miniaturize and reduce the amount of hair in the anagen phase, leading to male-pattern baldness [142].

Men with a deficiency in type 2 5α-reductase display little or no beard growth and do not develop androgenetic alopecia; moreover, finasteride inhibition of the enzyme slows or reverses the progression of alopecia [143]. In male-pattern balding, the expression of type 2 5α-reductase is higher in dermal papilla cells from sites of androgenetic alopecia and beard than those from other sites; AR expression is also 30 % higher in sites of alopecia; and the AR coactivator Hic-5/ARA55 is more highly expressed in dermal papilla cells of hair follicles from sites of androgenetic alopecia and beard [58, 144]. The consequence is heightened sensitivity to DHT.

DHT stimulates the synthesis of transforming growth factor-β2 (TGF-β2) in dermal papilla cells. TGF-β2 in turn suppresses the proliferation of epithelial cells and stimulates the synthesis of certain caspases, which triggers the elimination of epithelial cells through apoptosis. These sequential events contribute to the shortening of the anagen phase of the hair cycle and premature entry into the catagen phase [145].

Female-pattern hair loss is more diffuse and usually involves the frontal and parietal scalp areas. It is independent of androgen levels, often begins after age 30, and is more prevalent after menopause. Women may be protected from developing androgenetic alopecia because their frontal and occipital hair follicles have more than three times lower 5α-reductase activity and 40 % lower AR levels [58, 146, 147]. This reduces the potential impact of DHT on the hair cycle in women. Moreover, scalp hair follicles in the frontal and occipital area express up to six times more aromatase activity in women than in men [58, 148]. This suggests that estrogen formation from testosterone also acts as a protective factor.

Estrogens also are potent modulators of hair growth: for example, during pregnancy, high systemic estrogen levels prolong the anagen phase, whereas plummeting postpartum levels cause excess numbers of anagen follicles to enter the telogen phase simultaneously, leading to hair loss [149]. In Europe, estrogens are used to treat androgenetic alopecia in women.

The estrogen signaling pathways for hair growth in the two genders are the subject of active research. Human hair follicles in culture express ERβ, but the distribution pattern is gender specific [150]. In men, ERβ resides predominantly in nuclei of matrix keratinocytes, whereas in women, the receptor resides in the fibroblasts of the dermal papilla of anagen hair follicles and in the bulge region of the outer root sheath, the site of stem cells involved in hair renewal. Hence, in women, estrogen receptor activation occurs at the target sites for hair growth. In addition, estradiol treatment diminishes the amount of DHT formed from testosterone in the epithelial part of the hair follicle of women. Estradiol induces aromatase activity at this site, which converts testosterone and androstenedione to estrogens [148] and limits androgenic effects. Aromatase is found in the outer root sheath of anagen hair follicles and sebaceous glands, but rarely in telogen hair follicles [58].

11.4.8 Wound Healing

Aged skin is more fragile. One of the most striking structural changes in aging skin is the flattening of the dermoepidermal junction, which reduces the connecting surface area between the two layers and makes the skin more vulnerable to shear forces [106]. Repair of injury is also affected by age. Epidermal turnover slows by 30–50 % between the third and eighth decades, and the capacity for re-epithelialization (wound healing) declines [107]. In the aged, wound healing is slower to start and slower to proceed. Moreover, the tensile strength of healing wounds decreases after age 70; for example, the risk of postoperative wound reopening increases dramatically in people over 80 compared to those in their 30s [87].

Men have slower rates of wound healing at all ages than women, and being an older man is a significant risk factor for impaired healing [151, 152]. For example, men exhibit impaired healing of chronic venous leg ulcers relative to women [153]; women have survival advantages in response to trauma, and their mortality following sepsis is 26 % compared to 70 % for men [154].

A shift in the balance of circulating estrogens and androgens and gender differences in the response to the hormones contribute to delayed wound healing in older adults. Wound-edge keratinocytes, infiltrating inflammatory cells, and dermal fibroblasts express AR [155]. Androgens depress wound healing by increasing local inflammation and promoting excessive proteolysis (reviewed in [108]). Under the influence of androgens, the inflammatory response does not resolve efficiently, and restorative matrix accumulation is delayed. Secondly, circulating androgens stimulate matrix degradation. In animal models, for example, castration reduces the levels of matrix metalloproteinases in wounds, thereby reducing matrix degradation and enabling the deposition of type I collagen and fibronectin to rise [156]. This process may be significant to impaired wound healing in the elderly, as the activity of matrix metalloproteinases in wounds is higher in older people of both sexes than in younger adults [69]. Older adults also display defective induction of tissue inhibitors of metalloproteinases (TIMP-1 and TIMP-2) that promote healing. DHT inhibits wound closure by retarding the migration of epidermal keratinocytes [157].

By contrast, estrogens are critical promoters of wound healing. Recent studies using a microarray-based approach revealed that differences in gene expression in wounds of both older men and younger people are almost exclusively estrogen-regulated [158]. A total of 83 % of downregulated probe sets and 80 % of upregulated probe sets in wounds were estrogen-regulated. These findings implicate estrogen as central to the wound healing process.

Estrogens both inhibit inflammation and promote deposition of matrix components. Topical estrogen treatment reduces neutrophil infiltration, increases the accumulation of type I collagen and fibronectin, decreases fibronectin degradation, and increases wound strength in both sexes [151]. Estrogen has a mitogenic effect on keratinocytes, increasing the rate of re-epithelialization of wounds [159]. In vitro, estradiol promotes angiogenesis of endothelial cell monolayers [160]. In postmenopausal women with impaired wound healing, estrogen treatment accelerates re-epithelialization and increases local collagen deposition [159]. In elderly men, however, the response to estrogen is lower than in women.

In animal models, some of the anti-inflammatory action of estrogens is mediated through the regulation of macrophage activation. After ovariectomy, which depletes circulating ovarian hormones, macrophages were activated in a classical manner, promoting inflammation; however, estrogen or progesterone supplementation shunted macrophage activation through an alternative pathway, driving wound repair, angiogenesis, and remodeling [161].

The multifunctional cytokine macrophage inhibitory factor (MIF) is a candidate proinflammatory cytokine involved in hormonal regulation of wound healing. MIF is expressed during wound healing by infiltrating neutrophils, endothelial cells, and the proliferating epidermis. Estrogen regulates the expression of MIF. MIF expression is markedly higher in wounds of estrogen-deficient mice, but in mice lacking the MIF gene, the wound inflammation associated with estrogen deficiency is reversed [162]. In postmenopausal women, systemic and wound production of MIF increases but is normalized by topical estrogen treatment or systemic HRT [163].

Recent evidence from mice with specific genetic deletions indicates that estrogen promotes wound healing in the skin through ERβ but not ERα. Estrogen treatment actually delayed wound healing in mice deficient in ERβ in the skin [164]. However, estrogen agonists to both ERβ and ERα were anti-inflammatory during skin repair. This indicates that the anti-inflammatory effects of estrogens are decoupled from the effects on overall re-epithelialization.

DHEA also influences wound repair. Systemic DHEA protects against chronic venous ulcers in older adults of both sexes compared to age-matched controls [110]. Exogenous DHEA also improved wound healing in aged mice [110]. In ovariectomized mice, subcutaneous DHEA restored the rate of wound healing, likely through local conversion to estrogens [110].

11.5 Summary

The sex steroids are intricately involved in supporting skin structure and function. The serum concentrations of the sex steroids differ in men and women and are affected differently by age in each sex. The concentration of the sex hormone precursors, DHEA and DHEAS, decline dramatically with age in both sexes, but more so in women. The pronounced decline in women is significant, as DHEA is the predominant, if not sole, source of androgen and estrogen synthesis following menopause. In men, serum concentrations of testosterone decline slowly with age, but remain higher in older men than in postmenopausal women. Similarly, levels of the highly potent androgen DHT are higher in older men than in women. Aging does not significantly affect estradiol levels in men, but following menopause, circulating levels of estradiol drop to miniscule levels: hence, estrone, the weaker estrogen formed from DHEA in peripheral tissue, becomes the sole source of estrogens in postmenopausal women.

These profiles impact gender differences in aging skin. Although both androgens and estrogens promote collagen deposition, the marked estradiol deficiency in postmenopausal women results in thinner, drier skin with a lower collagen content and reduced elasticity. By contrast, wound healing is compromised to a greater degree in older men than in older women, placing older men at greater risk of skin injury. This excess risk could be a consequence of the higher concentration of circulating androgens in older men than in women. Sebum production, which is affected by the interplay of growth factors and the sex steroids, changes minimally with age in men and only gradually in women. Senile sebaceous gland hypertrophy is a compensatory mechanism against the decrease in sebum secretion with age [139].

The formation and action of the sex steroids within the skin is also important. Local differences in the synthesis and receptor-mediated action of androgens and estrogens influence their effects on sweat glands and hair follicles. Sweat glands are androgen targets: they express 5α-reductase (which converts testosterone to DHT) and AR, through which these hormones act. Hence, although the sweat response declines with age overall, evidence exists that men sweat to a greater degree than women at all ages.

Hair follicles are targets of action of both androgens and estrogens. DHT causes hair follicles of genetically susceptible men to miniaturize and reduces the number of follicles in the growth phase, leading to male-pattern baldness (androgenetic alopecia). In women, the impact of DHT is limited because their scalp hair follicles express lower levels of 5α-reductase and AR and higher levels of aromatase, which converts testosterone to estrogen. Estrogen promotes hair growth through action on the ERβ receptor, which is present at sites of hair renewal in the follicles of women but not of men. In short, declines in the circulating levels of sex steroids, changes in the relative levels of androgens and estrogens in older men and women, and the expression of key steroidogenic enzymes and receptors within the skin itself work in concert to influence the salient gender differences in aging skin.

References

1. Zouboulis CC, Makrantonaki E. Clinical aspects and molecular diagnostics of skin aging. Clin Dermatol. 2011;29(1):3–14. doi:10.1016/j.clindermatol.2010.07.001.
2. Labrie F, Belanger A, Cusan L, Candas B. Physiological changes in dehydroepiandrosterone are not reflected by serum levels of active androgens and estrogens but of their metabolites: intracrinology. J Clin Endocrinol Metab. 1997;82(8):2403–9.
3. Ravaglia G, Forti P, Maioli F, Boschi F, Bernardi M, Pratelli L, Pizzoferrato A, Gasbarrini G. The relationship of dehydroepiandrosterone sulfate (DHEAS) to endocrine-metabolic parameters and functional status in the oldest-old. Results from an Italian study on healthy free-living over-ninety-year-olds. J Clin Endocrinol Metab. 1996;81(3):1173–8.
4. Feldman HA, Longcope C, Derby CA, Johannes CB, Araujo AB, Coviello AD, Bremner WJ, McKinlay JB. Age trends in the level of serum testosterone and other hormones in middle-aged men: longitudinal results from the Massachusetts male aging study. J Clin Endocrinol Metab. 2002;87(2):589–98.
5. Kaaks R, Berrino F, Key T, Rinaldi S, Dossus L, Biessy C, Secreto G, Amiano P, Bingham S, Boeing H, Bueno de Mesquita HB, Chang-Claude J, Clavel-Chapelon F, Fournier A, van Gils CH, Gonzalez CA, Gurrea AB, Critselis E, Khaw KT, Krogh V, Lahmann PH, Nagel G, Olsen A, Onland-Moret NC, Overvad K, Palli D, Panico S, Peeters P, Quiros JR, Roddam A, Thiebaut A, Tjonneland A, Chirlaque MD, Trichopoulou A, Trichopoulos D, Tumino R, Vineis P, Norat T, Ferrari P, Slimani N, Riboli E. Serum sex steroids in premenopausal women and breast cancer risk within the European Prospective Investigation into Cancer and Nutrition (EPIC). J Natl Cancer Inst. 2005;97(10):755–65. doi:10.1093/jnci/dji132.
6. Burger HG, Dudley EC, Cui J, Dennerstein L, Hopper JL. A prospective longitudinal study of serum testosterone, dehydroepiandrosterone sulfate, and sex hormone-binding globulin levels through the menopause transition. J Clin Endocrinol Metab. 2000;85(8):2832–8.
7. Burger HG. Androgen production in women. Fertil Steril. 2002;77 Suppl 4:S3–5.
8. Labrie F, Belanger A, Luu-The V, Labrie C, Simard J, Cusan L, Gomez JL, Candas B. DHEA and the intracrine formation of androgens and estrogens in peripheral target tissues: its role during aging. Steroids. 1998;63(5–6):322–8.
9. Harman SM, Metter EJ, Tobin JD, Pearson J, Blackman MR. Longitudinal effects of aging on serum total and free testosterone levels in healthy men. Baltimore longitudinal study of aging. J Clin Endocrinol Metab. 2001;86(2):724–31.
10. Laughlin GA, Barrett-Connor E, Kritz-Silverstein D, von Muhlen D. Hysterectomy, oophorectomy, and endogenous sex hormone levels in older women: the Rancho Bernardo Study. J Clin Endocrinol Metab. 2000;85(2):645–51.
11. Gapstur SM, Gann PH, Kopp P, Colangelo L, Longcope C, Liu K. Serum androgen concentrations in young men: a longitudinal analysis of associations with age, obesity, and race. The CARDIA male hormone study. Cancer Epidemiol Biomarkers Prev. 2002;11(10 Pt 1):1041–7.
12. Sinha-Hikim I, Arver S, Beall G, Shen R, Guerrero M, Sattler F, Shikuma C, Nelson JC, Landgren BM, Mazer NA, Bhasin S. The use of a sensitive equilibrium dialysis method for the measurement of free testosterone levels in healthy, cycling women and in human immunodeficiency virus-infected women. J Clin Endocrinol Metab. 1998;83(4):1312–8.
13. Labrie F, Cusan L, Gomez JL, Martel C, Berube R, Belanger P, Belanger A, Vandenput L, Mellstrom D, Ohlsson C. Comparable amounts of sex steroids are made outside the gonads in men and women: strong lesson for hormone therapy of prostate and breast cancer. J Steroid Biochem Mol Biol. 2009;113(1–2):52–6. doi:10.1016/j.jsbmb.2008.11.004.
14. Secreto G, Toniolo P, Pisani P, Recchione C, Cavalleri A, Fariselli G, Totis A, Di Pietro S, Berrino F. Androgens and breast cancer in premenopausal women. Cancer Res. 1989;49(2):471–6.
15. Secreto G, Toniolo P, Berrino F, Recchione C, Cavalleri A, Pisani P, Totis A, Fariselli G, Di Pietro S. Serum and urinary androgens and risk of breast cancer in postmenopausal women. Cancer Res. 1991;51(10):2572–6.
16. Vermeulen A, Kaufman JM, Goemaere S, van Pottelberg I. Estradiol in elderly men. Aging Male. 2002;5(2):98–102.
17. Legrain S, Girard L. Pharmacology and therapeutic effects of dehydroepiandrosterone in older subjects. Drugs Aging. 2003;20(13):949–67.
18. Labrie F. DHEA, important source of sex steroids in men and even more in women. Prog Brain Res. 2010;182:97–148. doi:10.1016/s0079-6123(10)82004-7.
19. Belanger A, Candas B, Dupont A, Cusan L, Diamond P, Gomez JL, Labrie F. Changes in serum concentrations of conjugated and unconjugated

steroids in 40- to 80-year-old men. J Clin Endocrinol Metab. 1994;79(4):1086–90.
20. Orentreich N, Brind JL, Rizer RL, Vogelman JH. Age changes and sex differences in serum dehydroepiandrosterone sulfate concentrations throughout adulthood. J Clin Endocrinol Metab. 1984;59(3):551–5.
21. Sulcova J, Hill M, Hampl R, Starka L. Age and sex related differences in serum levels of unconjugated dehydroepiandrosterone and its sulphate in normal subjects. J Endocrinol. 1997;154(1):57–62.
22. Laughlin GA, Barrett-Connor E. Sexual dimorphism in the influence of advanced aging on adrenal hormone levels: the Rancho Bernardo Study. J Clin Endocrinol Metab. 2000;85(10):3561–8.
23. Mazat L, Lafont S, Berr C, Debuire B, Tessier JF, Dartigues JF, Baulieu EE. Prospective measurements of dehydroepiandrosterone sulfate in a cohort of elderly subjects: relationship to gender, subjective health, smoking habits, and 10-year mortality. Proc Natl Acad Sci U S A. 2001;98(14):8145–50. doi:10.1073/pnas.121177998.
24. Labrie F, Martel C, Balser J. Wide distribution of the serum dehydroepiandrosterone and sex steroid levels in postmenopausal women: role of the ovary? Menopause. 2011;18(1):30–43. doi:10.1097/gme.0b013e3181e195a6.
25. Moghissi E, Ablan F, Horton R. Origin of plasma androstanediol glucuronide in men. J Clin Endocrinol Metab. 1984;59(3):417–21.
26. Vermeulen A. The hormonal activity of the postmenopausal ovary. J Clin Endocrinol Metab. 1976;42(2):247–53.
27. Overlie I, Moen MH, Morkrid L, Skjaeraasen JS, Holte A. The endocrine transition around menopause – a five years prospective study with profiles of gonadotropines, estrogens, androgens and SHBG among healthy women. Acta Obstet Gynecol Scand. 1999;78(7):642–7.
28. Nagamani M, Urban RJ. Expression of messenger ribonucleic acid encoding steroidogenic enzymes in postmenopausal ovaries. J Soc Gynecol Investig. 2003;10(1):37–40.
29. Havelock JC, Rainey WE, Bradshaw KD, Carr BR. The post-menopausal ovary displays a unique pattern of steroidogenic enzyme expression. Hum Reprod. 2006;21(1):309–17. doi:10.1093/humrep/dei373.
30. Couzinet B, Meduri G, Lecce MG, Young J, Brailly S, Loosfelt H, Milgrom E, Schaison G. The postmenopausal ovary is not a major androgen-producing gland. J Clin Endocrinol Metab. 2001;86(10):5060–6.
31. Longcope C, Franz C, Morello C, Baker R, Johnston Jr CC. Steroid and gonadotropin levels in women during the peri-menopausal years. Maturitas. 1986;8(3):189–96.
32. Horton R, Tait JF. Androstenedione production and interconversion rates measured in peripheral blood and studies on the possible site of its conversion to testosterone. J Clin Invest. 1966;45(3):301–13. doi:10.1172/JCI105344.
33. Gray A, Feldman HA, McKinlay JB, Longcope C. Age, disease, and changing sex hormone levels in middle-aged men: results of the Massachusetts Male Aging Study. J Clin Endocrinol Metab. 1991;73(5):1016–25.
34. Morley JE, Kaiser FE, Perry 3rd HM, Patrick P, Morley PM, Stauber PM, Vellas B, Baumgartner RN, Garry PJ. Longitudinal changes in testosterone, luteinizing hormone, and follicle-stimulating hormone in healthy older men. Metabolism. 1997;46(4):410–3.
35. Wu FC, Tajar A, Pye SR, Silman AJ, Finn JD, O'Neill TW, Bartfai G, Casanueva F, Forti G, Giwercman A, Huhtaniemi IT, Kula K, Punab M, Boonen S, Vanderschueren D. Hypothalamic-pituitary-testicular axis disruptions in older men are differentially linked to age and modifiable risk factors: the European Male Aging Study. J Clin Endocrinol Metab. 2008;93(7):2737–45. doi:10.1210/jc.2007-1972.
36. Bremner WJ, Vitiello MV, Prinz PN. Loss of circadian rhythmicity in blood testosterone levels with aging in normal men. J Clin Endocrinol Metab. 1983;56(6):1278–81.
37. Judd HL, Yen SS. Serum androstenedione and testosterone levels during the menstrual cycle. J Clin Endocrinol Metab. 1973;36(3):475–81.
38. Burger HG, Dudley EC, Hopper JL, Groome N, Guthrie JR, Green A, Dennerstein L. Prospectively measured levels of serum follicle-stimulating hormone, estradiol, and the dimeric inhibins during the menopausal transition in a population-based cohort of women. J Clin Endocrinol Metab. 1999;84(11):4025–30.
39. Luu-The V, Dufort I, Pelletier G, Labrie F. Type 5 17beta-hydroxysteroid dehydrogenase: its role in the formation of androgens in women. Mol Cell Endocrinol. 2001;171(1–2):77–82.
40. Baird DT, Horton R, Longcope C, Tait JF. Steroid dynamics under steady-state conditions. Recent Prog Horm Res. 1969;25:611–64.
41. MacDonald PC, Madden JD, Brenner PF, Wilson JD, Siiteri PK. Origin of estrogen in normal men and in women with testicular feminization. J Clin Endocrinol Metab. 1979;49(6):905–16.
42. Saez JM, Morera AM, Dazord A, Bertrand J. Adrenal and testicular contribution to plasma oestrogens. J Endocrinol. 1972;55(1):41–9.
43. Nankin HR, Pinto R, Fan DF, Troen P. Daytime titers of testosterone, LH, estrone, estradiol, and testosterone-binding protein: acute effects of LH and LH-releasing hormone in men. J Clin Endocrinol Metab. 1975;41(2):271–81.
44. Khosla S, Melton 3rd LJ, Atkinson EJ, O'Fallon WM. Relationship of serum sex steroid levels to longitudinal changes in bone density in young versus elderly men. J Clin Endocrinol Metab. 2001;86(8):3555–61.
45. van den Beld AW, de Jong FH, Grobbee DE, Pols HA, Lamberts SW. Measures of bioavailable serum

testosterone and estradiol and their relationships with muscle strength, bone density, and body composition in elderly men. J Clin Endocrinol Metab. 2000;85(9):3276–82.
46. Leifke E, Gorenoi V, Wichers C, Von Zur MA, Von Buren E, Brabant G. Age-related changes of serum sex hormones, insulin-like growth factor-1 and sex-hormone binding globulin levels in men: cross-sectional data from a healthy male cohort. Clin Endocrinol (Oxf). 2000;53(6):689–95.
47. Vermeulen A, Goemaere S, Kaufman JM. Testosterone, body composition and aging. J Endocrinol Invest. 1999;22(5):110–6.
48. Vermeulen A, Goemaere S, Kaufman JM. Sex hormones, body composition and aging. Aging Male. 1999;2:8–11.
49. Zouboulis CC, Chen WC, Thornton MJ, Qin K, Rosenfield R. Sexual hormones in human skin. Horm Metab Res. 2007;39(2):85–95. doi:10.1055/s-2007-961807.
50. Makrantonaki E, Zouboulis CC. Androgens and ageing of the skin. Curr Opin Endocrinol Diabetes Obes. 2009;16(3):240–5. doi:10.1097/MED.0b013e32832b71dc.
51. Chen W, Tsai SJ, Sheu HM, Tsai JC, Zouboulis CC. Testosterone synthesized in cultured human SZ95 sebocytes derives mainly from dehydroepiandrosterone. Exp Dermatol. 2010;19(5):470–2. doi:10.1111/j.1600-0625.2009.00996.x.
52. Fritsch M, Orfanos CE, Zouboulis CC. Sebocytes are the key regulators of androgen homeostasis in human skin. J Invest Dermatol. 2001;116(5):793–800. doi:10.1046/j.0022-202x.2001.doc.x.
53. Thornton MJ, Nelson LD, Taylor AH, Birch MP, Laing I, Messenger AG. The modulation of aromatase and estrogen receptor alpha in cultured human dermal papilla cells by dexamethasone: a novel mechanism for selective action of estrogen via estrogen receptor beta? J Invest Dermatol. 2006;126(9):2010–8. doi:10.1038/sj.jid.5700344.
54. Chen W, Thiboutot D, Zouboulis CC. Cutaneous androgen metabolism: basic research and clinical perspectives. J Invest Dermatol. 2002;119(5):992–1007. doi:10.1046/j.1523-1747.2002.00613.x.
55. Milewich L, Sontheimer RD, Herndon Jr JH. Steroid sulfatase activity in epidermis of acne-prone and non-acne-prone skin of patients with acne vulgaris. Arch Dermatol. 1990;126(10):1312–4.
56. Deplewski D, Rosenfield RL. Role of hormones in pilosebaceous unit development. Endocr Rev. 2000;21(4):363–92.
57. Samson M, Labrie F, Zouboulis CC, Luu-The V. Biosynthesis of dihydrotestosterone by a pathway that does not require testosterone as an intermediate in the SZ95 sebaceous gland cell line. J Invest Dermatol. 2010;130(2):602–4. doi:10.1038/jid.2009.225.
58. Sawaya ME, Price VH. Different levels of 5alpha-reductase type I and II, aromatase, and androgen receptor in hair follicles of women and men with androgenetic alopecia. J Invest Dermatol. 1997;109(3):296–300.
59. Thornton MJ, Taylor AH, Mulligan K, Al-Azzawi F, Lyon CC, O'Driscoll J, Messenger AG. The distribution of estrogen receptor beta is distinct to that of estrogen receptor alpha and the androgen receptor in human skin and the pilosebaceous unit. J Investig Dermatol Symp Proc. 2003;8(1):100–3. doi:10.1046/j.1523-1747.2003.12181.x.
60. Zouboulis CC, Degitz K. Androgen action on human skin – from basic research to clinical significance. Exp Dermatol. 2004;13 Suppl 4:5–10. doi:10.1111/j.1600-0625.2004.00255.x.
61. Thornton MJ, Taylor AH, Mulligan K, Al-Azzawi F, Lyon CC, O'Driscoll J, Messenger AG. Oestrogen receptor beta is the predominant oestrogen receptor in human scalp skin. Exp Dermatol. 2003;12(2):181–90.
62. Haczynski J, Tarkowski R, Jarzabek K, Slomczynska M, Wolczynski S, Magoffin DA, Jakowicki JA, Jakimiuk AJ. Human cultured skin fibroblasts express estrogen receptor alpha and beta. Int J Mol Med. 2002;10(2):149–53.
63. Haczynski J, Tarkowski R, Jarzabek K, Wolczynski S, Magoffin DA, Czarnocki KJ, Ziegert M, Jakowicki J, Jakimiuk AJ. Differential effects of estradiol, raloxifene and tamoxifen on estrogen receptor expression in cultured human skin fibroblasts. Int J Mol Med. 2004;13(6):903–8.
64. Jee SH, Lee SY, Chiu HC, Chang CC, Chen TJ. Effects of estrogen and estrogen receptor in normal human melanocytes. Biochem Biophys Res Commun. 1994;199(3):1407–12. doi:10.1006/bbrc.1994.1387.
65. Nading MA, Nanney LB, Boyd AS, Ellis DL. Estrogen receptor beta expression in nevi during pregnancy. Exp Dermatol. 2008;17(6):489–97. doi:10.1111/j.1600-0625.2007.00667.x.
66. Seidenari S, Pagnoni A, Di Nardo A, Giannetti A. Echographic evaluation with image analysis of normal skin: variations according to age and sex. Skin Pharmacol. 1994;7(4):201–9.
67. Waller JM, Maibach HI. Age and skin structure and function, a quantitative approach (I): blood flow, pH, thickness, and ultrasound echogenicity. Skin Res Technol. 2005;11(4):221–35. doi:10.1111/j.0909-725X.2005.00151.x.
68. McCallion R, Li Wan Po A. Dry and photo-aged skin: manifestations and management. J Clin Pharm Ther. 1993;18(1):15–32.
69. Ashcroft GS, Horan MA, Herrick SE, Tarnuzzer RW, Schultz GS, Ferguson MW. Age-related differences in the temporal and spatial regulation of matrix metalloproteinases (MMPs) in normal skin and acute cutaneous wounds of healthy humans. Cell Tissue Res. 1997;290(3):581–91.
70. Azzi L, El-Alfy M, Martel C, Labrie F. Gender differences in mouse skin morphology and specific effects of sex steroids and dehydroepiandrosterone. J Invest Dermatol. 2005;124(1):22–7. doi:10.1111/j.0022-202X.2004.23545.x.

71. Markova MS, Zeskand J, McEntee B, Rothstein J, Jimenez SA, Siracusa LD. A role for the androgen receptor in collagen content of the skin. J Invest Dermatol. 2004;123(6):1052–6. doi:10.1111/j.0022-202X.2004.23494.x.
72. Lee KS, Oh KY, Kim BC. Effects of dehydroepiandrosterone on collagen and collagenase gene expression by skin fibroblasts in culture. J Dermatol Sci. 2000;23(2):103–10.
73. Shin MH, Rhie GE, Park CH, Kim KH, Cho KH, Eun HC, Chung JH. Modulation of collagen metabolism by the topical application of dehydroepiandrosterone to human skin. J Invest Dermatol. 2005;124(2):315–23. doi:10.1111/j.0022-202X.2004.23588.x.
74. Fisher GJ, Varani J, Voorhees JJ. Looking older: fibroblast collapse and therapeutic implications. Arch Dermatol. 2008;144(5):666–72. doi:10.1001/archderm.144.5.666.
75. Varani J, Dame MK, Rittie L, Fligiel SE, Kang S, Fisher GJ, Voorhees JJ. Decreased collagen production in chronologically aged skin: roles of age-dependent alteration in fibroblast function and defective mechanical stimulation. Am J Pathol. 2006;168(6):1861–8. doi:10.2353/ajpath.2006.051302.
76. Brincat M, Kabalan S, Studd JW, Moniz CF, de Trafford J, Montgomery J. A study of the decrease of skin collagen content, skin thickness, and bone mass in the postmenopausal woman. Obstet Gynecol. 1987;70(6):840–5.
77. Brincat M, Moniz CF, Kabalan S, Versi E, O'Dowd T, Magos AL, Montgomery J, Studd JW. Decline in skin collagen content and metacarpal index after the menopause and its prevention with sex hormone replacement. Br J Obstet Gynaecol. 1987;94(2):126–9.
78. Pierard GE, Letawe C, Dowlati A, Pierard-Franchimont C. Effect of hormone replacement therapy for menopause on the mechanical properties of skin. J Am Geriatr Soc. 1995;43(6):662–5.
79. Pierard-Franchimont C, Cornil F, Dehavay J, Deleixhe-Mauhin F, Letot B, Pierard GE. Climacteric skin ageing of the face–a prospective longitudinal comparative trial on the effect of oral hormone replacement therapy. Maturitas. 1999;32(2):87–93.
80. Elias PM, Ghadially R. The aged epidermal permeability barrier: basis for functional abnormalities. Clin Geriatr Med. 2002;18(1):103–20. vii.
81. Ghadially R, Brown BE, Sequeira-Martin SM, Feingold KR, Elias PM. The aged epidermal permeability barrier. Structural, functional, and lipid biochemical abnormalities in humans and a senescent murine model. J Clin Invest. 1995;95(5):2281–90. doi:10.1172/JCI117919.
82. Reed JT, Ghadially R, Elias PM. Skin type, but neither race nor gender, influence epidermal permeability barrier function. Arch Dermatol. 1995;131(10):1134–8.
83. Kao JS, Garg A, Mao-Qiang M, Crumrine D, Ghadially R, Feingold KR, Elias PM. Testosterone perturbs epidermal permeability barrier homeostasis. J Invest Dermatol. 2001;116(3):443–51. doi:10.1046/j.1523-1747.2001.01281.x.
84. Tsutsumi M, Denda M. Paradoxical effects of beta-estradiol on epidermal permeability barrier homeostasis. Br J Dermatol. 2007;157(4):776–9. doi:10.1111/j.1365-2133.2007.08115.x.
85. Hanley K, Rassner U, Jiang Y, Vansomphone D, Crumrine D, Komuves L, Elias PM, Feingold KR, Williams ML. Hormonal basis for the gender difference in epidermal barrier formation in the fetal rat. Acceleration by estrogen and delay by testosterone. J Clin Invest. 1996;97(11):2576–84. doi:10.1172/JCI118706.
86. Roskos KV, Guy RH. Assessment of skin barrier function using transepidermal water loss: effect of age. Pharm Res. 1989;6(11):949–53.
87. Fenske NA, Lober CW. Structural and functional changes of normal aging skin. J Am Acad Dermatol. 1986;15(4 Pt 1):571–85.
88. Jackson SM, Williams ML, Feingold KR, Elias PM. Pathobiology of the stratum corneum. West J Med. 1993;158(3):279–85.
89. Pierard-Franchimont C, Letawe C, Goffin V, Pierard GE. Skin water-holding capacity and transdermal estrogen therapy for menopause: a pilot study. Maturitas. 1995;22(2):151–4.
90. Uzuka M, Nakajima K, Ohta S, Mori Y. The mechanism of estrogen-induced increase in hyaluronic acid biosynthesis, with special reference to estrogen receptor in the mouse skin. Biochim Biophys Acta. 1980;627(2):199–206.
91. Sobel H, Hewlett MJ, Hrubant HE. Collagen and glycosaminoglycans in skin of aging mice. J Gerontol. 1970;25(2):102–4.
92. Grosman N, Hvidberg E, Schou J. The effect of oestrogenic treatment on the acid mucopolysaccharide pattern in skin of mice. Acta Pharmacol Toxicol (Copenh). 1971;30(5):458–64.
93. Sudel KM, Venzke K, Mielke H, Breitenbach U, Mundt C, Jaspers S, Koop U, Sauermann K, Knussman-Hartig E, Moll I, Gercken G, Young AR, Stab F, Wenck H, Gallinat S. Novel aspects of intrinsic and extrinsic aging of human skin: beneficial effects of soy extract. Photochem Photobiol. 2005;81(3):581–7. doi:10.1562/2004-06-16-RA-202.
94. Ohta H, Makita K, Kawashima T, Kinoshita S, Takenouchi M, Nozawa S. Relationship between dermato-physiological changes and hormonal status in pre-, peri-, and postmenopausal women. Maturitas. 1998;30(1):55–62.
95. Dufour A, Candas V. Ageing and thermal responses during passive heat exposure: sweating and sensory aspects. Eur J Appl Physiol. 2007;100(1):19–26. doi:10.1007/s00421-007-0396-9.
96. Foster KG, Ellis FP, Dore C, Exton-Smith AN, Weiner JS. Sweat responses in the aged. Age Ageing. 1976;5(2):91–101.
97. Green JM, Bishop PA, Muir IH, Lomax RG. Gender differences in sweat lactate. Eur J Appl Physiol. 2000;82(3):230–5.
98. Yosipovitch G, Reis J, Tur E, Sprecher E, Yarnitsky D, Boner G. Sweat secretion, stratum corneum

hydration, small nerve function and pruritus in patients with advanced chronic renal failure. Br J Dermatol. 1995;133(4):561–4.
99. Baulieu EE, Thomas G, Legrain S, Lahlou N, Roger M, Debuire B, Faucounau V, Girard L, Hervy MP, Latour F, Leaud MC, Mokrane A, Pitti-Ferrandi H, Trivalle C, de Lacharriere O, Nouveau S, Rakoto-Arison B, Souberbielle JC, Raison J, Le Bouc Y, Raynaud A, Girerd X, Forette F. Dehydroepiandrosterone (DHEA), DHEA sulfate, and aging: contribution of the DHEAge Study to a sociobiomedical issue. Proc Natl Acad Sci U S A. 2000;97(8):4279–84.
100. Makrantonaki E, Vogel K, Fimmel S, Oeff M, Seltmann H, Zouboulis CC. Interplay of IGF-I and 17beta-estradiol at age-specific levels in human sebocytes and fibroblasts in vitro. Exp Gerontol. 2008;43(10):939–46. doi:10.1016/j.exger.2008.07.005.
101. Makrantonaki E, Zouboulis CC. Testosterone metabolism to 5alpha-dihydrotestosterone and synthesis of sebaceous lipids is regulated by the peroxisome proliferator-activated receptor ligand linoleic acid in human sebocytes. Br J Dermatol. 2007;156(3):428–32. doi:10.1111/j.1365-2133.2006.07671.x.
102. Sator PG, Schmidt JB, Sator MO, Huber JC, Honigsmann H. The influence of hormone replacement therapy on skin ageing: a pilot study. Maturitas. 2001;39(1):43–55.
103. Makrantonaki E, Adjaye J, Herwig R, Brink TC, Groth D, Hultschig C, Lehrach H, Zouboulis CC. Age-specific hormonal decline is accompanied by transcriptional changes in human sebocytes in vitro. Aging Cell. 2006;5(4):331–44. doi:10.1111/j.1474-9726.2006.00223.x.
104. Pochi PE, Strauss JS, Downing DT. Age-related changes in sebaceous gland activity. J Invest Dermatol. 1979;73(1):108–11.
105. Paus R, Cotsarelis G. The biology of hair follicles. N Engl J Med. 1999;341(7):491–7. doi:10.1056/NEJM199908123410706.
106. Grove GL. Physiologic changes in older skin. Clin Geriatr Med. 1989;5(1):115–25.
107. Holt DR, Kirk SJ, Regan MC, Hurson M, Lindblad WJ, Barbul A. Effect of age on wound healing in healthy human beings. Surgery. 1992;112(2):293–7; discussion 297–8.
108. Gilliver SC, Ashworth JJ, Ashcroft GS. The hormonal regulation of cutaneous wound healing. Clin Dermatol. 2007;25(1):56–62. doi:10.1016/j.clindermatol.2006.09.012.
109. Ashcroft GS, Horan MA, Ferguson MW. Aging is associated with reduced deposition of specific extracellular matrix components, an upregulation of angiogenesis, and an altered inflammatory response in a murine incisional wound healing model. J Invest Dermatol. 1997;108(4):430–7.
110. Mills SJ, Ashworth JJ, Gilliver SC, Hardman MJ, Ashcroft GS. The sex steroid precursor DHEA accelerates cutaneous wound healing via the estrogen receptors. J Invest Dermatol. 2005;125(5):1053–62. doi:10.1111/j.0022-202X.2005.23926.x.
111. Escoffier C, de Rigal J, Rochefort A, Vasselet R, Leveque JL, Agache PG. Age-related mechanical properties of human skin: an in vivo study. J Invest Dermatol. 1989;93(3):353–7.
112. Shuster S, Black MM, McVitie E. The influence of age and sex on skin thickness, skin collagen and density. Br J Dermatol. 1975;93(6):639–43.
113. de Rigal J, Escoffier C, Querleux B, Faivre B, Agache P, Leveque JL. Assessment of aging of the human skin by in vivo ultrasonic imaging. J Invest Dermatol. 1989;93(5):621–5.
114. Boss GR, Seegmiller JE. Age-related physiological changes and their clinical significance. West J Med. 1981;135(6):434–40.
115. Maheux R, Naud F, Rioux M, Grenier R, Lemay A, Guy J, Langevin M. A randomized, double-blind, placebo-controlled study on the effect of conjugated estrogens on skin thickness. Am J Obstet Gynecol. 1994;170(2):642–9.
116. Chen L, Dyson M, Rymer J, Bolton PA, Young SR. The use of high-frequency diagnostic ultrasound to investigate the effect of hormone replacement therapy on skin thickness. Skin Res Technol. 2001;7(2):95–7.
117. Brincat M, Versi E, Moniz CF, Magos A, de Trafford J, Studd JW. Skin collagen changes in postmenopausal women receiving different regimens of estrogen therapy. Obstet Gynecol. 1987;70(1):123–7.
118. Brincat MP, Baron YM, Galea R. Estrogens and the skin. Climacteric. 2005;8(2):110–23. doi:10.1080/13697130500118100.
119. Verdier-Sevrain S, Bonte F, Gilchrest B. Biology of estrogens in skin: implications for skin aging. Exp Dermatol. 2006;15(2):83–94. doi:10.1111/j.1600-0625.2005.00377.x.
120. Thompson Z, Maibach HI. Biological effects of estrogen on skin. In: Farage MA, Miller KW, Maibach HI, editors. Textbook of aging skin. Berlin: Springer; 2010. p. 361–7.
121. Henry F, Pierard-Franchimont C, Cauwenbergh G, Pierard GE. Age-related changes in facial skin contours and rheology. J Am Geriatr Soc. 1997;45(2):220–2.
122. Creidi P, Faivre B, Agache P, Richard E, Haudiquet V, Sauvanet JP. Effect of a conjugated oestrogen (Premarin) cream on ageing facial skin. A comparative study with a placebo cream. Maturitas. 1994;19(3):211–23.
123. Sumino H, Ichikawa S, Abe M, Endo Y, Ishikawa O, Kurabayashi M. Effects of aging, menopause, and hormone replacement therapy on forearm skin elasticity in women. J Am Geriatr Soc. 2004;52(6):945–9. doi:10.1111/j.1532-5415.2004.52262.x.
124. Rittie L, Kang S, Voorhees JJ, Fisher GJ. Induction of collagen by estradiol: difference between sun-protected and photodamaged human skin in vivo. Arch Dermatol. 2008;144(9):1129–40. doi:10.1001/archderm.144.9.1129.

125. Shuster S, Black MM, Bottoms E. Skin collagen and thickness in women with hirsuties. Br Med J. 1970;4(5738):772.
126. Ozasa H, Tominaga T, Nishimura T, Takeda T. Evidence for receptor-dependent response to dihydrotestosterone in cultured human fibroblasts. Endokrinologie. 1981;77(2):129–36.
127. Dunn LB, Damesyn M, Moore AA, Reuben DB, Greendale GA. Does estrogen prevent skin aging? Results from the First National Health and Nutrition Examination Survey (NHANES I). Arch Dermatol. 1997;133(3):339–42.
128. Fuchs KO, Solis O, Tapawan R, Paranjpe J. The effects of an estrogen and glycolic acid cream on the facial skin of postmenopausal women: a randomized histologic study. Cutis. 2003;71(6):481–8.
129. Schmidt JB, Binder M, Demschik G, Bieglmayer C, Reiner A. Treatment of skin aging with topical estrogens. Int J Dermatol. 1996;35(9):669–74.
130. Callens A, Vaillant L, Lecomte P, Berson M, Gall Y, Lorette G. Does hormonal skin aging exist? A study of the influence of different hormone therapy regimens on the skin of postmenopausal women using non-invasive measurement techniques. Dermatology. 1996;193(4):289–94.
131. Rogers J, Harding C, Mayo A, Banks J, Rawlings A. Stratum corneum lipids: the effect of ageing and the seasons. Arch Dermatol Res. 1996;288(12):765–70.
132. Sobel H, Cohen RA. Effect of estradion on hyaluronic acid in the skin of aging mice. Steroids. 1970;16(1):1–3.
133. Jemec GB, Serup J. Scaling, dry skin and gender. A bioengineering study of dry skin. Acta Derm Venereol Suppl Stockh. 1992;177:26–8.
134. Sato T, Sonoda T, Itami S, Takayasu S. Predominance of type I 5alpha-reductase in apocrine sweat glands of patients with excessive or abnormal odour derived from apocrine sweat (osmidrosis). Br J Dermatol. 1998;139(5):806–10.
135. Kenney WL, Anderson RK. Responses of older and younger women to exercise in dry and humid heat without fluid replacement. Med Sci Sports Exerc. 1988;20(2):155–60.
136. Akamatsu H, Zouboulis CC, Orfanos CE. Control of human sebocyte proliferation in vitro by testosterone and 5-alpha-dihydrotestosterone is dependent on the localization of the sebaceous glands. J Invest Dermatol. 1992;99(4):509–11.
137. Roh M, Han M, Kim D, Chung K. Sebum output as a factor contributing to the size of facial pores. Br J Dermatol. 2006;155(5):890–4. doi:10.1111/j.1365-2133.2006.07465.x.
138. Zouboulis CC. Acne and sebaceous gland function. Clin Dermatol. 2004;22(5):360–6. doi:10.1016/j.clindermatol.2004.03.004.
139. Zouboulis CC, Boschnakow A. Chronological ageing and photoageing of the human sebaceous gland. Clin Exp Dermatol. 2001;26(7):600–7.
140. Jahoda CA, Horne KA, Oliver RF. Induction of hair growth by implantation of cultured dermal papilla cells. Nature. 1984;311(5986):560–2.
141. Asada Y, Sonoda T, Ojiro M, Kurata S, Sato T, Ezaki T, Takayasu S. 5 alpha-reductase type 2 is constitutively expressed in the dermal papilla and connective tissue sheath of the hair follicle in vivo but not during culture in vitro. J Clin Endocrinol Metab. 2001;86(6):2875–80.
142. Rebora A. Pathogenesis of androgenetic alopecia. J Am Acad Dermatol. 2004;50(5):777–9. doi:10.1016/j.jaad.2003.11.073.
143. Drake L, Hordinsky M, Fiedler V, Swinehart J, Unger WP, Cotterill PC, Thiboutot DM, Lowe N, Jacobson C, Whiting D, Stieglitz S, Kraus SJ, Griffin EI, Weiss D, Carrington P, Gencheff C, Cole GW, Pariser DM, Epstein ES, Tanaka W, Dallob A, Vandormael K, Geissler L, Waldstreicher J. The effects of finasteride on scalp skin and serum androgen levels in men with androgenetic alopecia. J Am Acad Dermatol. 1999;41(4):550–4.
144. Inui S, Itami S. Molecular basis of androgenetic alopecia: from androgen to paracrine mediators through dermal papilla. J Dermatol Sci. 2011;61(1):1–6. doi:10.1016/j.jdermsci.2010.10.015.
145. Hibino T, Nishiyama T. Role of TGF-beta2 in the human hair cycle. J Dermatol Sci. 2004;35(1):9–18. doi:10.1016/j.jdermsci.2003.12.003.
146. Price VH. Androgenetic alopecia in women. J Investig Dermatol Symp Proc. 2003;8(1):24–7. doi:10.1046/j.1523-1747.2003.12168.x.
147. Rosenfield RL. Hirsutism and the variable response of the pilosebaceous unit to androgen. J Investig Dermatol Symp Proc. 2005;10(3):205–8. doi:10.1111/j.1087-0024.2005.10106.x.
148. Hoffmann R, Niiyama S, Huth A, Kissling S, Happle R. 17alpha-estradiol induces aromatase activity in intact human anagen hair follicles ex vivo. Exp Dermatol. 2002;11(4):376–80.
149. Oh HS, Smart RC. An estrogen receptor pathway regulates the telogen-anagen hair follicle transition and influences epidermal cell proliferation. Proc Natl Acad Sci U S A. 1996;93(22):12525–30.
150. Conrad F, Ohnemus U, Bodo E, Biro T, Tychsen B, Gerstmayer B, Bosio A, Schmidt-Rose T, Altgilbers S, Bettermann A, Saathoff M, Meyer W, Paus R. Substantial sex-dependent differences in the response of human scalp hair follicles to estrogen stimulation in vitro advocate gender-tailored management of female versus male pattern balding. J Investig Dermatol Symp Proc. 2005;10(3):243–6. doi:10.1111/j.1087-0024.2005.10115.x.
151. Ashcroft GS, Greenwell-Wild T, Horan MA, Wahl SM, Ferguson MW. Topical estrogen accelerates cutaneous wound healing in aged humans associated with an altered inflammatory response. Am J Pathol. 1999;155(4):1137–46. doi:10.1016/S0002-9440(10)65217-0.
152. Fimmel S, Zouboulis CC. Influence of physiological androgen levels on wound healing and immune status in men. Aging Male. 2005;8(3–4):166–74. doi:10.1080/13685530500233847.
153. Taylor RJ, Taylor AD, Smyth JV. Using an artificial neural network to predict healing times and

risk factors for venous leg ulcers. J Wound Care. 2002;11(3):101–5.
154. Schroder J, Kahlke V, Staubach KH, Zabel P, Stuber F. Gender differences in human sepsis. Arch Surg. 1998;133(11):1200–5.
155. Ashcroft GS, Mills SJ. Androgen receptor-mediated inhibition of cutaneous wound healing. J Clin Invest. 2002;110(5):615–24. doi:10.1172/jci15704.
156. Gilliver SC, Ruckshanthi JP, Atkinson SJ, Ashcroft GS. Androgens influence expression of matrix proteins and proteolytic factors during cutaneous wound healing. Lab Invest. 2007;87(9):871–81. doi:10.1038/labinvest.3700627.
157. Gilliver SC, Ruckshanthi JP, Hardman MJ, Zeef LA, Ashcroft GS. 5alpha-dihydrotestosterone (DHT) retards wound closure by inhibiting re-epithelialization. J Pathol. 2009;217(1):73–82. doi:10.1002/path.2444.
158. Hardman MJ, Ashcroft GS. Estrogen, not intrinsic aging, is the major regulator of delayed human wound healing in the elderly. Genome Biol. 2008;9(5):R80. doi:10.1186/gb-2008-9-5-r80.
159. Ashcroft GS, Dodsworth J, van Boxtel E, Tarnuzzer RW, Horan MA, Schultz GS, Ferguson MW. Estrogen accelerates cutaneous wound healing associated with an increase in TGF-beta1 levels. Nat Med. 1997;3(11):1209–15.
160. Morales DE, McGowan KA, Grant DS, Maheshwari S, Bhartiya D, Cid MC, Kleinman HK, Schnaper HW. Estrogen promotes angiogenic activity in human umbilical vein endothelial cells in vitro and in a murine model. Circulation. 1995;91(3):755–63.
161. Routley CE, Ashcroft GS. Effect of estrogen and progesterone on macrophage activation during wound healing. Wound Repair Regen. 2009;17(1):42–50. doi:10.1111/j.1524-475X.2008.00440.x.
162. Ashcroft GS, Mills SJ, Lei K, Gibbons L, Jeong MJ, Taniguchi M, Burow M, Horan MA, Wahl SM, Nakayama T. Estrogen modulates cutaneous wound healing by downregulating macrophage migration inhibitory factor. J Clin Invest. 2003;111(9):1309–18. doi:10.1172/JCI16288.
163. Hardman MJ, Waite A, Zeef L, Burow M, Nakayama T, Ashcroft GS. Macrophage migration inhibitory factor: a central regulator of wound healing. Am J Pathol. 2005;167(6):1561–74. doi:10.1016/S0002-9440(10)61241-2.
164. Campbell L, Emmerson E, Davies F, Gilliver SC, Krust A, Chambon P, Ashcroft GS, Hardman MJ. Estrogen promotes cutaneous wound healing via estrogen receptor beta independent of its antiinflammatory activities. J Exp Med. 2010;207(9):1825–33. doi:10.1084/jem.20100500.

Hair Changes Caused by Aging

Caroline Romanelli, Ellem T.S. Weimann,
Felipe B.C. Santos, and Adilson Costa

Contents

12.1	**Physiology of the Hair Follicle**	151
12.1.1	Embryology	151
12.1.2	Anatomy	152
12.2	**Growth Cycle**	153
12.2.1	Growth (Anagen)	153
12.2.2	Cessation (Catagen)	154
12.2.3	Rest (Telogen)	155
12.3	**Physiology of Aging**	155
12.3.1	Changes in Scalp Hair Caused by Aging	155
12.3.2	Canities	156
12.4	**Androgenetic Alopecia**	158
12.4.1	Concept and Etiopathogenesis	158
12.4.2	Diagnosis	159
12.4.3	Treatment	160
References		161

12.1 Physiology of the Hair Follicle

12.1.1 Embryology

The development of the hair follicle begins between the 8th and 12th week of gestation as dermal condensations of fetal skin which appear at regular intervals, initially in the eyebrows, chin, and upper lip. Subsequently, it is extended caudally and ventrally in waves. It appears that the stimulus which initiates and maintains the process in the fetus originates from within the mesenchymal tissue of the human dermis. This specialized mesenchyme also regulates the epidermal placoid scales' subsequent penetration in the dermis, causing the hair follicles to widen like a cord of epithelial cells, in an open angle with the epidermis. The eventual location of this specialized connective tissue is situated as a condensation below the deepest part of the epithelial invagination, resulting in the dermal papilla of the hair bulb (Fig. 12.1). The follicles do not form in the absence of mesenchymal influence. The erector muscle of the follicle originates independently of the hair follicle [1].

During the second quarter, the peripheral epithelial cells are separated from the central epithelial cells in the hair bulb, thus forming the outer root sheath. The centrally located cells are situated above the dermal papilla and are later differentiated in the inner root sheath and in the hair shaft with its cuticle, cortex, and medulla. All hair follicles are formed during the period of

C. Romanelli, MD (✉) • E.T.S. Weimann, MD
F.B.C. Santos, MD • A. Costa, MD, MSc, PhD
Department of Dermatology, Pontifical Catholic
University of Campinas, 145 Dona Presciliana Soares,
Apt. 92, Campinas, São Paulo 13025-080, Brazil
e-mail: dracarolineromanelli@yahoo.com.br;
tatianisouza03@yahoo.com.br;
felipe_med34@yahoo.com.br;
adilson_costa@hotmail.com

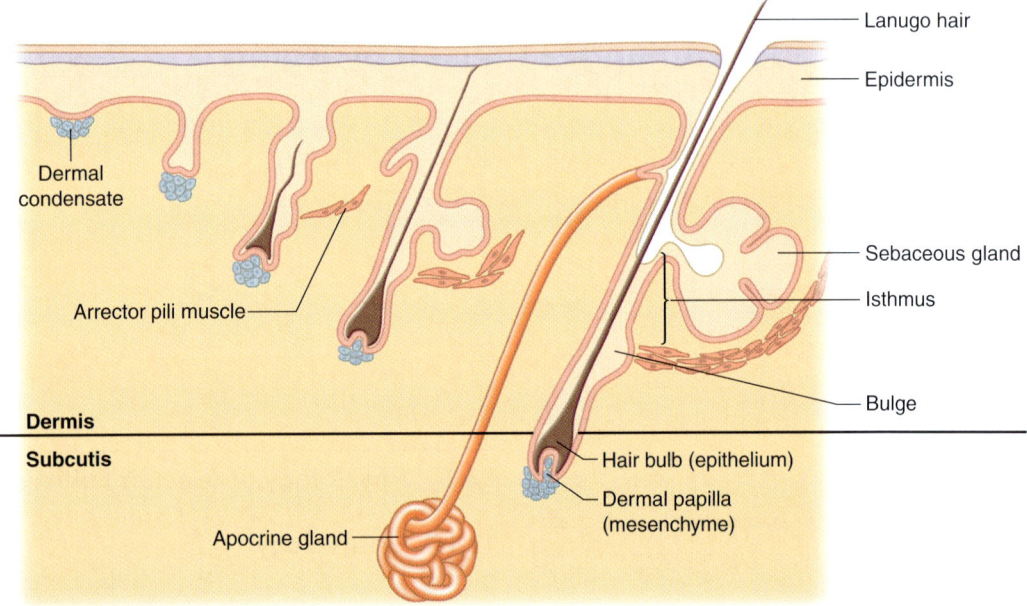

Fig. 12.1 Fetal development of the hair follicle

embryonic life, and in humans additional follicles are not formed after birth. The maximum density of hair follicles on the scalp is found in newborns and gradually decreases with age until adulthood [2]. There are two types of hair: (1) the vellus, a thin and light hair that after birth replaces the fetal or lanugo hair, and (2) the terminal hair, thicker and pigmented hair that includes the scalp, face, eyelids, trunk, armpits, groin, and extremities [3].

The melanocytes are the cells responsible for the pigmentation of the hair and are embryologically derived from a germinal population of melanoblasts originating from within the neural crest cells, shortly after neural tube closure [4]. The melanoblasts migrate from the neural crest stem, following a dorsolateral path between the dermatome of the somites and the ectoderm, to their destination in the basal layer of the epidermis or the hair follicle [5]. Other melanocytes, which are derived from the neural crest, migrate to areas around the eye and the *stria vascularis* in the inner ear. A cell subpopulation differs from the neuroectoderm in situ to become the retinal pigment epithelium. In addition, some melanocytes migrate to the leptomeninges and the mucosa (Fig. 12.2).

12.1.2 Anatomy

Schematically, the hair follicle is divided into two segments (Fig. 12.3): the upper segment, which is a permanent part of the follicle and extends from the insertion point of the arrector pili muscle of the follicle up to the skin surface. The upper segment is comprised of two subdivisions: the isthmus, which comes from the insertion point of the arrector pili muscle up to the opening of the sebaceous gland in the hair follicle, and the infundibulum, which extends from the opening of the sebaceous gland to the skin surface. The opening of the infundibulum on the skin surface is called the follicular ostium or acrotrichum [6].

The part of the hair follicle between the insertion point of the arrector pili muscle to the base of the bulb is called the inferior segment or transient follicle and as is the case in the upper segment is divided into two parts: (1) a stem that extends from the insertion point of the arrector pili muscle to the Adamson's fringe (the transition region between the "fully cornified" cells, i.e., dead cells, which constitute the hair shaft, and (2) the bulb, which corresponds to the region of Adamson's fringe, up to the base of the follicle. The bulb base, shaped as a "cup," contains the

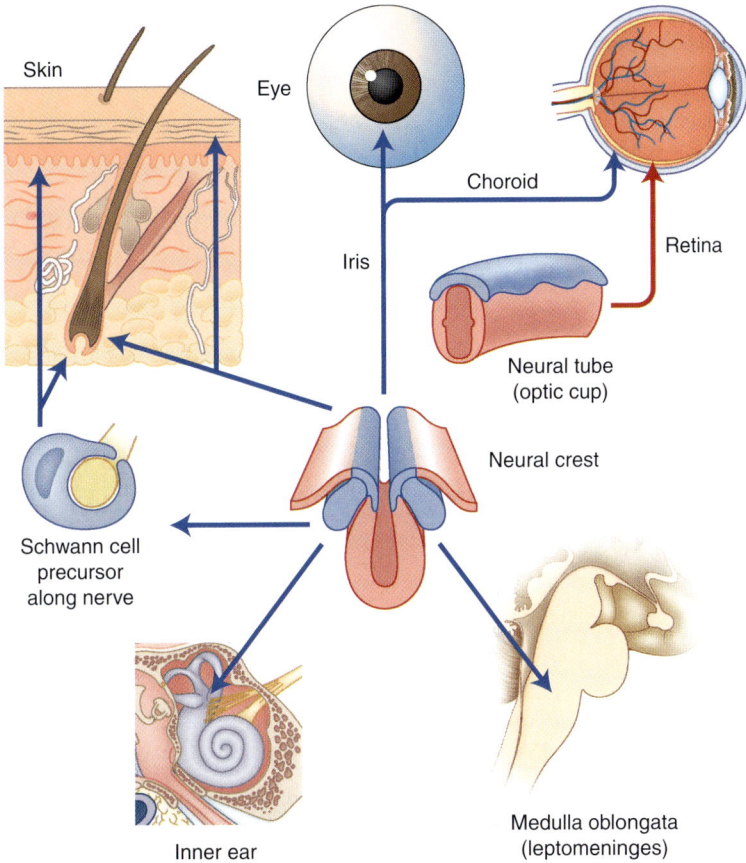

Fig. 12.2 Migration of melanocytes from the neural crest

matrix and involves the dermal papilla. The dermal papilla is the only part of the lower segment that is not transitory. It is in the lower or transient segment that the basic physiology of the hair occurs, i.e., the biological cycle of the hair follicle [6].

12.2 Growth Cycle

In humans, hair loss occurs in a continuous and asynchronous manner, due to the interaction of numerous growth factors, including cytokines, hormones, neurotransmitters, and their receptors. The hair cycling affects the terminal follicles and the vellus hair, drastically modifying the morphology of the lower segment of the follicle, in addition to connective tissue, blood vessels, nerves, and the cell populations connected with the hair follicle [7]. The hair cycle is divided into three phases (Fig. 12.4):

12.2.1 Growth (Anagen)

It is the longest phase of active growth, enduring from 2 to 7 years, and which may result in hair 12 to 80 cm long. This phase is divided into six phases – I to VI. Its duration varies from one area to another on the body and is the most important determining factor to define the length of the hair. This process may continue for several years in the scalp and only endures a few weeks in the hair follicles of the extremities [1]. The hair bulb of the follicles in the anagen phase presents an abundant production of melanin and an intense mitotic activity that may result in stem growth of about 1 cm per month or 0.35 mm per day. The hairs, which grow more rapidly in humans, are those found in the follicles of the chin, about 0.38 mm/day [8]. About 80–100 % of the hair follicles are in the anagen phase. Due to the fact that intense mitotic activity occurs during this phase, the DNA and melanin synthesis is the

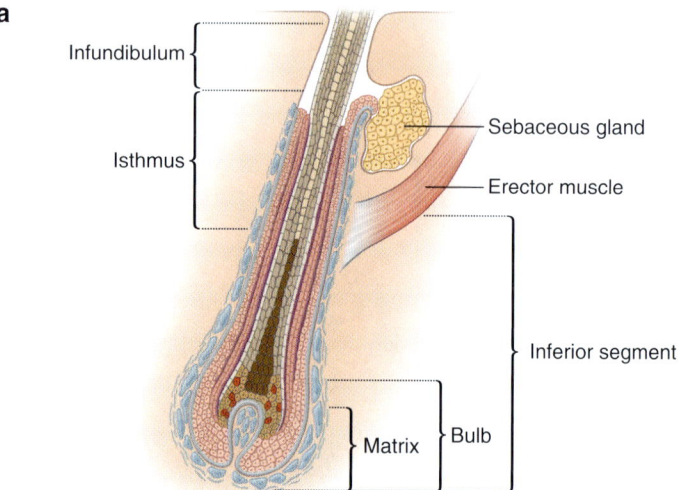
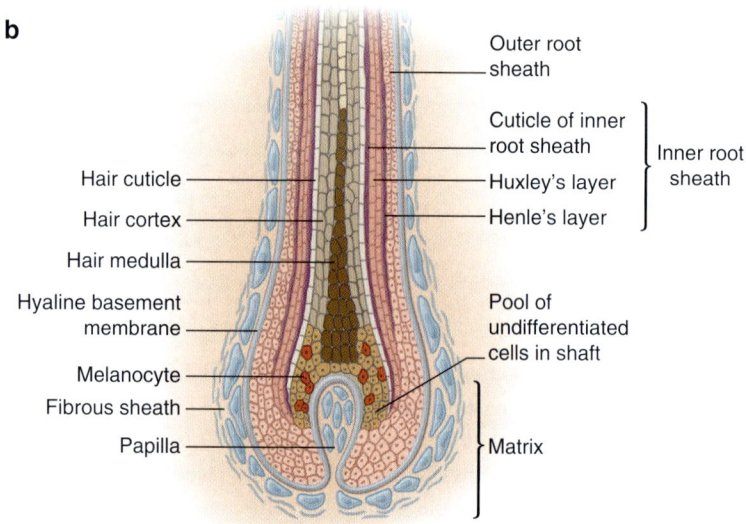

Fig. 12.3 (**a**) Hair follicle. Longitudinal section showing the three sections: the infundibulum, the isthmus, and the inferior segment. (**b**) Hair bulb. The outer and inner root sheaths mold and protect the growing hair shaft. The hair shaft consists of the medulla, hair cortex, and cuticle

phase which is most susceptible to hormonal changes, medications, and toxics in general. It is the only phase during which hair pigmentation occurs as a result of the internalization of bulbar melanocytes, keratinocytes, and fibroblasts of the dermal papilla [1].

12.2.2 Cessation (Catagen)

During this phase, the inferior segment of the follicle regresses sharply due to massive apoptosis of the follicular epithelium, with a remarkable reduction of it in size. This is the shortest phase in the hair cycle and lasts only 2–3 weeks. Consequently, only between 1 and 2 % of follicles develop in this phase and follicles may therefore rarely be encountered in biopsies of the scalp. A horizontal cut of this hair is characterized by oval- or round-shaped hair follicles, abundant apoptosis, and an absence of mitotic activity and melanin pigment production. Forced traction induces the catagen phase. The best time to perform biopsies in order to observe

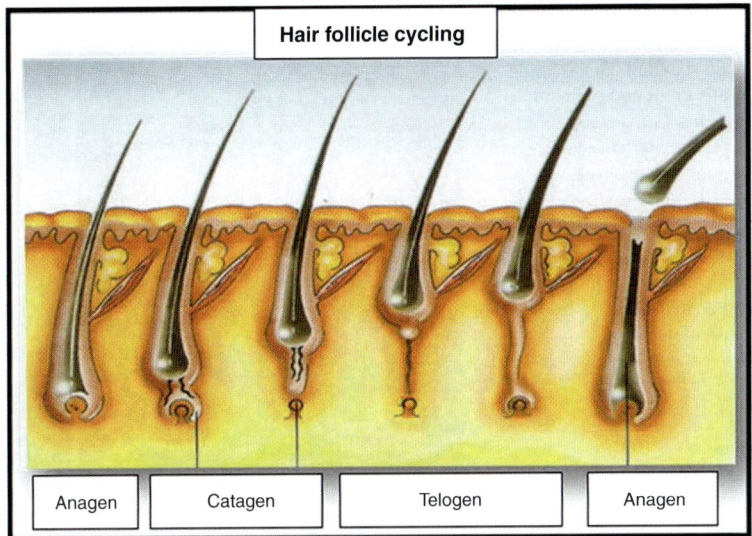

Fig. 12.4 Hair follicle cycling

this phenomenon is when biopsies are performed 2–3 months after the occurrence of a traumatic event [1].

12.2.3 Rest (Telogen)

This phase lasts for about 100 days. Between 10 and 20 % of all hair grow during this phase. On the scalp, about 100 hair follicles in the telogen phase are lost per day. Follicles on the chest and extremities have a more frequent and lasting telogen phase than the hair follicles of the scalp. This phase is the final phase of involution of the inferior segment of the hair follicle. Development during this phase consists of two other stages that represent the final components of the telogen phase and that may not be easily detected in routine histological studies:

1. *Exogenous* (*Teloptose*): hair loss without traction occurs spontaneously each day (approximately 100).
2. *Xenogenous*: the time interval after the exogenous stage in which the hair follicle remains empty before a new follicle in the anagen phase starts to grow. The frequency and the duration of loss of hair follicles during this phase increase in women and men with androgenetic alopecia [1].

12.3 Physiology of Aging

12.3.1 Changes in Scalp Hair Caused by Aging

According to Accursio [34], the hair aging process includes canities (loss of hair color) and a reduction in the number of hair follicles. Remaining hair is smaller in diameter and grows slower. The resulting baldness is primarily androgenetic [9]. The rate of hair growth varies during human aging.

The onset and progression of hair whitening strongly correlate with chronological age and occurs in various degrees in all individuals, regardless of gender and race. The age of onset is genetically inheritable and controllable. Thus, the age range for Caucasians is, on average, around 30; for Asians after 30; and for Africans, on average, at 40. In fact, premature graying only occurs before the age of 20 in Caucasians, before the age of 25 in Asians, and before the age of 30 in Africans [10].

The darker the hair, the earlier it may turn gray. Scalp hair first turns gray at the temples, spreading to the vertex and subsequently across the head. The occipital region is the last to be affected [11]. The epidermal melanocyte units become less stable and reduce by 10–20 % in its pigment production by the epidermal melanocytes (whether in sun-exposed skin or not) in each decade after the age of 30.

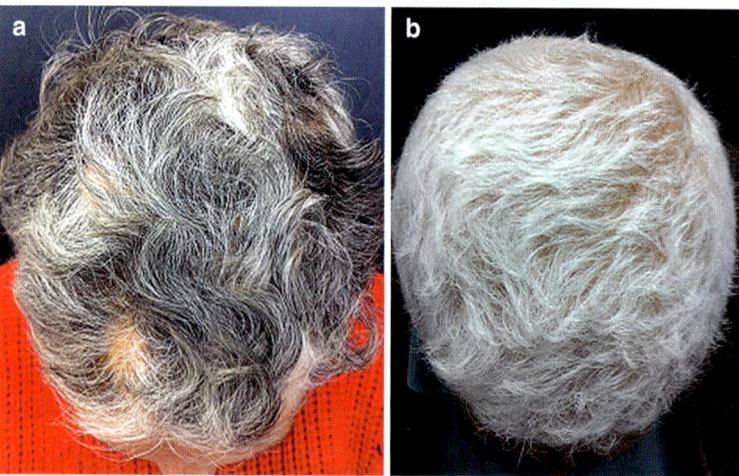

Fig. 12.5 (**a**) Macroscopic view of graying of the scalp showing admixture of *white*, *gray*, and pigmented hair in a woman. (**b**) Total depigmented hair (canities) in a man (Reprinted with permission from Tobin [11]. © 2008 The Author. *Journal compilation*. © 2008 Society of Cosmetic Scientists and the Société Française de Cosmétologie)

The bulb melanocytes on the scalp engage in greater activity during the years of youth when the follicular melanin unit only experiences aging during a few of its growth cycles [13]. There is empirical evidence to suggest that the capacity of the reservoir of stem cells in the hair follicle may be limited in adults. Repeated removal of the vibrissae of mice possibly caused in an increase of gray hair [14].

Follicular melanocytes differ from epidermal melanocytes by their larger size and longer dendrites and only relate to four to five keratinocytes, as opposed to 36–40 in the case of epidermal melanocytes [15]. Just as the close correlation between keratinocytes and melanocytes in the epidermal melanin units of the skin, the likelihood exists that the hair bulb melanocytes in the follicular melanin unit also influence their neighboring pre-cortical keratinocytes in many ways [12]. For example, the transfer of melanin to the keratinocytes appears to reduce potential of late proliferation and may actually stimulate their differentiation. This suspended proliferation interrupted modulation of keratinocytes, in association with melanin, appears to cause a slight increase in gray and white hair follicles. In fact, white facial hair appears to grow faster than the adjacent hair with color in vivo [16]. Furthermore, white hair follicles display a high degree of elongation of the hair fiber in vitro compared to pigmented hair follicles [17].

12.3.2 Canities

Canities (hair color loss) results from a marked reduction in the melanogenic activity of melanocytes in the hair bulb of hair follicles in the anagen phase. The depigmented follicles emerge on the skin surface already as white hair (Fig. 12.5). "Gray" hair may only be illusory, and in many cases the appearance of gray stems from the mixture of white and pigmented hair. However, gray follicles can also affect individual hair follicles during a short growth stage in anagen phase VI, during which a gradual loss of pigmentation along the stem occurs. In these true gray hair follicles, melanin granules can quickly be detected within the pre-cortex and capillary fiber [11]. These gray follicles display a reduced but detectable dopamine oxidation reaction (an indication of the tyrosinase activity), whereas white hair bulbs appear greatly reduced [18].

The extremely low turnover of melanocytes in the epidermis (even after sun exposure) may indicate that the epidermal melanocytes are cells that live a relatively long life. This may be a result of the high concentration of Bcl-2 (anti-apoptotic protein) in epidermal melanocytes, which may allow these cells to survive exogenous aggressions, including the influence of reactive oxygen species (ROS) and the endogenous oxidative stress generated during the actual melanogenesis [19]. In instances where this protein is deficient, loss of melanocytes is accelerated through apoptosis when the follicle enters the telogen phase.

There appears to be a loss of dopamine-positive melanocytes with the onset of age across the body surface, not only on the skin (epidermis and hair follicles) but also on the nevi and eyes. However, this pigment reduction is gradual in the epidermis and more dramatic in the hair follicle. Under these conditions, different subpopulations of melanocytes are regulated by different melanogenic clocks. The dominant factor appears to be hereditary and many canities seem to be inherited in an autosomal dominant pattern; this would explain all blood relatives who have gray hair at an early age [20].

The replicative potential loss of melanocytes in vitro is not only associated with increased age of the donor but also with the extensive manipulation of melanin within the cell [21]. The loss of proliferative capacity in hyperpigmented cells appears to result from its inability to activate the mitogen-activated protein (MAP) kinase that is required for proliferation [22]. Upon reaching senescence, melanocytes also express increased levels of inhibitors of cyclin-dependent kinases, which inhibit the cell cycle [23].

Bath et al. [38] demonstrated in an epidemiological study on premature graying, in which serum levels of iron, ferritin, the total capacity of iron binding (TIBC), vitamin D3, calcium, and vitamin B12 were measured, that levels of ferritin, calcium, and vitamin D3 were found to be lower in said case studies, compared with controlled groups. While analyzing the level of vitamin D3, there were a statistically significant number of patients with deficiency (45.7 % vs. 20 %) and failure (54.3 % vs. 45.7 %), compared with controlled groups. In this study, there were no significant differences between patients and controlled group individuals in relation to hemoglobin, TIBC, iron serum, and vitamin B12.

The accumulation of oxidative damage is an important factor in order to determine the rate of aging, although it is unclear whether or not it is the primary cause. The ROS causes damage to the DNA structure and this may lead to an accumulation of mutations which may induce the oxidative stress and thereby activate antioxidant mechanisms. It is likely that these mechanisms within the melanocytes of hair follicles become impaired with age [24].

Kauser et al. illustrated that it is possible to successfully transfer the phenotype of melanocytes present in aged hair follicles of the skin ex vivo to the culture of cells in vitro. It also suggested that the expression/activity of catalase is an important effector of senile melanocyte responses. The data collected support the theory that the susceptibility of these melanocytes to oxidative stress over time can be a major factor in the loss of hair pigment, the overall reduction in follicle melanocytes, and ultimately the increase in number of white hair [37].

Research conducted by Arck et al. [17] suggests that the melanin unit of aged hair follicles is, in fact, related to the increased apoptosis levels of melanocytes and oxidative stress. This research also demonstrated that the common deletion in mitochondrial DNA (associated with oxidative stress) occurred more prominently in graying hair follicles compared to those with normal pigmentation.

The involvement of reactive oxygen species in the histopathology of canities is confirmed by observing that the melanocytes in gray and white hair bulbs can be vacuolated. This is a common cellular response to increased oxidative stress. Similar cellular characteristics are also seen in melanocytes in vitiligo, where millimolar levels of the oxidant H_2O_2 damage the epidermal melanocytes [25].

Wood et al. [36] demonstrated, through an in vivo study, the presence of concentrations of 10^{-3} M of H_2O_2 in completely white and gray hair; however, in pigmented brown hair, H_2O_2 was not detected. Based on these findings, they concluded that gray/white hair presents a massive concentration of H_2O_2, associated with the oxidation of amino acid residues (methionine, tryptophan, and cysteine), mediated by H_2O_2, and demonstrated by the oxidation of the tyrosinase in spectrophotometry (Fig. 12.6).

Fig. 12.6 H_2O_2 prevents Met-S=O repair in tyrosinase. Evidence that tyrosinase activity is interrupted as a result of oxidation of Met (methionine) 374 in the enzyme active site by these ROS. The resulting Met-S_O cannot be repaired because methionine sulfoxide reductases A and B (MSRA and MSRB) are also deactivated by H_2O_2, as evidenced by low enzyme activities in gray hair follicle extracts, or they can originate from low protein levels. The same scenario applies to catalase. Combined, a shift in the H_2O_2 redox balance can significantly alter melanogenesis in the human hair follicle

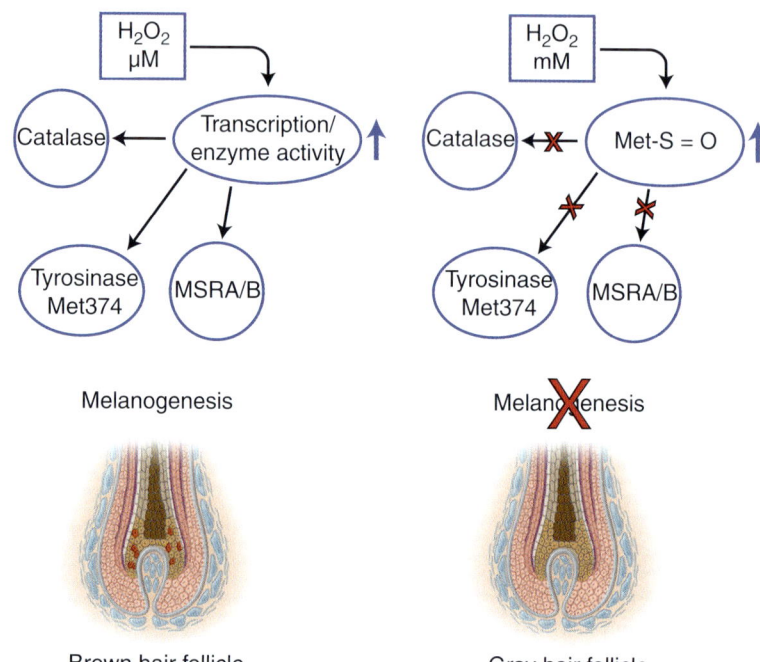

12.4 Androgenetic Alopecia

12.4.1 Concept and Etiopathogenesis

Hair loss is a common genetic condition, caused by the action of circulating androgens. There is progressive loss and thinning of the hair, with clinical condition easily recognized by the anterior and middle temporal recess of hair follicles on the scalp. The etiopathogenesis is multifactorial, since it involves factors of genetic and hormonal nature [35].

In relation to the genetic factor, androgenetic alopecia is caused by a single autosomal and dominant gene with reduced penetrance in females. It is considered a classic example of polygenic origin [26]. Hormone changes start at puberty, when androgens acting within the follicles, genetically programmed and located in the frontoparietal region, lead to the transformation of the miniaturized terminal. Consequently, the hair is biologically modified, with a progressive decrease in the time of the anagen phase after several cycles [27].

The hormonal factor manifests in places where the pilosebaceous androgen-dependent unit (hair follicle and sebaceous gland) has specific receptors. In men, testosterone is the androgen in higher concentration. It is secreted by the testicles and adrenal glands and metabolized by the 5-alpha-reductase in the liver, skin, prostate gland, and scalp to dihydrotestosterone (DHT). In women, the androstenedione is the principal androgen. It precedes the production of testosterone [28].

The etiopathogenesis of androgenetic alopecia has the following sequence: the hair contains 5-alpha-reductase type II, which acts on the peripheral conversion of free testosterone into DHT in genetically predisposed men, leading to baldness. Thus, the bald area has increased amounts of DHT and the miniaturization and/or reduction of hair follicles. Hence, men with genetic deficiency of 5-alpha-reductase type II do not present androgenetic alopecia [27].

Inside the hair follicle cells, testosterone and androstenedione can suffer the action of an enzyme aromatase cytochrome P450, which transforms the follicles into estradiol. It is through the functioning of this mechanism that the amount of testosterone and intracellular DHT decreases, leading to the protection of the follicle and no predisposition to baldness [29]. In men, hair follicles located in the frontal region have

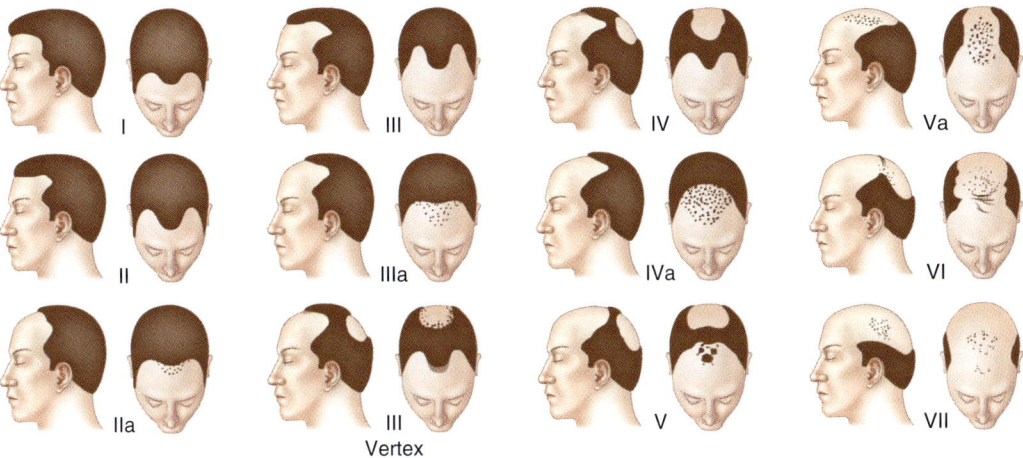

Fig. 12.7 Hamilton-Norwood classification of male pattern baldness

half the amount of aromatase in relation to the occipital region. The opposite scenario is found in women, who have six times more aromatase in the frontal region than men with androgenetic alopecia. This high level of aromatase results in an increased conversion of testosterone to estradiol and estrone, and consequently, the conversion of testosterone into DHT reduces [30].

In light of the above, women with androgenetic alopecia maintain a frontal line with thinning, but not receding hair. It is likely that these differences determine the typical patterns of baldness in men and women. The androgenetic alopecia in women, due to cutaneous hyperandrogenism, may appear as a result of the following hormonal factors, whether isolated or combined with each other: increased glandular secretion of androgens by the ovaries, adrenals, or both; changes in blood levels of sex hormone-binding globulin (SHBG); greater peripheral sensitivity of androgen receptors of the pilosebaceous units; and increased conversion of free testosterone to DHT in the tissues by raising the rate of 5-alpha-reductase [27].

12.4.2 Diagnosis

Androgenetic alopecia can be divided into two types: androgenetic alopecia in men or male pattern baldness and androgenetic alopecia in women or female pattern baldness.

12.4.2.1 Androgenetic Alopecia in Men: Classification

This is also called Hippocratic or classic pattern. The progression and various patterns of hair loss are classified by the system of classification of male pattern baldness named Hamilton-Norwood, in eight types of progression (Fig. 12.7).

The frontotemporal triangular retraction normally occurs in most young men (type I) and in women after puberty. The first sign that a person is becoming bald is the increasing frontotemporal retraction, accompanied by a retraction of the frontal medial portion (type II). This is followed by hair loss in the round area of the vertex, followed by a decrease in hair density, sometimes rapidly, over the top of the scalp (types III to VII) [31].

In cases of androgenetic alopecia in men, there is no need for laboratory tests, unless there is suspicion of systemic disease, such as anemia, hypothyroidism, and other collagen diseases. Serum levels of androgens in bald men remain equal to those of men who are not bald, reinforcing the theory that the pathophysiological mechanism of this change is peripheral and genetic [27].

12.4.2.2 Female Pattern Hair Loss: Classification

Ludwig in 1977 classified this pattern noticeable by virtue of the progressive thinning of hair in the central area of the scalp, without retraction of the

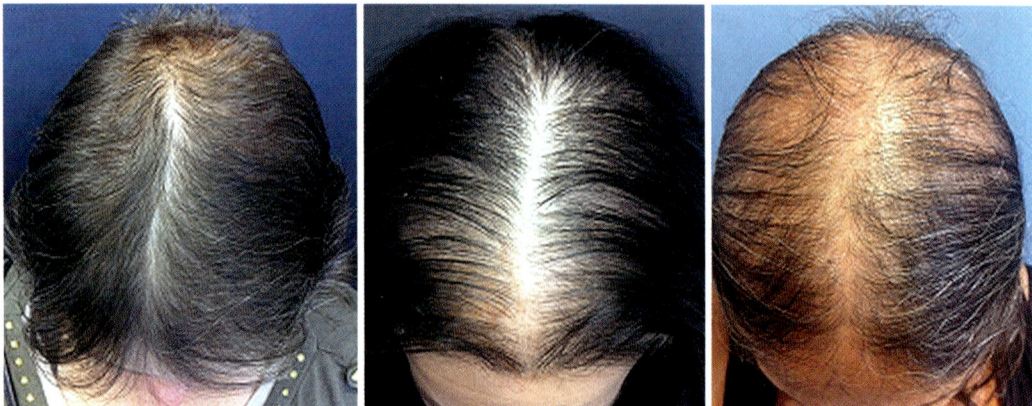

Fig. 12.8 Ludwig pattern. Evolution of female androgenetic alopecia (Reprinted with permission from Ludwig [39]. Copyright © 2006, John Wiley and Sons)

implant line in the frontal region. There are three types of evolution: Type I, mild form with thinning of the middle portion; Type II, moderate; and Type III, severe (Fig. 12.8) [27].

Androgens only lead to female baldness – both in menopausal women and women in gestational age – if they present strong genetic predisposition. In those women with fewer genetic traits, hair loss will only occur when androgen production is increased or when drugs with androgenic activity are taken, as is the case of some anovulatory containing progestogen [27].

12.4.3 Treatment

The main objective is to reverse and/or stabilize the process of miniaturization. In hormonal terms, the goal is to reduce androgen activity in the follicles; to block the conversion of testosterone into DHT, with 5-alpha-reductase inhibitor; and to block the androgen receptor protein or transform androgens into estrogens.

The strategy for the treatment of men androgenetic alopecia is based on the following aspects: (1) presence of miniaturized hair, (2) extent of hair loss, and (3) patient's preference for topical or systemic drug. As for surgery, age, willingness, and financial cost have to be considered.

For men with mild to moderate loss, according to Norwood-Hamilton types II to V (see Fig. 12.7), the therapeutic option includes a solution of 2–5 % minoxidil or oral finasteride of 1 mg/day. These can be used individually or combined for at least 1 year. At the end of this period, if the hair loss stabilizes or improves, this therapy should be maintained indefinitely. If there is no response, and for patients with severe or nearly complete loss, the options are scarce and may include hair transplant, the implant of expanders, or the use of hairpieces. Whether or not the patient chooses a treatment, protection of the scalp against solar radiation due to carcinogenic effects should be indicated [27].

For women with female pattern hair loss, the strategy depends on the presence of miniaturized hair and its density. For those women with type I to II (Ludwig classification) female pattern hair loss, a 2 or 5 % minoxidil solution should be used for at least 1 year. At the end of this period, if the hair loss is not stable, androgenic blockers should be administered, such as spironolactone, cyproterone acetate, or finasteride. If the occipital region is a good donor area, a hair transplant could be an option. Should the patient present a type III female pattern hair loss, the topical and/or systemic therapy will be ineffective and may require an evaluation for purposes of a transplant [27].

In female pattern hair loss, there is ongoing discussion about the possible associations with hormonal disturbances in the pathophysiology of the disease; however, there is yet no consensus on this. Notwithstanding the aforesaid, it would still be advisable to run laboratory and imaging tests, especially in young patients with an advanced degree of androgenetic alopecia.

Recent advances have shown that caffeine has beneficial effects on patients with androgenetic alopecia. The proposed mechanism for this would be the phosphodiesterase inhibition through caffeine, which increases the serum levels of cyclic adenosine monophosphate (cAMP) and subsequently promotes the proliferation by stimulation of the cell metabolism [32]. Recent studies analyzing the follicular penetration of caffeine in topical hair follicles showed that the follicles can be a quick route of drug delivery for topical drugs [33].

References

1. Restrepo R. Anatomía microscópica del folículo piloso. Rev Asoc Colomb Dermatol. 2010;18:123–38.
2. Hardy MH. The secret life of the hair follicle. Trends Genet. 1992;8:55–61.
3. Sampaio SAP, Rivitti EA. Dermatologia. 3rd ed. São Paulo: Artes Médicas; 2007. Rev. ampl.
4. Nordlund JJ. The lives of pigmented cells. Dermatol Clin. 1986;4:407–18.
5. Erickon CA. From the crest to the periphery: control of pigment cell migration and lineage segregation. Pigment Cell Res. 1993;6:336–47.
6. Belda Júnior W, Chiacchio N, Di e Criado PR. Tratado de Dermatologia, vol. 1. São Paulo: Atheneu; 2010. p. 970–1.
7. Krause K, Foitzik K. Biology of the hair follicle: the basics. Semin Cutan Med Surg. 2006;25:2–10.
8. Myers RJ, Hamilton JB. Regeneration and rate of growth of hairs in man. Ann NY Acad Sci. 1951;53:562–8.
9. Pelfini C, Cerimele D, Pisanu G. Aging of the skin and hair growth in man. In: Montagna W, Dobson RL, editors. Advances in biology of the skin – hair growth, vol. 9. Oxford, UK: Pergamon; 1969. p. 153–60.
10. Tobin DJ, Paus R. Graying: gerontobiology of the hair follicle pigmentary unit. Exp Gerontol. 2001;36(1):29–54.
11. Tobin DJ. Human hair pigmentation – biological aspects. Int J Cosmet Sci. 2008;30:233–57.
12. Whiteman DC, Parsons PG, Green AC. Determinants of melanocyte density in adult human skin. Arch Dermatol Res. 1999;291:511–6.
13. Keogh EV, Walsh RJ. Rate of graying of human hair. Nature. 1965;207:877–8.
14. Ibrahim L, Wright EA. The long term effect of repeated puckings on the function of the mouse vibrissal follicles. Br J Dermatol. 1978;99:371–6.
15. Goldsmith LA. Physiology, biochemistry and molecular biology of the skin. New York: Oxford University Press; 1991. p. 320–4.
16. Nagl W. Different growth rates of pigmented and white hair in the beard: differentiation vs. proliferation? Br J Dermatol. 1995;132:94–7.
17. Arck PC, Overall R, Spatz K, Liezman C, Handjiski B, Klapp BF, et al. Towards a "free radical theory of graying": melanocyte apoptosis in the aging human hair follicle is an indicator of oxidative stress induced tissue damage. FASEB J. 2006;20:1567–9.
18. Slominski A, Wortsman J, Plonka PM, Schallreuter KU, Paus R, Tobin DJ. Hair follicle pigmentation. J Invest Dermatol. 2005;124:13–21.
19. Tobin DJ. Aging of the hair follicle pigmentation system. Int J Trichol. 2009;1:83–93.
20. Nishimura EK, Granter SR, Fisher DE. Mechanisms of hair graying: incomplete melanocyte stem cell maintenance in the niche. Science. 2005;307(5710):720–4.
21. Bennett DC. Differentiation in mouse melanoma cells: initial reversibility and an on-off stochastic model. Cell. 1983;34:445–53.
22. Medrano EE, Yang F, Boissy R, Farooqui J, Shah V, Matsumoto K, et al. Terminal differentiation and senescence in the human melanocyte: repression of tyrosine-phosphorylation of the extracellular signal-regulated kinase 2 selectively defines the tow phenotypes. Mol Biol Cell. 1994;5(4):497–509.
23. Bennett DC. Human melanocyte senescence and melanoma susceptibility genes. Oncogene. 2003;22(20):3063–9.
24. Kauser S, Westgate G, Green M, Tobin DJ. Age-associated down-regulation of catalase in human scalp hair follicle melanocytes. Pigment Cell Res. 2008;20(5):432–22.
25. Tobin DJ, Swanson NN, Pittelkow MR, Peters EM, Schallreuter KU. Melanocytes are not absent in lesional skin of long duration vitiligo. J Pathol. 2000;191:407–16.
26. Sawaya ME, Hordinsky MK. Advances in alopecia areata and androgenetic alopecia. Arch Dermatol. 1992;7:211–26.
27. Rutowitsch MS, Antônio JR, Steinner D, et al. Alopecia Androgenética. An Bras Dermatol. 1999;74(6):561–72.
28. Bardin CW, Paulsen CA. Textbook of endocrinology. 2. Philadelphia: Saunders; 1981.
29. Pereira JM. Alopecia androgenética difusa na mulher. Rev Bras Med. 1998;55:87–93.
30. Shapiro J, Price V. Hair regrowth. Therapeutic agents. Dermatol Clin. 1998;16:341–56.
31. Habif TP. Clinical dermatology: a color guide to diagnosis and therapy. Philadelphia: Elsevier; 2010. s.l.
32. Fischer TW, Hipler UC, Elsner P. Effect of caffeine and testosterone on the proliferation of human hair follicles n vitro. Int J Dermatol. 2007;46:27–35.

33. Otberg N, Patzelt A, Rasulev U, Hagemeister T, Linscheid M, Sinkgraven R, et al. The role of hair follicles in the percutaneous absorption of caffeine. Br J Clin Pharmacol. 2007;65:88–92.
34. Accursio CSC. Alterações da pele na terceira idade. Rev Bras Med. 2001;58(9):646–58.
35. Bolognia JL, Jorizzo JL, Schaffer JV. Dermatology. Philadelphia: Elsevier; 2012. ISBN 9780723435716.
36. Wood JM, Decker H, Hartmann H, Chavan B, Rokos H, Spencer JD, et al. Senile hair graying: H_2O_2 – mediated oxidative stress affects human hair color by blunting methionine sulfoxide repair. FASEB J. 2009;23:265–75.
37. Kauser S, Westgate GE, Green MR, Tobin DJ. Human hair follicle and epidermal melanocytes exhibit striking differences in their aging profile which involves catalase. J Invest Dermatol. 2011;131:979–82.
38. Bath RM, Sharma R, Pinto AC, Dandekeri S, Martis J. Epidemiological and Investigative Study of Premature Graying of Hair in Higher Secondary and Pre-University School Children. Int J Trichology. 2013;5(1):17–21.
39. Ludwig E. Classification of the types of androgenetic alopecia (common baldness) occurring in the female sex. Br J Dermatol. 2006;97(3):247–54.

Changes in Nails Caused by Aging

Ana Carolina B.B. Arruda, Aline S. Talarico, Felipe B.C. Santos, and Adilson Costa

Contents

13.1	**Normal Nail Biology**	163
13.1.1	Anatomy	163
13.1.2	Physiology	164
13.2	**Changes with Aging**	165
13.3	**The Most Common Disorders in Aged Nails**	166
13.3.1	Brittle Nails	166
13.3.2	Onychodystrophy Caused by Biomechanical Defect and Trauma	167
13.3.3	Infections and Infestations	168
13.3.4	Pachyonychia	169
13.3.5	Onychocryptosis	170
13.3.6	Splinter Hemorrhages and Subungual Hematomas	170
13.3.7	Neoplasms of the Nail Apparatus	170
References		171

A.C.B.B. Arruda, MD (✉)
A.S. Talarico, MD • F.B.C. Santos, MD
A. Costa, MD, MSc, PhD
Department of Dermatology, Pontifical Catholic University of Campinas, Av John Boyd Dunlop, Campinas, Sao Paulo 13060-904, Brazil
e-mail: dermato@hmcp.puc-campinas.edu.br; acbbazan@yahoo.com.br; alinetalarico@hotmail.com; felipe_med34@yahoo.com.br; adilson_costa@hotmail.com

13.1 Normal Nail Biology

13.1.1 Anatomy

The formation process of the nail apparatus starts in the ninth week of pregnancy. The human nail comprises a corneum product, the nail plate, and four specialized tissues, namely, the proximal nail fold, the matrix, the nail bed, and the hyponychium.

The nail plate is the result of maturation and keratinization of the epithelium of the nail matrix and consists of keratinized cells, without a core and closely bonded, providing its hard and translucent characteristic. A nail's pink color is ascribable to the transparent display of a vascularized nail bed. The physical characteristics of the nail plate and its growth depends on the conditions of the nail matrix and its surrounding tissues, including the distal phalanx, which provides shape to the nail and in pathological conditions, may lead to nail abnormalities.

The cuticle, formed by the stratum corneum of the proximal nail fold, is closely adhered/attached to the surface of the nail and is responsible for protecting the nail matrix against the penetration of harmful environmental agents.

The nail matrix is divided into the proximal part, the portion that produces the dorsal nail plate (top two thirds of the nail plate), and the distal part, which is responsible for producing the ventral nail plate (bottom third of the nail plate). In some fingernails, it is possible to see a whitish crescent-shaped base in the proximal part of the nail plate, known as the lunula ("small moon"), which corresponds to the distal matrix that is not covered by the proximal nail fold.

The matrix also contains quiescent melanocytes which, in some pathological or physiological conditions, can be activated to produce melanin, which it then transfers to the surrounding keratinocytes. The formation of melanonychia – the black or brown pigmentation of the normal nail plate – can be detected clinically, usually as a single longitudinal band or, less frequently, as multiple bands or as covering the whole nail.

The nail bed extends from the distal margin of the lunula to the hyponychium and, due to the transparency of the nail plate, may appear fully visible. Its keratinization occurs without the formation of the granular layer and contains a thin layer that is closely attached to the ventral portion of the nail plate.

The hyponychium corresponds to the anatomical area situated between the nail bed and the distal groove, within which the nail plate stands out from the underlying tissues. Its keratinization occurs with formation of the granular layer, different from that of the nail bed. It is usually covered by the nail plate, but in certain pathologies, such as in nail biting, it can become exposed (Fig. 13.1).

The vascularity of the nail apparatus occurs through the digital arteries, which run along the sides of the fingers and give rise to branches that supply both the matrix and proximal nail fold, as the arcs that supply the matrix and the nail bed. Thus, the matrix features two different sources of irrigation. In the nail bed, glomus bodies are present which are encapsulated neurovascular structures containing one to four arteriovenous anastomoses and nerve endings. Their apparent role is to regulate the vascular supply to the digits at low temperatures.

The innervation of the nail apparatus occurs via sensory nerves originating from the dorsal branches of the digital nerves, which run along the digital blood vessels.

13.1.2 Physiology

The nail plate is mainly composed of keratin (filamentous protein with low sulfur content), arranged in an amorphous matrix. Other components are water, lipids, and trace elements (primarily iron, zinc, and calcium). The keratins may be hard (80–90 % of the composition) or mild (10–20 %), and the percentage variation of their subtypes is what determines their characteristics, such as hardness and strength. The water content of the nail is variable, which is a characteristic that occurs as a result of the porosity of the nail. This means it can be hydrated and dehydrated. When the concentration falls below 16 %, the nails become brittle, and when higher than 30 %, the nail becomes opaque and flexible. Lipids are responsible for less than 5 % of the composition

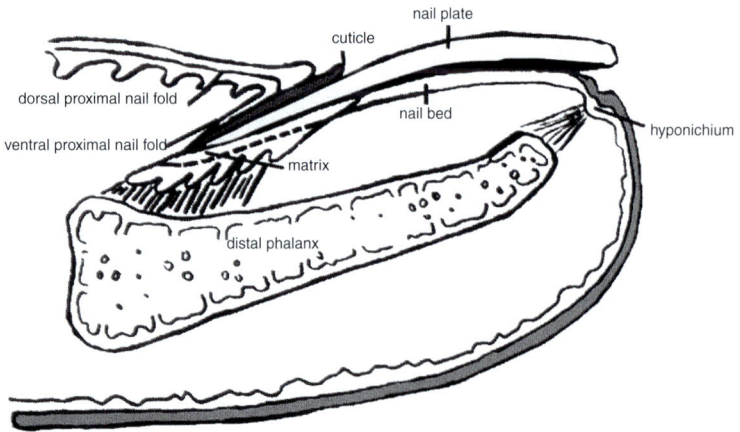

Fig. 13.1 Nail's anatomy (Publication authorized by Romiti et al. [30])

of the nail plate. They are under hormonal control and reduce after menopause [1, 2].

The double curvature of the nail plate along the longitudinal and transverse axes increases its resistance to stress mechanisms, especially mechanical stress.

The growth of the nail plate is continuous throughout life. On average, fingernails grow 3 mm/month and toenails grow 1 mm/month. Therefore, it takes approximately 100–180 days for full replacement of a fingernail and 12–18 months for the toenail. Due to this slow growth rate, diseases involving the nail matrix take a long time to heal and disappear [3].

The growth rate depends on the mitotic activity of the cells of the nail matrix. The nail matrix undergoes changes in and during the course of its life cycle: it has its peak around the person's 20s and 30s, with a dramatic decrease after the age of 50 [3]. Physiological and pathological conditions can influence nail growth. Nails grow faster in certain circumstances like pregnancy, trauma, psoriasis, nail biting, and oral intake of retinoids and itraconazole. On the other hand, nails grow slower in certain instances such as vascular diseases, malnutrition, peripheral neurological diseases, and during chemotherapy [1–3].

13.2 Changes with Aging

With aging, nails undergo changes in their normal characteristics which affect some factors such as growth rate, shape, color, and the composition of the nail plate, which changes occur in addition to an increase to their susceptibility to some diseases [4, 5]. The mechanisms leading to these changes are not yet fully understood, but are probably attributable to vascular dysfunction of the extremities and the effects of sun exposure [6].

The growth rate of nails – which is typically 3 mm/month for fingernails and 1 mm/month for toenails – falls by 0.5 % per year after the age of 25. In men and women, the thickness of the nail plate in toenails and fingernails also tends to decrease [4, 5]. The composition of the nail is altered, displaying a decrease in iron and increase in calcium. These are the only confirmed changes

Table 13.1 Physiological changes in nails, and its clinical representations, in aging process

Nail physiology		Changes with aging
Composition	Keratin (hard or light)	Iron decrease
	Water	Calcium increase
	Lipids	
	Trace elements (iron, zinc, and calcium)	
Growth	Fingernails, 3 mm/month	A decrease of 0.5 %/year
	Toenails, 1 mm/month	Drastic reduction of nail cell mitosis after the age of 50
	Maximum mitotic activity: person's 20s and 30s	

in nails resulting from the aging process [7]. The latter findings are corroborated by a study that analyzed the improvement in the quality of nails during calcium replacement in postmenopausal women. However, no significant difference in quality was detected when compared to the control group [8] (Table 13.1).

Histologically, in the course of the aging process, keratinocytes increase and more thickened blood vessels and degeneration of collagen tissue may be observed in the nail bed [9].

The contour of senile nails changes. This is characterized by a reduced longitudinal curvature and an increased transversal convexity. In this age group, it is common to see nails becoming flat and broad (platonychia), spoon shaped (koilonychia), or excessively curved (pincer nail deformity) [10, 11].

The texture also undergoes changes with advanced age. It gradually loses its soft characteristic and becomes more brittle, prone to cracking, and superficial or deep longitudinal striations [9, 11].

Aging of the nails is the most common cause of onychorrhexis (striations). Beau's lines (deep grooved lines that run from side to side on the fingernail) (Fig. 13.2) and nail pitting are texture changes commonly observed in the elderly. Other changes may include trachyonychia (increased roughness), cracks, and splitting (delamination of the nail plate) [5].

The nail color also undergoes some changes, the most common being a yellowish to grayish

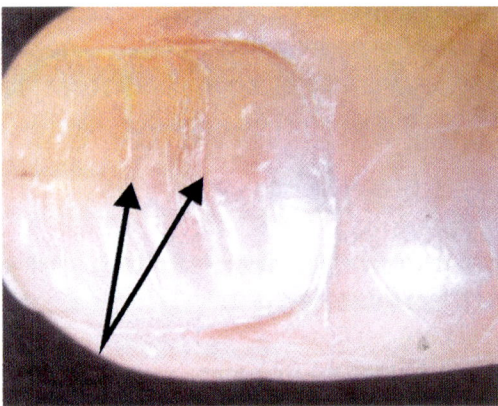

Fig. 13.2 Beau's lines (Publication authorized by Romiti et al. [31])

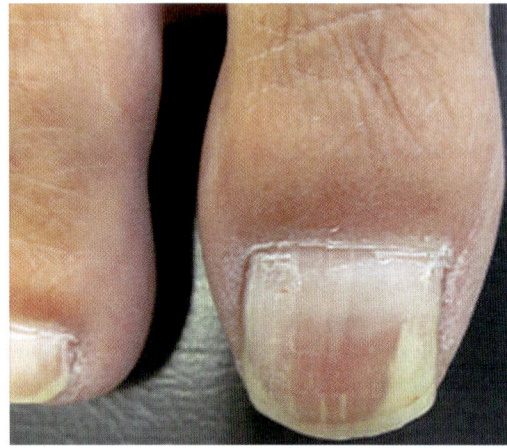

Fig. 13.3 Distal onycholysis (Image from Pontificia Universidade Catolica, Dermatology Department, Campinas, Brazil)

color, with a pale and opaque look. The lunula diminishes or disappears, without displaying any pathological characteristic [9].

Other color changes usually associated with some diseases have recently been defined in the observation of non-pathological changes in normally aging nails. Among these changes, the following are worth highlighting:

- Terry's nails: nails with white color on the proximal half and pinkish color in the distal area. This change was first described in the observation of cirrhotic patients, patients with congestive heart failure, and diabetic or malnourished adults [12].
- Neapolitan nails: these nails are seen in approximately 20 % of the elderly over the age of 70. They are characterized by three bands of color, like Neapolitan ice cream; the proximal area is white, the center has a normal pinkish color, and the free distal edge is opaque. This change is defined and is associated with skin changes and osteoporosis as well as probable etiology related to collagen change [13].

Some other suggestive pathological changes of the nail resulting from the aging condition of the nail apparatus may be regarded as idiopathic. Among these changes are onycholysis (detachment of the nail from the nail bed, starting from its distal and/or lateral attachment) (Fig. 13.3). This is very common in the elderly and may be idiopathic, secondary to trauma, or caused by decreased local circulation [5].

13.3 The Most Common Disorders in Aged Nails

Clinical nail disorders are listed in Table 13.2. Those which are observed during aging process in elderly people are approached in the next paragraphs.

13.3.1 Brittle Nails

The hardness of the nail plate is determined by the concentration of water in its composition. The normal water level is approximately 18 %. Concentrations below 16 % may cause the nail plate to become brittle and above 25 % to become too flexible [9]. Studies have shown that in individuals over the age of 60, fragile nails are more common. This is caused by trachyonychia (increased roughness and longitudinal fissures), onychoschizia (nail splitting, when the horizontal lamellar separates from the distal nail plate) (Fig. 13.4), and the irregularity of the free edge of the distal nail plate [4, 14, 15].

The main causes of brittle nails are hypohydration (which mainly occurs through regular household tasks with water), removal of cuticles, and use of agents that dehydrate the nail plate such as nail polish and nail polish removers.

Table 13.2 Morphological classification of nail changes

Change in nail plate consistency	Onychoschizia: cracks in free edge and peeling of nail plate
	Onychorrhexis: brittle, fragmented nails, with longitudinal cracks (grooves)
Change in nail plate thickness	Pachyonychia congenita: thickening of the nail plate
	Onychogryphosis: thickening of the nail plate, elongated and curved nail (known as "ram's horn nails")
Change in nail plate curvature	Pachyonychia congenita
	Onychogryphosis
	Koilonychia: inversion of the nail, which becomes concave (spoon shaped)
	Hippocratic nails (nail clubbing): watch-glass nails
	Platonychia: flat and broad nail
Change in nail plate surface	Onychorrhexis
	Beau's lines: grooved lines that run from side to side on the fingernail, resulting from the temporary interruption of nail matrix
	Punctures or cupuliform depressions on nails (nail pitting): thimble-shaped nails
	Median canaliform dystrophy of Heller: longitudinal splitting or canal formation in the midline of the nail. It begins in the proximal fold and progresses to the free edge as the matrix is affected
	Nail scratching: bright nails as polished by friction from scratching
Change in the adhesion of the nail plate to the nail bed	Onycholysis: separation of the nail plate from the bed
	Onychomadesis: shedding of the nails beginning at its proximal end
	Subungual keratosis: accumulation of keratin in the nail bed, away from the nail plate
	Nail pterygium: destruction of the nail matrix and nail bed with the formation of scars by the adhesion of the nail fold to the subungual epithelium

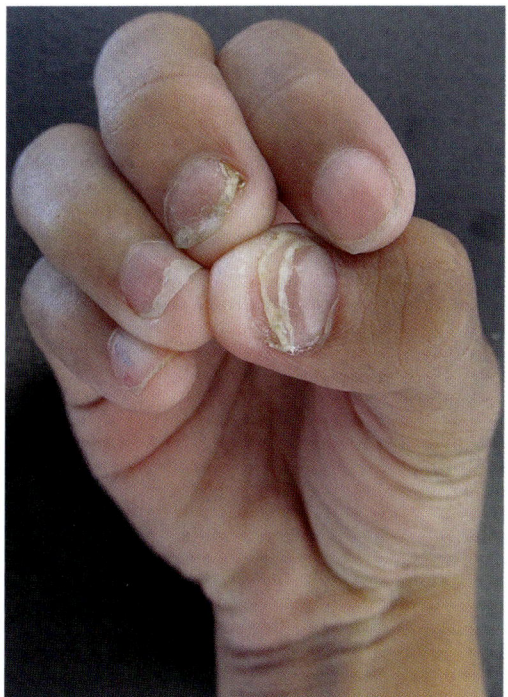

Fig. 13.4 Onychoschizia (first finger) and onycholysis (third finger) (Publication authorized by Romiti et al. [31])

The most affected nails are those of the first three fingers of the dominant hand [4, 14].

Treatment starts with the removal of the triggering factors and by adopting some local measures to hydrate the nail plate, cuticles, and the nail matrix, for instance, treatments involving immersion of the nails in warm water for 10–20 min before applying urea, lactic acid, and mineral oils, preferably under occlusion [4]. The systemic treatment with biotin, iron, thiamine, cysteine, and PABA is also effective [4, 16, 17]. In cases that may not be treatable by way of the aforesaid methods, weekly use of nail polish containing formaldehyde is recommended [4].

13.3.2 Onychodystrophy Caused by Biomechanical Defect and Trauma

Bone deformities in fingers or incompatible shoes, causing minor trauma, can lead to onychodystrophy (malformation), such as subungual

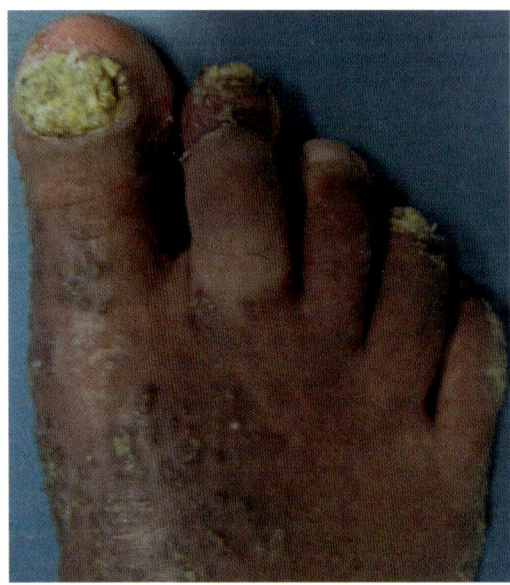

Fig. 13.5 Subungual hyperkeratosis (Publication authorized by Romiti et al. [31])

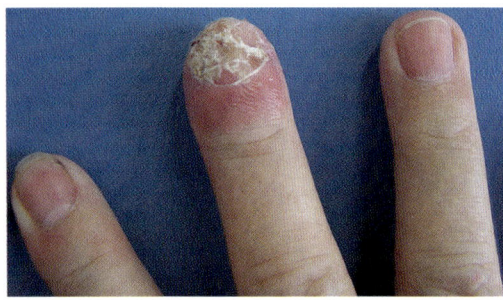

Fig. 13.6 Onychodystrophy by pustular psoriasis (Hallopeau's acrodermatitis) (Publication authorized by Romiti et al. [31])

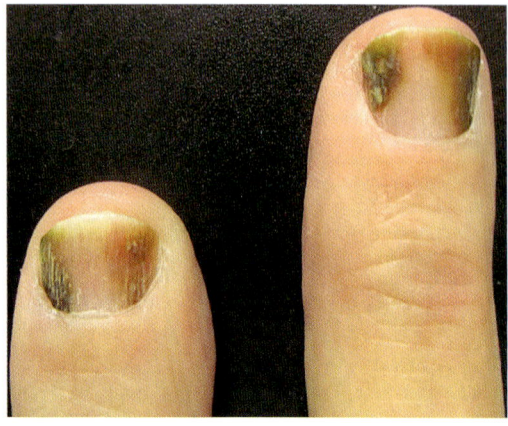

Fig. 13.7 Onychomycosis and *Pseudomonas* infection (Image from Pontificia Universidade Catolica, Dermatology Department, Campinas, Brazil)

hyperkeratosis (Figs. 13.5 and 13.6), onychocryptosis (ingrown nails), onycholysis, subungual hematoma, and thickening of the nail plate.

Treatment should always be aimed toward correcting orthopedic errors, advice on wearing appropriate shoes and insoles, as well as proper foot care [4, 9].

13.3.3 Infections and Infestations

Onychomycosis is a fungal infection of the nail, commonly detected at any age and which represents more than 50 % of diseases mentioned herein. Its prevalence increases with age, and about 40 % of the patients with onychomycosis are older than 60. The occurrence of this infection gradually increases as immune systems become weak, the likelihood of traumas higher, and foot care habits are barely employed due to the lower mobility present in this age group [18, 19].

In 90 % of cases, onychomycosis is due to dermatophytes (the *Trichophyton rubrum* accounts for 71 % of onychomycosis), but may also be caused by other fungi and yeasts. *Candida albicans* is a common type of fungus of the latter group, accounting for 5 % of fungal infections [20].

They are found in four different circumstances: distal subungual onychomycosis (the most common type), proximal subungual onychomycosis, white superficial onychomycosis, and candidal onychomycosis [20, 21] (Fig. 13.7).

The infection commonly begins through the invasion of the hyponychium and distal nail bed and is clinically detectable by a whitish opacification and distal onycholysis. In response to the infection, the nail bed causes hyperproliferation, with nail dystrophy, and the fungus spreads toward the floor plate [20–22].

Conversely, in proximal nail bed infections which are almost exclusively observed in HIV patients, there is a blank area near the lunula that extends distally. Thus, whenever proximal subungual onychomycosis is diagnosed, HIV tests should be run [20–22].

In the elderly, the toenails are most frequently affected. However, both fingernails and toenails can be affected simultaneously, more often the case than in other age groups [4].

The definitive diagnosis of onychomycosis is of utmost importance, as it is responsible for only 50 % of onychodystrophy. Laboratory tests should be performed before the start of oral antifungal therapies. Some diagnostic methods available are direct mycological examinations with KOH, cultures, and biopsies. These methods may be applied separately or together. The method with the highest sensitivity (98.8 %) is the histopathological analysis [20–23].

The treatment usually involves topical or systemic antifungal drugs and chemical or mechanical debridement of the affected nail plate. The choice of the most appropriate therapy depends on many factors, such as cost, adverse effects, the interaction between the respective drugs, the number and extent of nails affected, the etiologic agent, comorbidities, and the continuous-use medications of the patient.

The chemical debridement – compound with 40 % of urea – and the mechanical debridement are considered necessary ancillary treatments as these treatments decrease the amount of fungi in the nail plate, allow greater penetration of topical antifungal, and increase the bioavailability of systemic antifungal medications. Topically, the most widely used drugs are amorolfine and ciclopirox olamine, recommended for the treatment of patients with minor problems and those with contraindications to systemic therapy. These drugs usually require longer treatment periods and more discipline [24]. For patients with restricted access to systemic treatments, a new laser treatment may be an alternative, which has provided good results, but still needs further studies [25].

In systemic treatment, terbinafine has shown good results as a fungicidal against dermatophytes and non-dermatophytes and variable action against *Candida*. It is the most effective therapy available, according to studies, and offers better results than those obtained with fluconazole and itraconazole, in addition to presenting lower drug interaction and negligible interaction with cytochrome P450, which is responsible for some hepatic reactions. The main side effects of terbinafine are gastrointestinal. Its association with topical antifungal drugs increases the curing rate [26].

Paronychia is the term used to refer to the inflammation/infection of the nail matrix and may be classified as acute or chronic. Paronychia is an acute bacterial infection, particularly caused by *Staphylococcus aureus* or *Pseudomonas* sp., and is normally preceded by trauma. It is clinically presented as an erythema with painful swelling of the periungual area, sometimes with pus and typically affecting only one nail. Treatment involves topical or systemic antibiotics, preceded by significant drainage, if the abscess is local [27].

Chronic paronychia occurs after chemical or physical trauma that damages the cuticle and allows the penetration of irritants or allergens that cause an inflammation of the proximal nail fold and nail matrix. It usually presents a secondary infection caused by *Candida* sp. or gram-negative bacteria (*Proteus* sp. or *Klebsiella* sp.). Clinically, a discrete edema and erythema of the proximal and lateral folds may be observed, with no cuticle. The treatment is prolonged and requires keeping the nail and surrounding skin dry, without prolonged exposure to water. Topical antifungal, topical antiseptics (4 % thymol in alcohol), and topical or intralesional corticosteroids may be used, and in some cases, surgical excision of the hypertrophy of the proximal fold may be needed [27].

13.3.4 Pachyonychia

Pachyonychia manifests itself as hyperkeratosis, yellowing, and loss of translucency of the nail plate, with or without subungual hyperkeratosis. An association and complication of pachyonychia may occur with distal onycholysis, pain, subungual bleeding, and ulceration. In addition, pachyonychia may also increase the susceptibility to onychomycosis. The treatment consists of periodical, physical, or chemical debridement (40 % urea cream) [5, 6].

13.3.5 Onychocryptosis

Onychocryptosis occurs when part of the nail penetrates the adjacent side of the nail matrix due to the change of curvature of the nail plate, increased subcutaneous tissue, or hypertrophy of the lateral nail matrix. It clinically manifests itself as local inflammatory signs, often with the formation of granulation tissue, pain, increased sensitivity, and possible secondary infections [4, 9].

As a result of the decreased blood circulation and sensitivity in the elderly, secondary infections and gangrene are more commonly associated with onychocryptosis than in patients of other age groups [4, 9].

The main causes of onychocryptosis are incorrect nail clipping, unsuitable shoes with excessive pressure in the specific location, long fingers, and other deformities, including bone deformities, hyperhidrosis, and poor foot hygiene [11].

The treatment should target the acute symptoms, but also correct the causative factors that may be improved. Conservative treatment includes immersion in warm water and placing of cotton under the nail plate to attempt to correct its curvature. Treatments with topical or systemic antibiotics and curettage of granulomas may be adopted depending on clinical condition. In definitive treatments through surgical procedure, a partial avulsion of the affected side of the nail plate is performed, with subsequent matricectomy with phenolization, the latter being an optional procedure, with better cosmetic results achieved only with the avulsion and correction of precipitating factors [11].

13.3.6 Splinter Hemorrhages and Subungual Hematomas

Splinter hemorrhages may be secondary to systemic diseases, such as fat embolism, collagen diseases, and endocarditis. They appear in a reddish color and at the proximal third of the nail, or when secondary to trauma, they may be blackened and at the middle and distal thirds of the nail bed. This is the most common form of splinter hemorrhage observed in the elderly [11].

Subungual hematomas, which also have post-traumatic etiology, are red and painful when in the initial process and may evolve to dark blue staining. They normally follow the growth of nails and are continuously removed from the proximal nail fold, until they reach the free edge of the nail. In acute injuries, in order to reduce the intralesional pressure and reduce the pain, drainage can be performed with delicate local puncture. In cases of doubt or chronic evolution with no improvement, the diagnosis of melanomas should be removed [28].

13.3.7 Neoplasms of the Nail Apparatus

The incidence of malignancies of the nail apparatus, such as Bowen's disease and melanoma, tends to increase with advancing age and is usually encountered at higher incidences in the elderly [11].

Bowen's disease originates in the nail matrix and has multiple factors in its pathogenesis, including trauma, arsenic, exposure to x-rays, and chronic paronychia and infection by human papillomavirus (primarily HPVs 16, 34, and 35). It commonly affects the thumbs, and its presentation may vary. The most common is a hyperkeratotic ulcerated subungual or periungual lesion, associated with onycholysis and other less common manifestations such as striated melanonychia and erythronychia. The treatment of choice is the excision through Mohs micrographic surgery [29].

The melanoma of the nail apparatus usually affects the Japanese and Africans and classically presents a longitudinal groove of melanonychia, especially in the big toe, thumb, or index finger. Hutchinson's nail sign is characterized by a blackish pigmentation extension beyond the nail apparatus and represents the radial extension phase of the melanoma (Fig. 13.8). The early diagnosis increases the chances of cure. It is extremely important to consider this pathology in case of older patients with isolated striated melanonychia (Fig. 13.9). Following histopathological confirmation, treatment must follow the melanoma protocol [29].

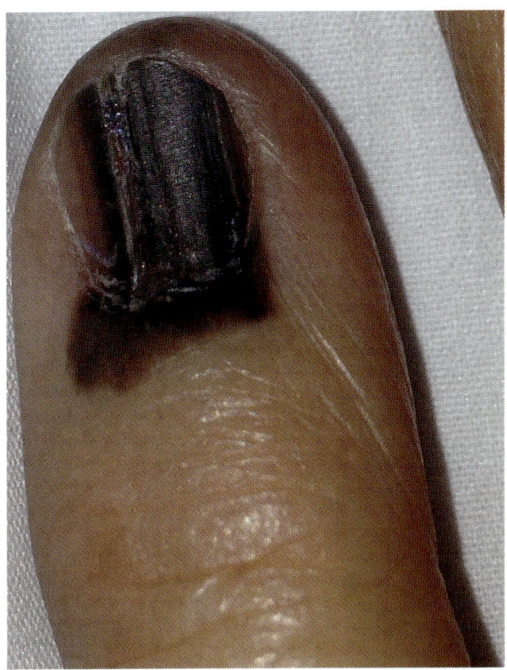

Fig. 13.8 Acral lentiginous melanoma and Hutchinson's sign (Image from Pontificia Universidade Catolica, Dermatology Department, Campinas, Brazil)

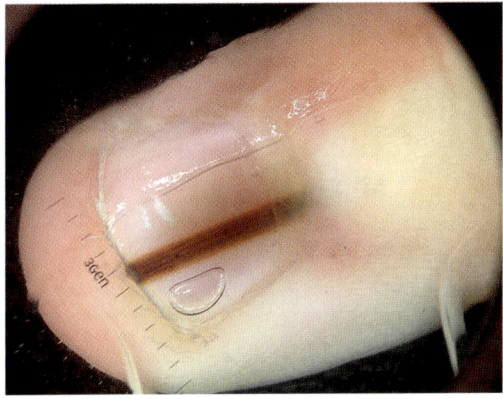

Fig. 13.9 Longitudinal melanonychia (Image from Pontificia Universidade Catolica, Dermatology Department, Campinas, Brazil)

References

1. Tosti A, Piraccini BM. Biologia das unhas e seus distúrbios. In: Fitzpatrick T, editor. Tratado de dermatologia. 5th ed. Rio de Janeiro: Revinter; 2005. p. 778–94. 87.
2. Tosti A, Piraccini BM, Jorge ARCD. Afecções da unhas. In: Junior WB, Di Chiacchio N, Criado PR, editors. Tratado de Dermatologia. Sao Paulo: Atheneu; 2010. p. 1045–70. 42.
3. Runne U, Orfano CE. The human nail. Structure, growth and pathological changes. Curr Prol Dermatol. 1981;9:102.
4. Cohen PR, Scher RK. Geriatric nail disorders: diagnosis and treatment. J Am Acad Dermatol. 1992;26(4):521–31.
5. Singh G, Haneef NS, Uday A. Nail changes and disorders among the elderly. Indian J Dermatol Venereol. 2005;71(6):386–92.
6. Abdullah L, Abbas O. Common nail changes and disorders in older people: diagnosis and management. Can Fam Physician. 2011;57(2):173–81.
7. Baran R, Dawber RP. The nail in childhood and old age. In: Baran R, Dawber RPR, editors. Diseases of the nails and their management. 2nd ed. Oxford: Blackwell Science; 1994. p. 81–96.
8. Reid IR. Calcium supplements and nail quality. N Engl J Med. 2000;343:1817.
9. Cohen PR, Scher RK. Aging. In: Hordinsky MK, Sawaya ME, Scher RK, editors. Atlas of hair and nails. Philadelphia: Churchill Livingstone; 2000. p. 213–25.
10. Dawber R, Bristow I, Turner W. Nail disorders. In: Text atlas of podiatric dermatology. London: Martin Dunitz Ltd; 2001. p. 105–31.
11. Cohen PR, Scher RK. Nail changes in the elderly. J Geriatr Dermatol. 1993;1:45–53.
12. Saraya T, Ariga M, Kurai D, Takeshita N, Honda K, Goto H. Terry's nails as a part of aging. Intern Med. 2008;47(6):567–8. Epub 2008 Mar 17.
13. Horan MA, Puxty JA, Fox RA. The white nails of old age (Neapolitan nails). J Am Geriatr Soc. 1982;30(12):734–7.
14. Baran R, Dawber RPR. Physical signs. In: Baran R, Dawber RP, editors. Diseases of the nails and their management. 2nd ed. Oxford: Blackwell Science; 1994. p. 35–80.
15. Wallis MS, Bowen WR, Guin JD. Pathogenesis of onychoschizia (lamellar dystrophy). J Am Acad Dermatol. 1991;24:44–8.
16. Hochman LG, Scher RK, Meyerson MS. Brittle nails: response to daily biotin supplementation. Cutis. 1993;51:303–5.
17. Colombo VE, Gerber F, Bronhofer M, Floersheim GL. Treatment of brittle fingernails and onychoschizia with biotin: scanning electron microscopy. J Am Acad Dermatol. 1990;23:1127–32.
18. Hemer A, Trau H, Davidovici B, Amichai B, Grunwald MH. Onychomycosis: rationalization of topical treatment. Isr Med Assoc J. 2008;10:415–6.
19. Araujo AJG, Bastos OMP, Souza MAJ, Oliveira JC. Occurrence of onychomycosis among patients attended in dermatology offices in the city of Rio de Janeiro. Brazil Ann Bras Dermatol. 2003;78:299–308.
20. Gupta AK, Ricci MJ. Diagnosing onychomycosis. Dermatol Clin. 2006;24(3):365–9.
21. De Berker D. Clinical practice. Fungal nail disease. N Engl J Med. 2009;360(20):2108–16.

22. Gupta AK, Taborda P, Taborda V, Gilmour J, Rachlis A, Salit I, et al. Epidemiology and prevalence of onychomycosis in HIV-positive individuals. Int J Dermatol. 2000;39(10):746–53.
23. Lilly KK, Koshnick RL, Grill JP, Khalil ZM, Nelson DB, Warshaw EM. Cost-effectiveness of diagnostic tests for toenail onychomycosis: a repeated-measure, single-blinded, cross-sectional evaluation of 7 diagnostic tests. J Am Acad Dermatol. 2006;55(4):620–6.
24. Effendy I, Lecha M, Feuilhade de Chauvin M, Di Chiacchio N, Baran R. European Onychomycosis Observatory. Epidemiology and clinical classification of onychomycosis. J Eur Acad Dermatol Venereol. 2005;1(19 Suppl):8–12.
25. Gupta A, Simpson F. Device-based therapies for onychomycosis treatment. Skin Ther Lett. 2012;17(9):4–9.
26. Verma S, Heffernan MP. Infecções fúngicas superficiais: dermatofitoses, onicomicoses, tinea nigra, piedra. In: Freedberg MI, Eisen AZ, Wolff K, Austen KF, Goldsmith LA, Katz SI, Fitzpatrick TB (editores). Fitzpatrick tratado de dermatologia. 5 ed. Rio de Janeiro: Revinter; 2005. pp. 1807–21.
27. Rigopoulos D, Larios G, Gregoriou S, Alevizos A. Acute and chronic paronychia. Am Fam Physician. 2008;77(3):339–46.
28. Huang YH, Ohara K. Medical pearl: subungual hematoma: a simple and quick method for diagnosis. J Am Acad Dermatol. 2006;54(5):877–8.
29. Perin C. Tumor of the nail unit. Part I: acquired localized longitudinal melanonychia and erythronychia. Am J Dermatol Pathol. 2013;35(6):621–36.
30. Arruda ACBB, Arruda LHF, Pontes LT. Psoríase ungueal. In: Romiti R. Compêndio de Psoríase. Rio de Janeiro: Elsevier; 2010. pp. 79–86.
31. Arruda ACBB, Arruda LHF, Pontes LT. Psoríase ungueal. In: Romiti R. Compêndio de Psoríase.2 ed. Rio de Janeiro: Elsevier; 2013. pp. 87–95.

Part II

Hormonal Change and Therapy

Atrophic Vaginitis in the Menopause

14

Ryan Sobel and Jack D. Sobel

Contents

14.1	**Pathophysiology**	175
14.2	**Clinical Manifestation**	176
14.3	**Laboratory Findings**	177
14.4	**Differential Diagnosis of Vaginal Atrophy**	177
14.5	**Treatment**	178
14.5.1	Additional Considerations in Treatment of Postmenopausal VVA and Atrophic Vaginitis	178
14.6	**Summary**	179
References		179

Vulvovaginal atrophy (VVA) is a chronic medical entity in both postmenopausal women and women during menopause transition secondary to decreased levels of circulating and consequent local vulvovaginal estrogen [1–3]. Atrophic vaginitis is considered by some to represent a more advanced form of vaginal atrophy in which evidence of vaginal inflammation supervenes with accompanying additional signs and symptoms. Traditionally, however, many authors have used the terms vaginal atrophy and atrophic vaginitis interchangeably.

It is estimated that up to 20–60 % of postmenopausal women experience symptoms of vaginal atrophy with 20–25 % of symptomatic women seeking medical treatment [2]. VVA and atrophic vaginitis are significantly increased in women taking aromatase inhibitors and some selective estrogen receptor modulators (SERMs, e.g., tamoxifen, raloxifene) [4].

The results of Women's Health Initiative (WHI) led to a dramatic decline in routine use of estrogen as preventative therapy for a variety of host maladies in postmenopausal women. With estrogen elimination the incidence of VVA has markedly increased.

R. Sobel, MD (✉)
Department of Obstetrics and Gynecology,
Jefferson Medical College, Jefferson University Hospitals,
834 Chestnut St., Suite 400, Philadelphia, PA 19107, USA
e-mail: ryan.sobel@jefferson.edu

J.D. Sobel, MD
Division of Infectious Diseases,
Department of Internal Medicine,
Detroit Medical Center, Wayne State University
School of Medicine, Detroit, MI, USA
e-mail: jsobel@med.wayne.edu

14.1 Pathophysiology

Estrogen components influence vulvovaginal physiology at several levels. The progressive decline in levels of endogenous estrogens is accompanied by a decrease in vaginal epithelial glycogen which serves as a major nutritional substrate both for epithelial cells per se and for vaginal microorganisms or flora (microbiota). Reduced glycogen substrate discourages the presence and population numbers of commensal protective bacteria, predominantly dominant *Lactobacillus* species which profoundly influence vaginal microbial communities. Accordingly with time, *Lactobacillus* numbers decline progressively and with significant consequences. Firstly decreased bacterial glycogenolysis results in decreased production of several organic acids but predominantly lactic acid, and consequently vaginal pH is altered with a progressive increase in pH above the normal acidic range (3.8–4.5). The normal acidic environment which fosters the presence of protective acidophilic *Lactobacillus* species is also an adversarial barrier to organisms originating from the neighboring gastrointestinal tract, specifically coliform bacteria. Accordingly, declining serum and local estrogen concentrations directly influence the healthy normal bacterial community or microbiome present in the vagina. The profoundly altered vaginal microbiome does not directly contribute to vaginal symptoms associated with vulvovaginal atrophy; hence, simply artificially reducing vaginal pH per se may not be an effective treatment modality for VVA. The role of estrogen in directly influencing microbial growth is poorly studied. Details of the vaginal microbiome associated with VVA are outside the scope of this review and are found elsewhere [5]. The microbiome of the atrophic vagina is mixed or heterogeneously devoid of *Lactobacillus* species, instead consisting of streptococci, staphylococci, and anaerobes such as *Prevotella* spp. and finally diphtheroids [6].

The second pathophysiologic consequence of declining estrogen relates to the stratified squamous epithelium lining of the vagina. Estrogen enhances maturation of basal epithelial cells, facilitating transition through parabasal cells to reach the mature larger squamous cells. In doing so the vaginal lining becomes considerably thickened and allows enhanced transudation of serum-derived fluid into the vaginal lumen. Accordingly, with decline in estrogenic effect, vaginal epithelium becomes progressively thinned, atrophic, more fragile, and accompanied by vaginal dryness reflecting the reduced transudation.

Declining estrogen also reduces function of both striated and smooth muscle, including bladder and pelvic floor. This contributes to bladder, rectum, uterus, and vault prolapse, as well as loss of muscle tone resulting in a patulous or dilated introitus. Bladder muscle and sphincter function progressively decline contributing to incontinence, post-voiding urine retention, and susceptibility to bladder bacterial infection.

There are no established definitions that separate atrophic vaginitis from VVA. The most prominent feature in addition to severity of symptoms and signs relates to presence of large numbers of polymorphonuclear leukocytes (PMNs) evident on saline microscopy suggesting an inflammatory process that is superimposed upon atrophy. The causes of PMN influx are unknown. No microorganisms are currently incriminated in their arrival, and some experts attribute the inflammatory component as secondary to minor/major trauma or friction that occurs with coitus especially in the presence of vaginal dryness.

14.2 Clinical Manifestation

The North American Menopause Society and International Menopause Society estimate that 10–50 % of postmenopausal women experience symptoms of VVA [7]. The earliest manifestation of estrogen deficiency, long before changes in pH, microbiota, and epithelial lining thinning, is vaginal dryness first recognized only during intercourse. Over time, dryness is progressive after making intercourse difficult, uncomfortable, painful, and even impossible [8].

Even in the absence of intercourse, VVA may be associated with irritation and itching. With worsening atrophy and thinning of the vulvovaginal lining, increased tenderness supervenes, thereafter the vaginal mucosa becomes friable, with petechiae, occasional ulceration, and postcoital bleeding. Vaginal elasticity is also lost. In spite of dryness, occasionally women are troubled by a thin watery discharge often necessitating use of pad. Infrequently, women will report new onset of genital malodor, not fishy but unpleasant in the presence or absence of discharge. Other symptoms include vulvovaginal pruritus and paresthesia. Urinary symptoms including burning on micturition, frequent urinary tract infections, and incontinence are also commonly present.

Physical findings include a dilated or later narrowed introitus, vestibular thinning, and prominent urethral caruncle often with petechiae. Diffuse vaginal epithelial surface thinning, pallor, and loss of rugae reflect vaginal atrophy with petechiae and ecchymoses, e.g., indicating advanced estrogen deficiency. Dyspareunia may also be the result of fissuring, ulceration, or stretching of the deep tissue surrounding a stenotic introitus or narrowed or shortened vagina. Vulvar findings include pubic hair loss, pendulous labia majora, less distinct labia minora, and less labial fat pad.

Unlike vasomotor manifestations such as hot flashes or night sweats, signs and symptoms of vaginal atrophy tend to increase over time [3]. Bachman et al. have emphasized that the aforementioned symptoms of vulvovaginal atrophy frequently overlap with those of female sexual dysfunction, i.e., reduced libido, arousal disorder, orgasmic disorders, and sexual pain disorder common in up to 50 % of postmenopausal women [3]. The role of reduced estrogen activity in the pathogenesis of these symptoms is suggested, given their higher frequency in women with concomitant vaginal atrophy. Postmenopausal women with sexual difficulties are significantly more likely to have VVA than women without.

14.3 Laboratory Findings

In the early phases, even in the presence of vaginal dryness, all commonly performed bedside laboratory tests performed on vaginal samples are normal. Established estrogen deficiency is associated with an elevated vaginal pH, in excess of 4.5, often 5–6. The amine or whiff test is always negative. Saline microscopy reveals absence of clue cells and typical *Lactobacillus* morphotype organisms reflecting altered vaginal flora (AVF). Most importantly, diagnosis requires the presence of parabasal cells, an essential marker of impaired epithelial cell maturation. Atrophic vaginitis is characterized by the further addition of increased numbers of PMNs.

Many clinicians use serum estradiol levels to diagnose estrogen-deficient vaginal atrophy; however, serum estradiol levels correlate poorly with the effects of local estrogen deficiency and add little to diagnosis, prognosis, and response to local estrogen replacement therapy.

14.4 Differential Diagnosis of Vaginal Atrophy

It should be emphasized that meaningful epithelial surface atrophy cannot occur without dramatic simultaneous changes in vaginal microbiota. Hence, a normal vaginal pH (pH <4.5) excludes the possibility or likelihood of estrogen deficiency-induced vaginal atrophy or atrophic vaginitis. Accordingly, the differential diagnosis includes only these entities with accompanying elevated vaginal pH. Bacterial vaginosis is easily excluded given its clinical picture of malodorous discharge, clue cells, positive amine tests, and absence of parabasal cells. Excluding chronic vaginal trichomoniasis is far more difficult, given the insensitivity of saline microscopy in identifying motile trichomonads. Moreover a recent epidemiologic study indicates increase numbers of postmenopausal women with unsuspected vaginal trichomoniasis [9]. Accordingly, it may be prudent to exclude trichomoniasis in postmenopausal women presenting with dyspareunia, elevated vaginal pH, increased PMNs with the vagina showing inflammation in mucosal friability, petechiae, and ecchymoses. The optimal test is *Trichomonas* PCR, DNA detection, or antigen detection.

Another entity requiring differentiating is desquamative inflammatory vaginitis (DIV). This not uncommon idiopathic inflammatory condition occurs predominantly in postmenopausal estrogen-deficient women [10]. Similarities include elevated pH, increased PMNs and parabasal cells on saline microscopy, and finally disrupted vaginal microbiota. However, DIV does not respond or reverse dramatically with estrogen therapy and can be easily ruled out. Similarly, rare causes of vaginitis including pemphigus and linear IgA disease can be excluded by this diagnostic test.

14.5 Treatment

Vulvovaginal atrophy and atrophic vaginitis respond dramatically to estrogen replacement [3, 11]. For many years, clinicians preferred systemic estrogen replacement prescribed orally or by the transcutaneous route [3, 7]. However, systemic estrogen therapy has fallen into disfavor and the use of well-tolerated intravaginal estrogen therapy has become favored [3, 7, 11, 12].

Most local vaginally administered estrogen creams or pessaries consist of estradiol and less frequently estriol. In terms of overall efficacy, all topical estrogen preparations are of similar efficacy in reversing vaginal atrophy and correcting atrophic vaginitis. A Cochrane analysis comparing 19 randomized controlled trials with 4,162 patients obtained a significant improvement of local estrogen therapy compared to placebo or moisturizing vaginal gel therapy. Significant reductions in vaginal pH, dryness, dyspareunia, and cytology patterns were so demonstrated [13–16]. Side effects with all topical formulations of estrogen are uncommon. Occasionally burning is reported with estradiol cream preparations [3, 13–15]. All forms of estrogen are associated with secondary attacks of vulvovaginal candidiasis especially in women with a past history of premenopausal *Candida* vaginitis.

All topical treatments are initially briefly administered daily and then reduced to approximately twice weekly regimens once the effects of estrogen deficiency are reversed. Complete reversal of vaginal atrophy can be expected in 4–6 weeks.

Another form of estrogen replacement therapy occurs as an estrogen-eluting intravaginal ring, which is replaced quarterly. These devices are extremely well tolerated and preferred by many women because of convenience and lack of messiness [15, 16].

In addition to efficacy, the safety of estrogen administered vaginally has been demonstrated. Although slightly controversial, risk of endometrial hyperplasia and carcinoma even in the absence of concomitant progesterone therapy is considered negligible [7]. Most clinicians do not use oral progestin with vaginal estrogen to reduce the risk of endometrial hyperplasia or cancer.

Alternative forms of hormone therapy include the use of intravaginal dehydroepiandrosterone [17–19]. Although not widely used, this combined androgenic/estrogenic stimulation appears effective in reversing vaginal atrophy and possibly improving sexual function [17–19]. Additional studies from other investigators would be reassuring.

14.5.1 Additional Considerations in Treatment of Postmenopausal VVA and Atrophic Vaginitis

While the safety and infrequency of local adverse effects of topical estrogens appear reassuring, there remains an important subpopulation of women in whom even topical or local therapy remains extremely controversial, viz., postmenopausal women with estrogen receptor-positive breast cancer [20]. While systemic estrogen is clearly contraindicated, the target for the controversy is local vaginal estrogen administration. Most oncologists remain rigidly opposed to their use, sentencing these women to continued vaginal symptoms, including dyspareunia and absence of meaningful sexual life. While all the topical low-dose estrogens achieve low concentrations of plasma estradiol only, with minimal risk of stimulating receptor-positive cancer cells, nevertheless, plasma levels are not zero and 100 % freedom of risk cannot be claimed for any of the currently available therapeutic products [21]. Even the recently introduced ospemifene, an estrogen agonist/antagonist with tissue-selective effects indicated for the treatment of moderate to severe dyspareunia due to VVA in the menopause, has not been studied in women with breast cancer [22, 23].

For women who are reluctant to use estrogen and those for whom use of estrogen is contraindicated, vaginal tablets of hyaluronic acid although inferior to estradiol should be considered [24–26]. Similarly, a vaginal pH-balanced gel relieved symptoms and improved vaginal health in breast cancer survivors who experienced menopause after cancer treatment [27].

See also Chap. 18.

14.6 Summary

In spite of simplicity of diagnosis, VVA and atrophic vaginitis remain underdiagnosed and undertreated. Barriers to increasing treatment availability have been identified, and with education, widespread treatment using either long-term available or more recently available products can alleviate widespread unnecessary suffering [28]. Multiple estrogen products both systemic and topical are now available, meeting the multivariable needs of women worldwide. Complications of local or topical estrogen therapy are relatively infrequent and safety can be assured. A major concern remains the unreasonable and inexplicable high cost of topical estrogen therapy including generic preparations.

References

1. MacBride MB, Rhodes DJ, Shuster LT. Vulvovaginal atrophy. Mayo Clin Proc. 2010;85:87–94.
2. Santoro N, Komi J. Prevalence and impact of vaginal symptoms among postmenopausal women. J Sex Med. 2009;6:2133–42.
3. Bachmann GA, Nevadunsky NS. Diagnosis and treatment of atrophic vaginitis. Am Fam Physician. 2000;61:3090–6.
4. Wills S, Ravipati A, Venuturumilli P, Kresge C, Folkerd E, Dowsett M, et al. Effects of vaginal estrogens on serum estradiol levels in postmenopausal breast cancer survivors and women at risk of breast cancer taking an aromatase inhibitor or a selective estrogen receptor modulator. J Oncol Pract. 2012;8:144–8.
5. Farage MA, Sobel JD. Vaginal flora in the menopause. In: Farage MA, Miller KW, Maibach HL, editors. Textbook of the aging skin. Heidelberg: Springer; 2010.
6. Brotman RM, Shardell MD, Gajer P, Fadrosh D, Chang K, Silver MI, et al. Association between the vaginal microbiota, menopause status, and signs of vulvovaginal atrophy. Menopause. 2014;21:450–8.
7. North American Menopause Society. The role of local vaginal estrogen for treatment of vaginal atrophy in postmenopausal women: position statement of The North American Menopause Society. Menopause. 2007;14(3 Pt 1):355–69.
8. Dennerstein L, Dudley EC, Hopper JL, Guthrie JR, Burger HG. A prospective population-based study of menopausal symptoms. Obstet Gynecol. 2000;96:351–8.
9. Ginocchio CC, Chapin K, Smith JS, Aslanzadeh J, Snook J, Hill CS, et al. Prevalence of Trichomonas vaginalis and coinfection with Chlamydia trachomatis and Neisseria gonorrhoeae in the United States as determined by the Aptima Trichomonas vaginalis nucleic acid amplification assay. J Clin Microbiol. 2012;50:2601–8.
10. Sobel JD, Reichman O, Misra D, Yoo W. Prognosis and treatment of desquamative inflammatory vaginitis. Obstet Gynecol. 2011;117:850–5.
11. Goodman MP. Are all estrogens created equal? A review of oral vs. transdermal therapy. J Womens Health (Larchmt). 2012;21:161–9.
12. Bachmann G, Bouchard C, Hoppe D, Ranganath R, Altomare C, Vieweg A, et al. Efficacy and safety of low-dose regimens of conjugated estrogens cream administered vaginally. Menopause. 2009;16:719–27.
13. Suckling J, Lethaby A, Kennedy R. Local oestrogen for vaginal atrophy in postmenopausal women. Cochrane Database Syst Rev. 2006;(18):CD001500.
14. Long CY, Liu CM, Hsu SC, Wu CH, Wang CL, Tsai EM. A randomized comparative study of the effects of oral and topical estrogen therapy on the vaginal vascularization and sexual function in hysterectomized postmenopausal women. Menopause. 2006;13:737–43.
15. Al-Baghdadi O, Ewies AA. Topical estrogen therapy in the management of postmenopausal vaginal atrophy: an up-to-date overview. Climacteric. 2009;12:91–105.
16. Krause M, Wheeler 2nd TL, Snyder TE, Richter HE. Local effects of vaginally administered estrogen therapy: a review. J Pelvic Med Surg. 2009;15:105–14.
17. Labrie F, Archer D, Bouchard C, Fortier M, Cusan L, Gomez JL, et al. Effect of intravaginal dehydroepiandrosterone (Prasterone) on libido and sexual dysfunction in postmenopausal women. Menopause. 2009;16:923–31.
18. Labrie F, Archer D, Bouchard C, Fortier M, Cusan L, Gomez JL, et al. Intravaginal dehydroepiandrosterone (Prasterone), a physiological and highly efficient treatment of vaginal atrophy. Menopause. 2009;16:907–22.
19. Labrie F, Archer D, Bouchard C, Fortier M, Cusan L, Gomez JL, et al. Serum steroid levels during 12-week intravaginal dehydroepiandrosterone administration. Menopause. 2009;16:897–906.
20. Moegele M, Buchholz S, Seitz S, Ortmann O. Vaginal estrogen therapy in postmenopausal breast cancer patients treated with aromatase inhibitors. Arch Gynecol Obstet. 2012;285:1397–402.

21. Labrie F, Cusan L, Gomez JL, Côté I, Bérubé R, Bélanger P, et al. Effect of one-week treatment with vaginal estrogen preparations on serum estrogen levels in postmenopausal women. Menopause. 2009;16:30–6.
22. Portman DJ, Bachmann GA, Simon JA, Ospemifene Study Group. Ospemifene, a novel selective estrogen receptor modulator for treating dyspareunia associated with postmenopausal vulvar and vaginal atrophy. Menopause. 2013;20:623–30.
23. Bachmann GA, Komi JO, Ospemifene Study Group. Ospemifene effectively treats vulvovaginal atrophy in postmenopausal women: results from a pivotal phase 3 study. Menopause. 2010;17:480–6.
24. Karaosmanoglu O, Cogendez E, Sozen H, Asoglu MR, Akdemir Y, Eren S. Hyaluronic acid in the treatment of postmenopausal women with atrophic vaginitis. Int J Gynaecol Obstet. 2011;113:156–7.
25. Ekin M, Yaşar L, Savan K, Temur M, Uhri M, Gencer I, et al. The comparison of hyaluronic acid vaginal tablets with estradiol vaginal tablets in the treatment of atrophic vaginitis: a randomized controlled trial. Arch Gynecol Obstet. 2011;283:539–43.
26. Chen J, Geng L, Song X, Li H, Giordan N, Liao Q. Evaluation of the efficacy and safety of hyaluronic acid vaginal gel to ease vaginal dryness: a multicenter, randomized, controlled, open-label, parallel-group, clinical trial. J Sex Med. 2013;10:1575–84.
27. Lee YK, Chung HH, Kim JW, Park NH, Song YS, Kang SB. Vaginal pH-balanced gel for the control of atrophic vaginitis among breast cancer survivors: a randomized controlled trial. Obstet Gynecol. 2011;117:922–7.
28. Chism LA. Overcoming resistance and barriers to the use of local estrogen therapy for the treatment of vaginal atrophy. Int J Womens Health. 2012;4:551–7.

Sensory Perception on the Vulva and Extragenital Sites

15

Miranda A. Farage, Kenneth W. Miller,
Denniz A. Zolnoun, and William J. Ledger

Contents

15.1	Introduction	181
15.2	Neural Pathways for the Sensation of Physical Stimuli	182
15.3	Quantitative Sensory Testing	182
15.4	Sensory Thresholds on Extragenital Sites	183
15.5	Sensory Perception on the Vulva	184
15.5.1	Quantitative Sensory Thresholds with Age and Menopausal Status	184
15.5.2	Subjective Reports of Vulvar Sensation in Controlled Trials of External Hygiene Products	191
15.6	Quantitative Sensory Testing and Vulvodynia	193
15.7	Discussion and Summary	194
	References	195

Portions of this chapter appeared in an open-access article by Farage et al., *The Open Women's Health Journal*, 2012 6: 6–18, and are reproduced under the terms of the Creative Commons Attribution License.

M.A. Farage, MSc, PhD (✉)
Clinical Innovative Sciences,
The Procter & Gamble Company,
6110 Center Hill Avenue,
Cincinnati, OH 45224, USA
e-mail: Farage.m@pg.com

K.W. Miller, PhD
Global Product Stewardship,
The Procter & Gamble Company, Cincinnati, OH, USA
e-mail: Miller.kw.1@pg.com

15.1 Introduction

Much of the research on sensory perception of the vulva has focused on the sexual response. This chapter focuses on the perception of various sensory stimuli by the vulva and vagina and the effects of age and other variables. Quantitative sensory testing (QST), which measures the perception thresholds of quantifiable stimuli such as temperature, touch, pressure, and vibration, provides quantitative estimates of sensory perception. Subjective sensory effects are more difficult to quantify, but comparative information on certain sensations (wetness, dryness, itch, burning, stinging) can be collected from prospective trials of external feminine hygiene products under controlled conditions. Although the research on vulvar sensation is very limited, objective QST and these surveys of subjective sensation provide complementary information about sensory perception on the vulva and the effects of variables such as age, the menstrual cycle, and menopause.

D.A. Zolnoun, MD, MPH
Department of Obstetrics and Gynecology,
Clinical Core and Pelvic Pain Research Center,
The Center for Neurosensory Disorder, The University of North Carolina at Chapel Hill, Chapel Hill, NC, USA
e-mail: Denniz_Zolnoun@med.unc.edu

W.J. Ledger, MD
Department of Obstetrics and Gynecology, Weill Medical College, New York, NY, USA
e-mail: wjledger@med.cornell.edu

15.2 Neural Pathways for the Sensation of Physical Stimuli

As background, the neural pathways that mediate sensation of stimuli applied to the skin or mucosa are reviewed briefly here. In glabrous and semiglabrous skin, the sensation of mechanical stimuli (touch, pressure, and vibration) and the sensations of temperature and pain are mediated by different parts of the nervous system. Touch, pressure, and vibration are detected by specialized mechanoreceptors. Specifically, rapidly adapting receptors (such as Meissner corpuscles and Pacinian corpuscles) detect transient light touch and transient deep pressure, respectively; slowly adapting receptors (such as Merkel cells and Ruffini receptors) respond to more sustained touch, such as sensing texture or shape. The sensory input from these mechanoreceptors is conducted by large myelinated fibers in the peripheral nerves and by the dorsal column of the spinal cord.

Temperature and pain are detected by free nerve endings in the skin. This sensory input is conducted by the small fiber system and its central connections in the spinothalamic tracts. Within the small fiber system, different fibers convey sensory impulses in response to temperature and pain: thinly myelinated fibers convey impulses from heat and cold receptors and unmyelinated fibers convey impulses from nociceptors that respond to painful or noxious stimuli. Sensory information transmitted along the spinal cord is ultimately processed via the thalamus to be interpreted by the cerebral cortex and cerebellum.

Several sensory nerves innervate the vulva and perineum (Fig. 15.1): the posterior femoral nerve innervates the latter aspect of the perineum posteriorly and the lateral margin of the vulva superiorly along the leg crease; the genitofemoral and ilioinguinal nerves (originating from L1 to L2) innervate the mons pubis and upper labia majora, approximately to the level of the urethra; and the perineal branch of the pudendal nerve (from sacral roots S2 to S4) is viewed by most clinicians as the primary source of vulvar innervation (lobes of the labia majora through the vestibule). A network of nerves over the dorsal aspect of the glans clitoris arises from the deeper pudendal nerve. Coverage of the vulva can also include the inferior cluneal nerve, which originates from S1 to S3. The correlation between these anatomical details and the characteristics of vulvar sensation and pain is an area of active research.

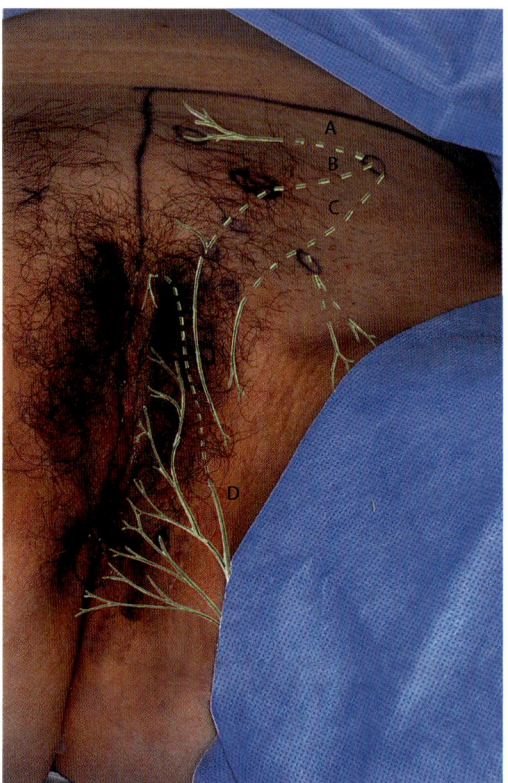

Fig. 15.1 Schematic of the innervation of the vulva. A: Anterior cutaneous branches of the iliohypogastric nerve; B: Anterior labial branches of the ilioinguinal nerve; C: Genitofemoral nerve (both the genital and femoral braches); D: Dorsal nerve of the clitoris (continuation of pudendal nerve shown as dashed lines deeper in the muscles of the urogenital diaphragm.) Note: the course of the specified nerves is delineated based on quantitative sensory testing and selective nerve block in this individual patient

15.3 Quantitative Sensory Testing

QST was traditionally used to quantify sensory function in healthy people and in patients at risk for neurological impairment [1]. It also serves as a tool to investigate factors that affect pain perception [2–4]. In QST, a measurable stimulus is applied to the skin and the subject or patient reports his or her perception of it. The method employs calibrated instruments to deliver known intensities of physical stimuli, for example, mild electric current (by means of surface electrodes), temperature (via electric thermodes with controlled surface temperatures), touch (using filaments whose bending force depends on diameter and length), pressure (exerted by spring-loaded devices), and vibration (using tuning forks or vibrators that deliver sinusoidal stimuli at a given frequency). Stimulus of a given intensity is applied, and the subject reports whether or not the stimulus is perceived (or, in pain studies, whether or not the stimulus elicits pain). The lowest intensity that is perceptible (or, if pertinent, painful) is the detection threshold.

Two general methods are employed to determine these thresholds: the method of limits and the method of levels. With the method of limits, the stimulus is progressively increased and the subject declares when it first becomes perceptible. With the method of levels, stimulus of a defined intensity is applied and then increased or decreased by specific increments depending on whether or not the subject perceives it (protocols may differ in terms of the number of consistent responses required to progress upward or downward in stimulus intensity).

With the method of limits, sensory information is processed neurologically at the same time as the stimulus intensity is being changed. The inherent response lag leads to a small error in threshold measurement; consequently, thresholds measured with the level of limits skew higher than those measured with the method of levels [5, 6]. Moreover, the rate of change of the stimulus affects thresholds obtained by the method of limits.

The method of levels is known as "forced-choice," as the subject must declare or "choose" whether or not the stimulus is perceived. Because this method takes longer and is more repetitive, error can result if the subjects become fatigued or distracted as the test proceeds.

Experimental variables such as the application site, the surface area of contact, the frequency of the stimulus (in the case of vibration), and the rate of change of stimulus intensity will affect the absolute value of thresholds measured. Consequently, the absolute values measured are a function of the experimental conditions employed and the lack of standardization complicates comparisons between experiments. Although this chapter reviews a number of published studies, it focuses on the relative thresholds assessed within experiments to draw conclusions about variables that affect sensory perception.

15.4 Sensory Thresholds on Extragenital Sites

Research on extragenital sites provides some general perspective on sensory perception thresholds. One general finding is that sensitivity to touch, vibration, and thermal stimuli varies by anatomical site. For example, the hands appear to be more sensitive to touch, and especially to vibration, than the feet [1, 7].

Besides the anatomical location itself, advancing age appears a most significant effect on perception of mechanical stimuli. For example, the sensitivity of the hands and feet to touch, skin indentation, and vibration declines with age. This decline becomes apparent by the fifth decade, progresses exponentially after age 65 or 70 [8, 9], and is more severe for the lower than the upper extremities [9, 10, 5]; the latter may reflect the longer distance of the neural pathway that the sensory input must travel.

By contrast, evidence for an age-related decline in the perception of thermal stimuli is inconsistent [5, 7, 8, 11]; some studies found an age-related decline, but several show no change. The disparate results may relate to the experimental conditions employed in each study: thermal stimuli are perceived more easily when a larger skin surface area is stimulated [11].

Gender differences in sensory perception have been found inconsistently. With respect to mechanical stimuli, several studies found no gender differences in perception thresholds on either the forehead [1], the hand and forearm [11], or the foot [10], regardless of age. However, a US study of 350 people found that, specifically among those aged over 50, women were more sensitive to vibration on the dorsum of the hands and feet than men [9]. A Taiwanese study among 484 subjects found vibratory thresholds to be lower in women than in men on the dorsum of foot, with no difference on the thenar eminence of the hand [5].

With respect to thermal stimuli, women exhibited higher sensitivity in a subset of studies. For example, a Dutch study found women to be more sensitive to thermal stimuli on the foot [7]; a Taiwanese study found women to be more sensitive to warm thresholds on both the hand and the dorsal surface of the foot [5]; and a British study found women to be more sensitive than men to heat and cold stimuli on the thenar eminence of the hand, the distal phalanx of the middle finger, and the dorsal surface of the forearm [11]. However, a North American study of 48 people found young men aged 19–31 to be more sensitive than women in the same age group to warm stimuli on the plantar surface of the feet, but found no difference on the thenar eminence of the hand [10]. The variability in results among different studies may relate to the range of the age groupings analyzed or to differences in the types of thermal probe employed.

In summary, anatomical sites vary in their sensitivity to sensory stimuli. Advancing age has been shown to reduce sensory perception of mechanical stimuli on extragenital sites, but limited evidence exists for age-related reductions in the perception of thermal stimuli. Some evidence exists that women are more sensitive than men to mechanical and thermal stimuli, but this may depend on the body site stimulated, the exposure conditions, and the age range of the subjects studied.

15.5 Sensory Perception on the Vulva

15.5.1 Quantitative Sensory Thresholds with Age and Menopausal Status

Published quantitative testing on vulvovaginal sensory thresholds is summarized in Table 15.1. Studies that compared vulvovaginal sensory perception to that of other anatomical sites suggest that the vulva and vagina are relatively less sensitive to sensory stimuli. For example, among 58 premenopausal women in the Netherlands, the labia majora, labia minora, and clitoris were less sensitive to mild electric current than the lower abdomen or the dorsum of the hand; the vaginal wall was the least sensitive site studied [12]. A Canadian study of 40 premenopausal women found the labium minus and the mucosa of the vulvar vestibule to be less sensitive than the forearm to filament touch and pressure, although the labium minus was more sensitive to pain than the forearm [13]. Similarly, a Canadian study of 13 premenopausal women found the vulvar vestibule to be less sensitive to filament touch and pressure than either the deltoid muscle, the forearm, or the thigh [14].

Several studies have examined vibratory thresholds on the vulva. A Swedish study found the clitoris to be less sensitive to the perception of vibration than the dorsum of the hand but more sensitive than the dorsum of the feet [15]. A study of vibratory thresholds performed in Turkey found that vulvar sites (labia majora and minora, clitoris, and vaginal introitus) were comparable in sensitivity to the first and second fingers and to the nipples. Of the various sites tested in that study, the ears and lips were the least sensitive to vibratory stimuli [16].

A few studies have compared sensory perception among different locations on the vulva. A US study among 17 premenopausal women found slightly lower sensitivity to touch on the perineum; comparable sensitivity on the labia majora, labia minora, and clitoris; and slightly higher sensitivity on the anal verge [17]. As noted earlier, a Dutch study reported that the vaginal wall was less sensitive to mild electric current than the labia majora, the labia minora, or the clitoris [12].

The vulvar vestibule may be more sensitive to touch than the labia. A Canadian study of 13 premenopausal women found the one o'clock position of the vulvar vestibule to be more sensitive to touch than the 6 or 9 o'clock positions or the inner aspect of the labium minus [14]. Similarly, a different study among 20 premenopausal

Table 15.1 Factors affecting vulvovaginal sensory thresholds

Population	N	Stimulus	Method	Anatomical location	Results	Comments	References
USA							
Healthy and neurologically impaired women	38	Pressure/touch	Pressure esthesiometer: Semmes-Weinstein monofilaments	Vulva/perineum	Significant loss of sensitivity to pressure/touch in postmenopausal women, hypoestrogenic women, women with vulvar atrophy, neurologically impaired women, and women with impaired sexual function	A clear effect of estrogen on vulvar sensitivity was demonstrated: menopause, nonuse of ERT, and vulvovaginal atrophy were associated with decreased sensitivity to pressure/touch	Doeland et al. [7]
	32 healthy		*Method of limits*: sequential application of pressure filaments to point of detection	Clitoral glans		Although the vulva has lower density of estrogen receptors than the vagina, effect of estrogen on touch sensitivity appears profound	
	5 impaired			Labium minus (right and left)			
	Premenopausal (17)			Perineum (right and left)			
	Postmenopausal (15)			Anal verge			
	6 with ERT			Average vulvar score (all sites)			
	9 without ERT						
	Normoestrogenic (premenopausal and postmenopausal women on ERT)						
	23 (*Hypoestrogenic*: postmenopausal women not on ERT)						
	Impaired sexual function (by questionnaire)						

(continued)

Table 15.1 Factors affecting vulvovaginal sensory thresholds (continued)

Population	N	Stimulus	Method	Anatomical location	Results	Comments	References
Postmenopausal hypoestrogenic women with lower genitourinary tract complaints (e.g., urinary incontinence, frequency, urgency, nocturia, vaginal atrophy)	39 (30 completed study)	Pressure/touch	*Protocol* RCT: topical application of estradiol cream to the vulvar vestibule and vagina, nightly for 2 weeks, 3× weekly for 2 weeks, and 2× weekly for 2 more weeks, with or without pelvic muscle biofeedback *Intervention groups* (1) Active cream with biofeedback, (2) active cream with sham biofeedback, (3) placebo cream with biofeedback, (4) placebo cream with sham biofeedback *Outcome measure* *Method of limits* (1) Von-Frey monofilament thresholds (mN) at the vulvar vestibule (2) Maximum intravaginal pressure	Vulvar vestibule Vaginal wall	Estradiol treatment significantly increased sensitivity of the vestibule to pressure/touch relative to placebo at 4 and 6 weeks. The greatest improvements occurred in women aged 70–79 years	Mechanism of estrogen action on sensory function of the vestibule not known. Potential sensorineural targets may be C fibers or Merkel cells	Foster et al. [19]
Women aged 20–78	58	Vibration	*Method of limits* Commercially available 120 Hz biothesiometer	Vulva Clitoris External urethral meatus Right and left perineum Medial right ankle	*Age* Vibratory sensation thresholds progressively increased with age at the vulva, clitoris, external urethral meatus, and ankle *Menopause* Sensitivity to vibration decreased after on genital sites but not on the ankle	Age affected both genital and peripheral sensation. Menopause affected genital sensation only	Connell et al. [16]
Examined variables of age, menopause, prior vaginal delivery, and history of neurological disorder	10 (aged 20–29) 13 (aged 30–39) 17 (aged 40–49) 8 (aged 50–59) 10 (aged 60–79)						

Israel					
Healthy women aged 18–78	89	Thermal (warm, cold)	Method of limits	Clitoris	Thermal thresholds with age	A smaller age effect on vibratory threshold was seen on the clitoris compared to the vagina	Vardi et al. [18]
			Thermal	Vagina	Sensitivity to warmth decreased with age at the clitoris but was constant on the anterior vagina	
			Cylindrical clitoral thermal probe, 25 mm diameter, with contact element on end; vaginal thermal probe with thermal contact on outer cylindrical surface (28 mm diameter)		Sensitivity to cold decreased with age at the anterior vagina but remained constant on the clitoris	
		Vibratory	Vibratory		Vibratory thresholds with age	
			Vibrameter, 100 Hz, amplitude 0–130 µm		Sensitivity to ascending vibration decreased with age on both the vagina and clitoris	
			Method of limits (linear change): 1 °C/s for thermal, 1 µm/s for vibratory			
Sweden						
Healthy women aged 27–44	Aged 35–45 $n = 95$ (examined once)	Vibration	Method of limits	Clitoris	Vibratory thresholds by site	No change in sensitivity with menstrual cycle	Helstrom and Lundberg [15]
			Commercially available 100 Hz vibrameter	Hands (dorsum)	The clitoris less sensitive than the hands but more sensitive than the feet	
	Aged 27–44 $n = 8$ (examined over the menstrual cycle)			Feet (dorsum)		

(continued)

Table 15.1 Factors affecting vulvovaginal sensory thresholds (continued)

Population	N	Stimulus	Method	Anatomical location	Results	Comments	References
Turkey							
Women with diabetes (aged 39–50) and without diabetes (aged 35–42)	30 with diabetes	Vibration	Method of limits	9 genital sites	Genital sites, the nipples and fingers did not differ in sensitivity; the ears and lips were least sensitive extragenital sites	Absolute threshold values are highly dependent on type of equipment used	Connell et al. [16]
Sexual function (questionnaire) and genital and extragenital sensory function assessed	20 without diabetes		Commercially available 120 Hz biothesiometer, 300 mm² surface area	Right and left labia majora, right and left labia minora, left and right side of clitoris, glans clitoris, and superior and inferior vaginal introitus	Women with diabetes were less sensitive to vibration at all anatomical sites tested		
			500 ms stimulus duration	14 extragenital sites Right and left nipple, upper and lower lip, right and left ear lobe, first and second fingers of right and left hand, first and second toes of right and left feet	In women with diabetes, genital sites with the greatest deficit in sensitivity to vibration were the vaginal introitus, followed by the labia minora and clitoris		
Netherlands							
Healthy women	60	Electric current	Method of limits	Genital sites	Genital sites less sensitive (ca. 1 mA) than extragenital sites	Absolute values depend on specific experimental conditions	Weijmar et al. [12]
Aged 18–60			Electrode	Vaginal wall (2–4 cm from introitus)	Vaginal wall least sensitive site. The 12-h position (upper vaginal wall) slightly more sensitive than other positions on vaginal tract circumference		
All but 2 were premenopausal			Range 0–30 mA 100 Hz 5 ms duration Threshold of perception of prickly sensation	Left and right labia majora Left and right labia minora Clitoris *Extragenital sites* Hand (dorsum) Left and right lower abdomen	Dorsum of the hand is more sensitive than the abdomen		

Canada					
Nulliparous premenopausal	26	Pressure/ touch	Modified von Frey filaments of suture material monofilaments calibrated to Semmes-Weinstein, plus three lower pressures	Vulvar vestibule (1, 3, 6, and 9 o'clock) and inner aspect of labium minus	Controls	In controls, the vulvar vestibule was less sensitive to punctate tactile stimuli than glabrous skin of the arm and leg. The labium minus most sensitive to touch. Pain thresholds similar at all body sites tested	Foster et al. [19]
	13 LPV		*Tactile thresholds by method of levels* (2-down, 1-up staircase method: 2 +ve responses to same stimulus needed to move to next lower, one −ve needed to move to next higher)		Thresholds higher at one o'clock position of the vestibule than at 6 and 9 o'clock positions or on the labium minus	In women with LPV, tactile and pain thresholds in vestibule dramatically lower: tactile sensation levels in controls caused pain in some women with LPV, and they perceived vestibular touch at levels imperceptible to controls	
Women with or without LPV	13 controls		*Pain thresholds by method of limits* (sequential pressure increase from tactile threshold)		*LPV* At all vestibular positions, *tactile thresholds* dramatically lower in LPV group: 6 o'clock most sensitive *Pain thresholds* significantly lower in LPV patients *Genital vs. extragenital sites* In controls, the vestibule at 1 o'clock less sensitive to touch than the deltoid, forearm, thigh; similar pain thresholds at all sites. In LPV group, vestibule more sensitive than the deltoid, and pain thresholds lower at all sites		

(continued)

Table 15.1 Factors affecting vulvovaginal sensory thresholds (continued)

Population	N	Stimulus	Method	Anatomical location	Results	Comments	References
Canada							
Premenopausal women aged 18–45 with or without LPV	40	Touch and pressure under erotic and neutral conditions (erotic film or travel film viewing)	*Tactile thresholds*	Vulvar vestibule (9 o'clock)	*Genital vs. extragenital sites*	Sexual arousal had no effect on extragenital sensation (forearm)	Payne et al. [13]
	20 LPV		Method of limits, using modified von Frey filaments	Inner aspect of labium minus	Forearm more sensitive to touch than genital sites	Forearm, though more sensitive to touch, was less sensitive to pain than the labia	
	20 controls		*Pain thresholds*	Volar surface of forearm	The vestibule more sensitive to touch than the labium minus	Data suggest dyspareunia in LPV patients not due to lack of arousal	
			Method of limits, using vulvalgesiometer (spring-based pressure device with cotton swab tip)		The labium minus more sensitive to pain than the forearm		
			Sexual arousal		*Controls vs. LPV*		
			Labial thermistor clip on the labium minus		LPV subjects more sensitive to touch and pain than healthy controls under both erotic and nonerotic conditions		

women found the 9 o'clock position of the vestibule to be more sensitive to touch than the labium minus [13].

As is the case at extragenital sites, vulvar sensitivity to mechanical stimuli deteriorates with age. A US study of 58 women aged 20–78 found that age affected both genital and peripheral sensation: vibratory thresholds increased progressively with age at the vulva, clitoris, external urethral meatus, perineum, and ankle [16]; on the vulva, the age effect first became apparent in the 30–39 age group. A study performed in Israel among 89 women aged 18–78 found that sensitivity to vibration decreased with age on the clitoris and on the anterior vagina, but that the effect of age on clitoral sensitivity was smaller [18]. The effect of age on vulvovaginal sensitivity to thermal stimuli was less straightforward: sensitivity to warmth decreased with age on the clitoris but remained constant on the anterior vagina; sensitivity to cold decreased with age on the anterior vagina but remained constant on the clitoris [18]. One small study examined the impact of the menstrual cycle on sensitivity to vibration and found no effects at the clitoris, the hands, or the feet [15].

Besides age, hormonal status appears to uniquely affect vulvar sensitivity: specifically, the decline in estrogen levels associated with menopause is a critical determinant of vulvar sensitivity to touch. The impact of estrogen status on the perception of punctate touch on the vulva and perineum was demonstrated in a study of 38 women divided into five comparison groups: (1) premenopausal and postmenopausal women; (2) normoestrogenic women (premenopausal women and postmenopausal women on estrogen replacement therapy) and hypoestrogenic women (postmenopausal women not on estrogen replacement therapy); (3) women with and without clinical signs of vulvar atrophy; (4) neurologically impaired women and healthy controls matched by age, parity, and estrogen status; and (5) women reporting sexual dysfunction and controls. Semmes-Weinstein monofilaments were used to apply different intensities of punctate pressure to the glans clitoris, bilateral sites on the labium minus and perineum, and the anal verge.

A clear effect of estrogen on vulvar sensitivity to punctate touch was demonstrated: menopause, nonuse of estrogen replacement therapy, and vulvar atrophy all were associated with decreased clitoral, labial, and overall vulvar sensitivity [17]. Indeed, thresholds to touch averaged over all vulvar sites (clitoris, labium minus, perineum, and anal verge) were 4.6-fold lower in normoestrogenic compared to hypoestrogenic women. Sexual dysfunction and neurological impairment also correlated with loss of vulvar sensitivity to touch.

Clinical trials of topical estrogen therapy support the conclusion that estrogen stimulation is needed to maintain vulvar sensory perception to touch. A prospective controlled trial examined the impact of topical estradiol cream applied to the vulvar vestibule and vaginal wall (either with or without biofeedback) in women with urogenital complaints aged 60 or older [19]. Topical estradiol cream was associated with a significant increase in vulvovaginal sensitivity to touch that improved as the duration of therapy progressed (specifically, after 4 weeks and 6 weeks of treatment). The greatest improvements occurred in women aged 70–79.

Notably, a US study of women aged 20–78 found that whereas age affected both genital and extragenital vibratory sensation, menopausal status affected genital sensation only [16]. Taken together, these data indicate that the perception of punctate touch and vibration on the vulva and vagina is dependent on estrogen status.

15.5.2 Subjective Reports of Vulvar Sensation in Controlled Trials of External Hygiene Products

Further perspective on vulvar sensation has been gained from prospective, randomized trials of external feminine hygiene products (menstrual pads, panty liners, and feminine wet wipes) in which participants reported sensory experiences of a more subjective quality. Over the past 26 years, dozens of randomized trials in various parts of the world have assessed observable vulvar irritation and subjective sensory effects associated with the use of such products (reviewed in [20, 21]). Women who use feminine hygiene products report a low frequency of vulvar sensory effects (such as rubbing, chaffing, burning, itch, or a moist, wet, sticky, or sweaty feeling). Generally speaking, the frequencies of such complaints range from a fraction of a percent to about 2 %, depending on the study. For example, in a trial of sanitary pads that differed solely in their surface covering conducted over two menstrual cycles, between 1 and 2 % of participants in each group reported any such effects after the first cycle; the frequency of reports dropped to between 0.4 and 1 % after the second cycle [22].

Subjective sensory effects are less quantifiable and more complex than the simple perception of a single physical stimulus: rubbing is the perception of a mechanical stimulus (touch) combined with friction; the sensation of wetness may be a combination of the perception of fluid contact combined with a sensation of cooling through heat transfer and evaporation; itching and burning are subjective pathological sensations. Nevertheless, the frequency of such effects in different groups of women also yields useful information on vulvar sensation.

A prospective trial of feminine wet wipes and dry toilet tissue conducted in France among groups of pre- and postmenopausal women provides perspective on the potential impact of menopause. The trial examined both clinically observable skin irritation and wetness and subjective sensory responses in 120 premenopausal women aged 18–45 (60 per product group) as well as in groups of 60 postmenopausal women aged 55–80 (30 per product group) who were not on hormone replacement therapy [23]. Participants used either the wet wipes or dry tissue for menstrual or post-urination cleansing for 28 consecutive days (beginning 2–4 days before the onset of menstrual flow in premenopausal women). Premenopausal women were assessed on days 2–4 of the cycle and 2–4 days prior to the onset of the menstrual period. Postmenopausal women were assessed on study days 14±2 and 28±2.

Objective vulvar erythema was either not observed, barely discernible, or slight, with no statistical difference in frequencies between product groups. Reported sensory effects included slight burning, itching, or stinging (in both product groups) and a wet or sticky sensation (reported in the wet wipe product group only).

The frequencies of vulvar burning and itching did not differ by menopausal status. A slight burning sensation was reported by 14 and 12.9 % of premenopausal and postmenopausal wet wipe users and by 1.8 and 3.4 % of pre- and postmenopausal tissue users, respectively. Slight itch was reported by 1.6 and 3.2 % of premenopausal and postmenopausal wet wipe users compared to 7 and 0 % of premenopausal and postmenopausal tissue users, respectively.

Interestingly, despite a clinically apparent and statistically significant increase in skin moisture on the labia majora and perineum of postmenopausal wet wipe users, the frequency of subjective reports of vulvar wetness was not significantly different between premenopausal and postmenopausal women in this product group (8 and 10 %, respectively). This observation suggests that the perception of heightened vulvar wetness may have been attenuated in postmenopausal women. Nevertheless, postmenopausal women significantly preferred wet wipes to dry tissue for comfort (84 % of postmenopausal compared to 54 % of premenopausal women rated the wet wipes excellent to very good for comfort.) The clinically observable increase in vulvar skin hydration in postmenopausal women may have contributed to their experience of greater comfort with the wet wipe product, particularly if the vulva was atrophic. The experience of "comfort" could reflect a summation of several sensory effects.

Stinging was the only sensory reaction for which reported frequencies differed by menopausal status. (Stinging is not an end point typically associated with dry articles: 2 % of premenopausal and 3 % of postmenopausal women in the toilet tissue group reported slight stinging.) Wet wipe users were more likely to report stinging, and premenopausal users reported a slight stinging sensation significantly more frequently than postmenopausal users (17 % vs. 9.6 %). This observation suggests that the sensory perception of sting on the vulva may be somewhat muted after menopause. The sensation of sting is of interest because dermatologists use the sting response to topically applied lactic acid as a surrogate marker for skin that is hyperreactive to wind, temperature, and chemical stimuli [24].

In summary, based on subjective reports in prospective trials of moistened wipes, sensations of sting and wetness appear to have been attenuated in postmenopausal women, but perceptions of burning and itching were unaffected by menopausal status. We speculate that the perception of burning and itching on the vulva may be conserved to a greater degree with age because these sensations play a role in signaling pathology (e.g., vulvovaginal infection, contact dermatitis, and systemic vulvar dermatoses). Indeed, some pathological conditions that accompanied by itch (e.g., lichen sclerosus) are more prevalent in older women.

15.6 Quantitative Sensory Testing and Vulvodynia

Vulvodynia, which refers to vulvar discomfort and pain of unexplained cause [25], is an issue of clinical significance. Generalized vulvodynia affects the entire vulva, whereas localized vulvodynia is restricted to a specific region. Localized provoked vestibulodynia (LPV), formerly known as vulvar vestibulitis syndrome [26], is a perplexing condition in which pain is provoked solely in the vulvar vestibule in response to touch or pressure (allodynia) with no associated clinical findings besides mild vestibular erythema. The most common and distressing symptoms, which lead women to seek medical attention, are painful intercourse (dyspareunia) or painful tampon insertion. The pain is usually described as sharp, burning, or lancing.

A diagnostic Q-tip test, in which light pressure is applied to the tissue in a clocklike pattern, most often reveals pain in the posterior vestibule around the opening of the Bartholin's glands (4 and 8 o'clock positions). A primary form of LVP is defined as having experienced pain from the first intercourse or tampon use, whereas secondary LPV emerges after an initial pain-free period. Whether these are different disease entities is unknown, but secondary LPV more often involves the entire vestibule (including the openings of the paraurethral glands) and is thought to be more recalcitrant to treatment. Interestingly, it has been reported that patients having focal pain at the 1 and 11 o'clock positions near the urethra have more intercourse pain upon deep penetration and during tampon insertion than patients with focal pain only at the 5 and 7 o'clock positions. Taken together, these observations suggest the possibility of different forms of pathogenesis manifesting as LPV [27].

Historically LPV was thought of as primarily a psychosocial syndrome, but mounting evidence suggests that it may be a neurological pain dysfunction with various precipitating causes (reviewed in [28, 29]). Indeed, under certain conditions (e.g., following experimentally induced vulvovaginal yeast infection), LPV can be reproduced in experimental animals [30].

Moreover, QST reveals that objective, quantifiable differences in pain perception exist in women with this condition. For example, women with LPV display increased pressure pain sensitivity not only on the vulva but also at peripheral sites [31]. In these patients, regions of the brain stimulated by painful stimulation of the vulva bear a similarity to those regions activated in other pain syndromes, such as neuropathic pain and fibromyalgia [32].

Vulvar touch and pain thresholds have been compared in women with and without LPV [13, 14]. A study with 13 nulliparous LPV patients and 13 controls found tactile and pain thresholds on the vestibule to be dramatically lower in patients than in healthy controls. Specifically, tactile thresholds were about fourfold lower and pain thresholds about sevenfold lower in LPV patients; moreover, levels of pressure that were perceived as touch by healthy controls caused pain in some LPV patients, and thresholds to touch in LPV patients were imperceptible to the controls [14].

Sexual arousal affects vulvar sensory perception differently in women with LPV. The sensitivity of the vulvar vestibule to touch and pressure was examined under neutral (travel film viewing) and erotic (erotic film viewing) conditions [13]. A labial thermistor applied to the labium minus registered the level of arousal. The forearm was found to be more sensitive to touch than genital sites (vestibule or labium minus) but less sensitive to pain. Among vulvar sites, the vestibule was more sensitive to touch than the labium minus.

Sexual arousal had no impact on the sensation threshold to touch on the forearm in either the patients or the controls, but increased vestibular sensitivity to touch. During sexual arousal, LPV patients were more sensitive to vulvar touch than healthy controls. Most notably, however, sexual arousal also increased vestibular sensitivity to pain in the LPV patients only; pain sensitivity of the vestibule remained unchanged in healthy women. These data indicate that LPV patients have measurably heightened sensitivity to both vestibular touch and pain and that dyspareunia in these patients is not necessarily due to a lack of sexual arousal but in fact may be exacerbated by it.

15.7 Discussion and Summary

QST has revealed that the vulva is less sensitive to mechanical stimuli (touch, pressure) than some peripheral sites (e.g., the hand, forearm, deltoid muscle, thigh, and abdomen). The relatively low sensitivity of the labia minora, vestibule, and vagina to mechanical stimuli in healthy women may represent an adaptation to the mechanical forces endured during sexual intercourse and childbirth.

As is observed on extragenital sites, vulvar sensitivity to punctate touch and vibration decreases with age. Moreover, the perception of these stimuli on the vulva deteriorates most profoundly after menopause but can be restored with topical estrogen supplementation. Conversely, estrogen was not shown to affect perception of these stimuli at extragenital sites.

One caveat is that the impact of estrogen status relates only to the perception of fine punctate pressure at defined locations on the vulva: the perception of other types of stimuli may not be affected by estrogen status in the same way. For example, the mechanical properties of vulvar tissue, vulvar skin barrier function, and vaginal lubrication are altered after menopause, and postmenopausal women report higher levels of subjective sensations, such as irritation and discomfort, associated with these atrophic vulvar changes [33, 34]. In addition, subjective sensations reported in controlled trials of hygiene products were differentially affected by menopausal status. The frequency of slight vulvar burning and itching in response to physical contact with wet wipes or dry tissue was unaffected, but the stinging response appeared to be muted in postmenopausal women. Hence, various pathways of vulvar sensation may be differentially affected by age or estrogen status.

Lastly, in contrast to healthy women, women with a pain dysfunction known as localized provoked vestibulodynia have a measurably heightened sensitivity to vestibular touch and pain: intensities of mechanical stimuli perceived as touch by healthy women elicit pain in these patients. QST studies have been helpful in quantifying and validating these differences under various conditions and in different subgroups of patients.

Despite these insights on vulvar sensory perception obtained from QST and subjective reports, systematic inquiry is hindered by the lack of standardized assessment methodologies for this morphologically complex tissue. Certain factors complicate the assessment. The glabrous and semiglabrous keratinized skin of the vulva is juxtaposed with areas of nonkeratinized mucosa, tissues that differ in their embryonic derivation and structure [35]. Stimulus of the labia, for example, may affect sensation in other vulvar regions, such as the clitoris or vulvar vestibule. Labial shape and thickness may affect the way the stimuli are applied or perceived. Hence, foundational work is needed to validate the experimental conditions used and to enable comparisons between experiments. Nevertheless, the challenge of assessing sensation on closely juxtaposed skin and mucosal sites that vary both anatomically and functionally is not unique to the vulva. Orofacial researchers also must account for these variables [36] and some of their approaches may be useful to the study of vulvar sensation. Future research will seek to standardize and validate the experimental conditions used to apply stimuli and monitoring the response in order to further investigate various anatomical, neurological, and dermatological factors that affect vulvar sensory perception.

References

1. Dyck PJ, Karnes J, O'Brien PC, Zimmerman IR. Detection thresholds of cutaneous sensation in humans. Peripher Neuropathy. 1993;1:706–28.
2. Sheffield D, Biles PL, Orom H, Maixner W, Sheps DS. Race and sex differences in cutaneous pain perception. Psychosom Med. 2000;62(4):517–23.
3. Wasner GL, Brock JA. Determinants of thermal pain thresholds in normal subjects. Clin Neurophysiol. 2008;119(10):2389–95.
4. Zatzick DF, Dimsdale JE. Cultural variations in response to painful stimuli. Psychosom Med. 1990;52(5):544–57.
5. Lin YH, Hsieh SC, Chao CC, Chang YC, Hsieh ST. Influence of aging on thermal and vibratory thresholds of quantitative sensory testing. J Peripher Nerv Syst. 2005;10(3):269–81.
6. Shy ME, Frohman EM, So YT, Arezzo JC, Cornblath DR, Giuliani MJ, Kincaid JC, Ochoa JL, Parry GJ, Weimer LH. Quantitative sensory testing: report of the Therapeutics and Technology Assessment Subcommittee of the American Academy of Neurology. Neurology. 2003;60(6):898–904.
7. Doeland HJ, Nauta JJ, van Zandbergen JB, van der Eerden HA, van Diemen NG, Bertelsmann FW, Heimans JJ. The relationship of cold and warmth cutaneous sensation to age and gender. Muscle Nerve. 1989;12(9):712–5.
8. Bartlett G, Stewart JD, Tamblyn R, Abrahamowicz M. Normal distributions of thermal and vibration sensory thresholds. Muscle Nerve. 1998;21(3):367–74.
9. Hilz MJ, Axelrod FB, Hermann K, Haertl U, Duetsch M, Neundorfer B. Normative values of vibratory perception in 530 children, juveniles and adults aged 3–79 years. J Neurol Sci. 1998;159(2):219–25.
10. Kenshalo Sr DR. Somesthetic sensitivity in young and elderly humans. J Gerontol. 1986;41(6):732–42.
11. Seah SA, Griffin MJ. Normal values for thermotactile and vibrotactile thresholds in males and females. Int Arch Occup Environ Health. 2008;81(5):535–43.
12. Weijmar Schultz WC, van de Wiel HB, Klatter JA, Sturm BE, Nauta J. Vaginal sensitivity to electric stimuli: theoretical and practical implications. Arch Sex Behav. 1989;18(2):87–95.
13. Payne KA, Binik YM, Pukall CF, Thaler L, Amsel R, Khalife S. Effects of sexual arousal on genital and non-genital sensation: a comparison of women with vulvar vestibulitis syndrome and healthy controls. Arch Sex Behav. 2007;36(2):289–300.
14. Pukall CF, Binik YM, Khalife S, Amsel R, Abbott FV. Vestibular tactile and pain thresholds in women with vulvar vestibulitis syndrome. Pain. 2002;96(1–2):163–75.
15. Helstrom L, Lundberg PO. Vibratory perception thresholds in the female genital region. Acta Neurol Scand. 1992;86(6):635–7.
16. Connell K, Guess MK, Bleustein CB, Powers K, Lazarou G, Mikhail M, Melman A. Effects of age, menopause, and comorbidities on neurological function of the female genitalia. Int J Impot Res. 2005;17(1):63–70.
17. Romanzi LJ, Groutz A, Feroz F, Blaivas JG. Evaluation of female external genitalia sensitivity to pressure/touch: a preliminary prospective study using Semmes-Weinstein monofilaments. Urology. 2001;57(6):1145–50.
18. Vardi Y, Gruenwald I, Sprecher E, Gertman I, Yartnitsky D. Normative values for female genital sensation. Urology. 2000;56(6):1035–40.
19. Foster DC, Palmer M, Marks J. Effect of vulvovaginal estrogen on sensorimotor response of the lower genital tract: a randomized controlled trial. Obstet Gynecol. 1999;94(2):232–7.
20. Farage MA, Elsner P, Maibach H. Influence of usage practices, ethnicity and climate on the skin compatibility of sanitary pads. Arch Gynecol Obstet. 2007;275(6):415–27.
21. Farage MA, Stadler A, Elsner P, Maibach HI. Safety evaluation of modern feminine hygiene pads: two decades of use. Female Patient. 2004;29:23–30.
22. Farage MA, Stadler A, Elsner P, Creatsas G, Maibach H. New surface covering for feminine hygiene pads: dermatological testing. Cutan Ocul Toxicol. 2005;24:137–46.
23. Farage MA, Stadler A, Chassard D, Pelisse M. A randomized prospective trial of the cutaneous and sensory effects of feminine hygiene wet wipes. J Reprod Med. 2008;53(10):765–73.
24. Muizzuddin N, Marenus KD, Maes DH. Factors defining sensitive skin and its treatment. Am J Contact Dermat. 1998;9(3):170–5.
25. Moyal-Barracco M, Lynch PJ. 2003 ISSVD terminology and classification of vulvodynia: a historical perspective. J Reprod Med. 2004;49(10):772–7.
26. Friedrich Jr EG. Vulvar vestibulitis syndrome. J Reprod Med. 1987;32(2):110–4.
27. Donders G, Bellen G. Characteristics of the pain observed in the focal vulvodynia syndrome (VVS). Med Hypotheses. 2012;78(1):11–4. doi:10.1016/j.mehy.2011.09.030.
28. Damsted-Petersen C, Boyer SC, Pukall CF. Current perspectives in vulvodynia. Womens Health (Lond Engl). 2009;5(4):423–36. doi:10.2217/whe.09.30.
29. Farage MA, Galask RP. Vulvar vestibulitis syndrome: a review. Eur J Obstet Gynecol Reprod Biol. 2005;123(1):9–16. doi:10.1016/j.ejogrb.2005.05.004.

30. Farmer MA, Taylor AM, Bailey AL, Tuttle AH, MacIntyre LC, Milagrosa ZE, Crissman HP, Bennett GJ, Ribeiro-da-Silva A, Binik YM, Mogil JS. Repeated vulvovaginal fungal infections cause persistent pain in a mouse model of vulvodynia. Sci Transl Med. 2011;3(101):101ra191. doi:10.1126/scitranslmed.3002613.
31. Giesecke J, Reed BD, Haefner HK, Giesecke T, Clauw DJ, Gracely RH. Quantitative sensory testing in vulvodynia patients and increased peripheral pressure pain sensitivity. Obstet Gynecol. 2004;104(1):126–33.
32. Pukall CF, Strigo IA, Binik YM, Amsel R, Khalife S, Bushnell MC. Neural correlates of painful genital touch in women with vulvar vestibulitis syndrome. Pain. 2005;115(1–2):118–27. doi:10.1016/j.pain.2005.02.020.
33. Johnston SL, Farrell SA, Bouchard C, Farrell SA, Beckerson LA, Comeau M, Johnston SL, Lefebvre G, Papaioannou A. The detection and management of vaginal atrophy. J Obstet Gynaecol Can. 2004;26(5):503–15.
34. Farage MA, Maibach H. Lifetime changes in the vulva and vagina. Arch Gynecol Obstet. 2006;273(4):195–202.
35. Sargeant P, Moate R, Harris JE, Morrison GD. Ultrastructural study of the epithelium of the normal human vulva. J Submicrosc Cytol Pathol. 1996;28(2):161–70.
36. Pigg M, Baad-Hansen L, Svensson P, Drangsholt M, List T. Reliability of intraoral quantitative sensory testing (QST). Pain. 2010;148(2):220–6.

Part III

Menopause and Genital Health

Gynaecological Problems Associated with Menopause

16

Aikaterini E. Deliveliotou

Contents

16.1 Introduction 199
16.2 **Aging Changes in the Female Reproductive System** 200
16.2.1 Ovaries 200
16.2.2 Uterus 200
16.2.3 Vagina and Vulva 200
16.3 **Gynecological Problems at Menopause** 201
16.3.1 Abnormal Bleeding 201
16.3.2 Ovarian Masses During Menopause 202
16.3.3 Screening for Cervical Cancer During Menopause 203
16.3.4 Vulvovaginal Atrophy 203
16.3.5 Recurrent Urinary Tract Infections (UTI) 204
16.3.6 Urinary Incontinence 204
16.4 **Sexual Activity in Menopause** 205
16.4.1 Decreased Libido and Sexual Satisfaction 205
16.5 **Summary** 206
References 207

A.E. Deliveliotou, MD, PhD
Department of Obstetrics and Gynaecology,
"Aretaieion" University Hospital of Athens'
Medical School, 121, Vasilissis Sofias Avenue,
Athens 11521, Greece
e-mail: kdeliveliotou@hotmail.com

16.1 Introduction

Aging is a reality of human beings that nobody can escape. The quest to understand the secrets of aging dates back to the dawn of civilization and reflects strongly the human desire to increase life expectancy and perpetuate an everlasting youthful look [1]. Reproductive aging plays a key role in this continuum, beginning in utero and ending with menopause. Simultaneously, the female reproductive system entirely changes over the course of life. The most salient changes are hormonally mediated and are linked to the onset of puberty, the menstrual cycle, pregnancy, and menopause [2].

Menopause is the most identifiable event of the perimenopausal period and should be characterized as an event rather than a period of time. The most widely used definition for natural menopause is defined by the World Health Organization as at least 12 consecutive months of amenorrhea not because of surgery or other obvious causes [3]. This cessation of menses resulting from the loss of ovarian function is a natural event, a part of the normal process of aging, and is physiologically correlated with the decline in estrogen production resulting from the loss of ovarian follicular function and therefore represents the end of a woman's reproductive life.

Gynecologic concerns in postmenopausal women are common. Although various conditions may affect genital health of all women in this age group, the prevalence of certain disorders, and also diagnostic approaches and treatment options, may vary significantly. The focus of this chapter is to describe the wide spectrum of genital problems and related symptoms seen throughout this period strictly associated with the concomitant important changes in the anatomy and physiology of the female reproductive tract.

16.2 Aging Changes in the Female Reproductive System

The female reproductive system undergoes characteristic age-related changes in morphology and physiology over the course of a lifetime [2, 4]. At birth, the genital tract exhibits the effects of residual maternal estrogens, while during puberty, it matures under the influence of adrenal and gonadal steroid hormones. During the reproductive years, the ovaries, uterus, and vagina respond to ovarian steroid hormone cycling and all tissues adapt to the needs of pregnancy and delivery.

The period of hormonal transition that precedes menopause – sometimes known as the menopausal transition period – is characterized by a varying degree of somatic changes that are the consequence of the significant alterations of ovarian function. During menopause, aging changes in the female reproductive system result mainly from declining estrogen levels and are considered to be rather a progressing process than a sudden event.

16.2.1 Ovaries

The biological basis of menopause and the years preceding is well established, being dependent on changes in ovarian structure and function. The biology underlying the transition to menopause includes not only the profound decline in follicle numbers of the ovary but also a significant increase in random genetic damage within the ovaries [5]. As a result, the ovaries undergo a major shrinkage, so that while premenopausal ovaries are 3–4 cm in size, after menopause they can be measured approximately 0.5–1.0 cm with a fairly smooth tan-white appearance [6]. The older one woman gets, the smaller her ovaries become, but they never disappear. Regarding ovarian function, throughout menopausal transition up to menopause, it is noticed that there is an increased prevalence of anovulatory cycles, leading progressively to definite cessation of ovarian function.

16.2.2 Uterus

After menopause the uterus becomes smaller, although the degree of shrinkage is less in the cervix than in the rest of the uterus [7]. The endometrium is no more affected by the monthly production of female hormones and becomes atrophic. The tissues that make up the cervix generally become thinner and less robust, and the transformation zone where the type of cervical lining changes tends to move higher and slightly inside the endocervical canal [8]. This change makes this zone more difficult to examine on a special visual exam of the cervix, called a colposcopy. The endocervical canal or opening into the uterus may also become narrower or even close completely, a situation called cervical stenosis. This is usually not a problem, because regular menstruation ceases once a woman has become menopausal, so menstrual flow no longer needs to drain out of the uterus.

The cervical glands and the cells that line the endocervical canal make mucus in response to the female hormones that are produced by the ovary during the menstrual cycle. After menopause, when a woman's ovaries stop making these hormones, these cells and glands produce less mucus, often leading to dryness in the vagina, where mucus normally acts as a lubricant.

16.2.3 Vagina and Vulva

Both the vagina and the external female genitalia (vulva) are affected by shifting levels of hormones (especially estrogen) during menopausal transition. Before menopause, when the vagina is well supplied with estrogen, its lining is thicker and has more folds, allowing it to stretch with intercourse and childbirth [9]. After menopause, when levels of estrogen are low, the vaginal lining gets thinner with fewer folds, which makes it less elastic or flexible. Concomitantly, the vaginal walls become atrophic, more easily irritated, and drier, as vaginal secretions are reduced, resulting in decreased lubrication [7]. Reduced levels of estrogen also result in an increase in vaginal pH, which makes the vagina less acidic, just as it was before puberty.

Along with vaginal atrophy, the tissues of the vulva become thinner and drier as well leading to a condition known as "vulvovaginal atrophy." Following menopause, pubic hair grays and becomes sparse, the labia majora loses subcutaneous fat, and the labia minora, vestibule, and vaginal epithelium atrophy [10, 11]. At the cytological level, estrogen-induced parakeratosis of vulvar stratum corneum is highest in the third decade of life, but rarely seen by the eighth decade [12]. At the same time, pubic muscles can lose tone resulting in the vagina, uterus, or urinary bladder falling out of their position (uterine prolapse, cystocele, rectocele).

16.3 Gynecological Problems at Menopause

Genital heath during menopause is directly related to aging changes of the female reproductive system beginning on the late reproductive stage, proceeding through the menopausal transition, and ending to late postmenopause. Despite the universality of "the change of life" during menopause, each woman's response to menopause may be different; as a result, management must be individualized to each woman's needs. A multiplicity of symptoms has been attributed to menopause. According to literature, at least 60 % of ladies suffer from mild symptoms and 20 % suffer severe symptoms and 20 % from no symptoms [8].

However, little distinction has been made between symptoms that result from a loss of ovarian function from the aging process or from the socioenvironmental stresses of the midlife years. It is particularly difficult to distinguish the effects of aging from those of the menopause. McKinlay has proposed a model requiring prospective observations (a cohort study) on a large number of subjects followed during the pre-, peri-, and postmenopausal periods to estimate the shape of the curve of data points on the variable of interest in order to distinguish better between the effects of aging and those of the menopause [13]. Another possibility is that cross-sectional studies include large numbers of women aged 45–55 in order to distinguish the differences in symptom frequency by menopausal status, while controlling for age.

Among the general symptoms commonly seen in menopause, those related to female genital health include menstrual cycle irregularity, vaginal dryness, recurrent vaginal infections, urine leakage and painful sexual intercourse, decreased interest in sex, and possibly decreased response to sexual stimulation.

16.3.1 Abnormal Bleeding

Menstrual irregularity occurs in more than one-half of all women during menopausal transition [14]. Uterine bleeding can be irregular, heavy, or prolonged. In most cases, this bleeding is related to anovulatory cycles. This disruption of normal menstrual flow has been attributed to a gradual decrease in the number of normally functioning follicles and is reflected by a gradual increase in early follicular-phase FSH levels [15]. The cessation of menstruation indicates that the amount of estrogen produced by the ovaries is no longer enough to promote endometrial proliferation and the absence of cyclic progesterone production is accompanied by the absence of withdrawal bleeding [16].

Although anovulation is one of the more common causes of abnormal uterine bleeding, pregnancy must always be considered. There are numerous reports of pregnancies in women in their late 40s who did not consider themselves fertile. In these women, abnormal bleeding may be the first indicator of an unexpected pregnancy [17].

Endometrial cancer should be suspected in any perimenopausal women with abnormal uterine bleeding. After menopause, the overall incidence of endometrial cancer is approximately 0.1 % of women per year, but in women with abnormal uterine bleeding, it is about 10 % [18, 19]. Malignant precursors such as complex endometrial hyperplasia become more common during the menopausal transition. Other causes that should be considered when a woman experiences abnormal uterine bleeding include cervical cancer, polyps, or leiomyomata.

With the advent of newer diagnostic modalities, vaginal ultrasonography has become an established first step in the evaluation of perimenopausal bleeding. An endometrial stripe <5 mm thick has been shown to be associated with an extremely low risk of endometrial hyperplasia or cancer [20–22]. A thickened or asymmetric endometrial lining or an obvious intrauterine lesion is an indication for more thorough evaluation [20].

Because early diagnosis is the most effective way to improve a woman's prognosis, perimenopausal women with abnormal uterine bleeding should undergo an endometrial biopsy to exclude a malignant condition. Although vaginal ultrasonography has changed the way patients with abnormal uterine bleeding are evaluated, endometrial biopsy continues to be the most accurate screening method available for these patients. Dilation and curettage in the operating room with adequate anesthesia should be reserved for patients with abnormal endometrial biopsies or for conditions that preclude performing an office biopsy, such as cervical stenosis. The addition of hysteroscopy to uterine curettage has greatly improved diagnostic accuracy in the evaluation of focal intrauterine lesions [23, 24]. It allows for visual inspection of the endometrial cavity and gives the physician the opportunity to perform directed biopsies [24]. Endometrial polyps or submucosal leiomyomas that are commonly seen in perimenopause can easily be identified by hysteroscopy.

Alternatively, in the absence of uterine pathology, intermittent doses of progestogen may be helpful for women who are having intermittent bleeding and who are not ovulating, while some women find it helpful to take nonsteroidal anti-inflammatory pain relievers such as ibuprofen and naproxen [25]. An intrauterine device, which secretes a low dose of the progestogen, levonorgestrel, can help control excess or unpredictable bleeding caused by irregular ovulation or hormonal problems.

16.3.2 Ovarian Masses During Menopause

With the increased use of imaging and the recognition by primary care doctors that ovarian cancers present with subtle symptoms, more ovarian masses are being detected in postmenopausal women. In screening studies, 5–20 % of women over the age of 50 with no other symptoms will have an ovarian mass detected on ultrasound [26]. However, only a percentage of these will prove to be ovarian cancer after surgery. Thus, it is important to distinguish ovarian cysts that can be monitored with repeat ultrasound studies from masses that need to be surgically evaluated due to their elevated risk of early ovarian cancer.

Transabdominal and transvaginal ultrasound have become a mainstay for the evaluation of pelvic masses due to their low cost and minimal invasiveness [27]. When reviewing ultrasound reports, there are five characteristics that are important in differentiating ovarian cysts with a low likelihood of harboring an ovarian cancer from masses with a higher risk. These characteristics are the size, the complexity of the cyst, the presence of solid areas, projections into the fluid called papillations, and the ovarian blood flow as measured by color Doppler assessment.

In postmenopausal women with simple ovarian cysts less than 5 cm, the risk of an ovarian cancer is very small (0–1 %) [28]. The risk for developing ovarian cancer in women with simple ovarian cysts less than 10 cm in diameter is extremely low. However, 10–40 % of complex cysts with solid areas and papillations will harbor a malignancy.

CA125 is a blood test that can be performed to help the physician to determine the risk of ovarian cancer [29]. The higher the level of

CA125, the more it is likely that an ovarian mass is malignant. However, CA125 is elevated above normal in only 50 % of patients with Stage 1 ovarian cancer and may miss half of the patients with a localized tumor. On the other hand, an elevated CA125 is nonspecific and can be elevated in the face of many common benign findings.

A magnetic resonance imaging (MRI) of the ovary is not diagnostic for cancer; however, it is very sensitive for benign ovarian masses such as dermoids or uterine fibroids that can be confused with ovarian masses. Thus, MRIs should be reserved for patients with indeterminate ultrasound findings who cannot have surgery because of the costs, the need for intravenous dye, and claustrophobia of the machine.

Treatment of ovarian cysts has been made more convenient with the introduction of laparoscopy in the 1980s. Simple cysts less than 5 cm in diameter without concerning features can safely be followed with repeated ultrasounds. Other ovarian masses should be referred to gynecologic oncologists for appropriate surgery, which may include laparoscopic removal of the ovaries with staging procedure if necessary.

16.3.3 Screening for Cervical Cancer During Menopause

Although a woman no longer has menstrual periods after menopause, it is still important for her to visit a gynecological specialist regularly, because an exam that includes a Papanicolaou smear can still detect many possible problems after menopause. In this test, a doctor obtains a tissue sample from the surface of the cervix. A Papanicolaou test can detect cervical cancer, which is the ninth leading cause of cancer deaths for American women and is more often diagnosed at a later stage in older women. This type of cancer is almost always caused by the human papillomavirus.

Other conditions that may be detected with a cervical exam include the presence of benign growths called polyps or other problems that can cause cervical bleeding.

16.3.4 Vulvovaginal Atrophy

Vaginal tissue and the tissues of the urethra and bladder base are known to be estrogen sensitive. Within 4–5 years after menopause, approximately one-third up to 50 % of postmenopausal women who are not taking hormone therapy experience symptoms of vaginal atrophy, a condition called postmenopausal atrophic vulvovaginitis [30]. When "-itis" is added to a word, it generally means inflammation. Inflammation of the vagina after menopause in a woman who is not using hormone therapy is called "atrophic vaginitis." This condition can include redness of the vagina and vaginal discharge. The symptoms of atrophic vulvovaginitis range in severity from mildly annoying to debilitating and include dryness, irritation, itching, burning, and dyspareunia (both with and outside of sexual activity) [31].

It is well known that the cells lining the cervix change the way they interact with each other after menopause, allowing less fluid from the underlying tissues to enter the cervical canal, further contributing to dryness in the vagina. Vaginal dryness can cause discomfort when it is severe, including a sensation of burning or itchiness or pain during sexual intercourse. As vaginal secretions decrease, reducing lubrication leads to increased coital discomfort. Thinned tissue is irritated more easily and may be more susceptible to infection. Atrophic vaginitis is associated with a rise in vaginal pH, which can lead to an increase in the prevalence of colonization by enteric organisms associated with more frequent infections, urinary tract infections, and worsening, irritative symptoms [11]. In addition to these physiologically induced changes, certain vulvar dermatoses, such as lichen sclerosus, are most prevalent in peri- and postmenopausal women [32].

When a woman does not have intercourse or other vaginal sexual activity on a regular basis following menopause, her vagina may also become shorter and narrower. Then when she does try to have intercourse, she is likely to experience pain, even if she uses a lubricant. That is because dry, fragile vulvovaginal tissues are susceptible to injury, tearing, and bleeding during intercourse or any penetration of the vagina. The resulting discomfort can be so great that the woman avoids intercourse and the condition worsens. Sometimes, even women who are not sexually active are bothered by vaginal dryness and the irritation that may accompany it.

These menopause-related vulvovaginal symptoms may occur early in the menopause transition or not until after several years of reduced estrogen levels. Furthermore, not all women develop troublesome vulvovaginal symptoms around menopause. But those women who do experience vulvovaginal symptoms should not automatically assume that reduced estrogen levels are the reason for these symptoms, as there are other possible causes.

Fortunately, the vast majority of the above symptoms are reversible with estrogen therapy [33]. The systemic dosage necessary for vaginal protection is somewhat higher than needed for bone protection, and thus, topical therapy by means of creams or vaginal rings may be advisable to limit systemic absorption. Unless systemic estrogen therapy is required for vasomotor instability, local estrogen therapy applied directly to the vagina in the form of creams, rings, and tablets can be used effectively to treat urogenital atrophy [34]. Vaginal estrogen cream or tablets can be used daily for approximately 2–3 weeks and then twice weekly after initial symptoms have improved and vaginal vascularization have increased [35]. Treatment is usually long term, because symptoms tend to recur when estrogen is discontinued. The twice weekly estrogen regimen can be used without supplemental progestin without an increase in endometrial thickness. The dosage should be kept low, however, because the well-vascularized vagina is extremely efficient in the absorption of steroids. The new low-dose vaginal ring may also be used without progestin protection of the endometrium. Vaginal estrogen frequently will improve symptoms of urinary frequency, dysuria, urgency, and post-void dribbling as well.

Alternatives to estrogen include vaginal moisturizers and lubricants. There is no evidence to support the use of agrimony, black cohosh, chaste tree, dong quai, witch hazel, or phytoestrogens for the treatment of atrophic vaginitis [34]. Additionally, regular sexual stimulation can help keep the vagina healthy by maintaining its elasticity.

16.3.5 Recurrent Urinary Tract Infections (UTI)

The incidence of urinary tract infection (UTI) is estimated to be 9 % in women older than 50 years [35]. Recurrent UTIs in healthy postmenopausal women are associated with urinary incontinence, cystocele, and increased post-void residual volumes. Other significant risk factors include at least one episode of UTI prior to menopause, urogenital surgery, and reduced urinary flow. From the Heart and Estrogen/Progestin Replacement Study (HERS) of postmenopausal women with coronary heart disease, additional risk factors included diabetes, vaginal itching, and vaginal dryness [36]. Changes in the vaginal environment after menopause such as the absence of lactobacilli, elevated vaginal pH, and increased rate of vaginal colonization with *Enterobacteriaceae* may also predispose to UTI. The intravaginal administration of estrogen has been shown to reduce the rate of recurrent UTI by normalizing the vaginal environment. Low-dose oral hormone therapy, with conjugated estrogen plus medroxyprogesterone acetate (MPA), does not reduce the frequency of UTIs in older women.

16.3.6 Urinary Incontinence

The prevalence of urinary incontinence in postmenopausal women is estimated to be in the range of 17–56 % [35]. Urinary incontinence is the eighth most prevalent chronic medical condition among women in the United States. Anatomic and physiologic alterations associated with aging and incontinence include thinning of the urethral mucosa, reversal of the proteoglycan-to-collagen ratio in the paraurethral connective tissue, decrease in urethral closure pressure, and changes in the normal urethrovesical angle. Many risk factors have been associated with incontinence. Menopause often is considered to be one of these risk factors, especially because a prevalence peak in midlife has been reported by many authors [37]. Epidemiologic studies generally have not found an increase in the prevalence of urinary incontinence in the menopausal transition. Urethral shortening associated with postmenopausal atrophic changes may result in urinary incontinence as well. Vaginal delivery is associated with transient postpartum incontinence, as well as an increased risk of incontinence later in life. Another risk factor for incontinence is an increased BMI, which is an especially important factor, because it is modifiable. Meta-analyses have found an association between hysterectomy and urinary incontinence, with an increase in incontinence of 60 % [38]. Considering that more than 600,000 hysterectomies are performed yearly in the United States and that approximately 40 % of women have undergone hysterectomy by age 60, these results are quite relevant. Women should be counselled about this relationship prior to undergoing hysterectomy. Other significant risk factors include history of UTI and depression.

Regarding the treatment, oral estrogen therapy has been shown to restore the genitourinary connective tissues to that of premenopausal women, as well as it seems to have little short-term clinical benefit in regard to urinary incontinence. Estrogen therapy may improve or cure stress urinary incontinence in more than 50 % of treated women, presumably by exerting a direct effect on urethral mucosa [39]. A trial of hormone therapy should be undertaken prior to a surgical approach in any woman with vaginal atrophy. Interestingly, oral estrogen therapy is associated consistently with an increased risk of incontinence in women aged 60 years and older in epidemiologic studies. This increase may reflect that women with more severe symptoms seek medical care and estrogen therapy more often than asymptomatic women. It is also possible that the local levels of estrogen in these studies was too low to benefit fully the urogenital system, given the data suggesting that higher systemic dosages may be needed for a vaginal effect.

16.4 Sexual Activity in Menopause

Sexual feelings and activities are a natural part of life. Sexual problems during menopause go usually unreported, as most women do not discuss their sexual problems with their health care providers. In a survey of US women ages 57–85, only 22 % reported that they had discussed sex with a physician since they had turned 50 [40].

Despite popular perceptions, many men remain sexually active well beyond midlife and into old age, and many women remain sexually active throughout menopause up to the late postmenopausal years [41]. This may be related to a decrease in the number of available male partners in an aging population. A recent telephone survey of 5,045 US adults ages 50 or older showed that many women have a high frequency of sexual activity well beyond midlife [40]. In fact, sexual activity declines with age in women, which is also the case for men as well [1]. Many studies have shown that men are more likely than women to be sexually active after midlife, and this difference widens with increasing age [42]. In addition, a large survey of US adults ages 57–85 found that more than one in three women (35 %) rated sex as "not at all important" to their lives, compared with only 13 % of men [40].

Taken together, scientific studies suggest that between a third and a half of peri- and postmenopausal women experience one or more sexual problems. The important question of how frequently these problems are bothersome to women has only recently been thoroughly examined, and studies often have varying findings because of differences in the way they are conducted. However, it is clear that while all sexual problems are more common in older women (ages 65 and over), distress from these problems is more widespread in women at midlife (ages 45–64) and declines in later years [43].

16.4.1 Decreased Libido and Sexual Satisfaction

A major concern for some women is a decrease in libido or sexual satisfaction that may occur with natural or surgical menopause. Vaginal changes associated with menopause may also contribute to decreased sexual satisfaction. Discomforts resulting from a lack of vaginal lubrication can lead to dyspareunia, bleeding, and decreased sexual comfort and pleasure, as described above. The role of androgens in libido before and after menopause is uncertain. Although testosterone levels have been reported to be lower in postmenopausal than in premenopausal women, circulating concentrations do not change at menopause, and free testosterone levels might actually increase for several months before they decrease to levels lower than those of premenopausal women [44]. In contrast, there is a marked drop in androgen levels following oophorectomy. In men, the relationship of androgens to libido is well established. For this reason, some clinicians have advocated androgen therapy in women experiencing decreased libido [45]. In women, however, the decrease in circulating androgens following menopause has not been shown to consistently alter libido. Available evidence suggests that sexual satisfaction among postmenopausal women is not decreased over time, making treatment with androgens controversial [46].

Sexual desire decreases with age in both sexes, but each individual is different. Although some experience a significant decline in desire, a few have increased interest, and others notice no change at all. Nevertheless, sexual problems are common for both women and men of all ages, with women being two to three times more likely than men to be affected by low desire. Low sexual desire is especially common in relationships of long duration. A clinical evaluation can help to identify any underlying medical or psychological causes of low sexual desire, which can then be treated as appropriate for each individual woman.

Given that vaginal atrophy can be treated easily with oral or vaginal estrogen therapy while vaginal dryness is usually improved significantly with the use of vaginal lubricants, this kind of treatment can considerably improve sexual satisfaction and libido. Vaginal moisturizers are available without a prescription. These can help with vulvar discomfort due to the drying and thinning of the tissues. Topical estrogen applied inside the vagina may help maintain the structure of the vaginal tissues by thickening the tissues and increasing moisture and sensitivity. At the same time it is very important to continue having regular vaginal sexual activity through menopause as it helps keep the vaginal tissues thick and moist and maintains the vagina's length and width. This helps keep sexual activity pleasurable as well. Getting regular exercise, eating healthy foods, and staying involved in activities and with friends and loved ones can help the aging process go more smoothly.

16.5 Summary

This chapter addresses several commonly encountered gynecologic issues in postmenopausal women, with particular attention given to aspects that must be considered when caring for women in this age group.

Menstrual cycle irregularity, vaginal dryness, recurrent vaginal infections, urine leakage and painful sexual intercourse, decreased interest in sex, and possibly decreased response to sexual stimulation are the commonest genital problems encountered around menopause.

Genital symptoms, though well tolerated by some women, may be particularly troublesome in others. Severe symptoms compromise overall quality of life for those experiencing them. There is under-reporting of symptoms among women due to sociocultural factors.

A thorough, regular evaluation of vulvovaginal health is recommended to all women at menopause and beyond, regardless of whether or not they have symptoms or are sexually active, just as it is for women of reproductive age. This should be emphasized since older women often neglect early symptoms of gynecologic diseases, some of which are potentially lethal.

With this in mind, the health care provider must be cognizant of not only gynecological problems that affect all women but also those disease processes which are either specific to or more prevalent in an older population. Early recognition of symptoms can help in the reduction of discomfort and fears among women.

References

1. United Nations. World population ageing: 1950–2050. New York: Population Division, Department of Economic and Social Affairs; 2001. Available at http://www.un.org/esa/population/publications/worldageing19502050/. Accessed 22 Sept 2009.
2. Farage MA, Maibach HI, Deliveliotou A, Creatsas G. Ch 3: Changes in the vulva and vagina throughout life. In: Farage MA, Maibach HI, editors. The vulva: anatomy, physiology and pathology. 1st ed. New York: Informa Health Care; 2006.
3. Research on the menopause. Report of a WHO Scientific Group. WHO Technical Report Series, No 670. Geneva: World Health Organization; 1981.
4. Storck S. A.D.A.M. Health Solutions, Ebix, Inc., Editorial Team: David Zieve, MD, MHA, David R. Eltz, Stephanie Slon, and Nissi Wang.
5. Hansen KR, Knowlton NS, Thyer AC, Charleston JS, Soules MR, Klein NA. A new model of reproductive aging: the decline in ovarian non-growing follicle number from birth to menopause. Hum Reprod. 2008;23(3):699–708.
6. Gougeon A, Ecochard R, Thalabard J. Age-related changes of the population of human ovarian follicles: increase in the disappearance rate of non-growing and early-growing follicles in aging women. Biol Reprod. 1994;50:653–63.
7. Erickson KL, Montagna W. New observations on the anatomical features of the female genitalia. J Am Med Womens Assoc. 1972;27:573.
8. Lobo RA. Ch 14: Menopause and care of the mature woman: endocrinology, consequences of estrogen deficiency, effects of hormone replacement therapy, treatment regimens. In: Katz VL, Lentz GM, Lobo RA, Gershenson DM, editors. Comprehensive gynecology. 6th ed. Philadelphia: Elsevier Mosby; 2012.
9. Farage MA, Maibach HI. Lifetime changes in the vulva and vagina. Arch Gynecol Obstet. 2006;273(4):195–202. doi:10.1007/s00404-005-0079-x.
10. Jones IS. A histological assessment of normal vulval skin. Clin Exp Dermatol. 1983;8:513.
11. Fischer BK, Margesson LJ. Normal anatomy of the vulva. In: Genital Skin Disorders. Diagnosis and Treatment. St. Louis: Mosby Publishing; 1998. p. 99.
12. Nauth HF, Boger A. New aspects of vulvar cytology. Acta Cytol. 1982;26:1.
13. McKinlay SM. Issues in design, measurement, and analysis for menopause research. Exp Gerontol. 1994;29:479–93.
14. Treloar AE. Menstrual cyclicity and the pre-menopause. Maturitas. 1981;3:249–64.
15. Buckler HM, Evans CA, Mamtora H, Burger HG, Anderson DC. Gonadotropin, steroid, and inhibin levels in women with incipient ovarian failure during anovulatory and ovulatory rebound cycles. J Clin Endocrinol Metab. 1991;72:116–24.
16. Hurd WW, Amesse LS, Randolph JF Jr. Ch. 29: Menopause. In: Berek JS, Novac's Gynecology. 13th ed. Baltimore: Lippincott Williams & Wilkins; 2002.
17. Whelan EA, Sandler DP, McConnaughey DR, Weinberg CR. Menstrual and reproductive characteristics and age at natural menopause. Am J Epidemiol. 1990;131:625–8.
18. Gambrell Jr R. Clinical use of progestins in the menopausal patient: dosage and duration. J Reprod Med. 1982;27:531–8.
19. Lidor A, Ismajovich B, Confino E, David MP. Histopathological findings in 226 women with postmenopausal uterine bleeding. Acta Obstet Gynecol Scand. 1986;65:41–3.
20. Goldstein SR, Zeltser I, Horan CK, Snyder JR, Schwartz LB. Ultrasonography-based triage for perimenopausal patients with abnormal uterine bleeding. Am J Obstet Gynecol. 1997;177:102–8.
21. Castelo-Branco C, Puerto B, Duran M, Gratacós E, Torné A, Fortuny A, Vanrell JA. Transvaginal sonography of the endometrium in postmenopausal women: monitoring the effect of hormone replacement therapy. Maturitas. 1994;19:59–65.
22. Cacciatore B, Ramsay T, Lehtovirta P, Ylöstalo P. Transvaginal sonography and hysteroscopy in postmenopausal bleeding. Acta Obstet Gynecol Scand. 1994;73:413–6.
23. Loffer FD. Hysteroscopy with selective endometrial sampling compared with D&C for abnormal uterine bleeding: the value of a negative hysteroscopic view. Obstet Gynecol. 1989;73:16–20.
24. Goldrath MH, Sherman AI. Office hysteroscopy and suction curettage: can we eliminate the hospital diagnostic dilatation and curettage? Am J Obstet Gynecol. 1985;152:220–9.
25. North American Menopause Society. Estrogen and progestogen use in postmenopausal women: 2010 position statement of The North American Menopause Society. Menopause. 2010;17(2):242–55.
26. Schüler S, Ponnath M, Engel J, Ortmann O. Ovarian epithelial tumors and reproductive factors: a systematic review. Arch Gynecol Obstet. 2013;287(6):1187–204.
27. Holtz D. Ovarian cysts and masses in menopause in menopause and you library women's health Source.., http://www.mainlinehealth.org/phy/Page.asp?out=html&familyName=Holtz&acceptPSpec=1&maxAge=100&mlhc=0&radius=5&PageID=PHY001207
28. Guzel AI, Kuyumcuoglu U, Erdemoglu M. Adnexal masses in postmenopausal and reproductive age women. J Exp Ther Oncol. 2011;9(2):167–9.
29. Koh SC, Huak CY, Lutan D, Marpuang J, Ketut S, Budiana NG, et al. Combined panel of serum human tissue kallikreins and CA-125 for the detection of epithelial ovarian cancer. J Gynecol Oncol. 2012;23(3):175–81.
30. Notelovitz M. Gynecologic problems of menopausal women: part 1. Changes in genital tissue. Geriatrics. 1978;33:24–30.
31. Keil K. Urogenital atrophy: diagnosis, sequelae, and management. Curr Womens Health Rep. 2002;2:305–11.
32. Kamarashev JA, Vassileva SG. Dermatologic diseases of the vulva. Clin Dermatol. 1997;15:53.

33. Raz R, Stamm WE. A controlled trial of intravaginal estriol in postmenopausal women with recurrent urinary tract infections. N Engl J Med. 1993;329:753–6.
34. Willhite LA, O'Connell MB. Urogenital atrophy: prevention and treatment. Pharmacotherapy. 2001; 21:464–80.
35. Cedars MI, Evans E. Chapter 41: Menopause In: Scott JR, Gibbs RS, Karlan BY, Haney AF, Danforth DN. Danforth's obstetrics and gynecology. 9th ed. Baltimore: Lippincott Williams & Wilkins; 2003.
36. Hulley S, Furberg C, Barrett-Connor E, Cauley J, Grady D, Haskell W, HERS Research Group, et al. Noncardiovascular disease outcomes during 6.8 years of hormone therapy: Heart and Estrogen/progestin Replacement Study follow-up (HERS II). JAMA. 2002;288(1):58–66.
37. Sherburn M, Guthrie JR, Dudley EC, O'Connell HE, Dennerstein L. Is incontinence associated with menopause? Obstet Gynecol. 2001;98:628–33.
38. Brown JS, Sawaya G, Thorn DH, Grady D. Hysterectomy and urinary incontinence: a systematic review. Lancet. 2000;356:535–9.
39. Bhatia NN, Bergman A, Karram MM. Effects of estrogen on urethral function in women with urinary incontinence. Am J Obstet Gynecol. 1989;160:176–81.
40. Schick V1, Herbenick D, Reece M, Sanders SA, Dodge B, Middlestadt SE, et al. Sexual behaviors, condom use, and sexual health of Americans over 50: implications for sexual health promotion for older adults. J Sex Med. 2010;Suppl 5: 315–29.
41. DeLamater J1, Karraker A. Sexual functioning in older adults. Curr Psychiatry Rep. 2009;11(1): 6–11.
42. Traupmann J. Does sexuality fade over time? A look at the question and the answer. J Geriatr Psychiatry. 1984;17:149–59.
43. DeLamater J1, Moorman SM. Sexual behavior in later life. J Aging Health. 2007;19(6):921–45.
44. Burger HG, Dudley EC, Cui J, Dennerstein L, Hopper JL. A prospective longitudinal study of serum testosterone, dehydroepiandrosterone sulfate, and sex hormone-binding globulin levels through the menopause transition. J Clin Endocrinol Metab. 2000;85:2832–8.
45. Greenblatt RB, Karpas A. Hormone therapy for sexual dysfunction. The only "true aphrodisiac". Postgrad Med. 1983;74:78–80.
46. Bachmann GA. Correlates of sexual desire in postmenopausal women. Maturitas. 1985;7:211–6.

Changes to Skin with Aging and the Effects of Menopause and Incontinence

17

Miranda A. Farage, Kenneth W. Miller,
Enzo Berardesca, Nabil A.M. Naja, Ghebre E. Tzeghai,
and Howard I. Maibach

Contents

17.1	Introduction	209
17.2	**Structural and Compositional Changes in Aging Skin**	210
17.2.1	Epidermis	210
17.2.2	Dermis	212
17.2.3	Hypodermis	213
17.3	**Functional and Physiological Changes in the Skin with Aging**	213
17.3.1	Barrier Function and Permeability	213
17.4	**Skin Sensitivity and Aging**	216
17.5	**The Skin and Menopause**	218
17.6	**Structural and Functional Changes in Female Genital Mucosa with Aging**	219
17.7	**Aging and Incontinence**	219
17.7.1	Effects of Incontinence on the Skin	219
17.7.2	Minimizing the Skin Effects of Incontinence	221
17.7.3	Incontinence and the Quality of Life	223
17.8	**Summary**	223
References		224

M.A. Farage, MSc, PhD (✉)
Clinical Innovative Sciences,
The Procter and Gamble Company,
6110 Center Hill Avenue, Cincinnati,
OH 45224, USA
e-mail: Farage.m@pg.com

17.1 Introduction

The skin is a sophisticated and dynamic organ comprising about 16–17 % of the body's weight [1]. It acts primarily as a barrier between the internal and external environment. However, the skin performs a wide variety of other functions, including: homeostatic regulation; prevention of percutaneous loss of fluid, electrolytes, and proteins; temperature maintenance; sensory perception; immune surveillance; and synthesis of vitamin D [2].

Like all other organ systems, skin is affected by aging. Aging involves intrinsic and extrinsic processes occurring in parallel [3]. Intrinsic

K.W. Miller, PhD
Global Product Stewardship, The Procter and Gamble Company, Cincinnati, OH, USA
e-mail: miller.kw.1@pg.com

E. Berardesca, MD
Clinical Dermatology, San Gallicano Dermatological Institute, Rome, Italy
e-mail: berardesca@berardesca.it

N.A.M. Naja, MD
Department of Geriatrics, Dar Alajaza Hospital,
Beirut, Lebanon
e-mail: nabilbnaja@gmail.com

G.E. Tzeghai, PhD
Quantitative Sciences and Innovation Corporate R&D, The Procter and Gamble Company,
Mason, OH, USA
e-mail: Tzeghai.ge@pg.com

H.I. Maibach, MD
Department of Dermatology, University of California, School of Medicine, San Francisco, CA, USA
e-mail: MaibachH@derm.ucsf.edu

aging proceeds in all organisms at genetically determined rates. It is caused primarily by the buildup of reactive oxygen species (ROS) as a by-product of cellular metabolism and by ROS-induced damage to critical cellular components like membranes, enzymes, and DNA [4]. Extrinsic aging results from environmental insults to the skin. The most important of these is exposure to ultraviolet radiation (photodamage), but other factors such as physical and psychological stress, smoking, alcohol intake, and poor nutrition also contribute [4, 5].

Normal changes that occur with aging can be complicated by the effects on the skin of urinary and fecal incontinence, conditions that affect a significant portion of the elderly population. Effects of occlusion, moisture, and the irritating materials in urine and feces can cause serious damage to the skin made more fragile through aging. This chapter reviews age-related and postmenopausal changes that occur in the skin and mucosa. In addition, it will review the impact of incontinence on these tissues.

17.2 Structural and Compositional Changes in Aging Skin

The skin is composed of three layers: epidermis, dermis, and hypodermis, or subcutaneous fat (Fig. 17.1). With aging, numerous changes have been described to the skin overall and to the individual layers of the skin. These structural, cellular, and compositional changes have a significant impact on its overall physiological functions.

17.2.1 Epidermis

This outer layer of the skin is composed primarily of keratinocytes, which account for ~90 % of the cells [1]. Melanocytes, Langerhans cells, and Merkel cells are also found. Thickness varies according to the individual and the anatomic site and averages from 50 to 100 mm (as reviewed by Farage et al. [2]). The epidermis fulfills two main

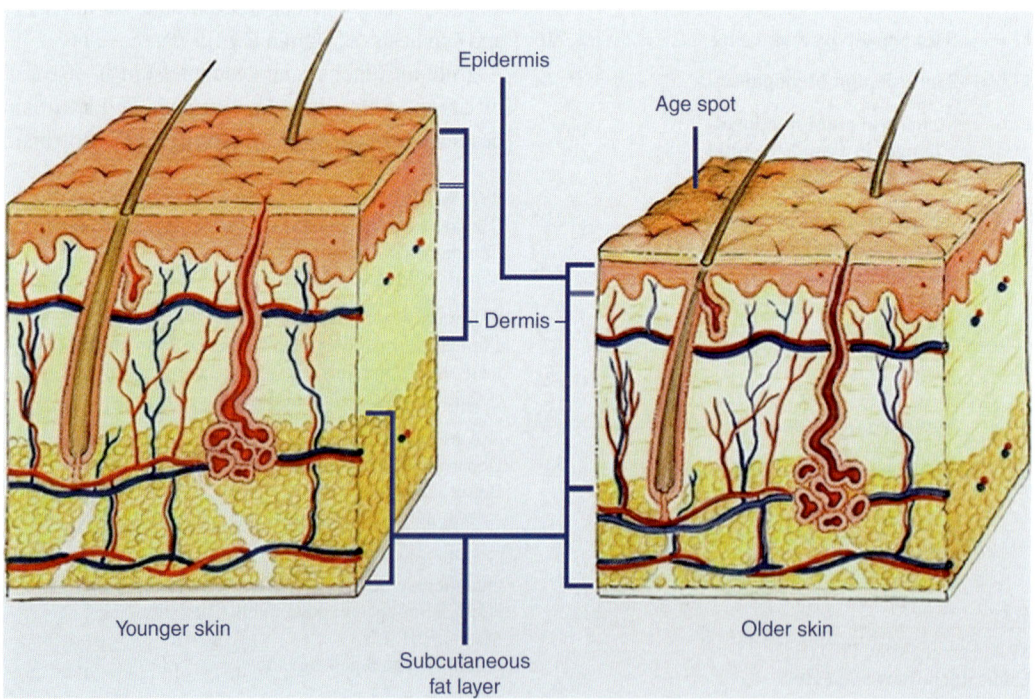

Fig. 17.1 Differences in structure between young and aged skin (Reproduced with permission from Farage [6])

functions: protecting the skin from external insult and maintaining hydration of internal tissues. Both functions are accomplished primarily by the outermost layer of the epidermis, the stratum corneum (SC). In healthy adults, water content of the viable portion of the epidermis is maintained at about 70 % [7].

Keratinocytes originate in a single layer of cells at the basement membrane (the layer between the dermis and the epidermis) and move upward. As they ascend and mature, they produce keratin and lipids, and the morphology alters. By the time they reach the SC, they are flattened cell bodies of keratinocytes, now called corneocytes. The SC averages 15 layers over most of the body but varies widely depending on body site. One body site with the fewest number of layers is the genital skin (6±2), followed by the face (9±2), neck (10±2), scalp (12±2), trunk (13±4), and extremities (15±4) [8]. In the thick palmoplantar skin of the palms and sole, the SC is in excess of 50 layers [8].

Corneocytes of the SC are covered by a highly cross-linked and cornified envelope, with strongly adhering lipids, i.e., ceramides, long-chain free fatty acids, and cholesterol [9]. These intercellular lipids, as well as sebum, natural moisturizing factor (NMF), organic acids, and inorganic ions, impart the water-holding capacity of the SC. The SC is comprised of about 50–60 % structural proteins, 20–25 % water, and 15–20 % lipids [10]. When the barrier function and water-retaining capacity of the SC are compromised, pathologic skin dryness can develop [11]. The skin is considered clinically dry when the moisture content of the SC falls below 10 % [12]. Dry skin is less flexible and is subject to cracking or fissuring.

17.2.1.1 Overall Structural Changes

Changes that occur to the epidermis with aging are summarized in Table 17.1. An important overall change is a thinning of the epidermis. Starting at about age 30, the epidermis decreases in thickness at about 6.4 % per decade [15]. Changes in epidermal thickness are most pronounced in exposed areas, such as the face, neck, upper part of the chest, and the extensor surface of the hands and forearms [34]. One contributor to the overall thinning of aged skin is a flattening of the dermal–epidermal junction due to a retraction of the rete pegs [15]. As a consequence of the reduced interdigitation between the dermis and epidermis, the skin becomes less resistant to shearing forces and more vulnerable to insult [20]. Furthermore, flattening of the dermal–epidermal junction results in a smaller contiguous surface between the two layers and reduces the supply of nutrients and oxygen to the epidermis [16]. This flattening also may limit basal cell proliferation, affect percutaneous absorption [15], and contribute to wrinkle formation [20].

17.2.1.2 Cellular Changes

With aging, epidermal cell numbers and the epidermal turnover rate decrease. The capacity for re-epithelialization diminishes [35]. Characteristic changes occur in each of the cell types in the epidermis (see Table 17.1). Basal layer cells, keratinocytes, and corneocytes decrease in number and become less uniform in size. A decrease in enzymatically active melanocytes results in uneven pigmentation in elderly skin, and a decrease in Langerhans cells leads to impairment of cutaneous immunity.

17.2.1.3 Compositional Changes

Water content of the SC decreases progressively with age and eventually falls below the level necessary for effective desquamation. This causes corneocytes to pile up and adhere to the skin surface, which accounts for the roughness, scaliness, and flaking that accompanies xerosis in aged skin.

Integrity of the SC barrier is dependent on an orderly arrangement of critical lipids [36]. The total lipid content of the aged skin decreases dramatically, and this alteration in the lipid barrier results in dryer skin [37]. Age-related changes in the amino acid composition [12] reduce the amount of cutaneous NMF, thereby decreasing the skin's water-binding capacity [11].

Table 17.1 Structural and compositional changes that occur in aging skin

		Observed effect of aging	References
Epidermis			
	Overall structural changes	Decrease in overall thickness	[13]
		Dermal–epidermal junction flattens	[14]
		Retraction of rete pegs	[15]
		Dermal papillae decrease in number and size	[16]
	Cellular changes	Epidermal cell numbers decrease	[17]
		Epidermal turnover rate decreases and morphology is less homogeneous	[18]
		Cells of the basal layer become less uniform in size	[19]
		Keratinocytes become shorter and fatter	[17]
		Corneocytes are fewer and larger	[20–23]
		Enzymatically active melanocytes decrease in number	[24]
		Langerhans cells in the epidermis decrease in number and display a more heterogeneous appearance	[18, 25]
	Compositional changes	Water content of aged skin is lower than that of younger skin	[11–13]
		The total lipid content decreases, particularly: ceramide 1 linoleate, ceramide 3, triglycerides, and the sterol ester fraction	[26, 27]
		Reduced amount of cutaneous NMF	[11]
Dermis			
	Overall structural changes	Decrease in overall thickness	[15]
		Structure of sweat glands becomes distorted, number of functional sweat glands decreases	[27]
		Number of blood vessels decreases	[28]
	Cellular changes	Fibroblasts decrease in number	[28]
		Mast cells decrease in number	[28]
		Number of nerve endings is reduced	[4]
		Pacinian and Meissner's corpuscles degenerate	[29]
	Compositional changes	Collagen synthesis decreases, and fibers and bundles are altered	[18, 30]
		Elastic fibers degrade	[12]
		Hyaluronic acid and glycosaminoglycans are depleted, reducing water-holding capacity	[16, 31]
		Interfibrillary ground substance decreases	[32]
Hypodermis			
		Overall volume decreases	[28]
		Distribution of subcutaneous fat changes	[33]

Adapted from Farage et al. [2]

17.2.2 Dermis

The dermis is a dense and irregular layer of connective tissue 2–3 mm thick that comprises most of the skin's thickness (see Fig. 17.1) [30]. The three major extracellular components of the dermis are collagen (which provides tensile strength), elastin (which provides elasticity and resilience), and hyaluronic acid (which provides water-holding capacity). Approximately 80 % of the dry weight of adult skin consists of collagen, and about 5 % of the dermis consists of elastin [30]. The dermis also contains much of the skin's vasculature, nerve fibers, and sensory receptors.

17.2.2.1 Overall Structural Changes

As with the epidermis, overall dermal thickness decreases with age at the same rate in both genders [12] (see Table 17.1). Loss of dermal collagen and elastin makes up most of the reduction in total skin thickness in elderly adults. The number of functional sweat glands and blood vessels decreases with aging.

17.2.2.2 Cellular Changes

Cellularity of the dermis generally decreases with aging as the number of fibroblasts and mast cells decreases. Perception of pressure and touch also decreases in aged skin as the number of Pacinian and Meissner's corpuscles degenerates.

17.2.2.3 Compositional Changes

All three major extracellular components of the dermis (collagen, elastin, and hyaluronic acid) are depleted in older skin. Collagen content decreases at about 2 % per year [18], due to both a decrease in collagen synthesis [28] and an increase in the degradation of collagen [38]. The relative proportions of collagen types are also disrupted in aged skin. The proportion of type I collagen to type III collagen in young skin is approximately 6:1, a ratio which drops significantly over the lifespan as type I collagen is selectively lost [39] and type III synthesis increases [40]. Collagen fibers become thicker and collagen bundles more disorganized than in younger skin [18]. Collagen cross-links stabilize resulting in a loss of elasticity.

Functional elastin declines in the dermis with age. Elastin becomes calcified, elastin fibers degrade [34], and turnover declines [28]. The amount of glycosaminoglycans (GAGs), an important contributor to the structure and water-holding capacity of the dermis, declines with age, as does the amount of hyaluronic acid produced by fibroblasts [16].

Loss of structural integrity of the dermis leads to increased rigidity and diminished elasticity [31], with a concomitant increase in vulnerability to shear force injuries [20]. These properties erode faster in women than in men [30]. The impact of these changes is dramatic: for example, when the skin is mechanically depressed, recovery occurs in minutes in young skin but takes over 24 h in skin of aged individuals [18].

17.2.3 Hypodermis

Hypodermis is a layer of loose connective tissue below the dermis (see Fig. 17.1). It contains the larger blood vessels of the skin, subcutaneous fat (for energy storage and cushioning), and areolar connective tissue. The hypodermis provides cushioning, insulation, and thermoregulation, and it stabilizes the skin by connecting the dermis to the internal organs.

Hypodermis loses much of its fatty cushion with age (see Table 17.1). The basement membrane, a very small fraction of the total skin thickness, actually increases in thickness with age [41]. Overall volume of subcutaneous fat typically diminishes with age, although the overall proportion of subcutaneous fat throughout the body increases until approximately age 70. Fat distribution changes as well, that is, in the face, hands, and feet, decrease, while a relative increase is observed in the thighs, waist, and abdomen. Physiological significance may be to increase thermoregulatory function by further insulating internal organs.

17.3 Functional and Physiological Changes in the Skin with Aging

Physiological changes that occur in aged skin are summarized in Table 17.2 and include changes in barrier function and permeability, vascularization and thermoregulation, irritant response, regenerative capacity and response to injury, immune response, biochemical changes, and neurosensory perception.

17.3.1 Barrier Function and Permeability

Baseline transepidermal water loss (TEWL), a measure of the functional capacity of the SC to maintain the moisture content of the skin, is lower in older patients compared to younger indicating a reduced capacity of the SC to maintain the moisture content of the skin [13, 48]. Recovery of baseline TEWL values after occlusion is also impaired in older skin [42].

Permeability of the skin is altered with aging. Penetration of permeants through the skin involves (1) absorption to the stratum corneum; (2) diffusion

Table 17.2 Functional and physiological changes that occur in aging skin

Observed effect of aging	References
Barrier function and permeability	
Lower baseline TEWL	[42]
Altered percutaneous absorption	[43]
Decreased vascularization	[44]
Decreased chemical clearance	[18]
Decreased sebum production	[18]
Increased vulnerability to mechanical trauma	[18]
Vascularization and thermoregulation	
Loss of vascularization	[15, 20]
Maximum level of blood flow diminished	[45]
Autonomic vasoconstriction delayed	[13, 15]
Decreased sweat production	[46]
Irritant response and regenerative capacity	
Lower inflammatory response (erythema and edema)	[47]
Altered response to irritants that elicit inflammation by different mechanisms	[13, 14, 20, 48, 49]
Attenuated response to sunburn	[20]
Decrease in inflammatory cells	[20]
Renewal time of stratum corneum increased by 50 %	[18]
Decreased wound healing	[18]
Reduced reepithelialization	[18]
Immune response	
Decreased number of Langerhans cells	[20]
Decreased number of circulating thymus-derived lymphocytes	[20]
Decreased risk and intensity of delayed hypersensitivity reactions	[50]
Biochemical changes	
Increase in pH after about age 70	[15]
Decreased vitamin D production	[51]
Reduced elasticity	[31]
Sensory and pain perception	
Increased itching	[52]
Loss in sensitivity, especially after age 50	[20]

Adapted from Farage et al. [2]

through the stratum corneum, epidermis, and papillary dermis; and (3) removal by microcirculation [13]. The first two steps depend on the integrity and hydration of the stratum corneum, which in turn is a function of the level and composition of intracellular lipids [13]. The final step depends on the integrity of the microcirculation [13]. Studies on percutaneous absorption in the aged have produced conflicting results (as reviewed in Farage et al. [2]) that may reflect compound- and body-site differences in the rates of percutaneous absorption.

Epidermal penetration of a substance is strongly associated with its hydrophobicity relative to the lipid content of the skin. Because aged skin is drier and has a lower lipid content than younger skin, it may be less amenable to penetration by hydrophilic moieties [43]. Diffusion to the dermis may be compromised by the flattening of the dermal–epidermal junctions. Reduced vascularization in older skin would impact the removal of penetrants by the microcirculation.

Permeability barrier of aged skin is more vulnerable to disruption. In a study in which loss of barrier integrity was achieved by tape-stripping, adults over 80 required only 18 strippings as compared to 31 strippings in young and middle-aged adults [53]. In the aged subjects, the time for recovery of barrier function was also dramatically increased. At 24 h, only 15 % of the older subjects had returned to baseline TEWL compared to 50 % of the younger group. Artificially induced water gradients produced by occlusion dissipated more slowly in older skin [42].

17.3.1.1 Vascularization and Thermoregulation

Overall, vascularity is lost in aged skin. Capillaries and small blood vessels regress and become more disorganized [20], blood vessel density diminishes [15], and a 30 % reduction in the number of venular cross sections per unit area of the skin surface occurs in non-exposed areas of the skin [20]. Capillaroscopic measurements using fluorescein angiography and native microscopy suggest a decrease in dermal papillary loops, which house the capillary network [15]. Although the pattern of blood flow through individual capillaries remains unchanged [45], the maximum level of blood flow diminishes as functional capillary plexi are lost.

A significant time delay in autonomic vasoconstriction in the aged (e.g., after postural changes, cold arm challenge, inspiratory gasp, body cooling) [13, 15] is well documented; this phenomenon is due primarily to declining function of the autonomic nervous system [13].

Eccrine sweating markedly decreased with age. Spontaneous sweating in response to dry heat was 70 % lower in healthy older subjects compared to young controls, due primarily to decreased output per gland [46].

17.3.1.2 Irritant Response and Regenerative Capacity

Inflammatory response to exogenous agents declines in people over 70 years old [13, 48]. It is slower and less intense, and some clinical signs of skin damage are absent [13, 47]. A comprehensive review of clinical assessments of the erythematous response in older people suggests that susceptibility to skin irritation generally decreases with age [54]. For example, a compilation of results of skin patch tests conducted among older people over a period of 4 years demonstrated a trend toward lower reactivity to four common irritants with age [55]. Specifically, older people exhibited significantly lower reactivity to two strong irritants (20 % sodium dodecyl sulfate and 100 % octanoic acid) and directionally lower reactivity (approaching statistical significance) to two milder irritants (100 % decanol and 10 % acetic acid). Elderly adults were less reactive to a range of skin irritants that elicit inflammation by clearly different mechanisms (references provided in Table 17.2). In addition, people aged 65–84 years were less reactive to stinging caused by 5 % sodium lauryl sulfate (SLS) than people aged 18–25 years [56].

Pretreatment with 0.25 % SLS also had less effect on skin barrier function in elderly people (mean age, 74.6 years) compared to younger adults (mean age, 25.9 years) [57]. Analysis of changes in TEWL after sodium lauryl sulfate (SLS) application to the skin confirmed that in aged skin, the irritation reaction is slower in postmenopausal women compared to premenopausal women [58]. Moreover, although blistering caused by ammonium hydroxide exposure is elicited more rapidly in older people, the time required to attain a full response is much longer than in younger ones [13].

Barrier function requires twice as long to restore in the aged as compared to younger individuals [59]. Repair of an impaired barrier requires the presence of the three main lipids in appropriate proportions, i.e., ceramides, cholesterol, and free fatty acids [60], as well as stratum corneum turnover; both of which are suboptimal in older subjects. In healthy skin, about one layer of corneocytes desquamates every day, so that the whole stratum corneum replaces itself about every 2 weeks [9]. In contrast, elderly stratum corneum may take twice as long [61].

Injury repair diminishes with age. Wound healing events begin later and proceed more slowly. For example, a wound area of 40 cm^2, which in 20-year-old subjects took 40 days to heal, required almost twice as long – 76 days – in those over 80 [18]. The risk of postoperative wound reopening increased 600 % in people in their mid-80s compared to those in their mid-30s [18]. Tensile strength of healing wounds decreased after the age of 70. Repair processes like collagen remodeling, cellular proliferation, and wound metabolism are all delayed in the aged. The rate at which fibroblasts initiated migration in vitro following wound initiation was closely related to the age of the cell lines [18].

17.3.1.3 Immune Response

The immune response of aged skin is generally diminished. Numbers of Langerhans cells in the epidermis decrease by about 50 % between the age of 25 and the age of 70 [18]. Total number of circulating lymphocytes decreases, as does the number of T cells and B cells [18], both of which lose functional capacity with age [62].

Delayed hypersensitivity reactions decrease with age: numerous reports have demonstrated a decrease in the capacity for allergic response [18, 50]. For example, healthy older subjects did not develop sensitivity to some known sensitizers and exhibited a lower frequency of positive reactions to standard test antigens compared to young adult controls [18].

17.3.1.4 Biochemical Changes

The surface pH of normal adult skin averages pH 5.5. This cutaneous acidity discourages bacterial colonization and contributes to the skin's moisture barrier as amino acids, salts, and other substances in the acid mantle absorb water [63]. The pH of the skin is relatively constant from childhood to approximately age 70 [15] then rises significantly. This rise is especially pronounced in lower limbs, possibly due to impaired circulation.

Vitamin D content of aged skin declines: synthesis of this compound slows because the dermis and epidermis have significantly reduced levels of its immediate biosynthetic precursor (7-dehydrocholesterol), which limits formation of the final product [51].

17.3.1.5 Neurosensory Perception

Itching is reported more frequently by older adults. However, pain perception declines and is delayed after age 50 [20]. Consequently, the risk of tissue injury rises, as the most obvious warning signals – pain, erythema, and edema – appear more slowly [20]. This, coupled with longer wound repair times, results in higher morbidity in the aged.

17.4 Skin Sensitivity and Aging

Based on objective assessments in patch tests and sting tests, as reviewed in a previous section, the inflammatory response to exogenous agents declines in the elderly. However, "sensitive skin" is subjective in nature. It is a condition of cutaneous hyper-reactivity that can result in exaggerated reactions to physical factors (e.g., weather extremes), chemical factors (e.g., cosmetics and other consumer products), and/or psychological or hormonal factors (e.g., stress or menstrual cycles) [64, 65]. It is commonly perceived as itching, burning, stinging, tingling, or a tight sensation. Often, there is no outward sign of irritation.

Prevalence of subjective, or self-assessed, sensitive skin in the general population has been the subject of a number of recent investigations using questionnaire-based surveys. Reported prevalence varies depending on the specific study population and the precise nature of the questions posed to the participants. Generally, the reported prevalence is about 40–60 % in the US and in European populations [65–70]. In two recent studies in China, the reported incidence was 15–20 % [71, 72]. One investigator suggested that the lower reported rates in China may be related in part to an unfamiliarity with the term and concept of "sensitive skin" among the Chinese population [72].

We previously reported the perceptions of skin sensitivity overall and at specific body sites among different age groups and genders through a questionnaire-based survey of 1,039 people in 2006 in Midwestern USA [67, 73–76]. Sixty-eight percent of the study population described themselves as having overall sensitive skin to some degree (Table 17.3): 77 % perceived their facial skin to be sensitive, 61 % perceived their body area to be sensitive, and 56 % perceived their genital area to be sensitive. Adverse reactions to products resulting in either visual signs (e.g., redness or swelling) or unpleasant sensations (e.g., burning, stinging, or itching) were cited as the reason for the perception of sensitive skin in about half of the responders. Extreme weather conditions were cited by about a third of the responders.

Other investigators reported on differences in the prevalence of sensitive skin among different age groups. Guinot et al. (2006) reported a decline in the reported incidence of sensitive skin in older subjects [69]. In a recent study conducted in China, the prevalence of "sensitive" and "very sensitive" skin decreased with age [72]. Misery et al. reported no significant difference between age groups and the proportion of the subjects claiming sensitive skin [65]. In our investigation, we found no age-related trends among subgroups of responding

Table 17.3 Perceptions of sensitive skin

	Question: Some people have skin that is more sensitive than others. How would you describe your skin?	Question: Please rate your skin in each of the following areas:		
	Overall rating of skin sensitivity	**Facial area**	**Body area**	**Genital area**
Sensitive (any degree)	**711 (68 %)**	**799 (77 %)**	**628 (61 %)**	**580 (56 %)**
Very sensitive	51 (5 %)	111 (11 %)	19 (2 %)	88 (9 %)
Moderately sensitive	239 (23 %)	245 (24 %)	189 (18 %)	140 (14 %)
Slightly sensitive	421 (41 %)	443 (43 %)	420 (41 %)	352 (34 %)
Not sensitive	328 (32 %)	234 (23 %)	407 (39 %)	451 (44 %)
Total number of subjects responding	1,039	1,033	1,035	1,031

Adapted from Farage [76]
Participants were questioned about how they would describe their skin; very sensitive, moderately sensitive, slightly sensitive, not sensitive. On a subsequent page of the questionnaire, participants were asked to rate the skin of three anatomical sites: facial area, body area, and genital area. Responses are shown above for the overall rating (number followed by percentage) and for the ratings at the three anatomical sites76

subjects in the perception of sensitive skin overall or sensitive skin at the specific sites of the face or body area (Fig. 17.2 a–c) [76]. However, age-related differences were apparent when asked about sensitivity of the skin of the genital area. The perception of sensitive genital skin rose directionally with age. Among the older subgroup of subjects (aged 50 or older), sensitivity of the skin of the genital area was significantly more likely to be reported compared to subjects in the <30 or 31–39 age subgroups (see Fig. 17.2d).

In several investigations, the prevalence of perceived sensitive skin is higher for women compared to men. Generally, the prevalence has been reported as 50–60 % for women and 30–40 % for men [65, 66, 69, 70]. We evaluated

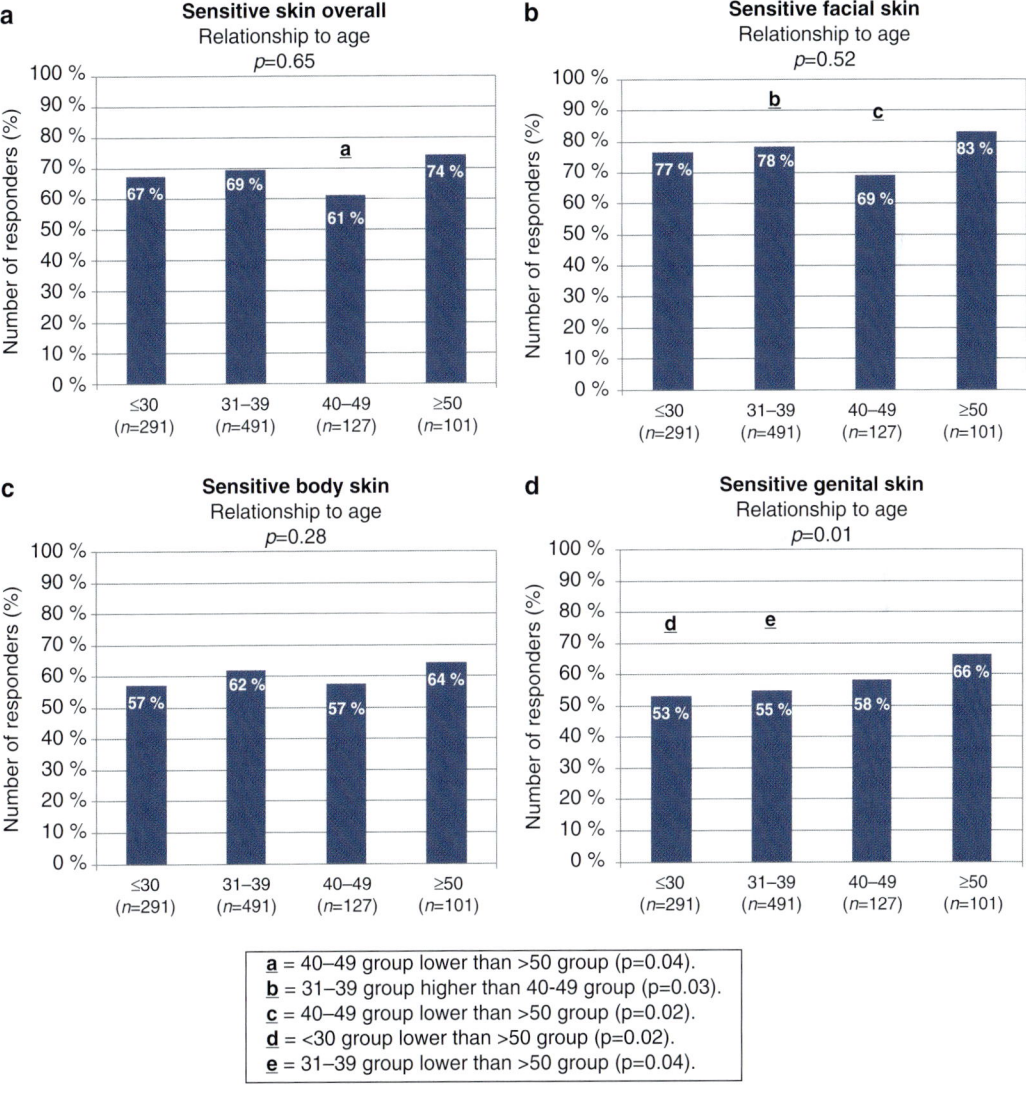

Fig. 17.2 Age group differences in perceptions of sensitive skin. The percentage of participants who claimed some degree of sensitivity overall (**a**) or sensitivity of the facial, body, or genital areas (**b–d**). Correlations between perceptions of sensitive skin and age were assessed by MH Chi-square. Paired age group comparisons were performed by Chi-square analysis. (**a**) On the bar of a – 40–49 group significantly lower than ≥50 group ($p=0.04$). (**b**) On the bar of b – 31–39 group significantly higher than 40–49 group ($p=0.03$). (**c**) On the bar of b – 40–49 group significantly lower than ≥50 group ($p=0.02$). (**d**) On the bar of d – ≤30 group significantly lower than ≥50 group ($p=0.02$). (**e**) On the bar of d – 31–39 group significantly lower than ≥50 group ($p=0.04$) (Adapted from Farage [76])

Table 17.4 Perceptions of sensitive skin by age and gender subgroups

		Responders with sensitive skin (%)					
		General			Face		
		Females	Males	p value	Females	Males	p value
All responders	Females, n=869	69.0 %	64.4 %	0.310	78.6 %	68.1 %	0.474
	Males n=163						
≤30	Females, n=261	66.7 %	73.3 %	0.461	77.8 %	66.7 %	0.173
	Males n=30						
31–39	Females, n=421	70.1 %	65.7 %	0.464	79.8 %	70.0 %	0.065
	Males n=70						
40–49	Females, n=83	62.7 %	59.1 %	0.695	72.3 %	63.6 %	0.315
	Males n=44)						
≥50	Females, n=84	78.6 %	52.9 %	0.036	84.5 %	76.5 %	0.478
	Males n=17						
Association between age and sensitive skin	p value	0.160	0.110		0.377	0.647	
		Body area			Genital area		
		Females	Males	p value	Females	Males	p value
All responders	Females, n=869	60.2 %	62.0 %	0.360	58.1 %	44.2 %	0.030
	Males, n=163						
≤30	Females, n=261	57.1 %	60.0 %	0.760	55.2 %	36.7 %	0.054
	Males, n=30						
31–39	Females, n=421	62.0 %	62.9 %	0.891	57.2 %	41.4 %	0.014
	Males, n=70						
40–49	Females, n=83	55.4 %	61.4 %	0.519	61.4 %	52.3 %	0.319
	Males, n=44)						
≥50	Females, n=84	65.5 %	58.8 %	0.602	70.2 %	47.1 %	0.065
	Males, n=17						
Association between age and sensitive skin	p value	0.263	0.926		0.012	0.173	

Responses were divided into age groups and gender comparisons were conducted using Chi-square analysis. In addition, data were evaluated for an association between age and sensitive skin using MH Chi-square

gender differences (Table 17.4) and found that the number of women who reported some degree of skin sensitivity overall (69.0 %) was higher than the number of men (64.4 %), but this difference did not reach significance ($p=0.310$) [67]. In addition, we found no gender differences in the prevalence of perceived sensitive skin of the face or body ($p=0.474$, $p=0.360$, respectively). However, a significantly higher proportion of women specifically perceived their genital skin to be sensitive (58.1 % of females and 44.2 % of males) ($p<0.030$). An analysis was conducted to determine if there was a significant association between age and perceived sensitive skin. No association was significant with the exception of sensitive skin of the genital area among women ($p=0.012$). The association of age and perceived genital skin sensitivity was not significant for men ($p=0.173$).

17.5 The Skin and Menopause

Menopause, and the effects of postmenopausal estrogen deficiency, can have profound effects on the skin. Estrogens affect several skin functions including hair growth, pigmentation, vascularity, elasticity, and water-holding capacity (as reviewed by Verdier-Sevrain et al. [77]). There is a strong correlation between skin collagen loss and estrogen deficiency due to menopause [30]. It has been demonstrated that the postmenopausal women have decreased amounts of types I and III collagen and a decreased type III/I ratio in comparison with premenopausal women [77]. Women with a premature menopause have accelerated degenerative changes in dermal elastic fibers [30]. In addition, decreased estrogens after menopause also affect the water-holding capacity of the skin. Estrogens clearly have a key role in skin aging, and menopause may accelerate the decline in skin appearance and function.

17.6 Structural and Functional Changes in Female Genital Mucosa with Aging

A constellation of symptoms emerges during the perimenopause (the transition period to menopause). Among these are changes to the genital mucosa (as reviewed in Ref. [78]). The vulva and vagina exhibit atrophy, with a reduction of subcutaneous fat in the labia majora and the labia minora, and vestibule and vaginal mucosa atrophy [79, 80]. At the cytological level, estrogen-induced parakeratosis of the vulvar stratum corneum is highest in the third decade of life, but rarely seen in the eighth decade [81].

It is commonly assumed that aged skin is intrinsically less hydrated, less elastic, more permeable, and more susceptible to irritation. However, assessments of the vulvar skin of pre- and postmenopausal women, using bioengineering techniques, did not reveal large age-related changes in these characteristics. The impact of the menopause on the water barrier function and friction coefficient of vulvar skin was negligible [82]. Vulvar skin is more permeable to hydrocortisone than forearm skin, but comparable testosterone penetration rates have been measured at both sites. In postmenopausal women, skin permeability to hydrocortisone drops on the forearm but not on the vulva, and no age-related differences in testosterone penetration were found at either site [83].

Exposed forearm skin was more susceptible than vulvar skin to the model irritant, aqueous SLS (1 % w/v). This agent caused more intense erythema on the forearms of premenopausal women but no visually discernible response on the vulva in either pre- or postmenopausal women [84].

17.7 Aging and Incontinence

As part of the aging process, the bladder becomes more irritable, holds less, and empties less efficiently [85]. These normal changes can produce incontinence, especially when accompanied by concomitant illnesses or medications, obstetrical injury, dementia, or changes in nutrition or hormonal status. Reported prevalence rates vary widely and tend to increase with age [86]. A community-based study of American women over 50 found that 48.4 % experienced urinary incontinence, 15.2 % suffered from fecal incontinence, and 9.4 % experienced both [87]. Studies have reported the prevalence of fecal incontinence in nursing homes to be as high as 50 % [88]. Incontinence can produce a host of adverse skin effects with dermatological complications.

17.7.1 Effects of Incontinence on the Skin

Urinary incontinence results in two conditions that can affect the skin in a number of ways, i.e., exposure to moisture and occlusion resulting from the use of incontinence pads or other containment devices. The skin effects of moisture and occlusion are summarized in Table 17.5. Both conditions contribute to increased skin pH. The pH of normal healthy skin ranges from 4.0 to 6.8, with an average of approximately 5.5 [106]. With exposure to excess moisture, pH can increase to as much as 7.5. With exposure to urine, pH can reach 8.0 [107]. Disruption of the normal acid mantle interferes with the production of lipids and enzymes critical for barrier integrity and with keratinization critical to the repair of damaged SC [107]. The acid mantle of the skin also provides significant resistance against dehydration and bacterial invasion [63]. Disruption of the acid mantle by incontinence allows for secondary infection [92] by organisms such as *Staphylococcus*, which is indigenous to perineal skin, and *Candida albicans*, which is a common resident of the gastrointestinal (GI) tract [107]. If fecal incontinence is also present, skin problems are further compounded. An increased pH promotes increased activity by fecal enzymes, i.e., lipases and proteases, which can directly decompose the skin constituents [108].

Moisture and occlusion both contribute to disruption in the function and integrity of the SC. Barrier permeability is effected [101]. Moist skin has a higher coefficient of friction, which can lead to an increased susceptibility to abrasion

Table 17.5 Dermatologic effects of occlusion and moisture

Parameter	Influence of occlusion	References	Influence of water	References
pH	Increases pH	[89]	Increase in pH	[90]
Bacterial counts	Increased	[91]	Increases susceptibility to bacterial colonization	[92, 93]
Function and integrity of stratum corneum	Increases TEWL and prevents recovery of elevated TEWL	[94]	Increases TEWL	[95, 96]
	Increases permeability, especially to nonpolar lipids	[89, 97]	Increases permeability to low-molecular-weight irritants	[93]
	Increases hydration of stratum corneum	[98]	Increases frictional coefficient, causing increased susceptibility to trauma	[92, 93]
	Inhibits barrier restoration	[99]	Increases risk of pressure ulcers	[63]
	Disrupts lipid organization and metabolism	[89]	Tends to increased cutaneous blood flow	[95, 96]
	Prevents expected increase in epidermal lipid synthesis	[94]	Increases risk of loss of skin integrity	[63, 93]
Visible changes	Deepens skin furrows	[98]	Increases erythema	[95, 96]
	Increases inflammation	[100]	Increases irritation	[101]
	Increases frequency of hydration dermatitis	[102]		
Cellular function	Carbon dioxide emission rate increased	[91]		
	Decreases mitotic activity	[103]		
	Inhibits DNA synthesis	[104]		
	Induces intercellular adhesion molecule 1	[100]		
	Increases CD3 + epidermal lymphocytes	[100]		
	Inhibits increase in epidermal cell proliferation	[105]		
	Reduces epidermal pool of IL-1α	[102]		
	Increases skin surface temperature	[101]		

Adapted from Farage et al. [106]

when skin is exposed to shear forces [108]. Occluded SC is more susceptible to erosion [91]. Visible changes indicative of increased inflammation have also been described.

Incontinence can develop into a cycle of skin damage resulting in incontinence-associated dermatitis (IAD). Among adults suffering from incontinence, the reported prevalence of IAD varies widely. In a recent review of the literature, the reported prevalence of IAD within adult populations in acute or long-term care facilities ranged from 5.7 to 27 % [109]. IAD has a multifactorial etiology [106]. It is initiated by the changes that can result from occlusion and exposure to moisture and feces (Fig. 17.3), leading to skin hydration, an increased pH, mechanical trauma to the SC, and a compromise of the skin barrier function. Further, skin damage is caused by chemical irritation from urine and feces, enzymatic degradation from fecal enzymes, and opportunistic colonization by pathogens. Without appropriate interventions, such as better control of moisture levels, the use of barrier creams, and medical treatment, the cycle continues and the condition of the skin can worsen progressively.

17.7.1.1 Urinary Incontinence and Sensitive Skin

A questionnaire-based study was conducted to determine the effect of incontinence on the perception of sensitive skin among 29 women aged 50 and older who experienced urinary incontinence [73, 76]. The participants completed a questionnaire probing perceptions of sensitive

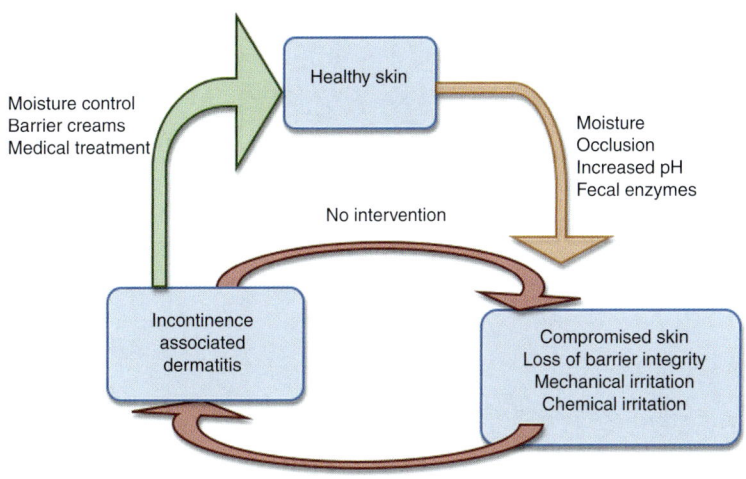

Fig. 17.3 Cycle of skin damage in incontinence-associated dermatitis (Adapted from Runeman [108])

skin at various body sites. Responses were compared to 42 age- and gender-matched controls. Those who experienced urinary incontinence were significantly more likely to perceive their skin to be sensitive in general (Table 17.6). Surprisingly, these individuals were not more likely to report skin sensitivity of the genital area (the expected site to be affected) or of the face or other body sites.

17.7.2 Minimizing the Skin Effects of Incontinence

Without appropriate interventions, the cycle of skin damage that often accompanies urinary and/or fecal incontinence worsens. Since aged skin is more susceptible to damage and slower to repair than younger skin, breaking the cycle of IAD can be even more challenging. The management of incontinence requires a multifaceting approach that includes the use of absorptive or containment products and a consistent skin care regimen of gentle perineal cleansing, moisturization, and the application of a skin protectant or moisture barrier [109].

17.7.2.1 Absorptive or Containment Products

Minimizing contact with moisture in incontinent individuals is key to maintaining healthy skin. Modern, "superabsorbent" polymers have been developed that effectively sequester moisture away from the skin producing a dryer environment [108]. Current advances are focused on developing improved designs to minimize the occlusive nature of incontinence control products incorporating breathable topsheet materials [110] and side panels [111], shaped absorbent pads to minimize exposure to the buttocks [112], and absorbent products with skin protectants [113].

17.7.2.2 Cleansing

Frequent cleansing is essential for individuals suffering from incontinence, but if done improperly, vigorous cleansing can have further detrimental effects on perineal skin. Too much friction can cause mechanical damage to already fragile skin. Gentle approach with a soft cloth is the best method. Perineal skin cleansing should be done with a product whose pH range reflects the acid mantle of healthy skin (pH between 5.4 and 5.9). No-rinse skin cleansers have been demonstrated to be an effective, gentle, and consistent means of perineal cleaning [109, 114].

17.7.2.3 Moisturization and Skin Protectants

Moisturizers contain a variety of different combination of substances that can have different effects on the skin [115]. Lipid-based emollients, such as petrolatum, lanolin, and dimethicone, can improve

Table 17.6 Comparison of incontinent group and matched controls, degree of sensitivity

		General		Face		Body		Genital	
		Number	Percentage	Number	Percentage	Number	Percentage	Number	Percentage
Incontinent >50	Total	29		29		29		29	
	Very sensitive	5	17.2 %	3	10.3 %	1	3.4 %	2	6.9 %
	Moderately…	12	41.4 %	12	41.4 %	9	31.0 %	8	27.6 %
	Slightly sensitive	7	24.1 %	10	34.5 %	10	34.5 %	15	51.7 %
	Not sensitive	5	17.2 %	4	13.8 %	9	31.0 %	4	13.8 %
Control >50	Total	42		41		41		41	
	Very sensitive	1	2.4 %	2	4.9 %	1	2.4 %	5	12.2 %
	Moderately…	10	23.8 %	13	31.7 %	9	22.0 %	6	14.6 %
	Slightly sensitive	21	50.0 %	19	46.3 %	17	41.5 %	17	41.5 %
	Not sensitive	10	23.8 %	7	17.1 %	14	34.1 %	13	31.7 %
MH Chi-square p value (Incontinent vs. control)			0.014		0.248		0.566		0.426

Adapted from Farage [76]

A subset of participants in this study consisted of 29 women in the age group of _50 who suffer from urinary incontinence. Responses were compared to a control group consisting of 42 women in the age group of _50 who were not suffering from incontinence. Analyses were conducted using MH Chi-square 76 barrier function [109] while at the same time preventing friction from diapers and bed linens. Topical administration of a petrolatum-based skin protectant has been demonstrated to improve skin condition and reduce diaper rash in babies [113]. The inclusion of protectants such as zinc oxide resulted in further improvement [116]. Humectants, such as glycerin, alpha-hydroxy acids, urea, and propylene glycol, are substances with water-attracting properties. Since one of the consequences of incontinence can be skin hydration, humectants are generally contra-indicated [109].

17.7.2.4 Medical Treatment for Infection

Interventions, such as the application of topical antibiotics, antimicrobials, and antifungals, should not be used routinely in treating IAD but should be employed only when an infection is actually present [109].

17.7.3 Incontinence and the Quality of Life

Incontinence of either urine or feces is a devastating development for older adults, carrying significant emotional, financial, and physical burden [117]. Urinary incontinence is associated with reduced social and personal interaction and a decrease in overall quality of life [118]. Incontinent elders commonly verbalize feelings of worthlessness and helplessness [119]. Patient coping strategies, in particular the avoidance of social activities due to the potential for embarrassment, can further compromise health [120]. Loss of bowel continence in the presence of essentially normal cognitive function is devastating, emotionally and often financially, for both patients and their families [88]. Incontinence often limits physical activity [118] and has been associated with depression and anxiety [121], a decline in social function [122], and compromised sexual function [123]. The issue of incontinence is often the deciding factor in the loss of independence for an older adult and is a common reason for nursing home admissions [119]. Incontinence is consistently associated with an increased risk of a debilitating, even fatal, fall in the elderly individual [124]. Thus, the effects of incontinence on emotional health, body image, social activity, and physical well-being are profound. Appropriate clinical management of incontinence is critical, not only to avoid the cutaneous sequelae of incontinence but to help seniors continue to lead vital active lives.

17.8 Summary

Over the last two centuries, medical progress has dramatically extended the human lifespan, more than doubling life expectancy across the world. Average global life expectancy has risen from about 25 (for both sexes) to 65 for men and 70 for women [46]. Women, whose average life expectancies exceed those of men, can now expect to spend more than one-third of their lifetimes in postmenopause [31]. More than 40 million postmenopausal women live in the USA today, comprising 17 % of the total population [36]. Many profound changes occur over a skin's lifetime; the human integument remains relatively functional when protected from excessive environmental insult. However, the skin of older adults is compromised in many ways. Structural changes lead to decreased elasticity and resilience as well as undesirable visible characteristics. Decreases in neurosensory capacity increase the risk of unrecognized injury. The intrinsic drying of the skin makes the skin itchy and increasingly uncomfortable. The decrease in the skin's ability to repair itself slows wound repair and re-epithelialization dramatically. Incontinence can further compromise older skin. The effects of occlusion and exposure to moisture and fecal material can disrupt the function and integrity of the skin. Left untreated, this can develop into a cycle of skin damage resulting in IAD and opportunistic colonization by pathogens. As the proportion of older adults in the industrialized world increases, understanding and caring for the problems of aged skin will improve the quality of life in those later years of life gained by medical advances.

References

1. McLafferty E, Hendry C, Alistair F. The integumentary system: anatomy, physiology and function of skin. Nurs Stand. 2012;27:35–42.
2. Farage MA, Miller KW, Maibach HI. Degenerative changes in aging skin. In: Farage MA, Miller KW, Maibach HI, editors. Textbook of aging skin. Berlin/Heidelberg: Springer-Verlag; 2010.
3. Ghersetich I, Troiano M, De Giorgi V, Lotti T. Receptors in skin ageing and antiageing agents. Dermatol Clin. 2007;25:655–62, xi.
4. Puizina-Ivic N. Skin aging. Acta Dermatovenerol Alp Panonica Adriat. 2008;17:47–54.
5. Callaghan TM, Wilhelm KP. A review of ageing and an examination of clinical methods in the assessment of ageing skin. Part I: cellular and molecular perspectives of skin ageing. Int J Cosmet Sci. 2008;30:313–22.
6. Farage MA, Miller KW, Elsner P, Maibach HI. Structural characteristics of the aging skin: a review. Cutan Ocul Toxicol. 2007;26:343–57.
7. Caspers PJ, Lucassen GW, Puppels GJ. Combined in vivo confocal Raman spectroscopy and confocal microscopy of human skin. Biophys J. 2003;85: 572–80.
8. Tagami H. Location-related differences in structure and function of the stratum corneum with special emphasis on those of the facial skin. Int J Cosmet Sci. 2008;30:413–34.
9. Tagami H. Functional characteristics of the stratum corneum in photoaged skin in comparison with those found in intrinsic aging. Arch Dermatol Res. 2008;300 Suppl 1:S1–6.
10. Mathias CG, Maibach HI. Perspectives in occupational dermatology. West J Med. 1982;137:486–92.
11. Jackson SM, Williams ML, Feingold KR, Elias PM. Pathobiology of the stratum corneum. West J Med. 1993;158:279–85.
12. McCallion R, Li Wan Po A. Dry and photo-aged skin: manifestations and management. J Clin Pharm Ther. 1993;18:15–32.
13. Harvell JD, Maibach HI. Percutaneous absorption and inflammation in aged skin: a review. J Am Acad Dermatol. 1994;31:1015–21.
14. Neerken S, Lucassen GW, Bisschop MA, Lenderink E, Nuijs TA. Characterization of age-related effects in human skin: a comparative study that applies confocal laser scanning microscopy and optical coherence tomography. J Biomed Opt. 2004;9:274–81.
15. Waller JM, Maibach HI. Age and skin structure and function, a quantitative approach (I): blood flow, pH, thickness, and ultrasound echogenicity. Skin Res Technol. 2005;11:221–35.
16. Sudel KM, Venzke K, Mielke H, Breitenbach U, Mundt C, Jaspers S, et al. Novel aspects of intrinsic and extrinsic aging of human skin: beneficial effects of soy extract. Photochem Photobiol. 2005;81: 581–7.
17. Suter-Widmer J, Elsner P. Age and irritation. In: Agner T, Maibach H, editors. The irritant contact dermatitis syndrome. Boca Raton: CRC Press; 1996. p. 257–61.
18. Fenske NA, Lober CW. Structural and functional changes of normal aging skin. J Am Acad Dermatol. 1986;15:571–85.
19. Bregegere F, Soroka Y, Bismuth J, Friguet B, Milner Y. Cellular senescence in human keratinocytes: unchanged proteolytic capacity and increased protein load. Exp Gerontol. 2003;38:619–29.
20. Grove GL. Physiologic changes in older skin. Clin Geriatr Med. 1989;5:115–25.
21. Verdier-Sevrain S, Bonte F. Skin hydration: a review on its molecular mechanisms. J Cosmet Dermatol. 2007;6:75–82.
22. Sauermann K, Jaspers S, Koop U, Wenck H. Topically applied vitamin C increases the density of dermal papillae in aged human skin. BMC Dermatol. 2004;4:13.
23. Long CC, Marks R. Stratum corneum changes in patients with senile pruritus. J Am Acad Dermatol. 1992;27:560–4.
24. Rees JL. The genetics of sun sensitivity in humans. Am J Hum Genet. 2004;75:739–51.
25. Wulf HC, Sandby-Moller J, Kobayasi T, Gniadecki R. Skin aging and natural photoprotection. Micron. 2004;35:185–91.
26. Rogers J, Harding C, Mayo A, Banks J, Rawlings A. Stratum corneum lipids: the effect of ageing and the seasons. Arch Dermatol Res. 1996;288:765–70.
27. Zettersten EM, Ghadially R, Feingold KR, Crumrine D, Elias PM. Optimal ratios of topical stratum corneum lipids improve barrier recovery in chronologically aged skin. J Am Acad Dermatol. 1997;37:403–8.
28. Duncan KO, Leffell DJ. Preoperative assessment of the elderly patient. Dermatol Clin. 1997;15:583–93.
29. Phillips T, Kanj L. Clinical manifestations of skin aging. In: Squier C, Hill MW, editors. The effect of aging in oral mucosa and skin. Boca Raton: CRC Press; 1994. p. 25–37.
30. Calleja-Agius J, Muscat-Baron Y, Brincat MP. Skin ageing. Menopause Int. 2007;13:60–4.
31. Brincat MP, Baron YM, Galea R. Estrogens and the skin. Climacteric. 2005;8:110–23.
32. Castelo-Branco C, Figueras F, Martinez de Osaba MJ, Vanrell JA. Facial wrinkling in postmenopausal women. Effects of smoking status and hormone replacement therapy. Maturitas. 1998;29:75–86.
33. Donofrio LM. Fat distribution: a morphologic study of the aging face. Dermatol Surg. 2000;26:1107–12.
34. Boss GR, Seegmiller JE. Age-related physiological changes and their clinical significance. West J Med. 1981;135:434–40.
35. Holt DR, Kirk SJ, Regan MC, Hurson M, Lindblad WJ, Barbul A. Effect of age on wound healing in healthy human beings. Surgery. 1992;112:293–7. Discussion 297-8.
36. Farage MA, Miller KW, Elsner P, Maibach HI. Intrinsic and extrinsic factors in skin ageing: a review. Int J Cosmet Sci. 2008;30:87–95.

37. Seyfarth F, Schliemann S, Antonov D, Elsner P. Dry skin, barrier function, and irritant contact dermatitis in the elderly. Clin Dermatol. 2011;29:31–6.
38. Ashcroft GS, Horan MA, Herrick SE, Tarnuzzer RW, Schultz GS, Ferguson MW. Age-related differences in the temporal and spatial regulation of matrix metalloproteinases (MMPs) in normal skin and acute cutaneous wounds of healthy humans. Cell Tissue Res. 1997;290:581–91.
39. Oikarinen A. The aging of skin: chronoaging versus photoaging. Photodermatol Photoimmunol Photomed. 1990;7:3–4.
40. Savvas M, Bishop J, Laurent G, Watson N, Studd J. Type III collagen content in the skin of postmenopausal women receiving oestradiol and testosterone implants. Br J Obstet Gynaecol. 1993;100:154–6.
41. Vazquez F, Palacios S, Aleman N, Guerrero F. Changes of the basement membrane and type IV collagen in human skin during aging. Maturitas. 1996;25:209–15.
42. Roskos KV, Guy RH. Assessment of skin barrier function using transepidermal water loss: effect of age. Pharm Res. 1989;6:949–53.
43. Roskos KV, Guy RH, Maibach HI. Percutaneous absorption in the aged. Dermatol Clin. 1986;4:455–65.
44. Gilchrest BA, Stoff JS, Soter NA. Chronologic aging alters the response to ultraviolet-induced inflammation in human skin. J Invest Dermatol. 1982;79:11–5.
45. Elias PM. Stratum corneum architecture, metabolic activity and interactivity with subjacent cell layers. Exp Dermatol. 1996;5:191–201.
46. Ohta H, Makita K, Kawashima T, Kinoshita S, Takenouchi M, Nozawa S. Relationship between dermato-physiological changes and hormonal status in pre-, peri-, and postmenopausal women. Maturitas. 1998;30:55–62.
47. Brincat M, Kabalan S, Studd JW, Moniz CF, de Trafford J, Montgomery J. A study of the decrease of skin collagen content, skin thickness, and bone mass in the postmenopausal woman. Obstet Gynecol. 1987;70:840–5.
48. Ghadially R. Aging and the epidermal permeability barrier: implications for contact dermatitis. Am J Contact Dermat. 1998;9:162–9.
49. Coenraads PJ, Bleumink E, Nater JP. Susceptibility to primary irritants: age dependence and relation to contact allergic reactions. Contact Dermatitis. 1975;1:377–81.
50. Robinson MK. Population differences in skin structure and physiology and the susceptibility to irritant and allergic contact dermatitis: implications for skin safety testing and risk assessment. Contact Dermatitis. 1999;41:65–79.
51. MacLaughlin J, Holick MF. Aging decreases the capacity of human skin to produce vitamin D3. J Clin Invest. 1985;76:1536–8.
52. Buckley C, Rustin MH. Management of irritable skin disorders in the elderly. Br J Hosp Med. 1990;44: 24–6. 28, 30-2.
53. Ghadially R, Brown BE, Sequeira-Martin SM, Feingold KR, Elias PM. The aged epidermal permeability barrier. Structural, functional, and lipid biochemical abnormalities in humans and a senescent murine model. J Clin Invest. 1995;95:2281–90.
54. Robinson MK. Age and gender as influencing factors in skin sensitivity. In: Berardesca E, Fluhr JW, Maibach HI, editors. Sensitive skin syndrome. New York: Taylor & Francis; 2006. p. 169–80.
55. Robinson MK. Population differences in acute skin irritation responses. Race, sex, age, sensitive skin and repeat subject comparisons. Contact Dermatitis. 2002;46:86–93.
56. Lejman E, Stoudemayer T, Grove G, Kligman AM. Age differences in poison ivy dermatitis. Contact Dermatitis. 1984;11:163–7.
57. Cua AB, Wilhelm KP, Maibach HI. Cutaneous sodium lauryl sulphate irritation potential: age and regional variability. Br J Dermatol. 1990;123:607–13.
58. Elsner P, Wilhelm D, Maibach HI. Sodium lauryl sulfate-induced irritant contact dermatitis in vulvar and forearm skin of premenopausal and postmenopausal women. J Am Acad Dermatol. 1990;23:648–52.
59. Grove GL, Kligman AM. Age-associated changes in human epidermal cell renewal. J Gerontol. 1983;38: 137–42.
60. Man MQM, Feingold KR, Thornfeldt CR, Elias PM. Optimization of physiological lipid mixtures for barrier repair. J Invest Dermatol. 1996;106:1096–101.
61. Baker H, Blair CP. Cell replacement in the human stratum corneum in old age. Br J Dermatol. 1968;80: 367–72.
62. Szewczuk MR, Campbell RJ. Loss of immune competence with age may be due to auto-anti-idiotypic antibody regulation. Nature. 1980;286:164–6.
63. Fiers SA. Breaking the cycle: the etiology of incontinence dermatitis and evaluating and using skin care products. Ostomy Wound Manage. 1996;42:32–4. 36, 38-40, passim.
64. Berardesca E, Farage M, Maibach H. Sensitive skin: an overview. Int J Cosmet Sci. 2013;35:2–8.
65. Misery L, Sibaud V, Merial-Kieny C, Taieb C. Sensitive skin in the American population: prevalence, clinical data, and role of the dermatologist. Int J Dermatol. 2011;50:961–7.
66. Misery L, Boussetta S, Nocera T, Perez-Cullell N, Taieb C. Sensitive skin in Europe. J Eur Acad Dermatol Venereol. 2009;23:376–81.
67. Farage MA. How do perceptions of sensitive skin differ at different anatomical sites? An epidemiological study. Clin Exp Dermatol. 2009;34:e521–30.
68. Saint-Martory C, Roguedas-Contios AM, Sibaud V, Degouy A, Schmitt AM, Misery L. Sensitive skin is not limited to the face. Br J Dermatol. 2008;158:130–3.
69. Guinot C, Malvy D, Mauger E, Ezzedine K, Latreille J, Ambroisine L, et al. Self-reported skin sensitivity in a general adult population in France: data of the SU.VI.MAX cohort. J Eur Acad Dermatol Venereol. 2006;20:380–90.
70. Willis CM, Shaw S, De Lacharriere O, Baverel M, Reiche L, Jourdain R, et al. Sensitive skin: an epidemiological study. Br J Dermatol. 2001;145:258–63.

71. Farage MA, Mandl CP, Berardesca E, Maibach HI. Sensitive skin in China. J Cosmetics Dermatol Sci Appl. 2012;2:184–95.
72. Xu F, Yan S, Wu M, Li F, Sun Q, Lai W, Shen X, Rahhali N, Taieb C, Xu J. Self-declared sensitive skin in China: a community-based study in three top metropolises. J Eur Acad Dermatol Venereol. 2012;27:370.
73. Farage MA. Perceptions of sensitive skin: women with urinary incontinence. Arch Gynecol Obstet. 2009;280:49–57.
74. Farage MA. Does sensitive skin differ between men and women? Cutan Ocul Toxicol. 2010;29:153–63.
75. Farage MA. Perceptions of sensitive skin of the genital area. In: Surber C, Elsner P, Farage MA, editors. Topical applications and the mucosa. Basel: Karger; 2011. p. 142–54.
76. Farage MA. Perceptions of sensitive skin with Age. In: Farage MA, Miller KW, Maibach HI, editors. Textbook of aging skin. Berlin/Heidelberg: Springer-Verlag; 2010. p. 1027–46.
77. Verdier-Sevrain S, Bonte F, Gilchrest B. Biology of estrogens in skin: implications for skin aging. Exp Dermatol. 2006;15:83–94.
78. Farage MA, Maibach HI. Morphology and physiological changes of genital skin and mucosa. In: Surber C, Elsner P, Farage MA, editors. Topical applications and the mucosa. Basel: Karger; 2011. p. 9–19.
79. Jones IS. A histological assessment of normal vulval skin. Clin Exp Dermatol. 1983;8:513–21.
80. Erickson KL, Montagna W. New observations on the anatomical features of the female genitalia. J Am Med Womens Assoc. 1972;27:573–81.
81. Nauth HF, Boger A. New aspects of vulvar cytology. Acta Cytol. 1982;26:1–6.
82. Elsner P, Wilhelm D, Maibach HI. Frictional properties of human forearm and vulvar skin: influence of age and correlation with transepidermal water loss and capacitance. Dermatologica. 1990;181:88–91.
83. Oriba HA, Bucks DA, Maibach HI. Percutaneous absorption of hydrocortisone and testosterone on the vulva and forearm: effect of the menopause and site. Br J Dermatol. 1996;134:229–33.
84. Elsner P, Wilhelm D, Maibach HI. Effect of low-concentration sodium lauryl sulfate on human vulvar and forearm skin. Age-related differences. J Reprod Med. 1991;36:77–81.
85. Farage MA, Miller KW, Berardesca E, Maibach HI. Incontinence in the aged: contact dermatitis and other cutaneous consequences. Contact Dermatitis. 2007;57:211–7.
86. Dannecker C, Friese K, Stief C, Bauer R. Urinary incontinence in women: part 1 of a series of articles on incontinence. Dtsch Arztebl Int. 2010;107:420–6.
87. Roberts RO, Jacobsen SJ, Reilly WT, Pemberton JH, Lieber MM, Talley NJ. Prevalence of combined fecal and urinary incontinence: a community-based study. J Am Geriatr Soc. 1999;47:837–41.
88. Cooper ZR, Rose S. Fecal incontinence: a clinical approach. Mt Sinai J Med. 2000;67:96–105.
89. Rippke F, Schreiner V, Doering T, Maibach HI. Stratum corneum pH in atopic dermatitis: impact on skin barrier function and colonization with Staphylococcus Aureus. Am J Clin Dermatol. 2004;5:217–23.
90. Berg RW. Etiologic factors in diaper dermatitis: a model for development of improved diapers. Pediatrician. 1987;14 Suppl 1:27–33.
91. Aly R, Shirley C, Cunico B, Maibach HI. Effect of prolonged occlusion on the microbial flora, pH, carbon dioxide and transepidermal water loss on human skin. J Invest Dermatol. 1978;71:378–81.
92. Zimmerer RE, Lawson KD, Calvert CJ. The effects of wearing diapers on skin. Pediatr Dermatol. 1986;3:95–101.
93. Berg RW, Buckingham KW, Stewart RL. Etiologic factors in diaper dermatitis: the role of urine. Pediatr Dermatol. 1986;3:102–6.
94. Grubauer G, Elias PM, Feingold KR. Transepidermal water loss: the signal for recovery of barrier structure and function. J Lipid Res. 1989;30:323–33.
95. Andersen PH, Maibach HI. Skin irritation in man: a comparative bioengineering study using improved reflectance spectroscopy. Contact Dermatitis. 1995;33:315–22.
96. Nangia A, Andersen PH, Berner B, Maibach HI. High dissociation constants (pKa) of basic permeants are associated with in vivo skin irritation in man. Contact Dermatitis. 1996;34:237–42.
97. Zhai H. Effects of occlusion: percutaneous absorption. In: Bronaugh R, editor. Percutaneous absorption, drug- cosmetics-mechanisms-methodology. 4th ed. Boca Raton: Taylor and Francis; 2005. p. 235–45.
98. Zhai H, Maibach HI. Occlusion vs. skin barrier function. Skin Res Technol. 2002;8:1–6.
99. Taljebini M, Warren R, Mao-Oiang M, Lane E, Elias PM, Feingold KR. Cutaneous permeability barrier repair following various types of insults: kinetics and effects of occlusion. Skin Pharmacol. 1996;9:111–9.
100. Emilson A, Lindberg M, Forslind B, Scheynius A. Quantitative and 3-dimensional analysis of Langerhans' cells following occlusion with patch tests using confocal laser scanning microscopy. Acta Derm Venereol. 1993;73:323–9.
101. Zhai H, Maibach HI. Skin occlusion and irritant and allergic contact dermatitis: an overview. Contact Dermatitis. 2001;44:201–6.
102. Kligman A. Hydration injury to human skin. In: Van der Valk P, Maibach H, editors. The irritant contact dermatitis syndrome. Boca Raton: CRC Press; 1996. p. 187–94.
103. Fisher LB, Maibach HI, Trancik RJ. Variably occlusive tape systems and the mitotic activity of stripped human epidermis. Effects with and without hydrocortisone. Arch Dermatol. 1978;114:727–9.

104. Proksch E, Feingold KR, Man MQ, Elias PM. Barrier function regulates epidermal DNA synthesis. J Clin Invest. 1991;87:1668–73.
105. Proksch E, Brasch J, Sterry W. Integrity of the permeability barrier regulates epidermal Langerhans cell density. Br J Dermatol. 1996;134:630–8.
106. Farage MA, Miller KW, Berardesca E, Maibach HI. Cutaneous effects and sensitive skin with incontinence in the aged. In: Farage MA, Miller KW, Maibach HI, editors. Textbook of aging skin. Berlin: Springer-Verlag; 2010.
107. Gray M. Preventing and managing perineal dermatitis: a shared goal for wound and continence care. J Wound Ostomy Continence Nurs. 2004;31:S2–9. Quiz S10-2.
108. Runeman B. Skin interaction with absorbent hygiene products. Clin Dermatol. 2008;26:45–51.
109. Gray M, Beeckman D, Bliss DZ, Fader M, Logan S, Junkin J, et al. Incontinence-associated dermatitis: a comprehensive review and update. J Wound Ostomy Continence Nurs. 2012;39:61–74.
110. Farage MA, Wang B, Tucker H, Ogle J, Rodenberg C, Azuka CE, et al. Dermatological testing of an improved apertured film surface for feminine hygiene pads. Cutan Ocul Toxicol 2011.
111. Beguin AM, Malaquin-Pavan E, Guihaire C, Hallet-Lezy AM, Souchon S, Homann V, et al. Improving diaper design to address incontinence associated dermatitis. BMC Geriatr. 2010;10:86.
112. Sugama J, Sanada H, Shigeta Y, Nakagami G, Konya C. Efficacy of an improved absorbent pad on incontinence-associated dermatitis in older women: cluster randomized controlled trial. BMC Geriatr. 2012;12:22.
113. Odio MR, O'Connor RJ, Sarbaugh F, Baldwin S. Continuous topical administration of a petrolatum formulation by a novel disposable diaper. 2. Effect on skin condition. Dermatology. 2000;200:238–43.
114. Beeckman D, Woodward S, Gray M. Incontinence-associated dermatitis: step-by-step prevention and treatment. Br J Community Nurs. 2011;16:382–9.
115. Loden M. Role of topical emollients and moisturizers in the treatment of dry skin barrier disorders. Am J Clin Dermatol. 2003;4:771–88.
116. Baldwin S, Odio MR, Haines SL, O'Connor RJ, Englehart JS, Lane AT. Skin benefits from continuous topical administration of a zinc oxide/petrolatum formulation by a novel disposable diaper. J Eur Acad Dermatol Venereol. 2001;15 Suppl 1:5–11.
117. Farage MA, Miller KW, Berardesca E, Maibach HI. Psychosocial and societal burden of incontinence in the aged population: a review. Arch Gynecol Obstet. 2008;277:285–90.
118. DuBeau CE, Levy B, Mangione CM, Resnick NM. The impact of urge urinary incontinence on quality of life: importance of patients' perspective and explanatory style. J Am Geriatr Soc. 1998;46: 683–92.
119. Specht JK. 9 myths of incontinence in older adults: both clinicians and the over-65 set need to know more. Am J Nurs. 2005;105:58–68. Quiz 69.
120. Miller J, Hoffman E. The causes and consequences of overactive bladder. J Womens Health (Larchmt). 2006;15:251–60.
121. Avery JC, Stocks NP, Duggan P, Braunack-Mayer AJ, Taylor AW, Goldney RD, et al. Identifying the quality of life effects of urinary incontinence with depression in an Australian population. BMC Urol. 2013;13:11.
122. Melville JL, Delaney K, Newton K, Katon W. Incontinence severity and major depression in incontinent women. Obstet Gynecol. 2005;106: 585–92.
123. Aslan G, Koseoglu H, Sadik O, Gimen S, Cihan A, Esen A. Sexual function in women with urinary incontinence. Int J Impot Res. 2005;17:248–51.
124. Brown JS, Vittinghoff E, Wyman JF, Stone KL, Nevitt MC, Ensrud KE, et al. Urinary incontinence: does it increase risk for falls and fractures? Study of Osteoporotic Fractures Research Group. J Am Geriatr Soc. 2000;48:721–5.

Current and Emerging Treatment Options for Vulvovaginal Atrophy

18

Jill M. Krapf, Zoe Belkin, Frank Dreher, and Andrew T. Goldstein

Contents

18.1	**Introduction**	229
18.2	**Estrogen and Vulvovaginal Atrophy**	229
18.3	**Local Estrogens**	230
18.4	**Systemic Estrogens**	230
18.5	**Selective Estrogen Receptor Modulators**	231
18.6	**Tissue-Selective Estrogen Complexes**	231
18.7	**Local Androgens**	232
18.7.1	Dehydroepiandrosterone	232
18.8	**Oxytocin**	232
18.9	**Phytoestrogens**	233
18.10	**Nonhormonal Treatment Options**	233
18.11	**Summary**	234
References		234

J.M. Krapf
Department of Obstetrics and Gynecology,
George Washington University, Washington, DC, USA
e-mail: jkrapf@mfa.gwu.edu

Z. Belkin
Department of Obstetrics and Gynecology, George Washington University School of Medicine and Health Sciences, Washington, DC, USA
e-mail: zoe.belkin@gmail.com

F. Dreher (✉)
NEOGYN Inc., 101 Hudson Street,
Jersey City, NJ 07302, USA
e-mail: fdreher@yahoo.com

A.T. Goldstein, MD
Department of Obstetrics and Gynecology, Center for Vulvovaginal Diseases, Washington, DC, USA
e-mail: obstetrics@yahoo.com

18.1 Introduction

Vulvovaginal atrophy is estimated to affect 10–40 % of postmenopausal women, but only 25 % of symptomatic women seek medical attention. Although this condition can have a large impact on quality of life and sexual function, it is frequently underdiagnosed and undertreated. The symptoms of vulvovaginal atrophy include vaginal dryness, irritation, itching, dysuria, and dyspareunia. These symptoms are usually progressive and less likely to resolve without effective treatment [1, 2]. Treatment approaches for vulvovaginal atrophy focus on symptom reduction and hormonal restoration of affected tissues, often in conjunction with application of over-the-counter moisturizes and lubricants. Among the estrogen restoration treatments are local estrogen, selective estrogen receptor modulators (SERMs), tissue-selective estrogen complexes (TSECs), local androgens, dehydroepiandrosterone (DHEA), oxytocin, phytoestrogens, as well as nonhormonal options [1, 3, 4]. The aim of this chapter is to review current treatments for vulvovaginal atrophy and explore emerging strategies for care.

18.2 Estrogen and Vulvovaginal Atrophy

The symptoms of vulvovaginal atrophy are caused by loss of estrogen production with menopause [1]. After menopause, serum estrogen levels fall from about 120 to about 20 pg ml^{-1}. Decreased estrogen levels lead to transformation of the vulvovaginal epithelium from a thick appearance to one that is pale, thin, prone to inflammation, and increased friability [4, 5]. A large number of estrogen receptors are found in the vulvovaginal area, which indicates the important role of estrogen to maintain the structure and function of this area [6]. The decreased levels of estrogen that accompany menopause cause atrophy of the vulva and vagina. Concurrently, the vagina shortens, narrows, and becomes less elastic. Blood flow to the vagina decreases which causes it to become pale and thin, which results in decreased vaginal secretions and increased susceptibility to vaginal pain and trauma [4, 7]. The degree of vaginal dryness increases in severity as time after menopause progresses [7].

18.3 Local Estrogens

For women with vulvovaginal atrophy who lack other postmenopausal symptoms, local estrogen therapy is the treatment of choice [3]. Exogenous estrogen promotes the revascularization and thickening of the vaginal epithelium, resulting in increased lubrication and elasticity [5, 8, 9]. Moreover, local estrogen preparations have been shown to decrease symptoms of atrophy, including vaginal dryness, irritation, pruritus, and dyspareunia [1, 10, 11]. These treatments may also improve sexual desire, arousal, and orgasmic function through increased blood flow and lubrication [7]. Since the vulva is also affected, treatment of vulvovaginal atrophy should ideally involve both the vagina and the vulva [12]. Nevertheless, most treatments thus far have focused on the vagina.

Two estrogens, estradiol and conjugated estrogens, are currently approved in the United States for treatment of vaginal atrophy, vaginal dryness, and dyspareunia. The various formulations for vaginal use include creams, tablets, and hormone-releasing rings. Although all of these formulations are equally effective, some women prefer the 3-month vaginal ring due to increased comfort, satisfaction, and ease of use [13]. In addition, estriol, a lower potency estrogen, has recently been investigated for the treatment of vulvovaginal atrophy. A double-blind and placebo-controlled study in 167 women evaluated the efficacy and safety of 0.005 % estriol vaginal gel when used daily for 3 weeks and then twice weekly for up to 12 weeks. The estriol treatment group showed positive changes in vaginal maturation index (VMI), vaginal pH, vaginal dryness, and a global symptom score, whereas treatment-related adverse events were similar among groups [14]. For long-term local estrogen therapy, it is recommended that the smallest effective dose is utilized, with the goal of eventually tapering local estrogen to maintenance dosing once urogenital function has improved. Although it may be acceptable to continue treatment indefinitely, safety data for local estrogen beyond 1 year is currently not available [1, 15].

Endometrial hyperplasia is the main concern with the use of unopposed estrogen by woman with an intact uterus. Local low-dose estrogen formulations, however, have not been shown to increase the incidence of proliferative endometrium when compared with placebo [15]. Furthermore, in the opinion of the North American Menopause Society, endometrial surveillance and progestin therapy are not indicated in asymptomatic, low-risk women receiving low-dose vaginal estrogen [1]. Nevertheless, although local estrogen therapies may not significantly stimulate the endometrium, all cases of postmenopausal bleeding should be evaluated by ultrasound of endometrial thickness and endometrial sampling [16].

18.4 Systemic Estrogens

Systemic estrogen therapy is indicated for vulvovaginal atrophy if menopausal vasomotor symptoms are also experienced. In this case, a progestin is used to reduce the risk of endometrial cancer associated with unopposed systemic estrogen for patients with an intact uterus [15]. Despite reduced vasomotor-related discomfort, 40 % of women who use systemic hormone therapy still experience persistent vulvovaginal dryness [17]. Consequently, local estrogen may frequently be needed in conjunction with systemic treatment [3, 4].

18.5 Selective Estrogen Receptor Modulators

Certain selective estrogen receptor modulators (SERMs), which act as estrogen agonists/antagonists, are promising future treatments for vulvovaginal atrophy. Raloxifene and tamoxifen, commonly used in the setting of breast cancer and osteoporosis, are of the most well-known SERMs; however, they are not optimal for the treatment of vulvovaginal atrophy [18]. Instead, SERMs ospemifene (Osphena) and lasofoxifene (Oporia) are preferred due to their positive effects on vaginal epithelium and the progression of atrophy and symptoms, as demonstrated in placebo-controlled clinical trials [19, 20].

Ospemifene, which was initially developed as a treatment for postmenopausal osteoporosis, was found to have favorable estrogenic effects on the vaginal epithelium in phase I and II clinical trials. This SERM was approved by the US Food and Drug Administration (FDA) in early 2013 for the treatment of moderate to severe dyspareunia after completing a 12-week phase III trial in 826 postmenopausal women between the ages of 40 and 80 with vulvovaginal atrophy randomized to receive ospemifene 30 mg/day, 60 mg/day, or placebo orally [19]. Participants receiving 30 and 60 mg of ospemifene showed statistically significant improvement in VMI, vaginal pH, and vaginal dryness, while benefits for dyspareunia were only seen in the 60 mg/day group. The most frequently reported adverse event was hot flushes; no proliferative effects on endometrial tissue were observed [21]. In addition, ospemifene's antiestrogenic activity in several preclinical models of breast cancer makes this SERM a potential candidate for the treatment of women with breast cancer suffering from vulvovaginal atrophy [19]. Another SERM, lasofoxifene, shows promising results for treatment of vulvovaginal atrophy. A series of large multicenter studies with lasofoxifene (PEARL) evaluated the efficacy and safety of this medication for osteoporosis and vulvovaginal atrophy symptoms in postmenopausal women [22, 23]. Lasofoxifene significantly reduced the symptoms of moderate to severe vulvovaginal atrophy while improving VMI and vaginal pH over a 12-week treatment period [24]. Additional studies have supported these findings and have also revealed decrease in dyspareunia in postmenopausal women treated with lasofoxifene [25]. Whereas in those studies that did not reveal an elevated risk of endometrial cancer, five women developed endometrial hyperplasia, and an increased risk of both venous thromboembolism and pulmonary embolism was observed [23]. Lasofoxifene is currently not approved for use in the United States.

18.6 Tissue-Selective Estrogen Complexes

Tissue-selective estrogen complexes (TSECs) pair a SERM with estrogen(s) aiming to relieve hot flushes, treat vulvovaginal atrophy, and prevent bone loss, while protecting the endometrium and breasts [25, 26].

The SERM bazedoxifene paired with conjugated estrogens was evaluated in a multicenter, randomized double-blind, placebo- and active-controlled phase III study in 3,397 postmenopausal women with intact uteruses aged 40–75 years [27]. This study revealed that bazedoxifene combined with conjugated estrogens significantly reduced the frequency and severity of hot flushes at 3 months and improved vaginal atrophy with reduced incidence of dyspareunia at 24 months as compared to placebo, while the incidences of adverse events were similar. Another study in postmenopausal women demonstrated that the combination of bazedoxifene with conjugated estrogens was associated with less than 1 % rate of endometrial hyperplasia over 2 years with no difference in endometrial thickness between the bazedoxifene/conjugated estrogens and placebo groups [28].

The primary objective of a further trial was to compare the safety and efficacy of multiple doses of bazedoxifene/conjugated estrogens for the treatment of moderate to severe vulvovaginal atrophy associated with menopause [29]. In this trial with 625 postmenopausal women aged 40–65, vaginal pH and vulvovaginal atrophy symptoms significantly improved as compared with placebo in the group treated with the higher dose of bazedoxifene/conjugated estrogens for

12 weeks. Although the treatment groups did not report increased adverse events, there was a significantly higher incidence of vaginitis in the groups receiving bazedoxifene/conjugated estrogens as compared with placebo.

18.7 Local Androgens

Although the vagina has previously not been considered an androgen-dependent organ, studies suggest that androgens may have a direct effect on vaginal structure and function, independent from estradiol. Androgen receptors and aromatase have been identified in the vaginal epithelium, suggesting both direct and indirect effects of testosterone on vaginal tissue [30, 31]. In addition, less androgen receptor mRNA and proteins are expressed in the vaginal epithelium with increasing age and postmenopausal status. Furthermore, testosterone administration was shown to increase androgen receptor protein expression in both the vaginal mucosa and stroma [32].

An exploratory study examined the impact of vaginal testosterone alone on vaginal atrophy in 21 postmenopausal women with breast cancer on long-term aromatase inhibitor therapy [33]. After treatment with a vaginal testosterone cream daily for 28 days, the vaginal atrophy symptoms, including dryness and dyspareunia, improved significantly, and this improvement persisted after cessation of treatment. Since estradiol levels remained suppressed after the treatment, the authors concluded that a 4-week regimen with vaginal testosterone improved vaginal atrophy without the potential risks associated with elevated systemic estradiol levels.

18.7.1 Dehydroepiandrosterone

Dehydroepiandrosterone (DHEA) is an androgen that can be converted into many biologically active sex steroids, including estradiol and testosterone. Like estrogen and testosterone, levels of DHEA decline with age. Although a recent trial did not show a benefit of oral DHEA therapy for women, advantages of intravaginal DHEA on sexual function are emerging [25].

In postmenopausal women, intravaginal DHEA improved VMI scores and decreased vaginal pH after a few days, without significantly elevating circulating levels of estrogen [34]. Intravaginal DHEA was found to act on all three layers of the vagina, inducing mucification of the epithelium, increasing density of collagen fibers in the vaginal wall, and stimulating the muscle layer. Therefore, it may be speculated that intravaginal DHEA may be superior to intravaginal estradiol, which acts mainly on the superficial epithelial layer.

In a prospective phase III clinical trial with 126 postmenopausal women with moderate to severe vaginal atrophy in order to evaluate effects on sexual dysfunction, intravaginal DHEA applied daily for 12 weeks improved sexual desire/interest, arousal, orgasm, and pain with sexual activity [35]. In a follow-up study, 114 postmenopausal women with dyspareunia as the most bothersome symptom of vaginal atrophy were identified [36]. After 12 weeks of treatment with varied doses of intravaginal DHEA, VMI and pain severity score during sexual activity improved, whereas DHEA levels remained within normal postmenopausal ranges. This study suggests beneficial local effects of intravaginal DHEA without significant systemic absorption.

18.8 Oxytocin

Due to safety concerns related to estrogen therapy, alternative treatments including oxytocin are being explored to address vulvovaginal atrophy. Oxytocin, a peptide hormone well known for its role in female reproduction, has been shown to increase wound healing, mucosal blood flood, and secretion of several growth factors.

In a pilot study with 20 postmenopausal women with vaginal atrophy symptoms, the group receiving intravaginal oxytocin showed a significant improvement upon colposcopic examination [36]. Although 70 % of the treatment group demonstrated decreased vaginal atrophy and reported relief of symptoms, this result was not as significantly different from the placebo group. Larger studies are currently in progress to further evaluate oxytocin for the treatment for vaginal atrophy.

18.9 Phytoestrogens

Phytoestrogens, plant-derived xenoestrogens or dietary estrogens, are being explored as a possible alternative to hormonal therapy. Isoflavones, in particularly genistein and daidzein found in soybeans, are the most studied of the phytoestrogens. Whereas oral phytoestrogens do not have an effect on vaginal epithelium, intravaginal application seems to provide some benefit [37]. Significant improvement in genital symptoms, colposcopy scores, and VMI after 90 days of daily intravaginal administration of genistein was demonstrated in a randomized-control study with 62 postmenopausal women [38]. However, this improvement was also seen in the control group with a hyaluronic acid formulation.

A recent double-blind, randomized placebo-controlled study compared the efficacy of isoflavone vaginal gel to conjugated equine estrogen and placebo in treating vulvovaginal atrophy [39]. In this study, 90 postmenopausal women were treated for 12 weeks with either isoflavone vaginal gel 4 % (1 g/day), conjugated equine estrogen cream (0.3 mg/day), or placebo gel. Women treated with isoflavone gel showed a similar improvement compared to the estrogen group for vaginal dryness and dyspareunia; both differed significantly from the placebo group. Additionally, there was also a significant increase in VMI with isoflavone gel treatment. No changes in endometrial thickness or estradiol levels were observed in any of the study groups. Accordingly, the isoflavone vaginal gel might be an effective alternative in the treatment of vaginal atrophy and maybe be particularly beneficial to women who have contraindications or decline hormone therapy.

18.10 Nonhormonal Treatment Options

Women with vaginal dryness and sexual pain frequently seek relief with nonhormonal, over-the-counter vaginal lubricants and moisturizers [40, 41]. More specifically, vaginal lubricants are designed to reduce friction associated with sexual activity, whereas vaginal moisturizers are utilized to hydrate and replace normal vaginal secretions.

A few small prospective studies analyzed the efficacy of a commonly used polycarbophil-based vaginal moisturizer. This product was shown to improve vaginal moisture and elasticity, reducing the symptoms of itching, irritation, and dyspareunia [42, 43]. In addition, cytological studies indicated a positive effect on maturation of the vaginal epithelium [44].

In a multicenter, parallel-group clinical trial, 144 postmenopausal women with vaginal dryness were randomized to receive either a hyaluronic acid vaginal gel or estriol cream [45]. After a total of ten applications over 30 days, both the hyaluronic acid vaginal gel and estriol cream groups showed significant improvement in vaginal dryness, itching, burning, and dyspareunia. However, in contrast to the estrogen control group, there was no improvement in vaginal pH for women using hyaluronic acid.

Widely available vaginal pH-balanced gels, which contain lactic acid to promote lower vaginal pH, have also been studied as a nonhormonal alternative for the treatment of vaginal atrophy. A placebo-controlled study in 86 chemotherapy or endocrine-therapy-induced menopausal breast cancer survivors revealed a significant improvement in vaginal dryness, dyspareunia, pH, and VMI in the group receiving a pH-balanced vaginal gel as compared to the placebo group after 12 weeks. The most common side effects of the pH-balanced gels were vaginal irritation and burning sensation.

Protein and peptide growth factor products may be a promising, nonhormonal treatment alternative for vulvovaginal atrophy. A double-blind and randomized controlled clinical study revealed that vulvar cream developed specifically for the local treatment of women with vestibulodynia was more effective in reducing dyspareunia and erythema than the vehicle control [46]. Recent evidence suggests that vestibulodynia in women taking oral contraceptive pills can be associated with a thinned and fragile vulvar epithelia resulting from diminished estrogen and testosterone, which is clinically comparable to the vulvar epithelia in postmenopausal women [47]. Given these findings, protein and peptide growth factor products may also be helpful for postmenopausal women with vulvovaginal atrophy. This is currently being investigated in an exploratory study.

Consequently, many of the currently available nonhormonal treatment options may be viable alternatives to help with relief of the symptoms associated with vulvovaginal atrophy, in particular, for women contraindicated to estrogen use.

18.11 Summary

As women are living longer and healthier lives, the importance of vulvovaginal health and maintenance of intimacy is being highlighted in the popular media, is discussed on the Internet, and is finally making its way into the doctor's office. Therefore, as patients present to clinicians, it is essential for practitioners to be able to identify vulvovaginal atrophy, differentiate this condition from vulvar dermatoses, and subsequently provide acceptable treatment options based upon risk profile.

Treatment of vulvovaginal atrophy was once limited to either vaginal lubricants and moisturizers or estrogen-containing regimens, which many clinicians felt uncomfortable recommending due to safety concerns addressed in the Women's Health Initiative trials. Today, however, practitioners are becoming better equipped to offer a wider range of treatment options due to increased reassurance of safety for existing therapies and advances in novel treatment options.

References

1. North American Menopause Society. The role of local vaginal estrogen for the treatment of vaginal atrophy in postmenopausal women: 2007 position statement of The North American Menopause Society. Menopause. 2007;14:355–69.
2. Calleja-Agius J, Brincat MP. Urogenital atrophy. Climacteric. 2009;12(4):279–85.
3. North American Menopause Society. Estrogen and progestogen use in postmenopausal women: 2010 position statement of the North American Menopause Society. Menopause. 2010;17(2):242–55.
4. North American Menopause Society. The 2012 hormone therapy position statement of: The North American Menopause Society. Menopause. 2012;19(3):257–71.
5. Nachtigall L, Nachigall M, Goren J, Loweenstein J. Update on vaginal atrophy. Menopause Manag. 2005;14:17–9.
6. Castelo-Branco C, Cancelo MJ, Villero J, Nohales F, Julia MD. Management of post-menopausal vaginal atrophy and atrophic vaginitis. Maturitas. 2005;52: S46–52.
7. Goldstein I, Alexander JL. Practical aspects in the management of vaginal atrophy and sexual dysfunction in perimenopausal and postmenopausal women. J Sex Med. 2005;2 Suppl 3:154–65.
8. Bachmann G, Nevadunsky N. Diagnosis and treatment of atrophic vaginitis. Am Fam Physician. 2000; 61:3090–6.
9. Long CY, Liu CM, Hsu SC, Wu CH, Wang CL, Tsai EM. A randomized comparative study of the effects of oral and topical estrogen therapy on the vaginal vascularization and sexual function in hysterectomized postmenopausal women. Menopause. 2006;13:727–43.
10. Simon J, Nachtigall L, Gut R, Lang E, Archer DF, Utian W. Effective treatment of vaginal atrophy with an ultra-low-dose estradiol vaginal tablet. Obstet Gynecol. 2009;112:1053–60.
11. Al-Baghdadi O, Ewies AA. Topical estrogen therapy in the management of postmenopausal vaginal atrophy: an up-to-date overview. Climacteric. 2009;12:91–105.
12. Goldstein I. Hormonal factors in women's sexual pain disorders. In: Goldstein A, Pukall C, Goldstein I, editors. Female sexual pain disorders: evaluation and management. Blackwell-Wiley; Chichester, 2009. p. 180–95.
13. Barentsen R, van de Weijer PHM, Schram JHN. Continuous low dose estradiol released from a vaginal ring versus estriol vaginal cream for urogenital atrophy. Eur J Obstet Gynecol Reprod Biol. 1997;71:73–80.
14. Cano A, Estevez J, Usandizaga R, Gallo JL, Guinot M, Delgado JL, et al. The therapeutic effect of a new ultra low concentration estriol gel formulation (0.005% estriol vaginal gel) on symptoms and signs of postmenopausal vaginal atrophy: results from a pivotal phase III study. Menopause. 2012;19(10):1130–9.
15. Suckling J, Lethaby A, Kennedy R. Local estrogen for vaginal atrophy in postmenopausal women. Cochrane Database Syst Rev. 2006;4:CD001500.
16. Ibe C, Simon JA. Vulvovaginal atrophy: current and future therapies. J Sex Med. 2010;7:1042–50.
17. Johnston SL, Farrell SA, Bouchard C, Farrell SA, Beckerson LA, Comeau M, et al. The detection and management of vaginal atrophy. J Obstet Gynaecol Can. 2004;26:503–15.
18. Shelly W, Draper MW, Krishnan V, Wong M, Jaffe RB. Selective estrogen receptor modulators: an update on recent clinical findings. Obstet Gynecol Surv. 2008;63:163–81.
19. Wurz GT, Soe LH, DeGregorio MW. Ospemifene, vulvovaginal atrophy, and breast cancer. Maturitas. 2013;74:220–5.

20. Pickar JH. Emerging therapies for postmenopausal vaginal atrophy. Maturitas. 2013;75:3–6.
21. Bachmann GA, Komi JO. Ospemifene effectively treats vulvovaginal atrophy in postmenopausal women: results from a pivotal phase 3 study. Menopause. 2010;17:480–6.
22. Goldstein SR, Cummings SR, Eastell R, Ensrud K, Tan O, Bradshaw K, et al. Vaginal effects of lasofoxifene: 3-year results from the PEARL trial. Menopause. 2008;15:1228.
23. Goldstein SR, Neven P, Cummings S, Colgan T, Runowicz CD, Krpan D, et al. Postmenopausal evaluation and risk reduction with Lasofoxifene (PEARL) trial: 5-year gynecological outcomes. Menopause. 2011;18(1):17–22.
24. Tan O, Bradshaw K, Carr BR. Management of vulvovaginal atrophy-related sexual dysfunction in postmenopausal women: an up-to-date review. Menopause. 2012;19(1):109–17.
25. Archer DR. Tissue-selective estrogen complexes: a promising option for the comprehensive management of postmenopausal symptoms. Drugs Aging. 2010;27: 533–44.
26. Lobo RA, Pinkerton JV, Gass ML, Dorin MH, Ronkin S, Pickar JH, et al. Evaluation of bazedoxifene/conjugated estrogens for the treatment of menopausal symptoms and effects on metabolic parameters and overall safety profile. Fertil Steril. 2009;92:1025–38.
27. Pickar JH, Yeh IT, Bachmann G, Speroff L. Endometrial effects of a tissue-selective estrogen complex containing bazedoxifene/conjugated estrogens as a menopausal therapy. Fertil Steril. 2009;92:1018–24.
28. Kagan R, Williams RS, Pan K, Mirkin S, Pickar JH. A randomized, placebo- and active-controlled trial of bazedoxifene/conjugated estrogens for treatment of moderate to severe vulvar/vaginal atrophy in postmenopausal women. Menopause. 2010;17(2):281–9.
29. Berman JR, Almeida FG, Jolin J, Raz S, Chaudhuri G, Gonzalez-Cadavid NF. Correlation of androgen receptors, aromatase and 5-alpha reductase in the human vagina with menopausal status. Fertil Steril. 2003;79:925–31.
30. Traish AM, Kim N, Min K, Muarriz R, Goldstein I. Role of androgens in female genital sexual arousal: receptor expression, structure and function. Fertil Steril. 2002;77(4):S11–8.
31. Baldassarre M, Perrone AM, Giannone FA, Armillotta F, Battaglia C, Costantino A, et al. Androgen receptor expression in the human vagina under different physiological and treatment conditions. Int J Impot Res. 2013;25:7–11.
32. Witherby S, Johnson J, Demers L, Mount S, Littenberg B, Maclean CD, et al. Topical testosterone for breast cancer patients with vaginal atrophy related to aromatase inhibitors: a phase I/II study. Oncologist. 2011;16:424–31.
33. Labrie F, Cusan L, Gomez JL, Côté I, Bérubé R, Bélanger P, et al. Effect of intravaginal DHEA on serum DHEA and eleven of its metabolites in postmenopausal women. J Steroid Biochem Mol Biol. 2008;111:178–94.
34. Labrie F, Archer D, Bouchard C, Fortier M, Cusan L, Gomez JL, et al. Effect of intravaginal dehydroepiandrosterone (prasterone) on libido and sexual function in postmenopausal women. Menopause. 2009;16(5):923–31.
35. Labrie F, Archer D, Bouchard C, Fortier M, Cusan L, Gomez JL, et al. Intravaginal dehydroepiandrosterone (prasterone), a highly efficient treatment of dyspareunia. Climacteric. 2011;14:282–8.
36. Jonasson AF, Edwall L, Uvnas-Moberg K. Topical oxytocin reverses vaginal atrophy in postmenopausal women: a double-blind randomized pilot study. Menopause Int. 2011;17:120–5.
37. Bedell S, Nachtigall M, Naftolin F. The pros and cons of plant estrogens for menopause. J Steroid Biochem Mol Biol. 2013 (in press). Available at: http://www.sciencedirect.com/science/journal/aip/09600760. Accessed 11 Nov 2013.
38. Le Donne M, Caruso C, Manscuso A, Costa G, Iemmo R, Pizzimenti G, et al. The effect of vaginally administered genistein in comparison with hyaluronic acid on atrophic epithelium in postmenopause. Arch Gynecol Obstet. 2011;283:1319–23.
39. Lima SM, Yamada SS, Reis BF, Sostenes P, Postigo S, Galvão da Silva MA, Aoki T. Effective treatment of vaginal atrophy with isoflavone vaginal gel. Maturitas. 2013;74(3):252–8.
40. Stika CS. Atrophic vaginitis. Dermatol Ther. 2010;23: 514–22.
41. Sinha A, Ewies AA. Non-hormonal topical treatment of vulvovaginal atrophy: an up-to-date overview. Climacteric. 2013;16(3):305–12.
42. Nachtigall LE. Comparative study: Replens versus local estrogen in menopausal women. Fertil Steril. 1994;61:178–80.
43. Bygdeman M, Swahn ML. Replens versus dienoestrol cream in the symptomatic treatment of vaginal atrophy in postmenopausal women. Maturitas. 1996; 23(3):259–63.
44. Van der Laak JA, de Bie LM, de Leeuw H, de Wilde PC, Hanselaar AG. The effects of Replens on vaginal cytology in the treatment of postmenopausal atrophy: cytomorphology versus computerized cytometry. J Clin Pathol. 2002;55(6):446–51.
45. Chen J, Geng L, Song X, Li H, Giordan N, Liao Q. Evaluation of the efficacy and safety of hyaluronic acid vaginal gel to ease vaginal dryness: a multicenter, randomized, controlled, open-label, parallel-group, clinical trial. J Sex Med. 2013;10(6): 1575–84.
46. Donders GG, Bellen G. Cream with cutaneous fibroblast lysate for the treatment of provoked vestibulodynia: a double-blind randomized placebo-controlled crossover study. J Low Genit Tract Dis. 2012;16(4):427–36.
47. Burrows LJ, Basha M, Goldstein AT. The effects of hormonal contraceptives on female sexuality: a review. J Sex Med. 2012;9(9):2213–23.

Implications of the Vulvar Sensitive Skin Syndrome After Menopause

Paul R. Summers

Contents

19.1 Introduction: What Makes Skin Sensitive? 237
19.2 How Common Is Sensitive Skin? 238
19.3 Vulvar Characteristics That Predispose to Sensitivity 238
19.4 Recognizing the Vulvar Sensitive Skin Syndrome 239
19.5 Vulvar Spongiotic Dermatitis and Yeast Infection 240
19.6 Vulvar Sensitivity Changes After Menopause 242
19.7 Some Vulvar Sensitive Skin Treatment Concepts 243
19.8 Summary 245
References 245

P.R. Summers, MD
Department of Obstetrics and Gynecology,
University of Utah School of Medicine,
30 North 1900 East room 2B200,
Salt Lake City, UT 84132, USA
e-mail: paul.summers@hsc.utah.edu

19.1 Introduction: What Makes Skin Sensitive?

Sensitive skin syndrome can be defined as symptomatic epidermal reactivity to common environmental insults that normally would not cause a recognized reaction [1]. This disorder reflects provoked or unprovoked sensations of itching, burning, or pain, typically with little or no visible skin changes. Interestingly, the definition for the dermatologic concept of sensitive skin also matches the gynecologic concepts of vulvodynia and vestibulitis. For the dermatologist, a common site of concern is the face with exposure to cosmetics, but other body sites have been investigated [2]. The gynecologic research has focused exclusively on vulvar sensitivity and pain. Age, ethnicity, hormone status, atopic tendency, and a wide range of environmental factors influence skin sensitivity at all body sites [3].

The individual with sensitive skin may complain after environmental exposures that are generally tolerated without annoyance by most other individuals. An understanding of dermatopathology and skin physiology has placed the dermatologists at an advantage in efforts to determine the causes for sensitive skin. Although continued investigation is warranted, sensitive skin syndrome has been reasonably well defined by dermatologists as a valid disorder, often with meaningful therapeutic implications. Dermatopathology can be a helpful guide in many cases. The gynecologic concepts of vulvodynia and vestibulitis are reasonably well defined, but the pathophysiology remains poorly understood, and treatment attempts are often unsatisfactory. Dermatopathology has traditionally not been utilized by gynecologists in the evaluation of vulvar pain and sensitivity [4].

The concept of sensitive skin is generally related to the additive effect of several skin defects rather than to a specific dermatologic problem, as follows. (1) The skin barrier may be compromised. Persistent rubbing or abrasion can cause mechanical disruption of the barrier. Chemical irritants may cause epidermal injury, with each chemical irritant having its own characteristic form of insult. A rise in epidermal pH is associated with a compromise in barrier function [5, 6]. (2) Dermatitis, whether visible or not, increases skin sensitivity [7]. The most common pathologic manifestation of skin reactivity is spongiotic dermatitis. (3) The skin barrier may be normal, without evident dermatologic disease, but nerve sensitivity may be increased. Presumably, this may be a congenital matter, or it may be due to some recognized or postulated nerve trauma (allodynia). In some cases, pathology may disclose increased or elongated nerve endings. Therapy for sensitive skin syndrome requires recognition of the specific elements that apply in the individual case.

19.2 How Common Is Sensitive Skin?

A perception of sensitive skin may be the most prevalent dermatologic complaint. In a recent survey, 68.4 % reported sensitive skin generally [8, 9]. In this review, approximately three-quarters of participants described sensitive facial skin, and around one-half of participants noted sensitive genital skin. Common complaints included intolerance of cosmetics, medicated creams, abrasive clothing and undergarments, and menstrual or incontinence pads. Women with clinically diagnosed atopic dermatitis are significantly more likely to report skin sensitivity generally and in the genital area [10]. A familial tendency for sensitive skin is also evident [8].

19.3 Vulvar Characteristics That Predispose to Sensitivity

Normal conditions in the vulvar area contribute to a high risk for dermatitis related to an irritant or allergic reaction [11]. The high level of epithelial hydration, as reflected by increased vulvar transepidermal water loss, increases susceptibility to hydrophilic irritants [12]. Lipid content and degree of keratinization, as well as any tendency for maceration, influence epidermal hydration. Vulvar epithelium tends toward maceration. Vulvar epithelium demonstrates a 35 % higher friction coefficient in comparison with the forearm, which is considered the baseline site for many skin physiology studies [13]. The high friction coefficient reflects an increased risk for mechanical damage from rubbing, abrasive clothing, toilet paper, and from activities like running and bicycle riding. In contrast, the fingerprint on the palms of the hand and similar patterns on the soles of the feet demonstrate good flexibility with a low friction coefficient, appropriate to the expected rubbing and abrasion at those sites [14]. Vulvar skin is not well configured to tolerate rubbing from modern exposures to tight fitting synthetic garments, harsh toilet paper, and poorly manufactured feminine hygiene pads. The acid mantle of the skin, around a pH of 4–5.5, is important for proper skin barrier function. The normal vaginal pH of 4.5 reflects an ideal pH for optimal epithelial barrier function. Common vaginal infections, such as bacterial vaginosis or trichomonas, may result in a local rise in pH. Changes in vaginal barrier function associated with a rise in pH may have a secondary effect on the adjacent vulvar epithelium [15]. For incontinent women, continuous exposure to urine similarly may adversely affect the vulvovaginal epithelial surface pH.

Thus, the vulvar epithelium is naturally at high risk for development of dermatitis. A genetic tendency for fragile skin and a harsh vulvovaginal environment are determining factors. A dermatologic diagnosis is based largely upon pattern recognition. Unfortunately, early vulvar disease may be highly symptomatic, but may not demonstrate a characteristic rash. A medical history

Table 19.1 Special risk factors for vulvar sensitive skin syndrome

1. Normally high vulvar transepidermal water loss
2. Normally high vulvar friction coefficient
3. Naturally high vulvar skin hydration
4. Persistent exposure to environmental irritants, rubbing, etc
5. Tendency for spongiotic dermatitis
6. Further barrier compromise with secondary yeast infection

may help. Vulvar pruritus with a history of asthma, hay fever, eczema, or sinusitis may suggest a diagnosis of vulvar allergic dermatitis, often secondarily resulting in recurrent yeast or bacterial infection. Typically with little or no associated visual change, spongiotic dermatitis is the most commonly detected vulvar dermatopathology in women with sensitive skin [4]. When vulvar dermatopathology develops, the compromised skin barrier results in vulvar sensations of dry skin and increased sensitivity to adverse environmental factors. With a significant local source of genitorectal pathogens, vulvar dermatopathology is often secondarily infected, resulting in further enhanced barrier loss and sensitivity. See Table 19.1.

19.4 Recognizing the Vulvar Sensitive Skin Syndrome

The vulva is potentially sensitive to a wider range of irritants and allergens than other skin sites [16]. Sensitive skin syndrome on a woman's face may only reflect a transient reaction to cosmetics. In contrast, vulvar sensitivity is generally an ongoing, uninterrupted reaction to urine, abrasion from clothing or contact with tight fitting clothing, hard water, harsh toilet paper, pads or panty liners, and various medicated creams and lubricants. Unfortunately, these adverse vulvar insults are generally persistent and unavoidable, in contrast to the occasional use of cosmetics on the face. Adverse cosmetics on the face can be discontinued. Thus, the dermatologic concept of sensitive skin syndrome may actually have more significant application to the vulva than to other body sites. Considering the unfortunate disability associated with the resulting vulvar pain, the reasonably well-defined concepts that describe the dermatologic sensitive skin syndrome have great importance when applied to vulvar care. It is clinically significant and scientifically instructive to view vulvar itching, burning, and pain within the domain of the sensitive skin syndrome. As acknowledgment of the unique sensitivity of the vulva, it would be appropriate at least to recognize a dermatologic subcategory of *vulvar* sensitive skin syndrome. A specific vulvar sensitive skin syndrome is not currently identified by dermatologists or by gynecologists as a unique diagnosis. Dermatologists graciously accept the gynecologist's vulvodynia work as a separate entity, and gynecologists generally may not be aware of the sensitive skin syndrome in the dermatologist's realm. With this overlap in concepts, it is appropriate to view the dermatologist's sensitive skin syndrome as the equal counterpart to the gynecologist's vestibulitis and vulvodynia. Gynecologists have made some progress in refining the definitions of the vulvodynia and vestibulitis concepts, but a physical explanation and an adequate treatment remain evasive in the gynecology world. Fortunately, with the application of dermatopathology and a solid understanding of skin physiology, dermatologists are achieving significant progress in the area of sensitive skin research. If the concepts of vulvodynia and vestibulitis had never been established, it is likely that a dermatologic concept of vulvar sensitive skin syndrome would adequately address these gynecologic needs.

Organized research in vulvar sensitive and painful skin started in 1976 [17] for gynecologists, and sensitive skin research independently began prior to that same era for dermatologists. Definitions can be a challenge in both categories. Causation that may be difficult to confirm occasionally must be presumed, such as allodynia (neuropathic pain). Typical of the clinical challenge of sensitive skin diagnosis, allodynia is a diagnosis of exclusion. In rare cases, a direct clinical cause for neuropathic pain, such as trauma, is evident. A biopsy of sensitive skin is useful. Vulvar skin sensitivity that would be attributed otherwise to the generic concepts of vulvodynia or vestibulitis often shows dermatologic disease if evaluated by a dermatopathologist, rather than a surgical pathologist [4]. Advances in vulvodynia and vestibulitis have been handicapped by omission of dermatopathology. Vulvar biopsy may not be the first step for diagnosis, but it becomes helpful if therapy for the presumed clinical diagnosis fails. For cancer surveillance, it is important to biopsy any persistent vulvar ulcer, erosion, or white patch.

19.5 Vulvar Spongiotic Dermatitis and Yeast Infection

Toilet paper, rubbing of clothing, various medicated creams and spermicides, etc., can be constant, essentially unavoidable irritants to the vulvar epithelium. Considering the persistent exposure to potential irritants and the fragile nature of the vulvar epithelium, a high prevalence of spongiotic dermatitis would be expected. Actually, spongiotic dermatitis is a common finding throughout the lower female genital tract. A "reactive change" reported on a pap smear reflects spongiotic change on the cervix if a biopsy is obtained [18, 19]. This finding refers to flakes of epithelium in the Pap smear sample, associated with the spongiotic change. Small flakes of epithelium are a common asymptomatic finding in the vaginal saline wet preparation (Fig. 19.1), often numerous and thick in women with sensitive skin [20] (Fig. 19.2). It would be expected that all women will experience some degree of spongiotic vulvar dermatitis at one time or another. For some women with moderately fragile vulvar epithelium, this would be a common problem. For others it can be a persistent and severe problem, depending upon relative innate factors that influence fragile skin as well as the relative harshness of the environmental conditions. Flakes of desquamated epithelium in the vaginal saline wet preparation can be viewed as a marker for spongiotic change in the female genital area. Flaking skin compromises the vulvovaginal skin barrier, facilitates microbe adhesion, and further increases sensitivity to environmental irritants.

More than 40 antimicrobial substances have been identified that are actively produced by the skin. These antimicrobial peptides are present and active in the stratum corneum [21]. For the vulva, these peptides likely have a significant role in the prevention of infection from fecal contamination. Human beta defensin-2 and human beta defensin-3 are antimicrobial peptides in this

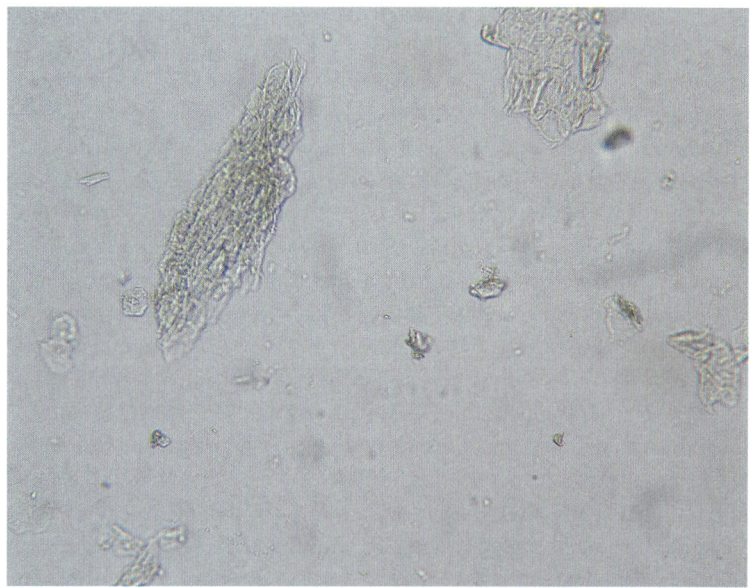

Fig. 19.1 High-power view of small skin flakes in an asymptomatic vaginal saline wet preparation

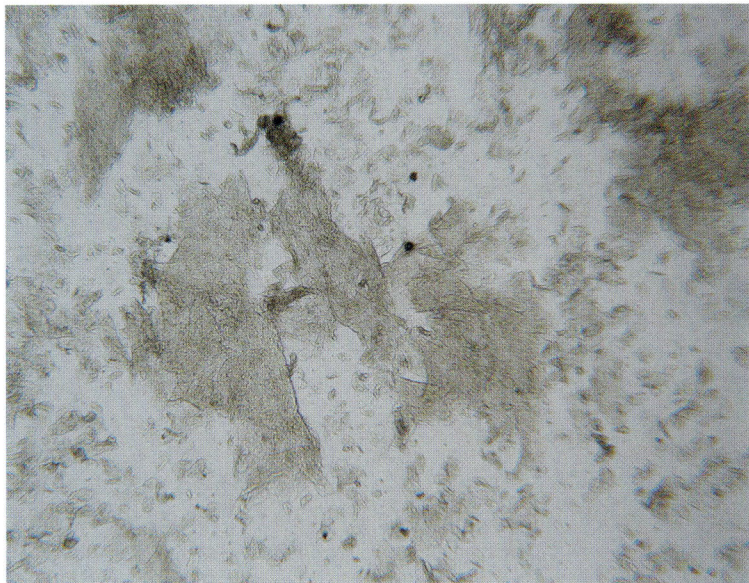

Fig. 19.2 Low-power view of numerous thick skin flakes in a vaginal saline wet preparation characteristic of symptomatic spongiotic dermatitis

category that demonstrate significant anti-yeast inhibitory action [22]. The production of these antimicrobial peptides is linked with the normal cell-mediated immune response. Thus, a compromise of cell-mediated immunity can contribute to increased skin colonization with yeast, related to a deficiency of these important skin peptides. As would be expected, there is downregulation of human beta defensin-2 and human beta defensin-3 in spongiotic dermatitis [23]. This decline is a likely cofactor for the development of a genital yeast infection for women with vulvar spongiotic dermatitis. Similarly, a strong association between Th2 cytokines in the vulvovaginal area and a risk for yeast infection has been well documented [24]. A rise in estrogen increases the rate of allergy in women after puberty and, to a greater extent, during pregnancy [25]. Histamine release associated with allergy can cause prostaglandin E2 production which downregulates the local Th1 response, increasing the risk for yeast infection [24, 26]. Allergic dermatitis further inhibits Langerhans cell Th1 function. The clustering of Langerhans cells in spongiotic dermatitis that causes the characteristic microvesicles reflects a shift of vulvar epithelial Langerhans cells away from Th1 response. This decline in Th1 response significantly increases the risk for vulvovaginal yeast infection. Thus, just as all women are likely to experience vulvar spongiotic dermatitis at least once, all women should expect to have a vulvovaginal yeast infection at least occasionally. Some women suffer constantly from vulvar spongiotic dermatitis and remain at constant risk for yeast infection. Factors related to spongiotic dermatitis are possibly the most frequent cause for recurrent vulvar yeast or bacterial infection.

Chronic epithelial inflammation can result in an increased population of epithelial nerve endings and elongated nerve endings, likely resulting in progressively increasing skin sensitivity. This increase in nerve sensitivity has been linked to neurotropic substances that are activated as part of the normal inflammatory response. Nerve growth factor has a well-studied role in this regard [27]. This progressive increase in elongated epithelial nerve endings has been described in spongiotic dermatitis [28]. Similarly, gynecologic research has shown increased nerve endings in biopsy samples from cases of vulvodynia and vestibulitis [29, 30]. Unfortunately, the gynecologic samples were not investigated for spongiotic change in these reported nerve sensitivity studies. It is highly likely that chronic vulvar spongiotic dermatitis progressively increases nerve ending-mediated vulvar skin sensitivity.

19.6 Vulvar Sensitivity Changes After Menopause

After menopause, the vulva remains vulnerable to rubbing, with a persisting high friction coefficient [13]. For the postmenopausal vulva, estrogen deficiency and chronological aging are the main detrimental factors. The associated decline in barrier function and the loss of immune reactivity combine to influence the sensitivity of postmenopausal vulvar skin. The decline in barrier function provides a new opportunity for irritants to harm the increasingly fragile epithelium. The concurrent loss of immune reactivity may decrease the ability of the vulvar epithelium to register a symptomatic reaction. Thus, the relative awareness of vulvar sensitivity after menopause results from the interplay of multiple predictable factors that will be somewhat unique to the individual. With the lack of estrogen stimulation, vulvar skin would be expected to heal and recover more slowly after any insult.

The influence of aging upon skin is well documented [5, 6]. With aging, there is a significant decline in lipid production. Epidermal cells produce the lipids that fill the intercellular space. Lipid production consists of a fixed ratio of cholesterol, ceramides, and free fatty acids. Both chronological aging and loss of estrogen play a role in the loss of intercellular lipids. The age-related loss of the normal calcium gradient in the skin is one factor that adversely influences lipid production. The normal mixture of polar and nonpolar lipids in the stratum corneum contributes significantly to the epidermal barrier [31]. The normal composition of intercellular lipids is important for normal skin hydration. The degree of estrogen-associated keratinization of the stratum corneum is also important to maintain normal skin hydration. With aging and estrogen deficiency, intercellular lipid production is not adequately upregulated after injury. Yet, this significant defect in postmenopausal vulvar stratum corneum composition may still remain asymptomatic in the absence of mechanical or chemical damage. Considering the persistent exposure to environmental irritants, the potential for postmenopausal vulvar skin barrier problems may be greater than other body sites.

Estrogen loss and chronological aging lead to an adverse rise in vulvar skin pH after menopause [5, 6]. The normal skin pH of 4–5.5 maintains limited skin permeability, promotes skin cell cohesion, and regulates desquamation [32, 33]. A rise in the vulvar skin pH adversely affects these elements of normal skin physiology. The integrity of vulvar epithelium is profoundly compromised by a rise in pH. The rise in pH is directly associated with deficient intercellular lipid content. Loss of intercellular lipids, disruption of cell cohesion, and abnormal desquamation facilitate entry of microbial pathogens as well as environmental irritants into the epithelium. Traditionally, some degree of antimicrobial action is attributed to the normally low stratum corneum pH. This surface antimicrobial action is lost with aging. This combination of defects results in a possibility of higher rates of vulvar epithelial microbe colonization or infection as well as a greater potential for irritant reaction.

Bone marrow–derived Langerhans cells are distributed unevenly throughout the body. The highest concentration of Langerhans cells in the female genital tract is found in normal vulvar skin [34]. The greatest prevalence of Langerhans cells in vulvar epithelium is found during the reproductive years [35]. With aging, there is a significant decline in Langerhans cell function, as well as a fall in Langerhans cell count by approximately 50 % [36]. With aging, there is a significant decline in cytokine response that is linked to the decline in Langerhans cell function [37]. Thus, Langerhans cell-mediated immune response can be significantly blunted in older persons.

There is a clinically important decline in cell-mediated immunity with aging. For women, estrogen deficiency plays a primary role in this immune shift. Prior to puberty, the rate of asthma is the same for young boys and girls [25]. After puberty, under the influence of onset of estrogen production, asthma and a tendency for allergy increase for young girls. This immune shift toward allergy is potentiated with the further rise in estrogen levels during pregnancy. Then, after menopause, there is a decline in asthma and allergic response in older women [25]. The tendency for asthma is restored with hormone replacement therapy after menopause [38]. Thus, the ability of the vulvar immune system to produce a spongiotic reaction to environmental allergens is blunted after menopause. After menopause, dermatologic conditions such as lichen sclerosus would be expected to persist, but there is a decline in relative prevalence of vulvar spongiotic dermatitis. There is also a lower rate of allergy-associated vulvovaginal yeast infection unless immune responsiveness is restored by topical application of estrogen. After menopause, the rate of vulvovaginal yeast infection is significantly lower [39].

Early-stage vulvar squamous cell carcinoma can be misinterpreted as sensitive skin or vulvodynia. Langerhans cells also have a significant role in cancer surveillance. The postmenopausal risk for vulvar carcinoma increases with the decline in Langerhans cell function. Defense against squamous cancer-associated human papillomavirus rests in the phagocytic action of Langerhans cells. Half of vulvar carcinomas are attributed to HPV infection, and half relate alone to poor malignant cell surveillance by Langerhans cells [40].

In summary, the final status of relative vulvar sensitivity after menopause reflects an interplay of many independent factors. Atrophic vulvovaginitis may be the most universal risk for vulvovaginal burning after menopause. Postmenopausal barrier compromise increases susceptibility to irritants, allergens, and microbes. Decreased skin reactivity, reflected by decline in cell-mediated immunity, lowers the chance for symptomatic vulvitis. The rate of yeast infection is lower after menopause, unless estrogen is restored to the vulvar epithelium. If vulvar vestibulitis and vulvodynia are viewed as surrogates for vulvar sensitive skin syndrome, it is not surprising that surveys of postmenopausal women have not revealed a significant rise in vulvodynia after menopause [41, 42]. Interestingly, in these vulvodynia studies, the populations reporting vulvar symptoms differ before and after menopause. In contrast, a sensitive skin survey reported an increasing rate of self-reported genital skin sensitivity with aging, with little or no corresponding increase at other body sites [9]. Approximately 70 % of postmenopausal women reported somewhat sensitive genital skin, contrasting with 50–60 % of premenopausal women. Hot weather and abrasive clothing were the factors most significantly associated with reported sensitive skin after menopause. Others have actually reported a general decrease in skin sensitivity with age [43]. Thus, menopausal effects on skin sensitivity must be multifactorial with several concurrent changes where there may be actually elements that compensate for developing defects. Vulvar sensitivity factors prior to menopause differ somewhat from sensitive skin factors after menopause. Which women with sensitive skin prior to menopause continue to suffer after menopause depends upon which factors dominate. Vulvar sensitivity to mechanical abrasion may decline after menopause, but can recur after estrogen replacement therapy [44]. The barrier compromise due to lichen sclerosus is likely to persist. If spongiotic dermatitis is the prominent factor, then menopause may provide some relief unless topical estrogen is applied. Postmenopausal estrogen deficiency alone introduces elements of barrier compromise that increase susceptibility, especially to hydrophilic irritants. See Table 19.2.

Table 19.2 Factors that increase or decrease the tendency for vulvar skin sensitivity after menopause

1. Loss of barrier function with decreased intercellular lipids
2. Loss of barrier function with elevated pH
3. Decline in immune reactivity of the skin, less ability of skin to have spongiotic reaction

19.7 Some Vulvar Sensitive Skin Treatment Concepts

Irritant avoidance is the mainstay of vulvar sensitive skin therapy. For some postmenopausal women with urinary incontinence, the increased vulvar exposure to ammonia and oxalate is a significant issue [45]. After voiding, rinsing off with a squirt bottle instead of wiping with abrasive toilet paper can avoid two irritants. In the base of medicated creams, a hydrophilic irritant such as propylene glycol is a greater concern than hydrophobic irritants like sodium lauryl sulfate [46]. Propylene glycol is unfortunately a constituent of most commercial vulvovaginal creams and lubricants. Propylene glycol is added to most topical gynecologic products as a humectant that increases absorption of the medication by humidifying the skin barrier. For the postmenopausal vulva, it is particularly important to avoid damage from aggressive cleansing, topical agents, and abrasion by clothing, panty liners, or incontinence pads which contribute to postmenopausal skin barrier compromise [11]. Most commercial topical gynecologic products can cause burning when applied to the sensitive pre- or postmenopausal vulvar skin. Ointments generally are better tolerated than creams. A compounding pharmacist typically can find a nonirritating base to compound products equivalent to commercial creams.

Although the ideal product to repair or establish a good skin barrier has not been developed yet, moisturizing oils can help to restore compromised skin. Daily application of solid vegetable oil can be helpful. Vegetable oil consists largely of linoleic acid, a ceramide fatty acid which should be skin friendly. Estradiol, compounded in a nonirritating base, can reverse estrogen deficiency, with the recognition that vulvar application of estrogen increases the risk of vulvovaginal yeast infection for the postmenopausal woman [47]. The compounding pharmacist can provide a 0.1 mg estradiol per gram product that is equivalent to the commercial cream. This can be compounded in a nonirritating base such as solid vegetable oil or some Vaseline-based cream for twice-daily application until atrophy symptoms resolve. The frequency of use can then be decreased, according to personal need. Unfortunately, estrogen cannot effectively reverse the effects of chronological aging. Continued topical application of estrogen can help to restore normal Langerhans cell function [48]. Oral estrogen replacement is less effective than topical application since oral doses are directed more toward control of hot flashes and maintenance of bone mass.

A prolonged course of a topical steroid such as 1 % hydrocortisone may be necessary for control of spongiotic dermatitis or lichen sclerosus. Anti-inflammatory therapy may also slow the progression of nerve ending proliferation in some chronic vulvar pain conditions [49]. Hydrocortisone suppresses keratinocyte release of nerve growth factor [50]. Transdermal absorption of the corticosteroid may be substantially greater after vulvar application in comparison with other body sites where barrier function is more favorable. Adrenal suppression becomes a possibility with vulvar topical application of a high-potency steroid such as clobetasol. In severe cases, the use of a high-potency steroid is justified. It is important to switch to a less potent agent when possible. Naturally, the potential risk of adverse cosmetic or systemic effects from the topical steroid must be balanced against the severity of the patient's vulvar symptoms.

Office microscopy is a helpful diagnostic adjunct. Inspection of vaginal secretions to identify microbial pathogens is the main focus of the wet prep. The cellular component of the sample is of equal importance in the evaluation of a woman with sensitive vulvar skin. Parabasal squamous cells may reflect either a lack of estrogen or an intense inflammatory response with rapid skin turnover (Fig. 19.3). Skin flakes support a diagnosis of spongiotic dermatitis or lichen sclerosus. Vaginal bacterial cultures are generally not useful since the standard culture swab only supports growth of a few of the numerous microbes that are present in the normal vaginal fluid. Microbes that grow in the swab sample may actually be minor participants in the vaginal microflora, falsely promoted by the nature of the culture medium. See Table 19.3.

Fig. 19.3 High-power view of numerous parabasal cells (*large cells*) and white blood cells (*small cells*) in atrophic vulvovaginitis (vaginal saline wet preparation)

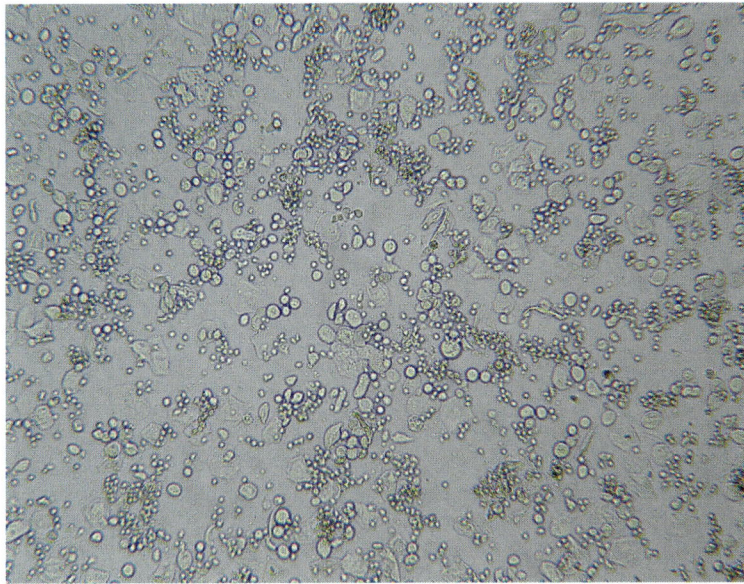

Table 19.3 Therapeutic considerations for vulvar sensitive skin after menopause

1. Topical estrogen restores intercellular lipids and improves barrier function
2. Topical estrogen restores lower pH
3. Topical estrogen restores skin reactivity and restores tendency for spongiotic dermatitis
4. Topical estrogen increases the risk for yeast infection
5. Vulvar skin remains reactive to propylene glycol in the topical estrogen products
6. Squirt bottle to rinse off urine after voiding can be helpful

19.8 Summary

Aging and estrogen deficiency compromise the skin barrier's defense mechanisms. Susceptibility to mechanical injury and chemical irritation increases. Menopause blunts the cell-mediated immune response to microbes and allergens. Healing after an insult is delayed. Skin disorders such as lichen sclerosus or allergic dermatitis may not be clinically obvious. A biopsy interpreted by a dermatopathologist is often helpful. Some conditions require the long-term use of topical steroid or estrogen ointments, as well as antimicrobial therapy. A compounding pharmacist may be necessary to find a base for the topical cream that does not irritate. Moisturizing the vulva with a nonirritating oil-based product is important in every case.

References

1. Berardesca E, Fluhr JW, Maibach HI. Sensitive skin syndrome. New York: Taylor & Francis; 2006.
2. Farage MA, Maibach HI. Sensitive skin: closing in on a physiological cause. Contact Dermatitis. 2010;62:137–49.
3. Farage MA, Robinson MK. Sensitive skin: intrinsic and extrinsic contributors. In: Lodin M, Maibach HI, editors. Treatment of dry skin. Berlin: Springer; 2012. p. 95–109.
4. Bowen AR, Vester A, Marsden L, Florell SR, Sharp H, Summers P. The role of vulvar skin biopsy in the evaluation of chronic vulvar pain. Am J Obstet Gynecol. 2008;199:467.e1–6.
5. Barland CO, Elias PM, Ghadially R. The aged epidermal permeability barrier: basis for functional abnormalities. In: Elias PM, Feingold KR, editors. Skin barrier. New York: Taylor & Francis; 2006.
6. Petersen MJ. Aging of the skin. In: Frienkel RK, Woodley DY, editors. The biology of the skin. New York: Parthenon Publishing; 2001.
7. Bettley FR. Non-specific irritant reactions in eczematous subjects. Br J Dermatol. 1964;76(3):116–9.

8. Farage MA. How do perceptions of sensitive skin differ at different anatomical sites? An epidemiological study. Clin Exp Dermatol. 2009;34:e521–30.
9. Farage MA. Perceptions of sensitive skin with age. In: Farage MA, Miller KW, Maibach HI, editors. Textbook of aging skin. New York: Springer; 2010. p. 1027–46.
10. Farage MA, Bowtell P, Katsarou A. Self-diagnosed sensitive skin in women with clinically diagnosed atopic dermatitis. Clin Med Derm. 2008;2:21–8.
11. Farage MA. Vulvar susceptibility to contact irritants and allergens: a review. Arch Gynecol Obstet. 2005;272:167–72.
12. Elsner P, Wilhelm D, Maibach HI. Physiological skin surface water loss dynamics of human vulvar and forearm skin. Acta Derm Venereol. 1990;70:141–4.
13. Elsner P, Wilhelm D, Maibach HI. Frictional properties of human forearm and vulvar skin: influence of age and correlation with transepidermal water loss and capacitance. Dermatologica. 1990;181:88–91.
14. Warman PH, Ennos AR. Fingerprints are unlikely to increase the friction of primate fingerpads. J Exp Biol. 2009;212:2016–22.
15. Linhares IM, Summers PR, Larsen B, Giraldo PC, Witkin SS. Contemporary perspectives on vaginal pH and lactobacilli. Am J Obstet Gynecol. 2011;204:120. e1–5.
16. Britz MB, Maibach HI. Human cutaneous vulvar reactivity to irritants. Contact Dermatitis. 1979;5:375–7.
17. Moyal-Barracco M, Lynch P. 2003 ISSVD terminology and classification of vulvodynia: a historical perspective. J Reprod Med. 2004;49:772–7.
18. Bonfiglio AR, Erozan TS. Gynecologic cytopathology. Philadelphia: Lippincott-Raven; 1997. p. 43.
19. Fu YS. Pathology of the uterine cervix and vulva. 2nd ed. Philadelphia: Saunders; 1989. p. 279–81.
20. Summers PR. Topical therapy for mucosal yeast infections. In: Surber C, Elsner P, Farage MA, editors. Topical applications and the mucosa. Basel: Karger; 2011. p. 51.
21. Braff MH, Bardan A, Nizet V, Gallo RL. Cutaneous defense mechanisms by antimicrobial peptides. J Invest Dermatol. 2005;125:9–13.
22. Garcia JC, Jaumann F, Schulz S, Krause A, Rodríguez-Jiménez J, Forssmann U, et al. Identification of a novel, multifunctional beta-defensin (human beta-defensin 3) with specific antimicrobial activity. Cell Tissue Res. 2001;306(2):257–64.
23. Nomura I, Goleva E, Howell MD, Hamid QA, Ong PY, Hall CF, et al. Cytokine milieu of atopic dermatitis, as compared to psoriasis, skin prevents induction of innate immune response genes. J Immunol. 2003;171:3262–9.
24. Witkin SS. Immunology of recurrent vaginitis. Am J Reprod Immunol Microbiol. 1987;15:34–7.
25. Balzano G, Fuschillo S, Melillo G, Bonini S. Asthma and sex hormones. Allergy. 2001;56(1):13–20.
26. Witkin SS, Linhares I, Girdo P, Jeremias J, Ledger WI. Individual immunity and susceptibility to female genital tract infection. Am J Obstet Gynecol. 2000; 183:252–6.
27. Dou YC, Hagstromer L, Emtestam L, Johansson O. Increased Nerve growth factor and its receptors in atopic dermatitis: an immunohistochemical study. Arch Dermatol Res. 2006;298:31–7.
28. Urashima R, Mihara M. Cutaneous nerves in atopic dermatitis. A histological, immunohistochemical, and electron microscopic study. Virchows Arch. 1998;432(4):363–70.
29. Bohm-Starke N, Hilliges M, Falconer C, Rylander E. Increased intraepithelial innervation in women with vulvar vestibulitis syndrome. Gynecol Obstet Invest. 1998;46:256–60.
30. Bohm-Starke N, Hilliges M, Falconer C, Rylander E. Neurochemical characterization of the vestibular nerves in women with vulvar vestibulitis syndrome. Gynecol Obstet Invest. 1999;48:270–5.
31. Schurer NY, Plewig G, Elias PM. Stratum corneum lipid function. Dermatologica. 1991;183:77–94.
32. Ohman H, Vahlquist A. In vivo studies concerning a pH gradient in human stratum corneum and upper epidermis. Acta Derm Venereol. 1994;74:375–9.
33. Denda M, Tsuchiya T, Elias PM, Feingold KR. Stress alters cutaneous permeability barrier homeostasis. Am J Physiol Regul Integr Comp Physiol. 2000;278:R367–72.
34. Edwards NJ, Morris HB. Langerhans' cells and lymphocyte subsets in the female genital tract. Br J Obstet Gynaecol. 1985;92:974–82.
35. Harper WF, McNicol EM. A histological study of normal vulval skin from infancy to old age. Br J Dermatol. 1977;96:249–53.
36. Gilchrest B, Murphy G, Soter N. Effect of chronological aging and ultraviolet light irradiation on Langerhans cells in human epidermis. J Invest Dermatol. 1982;79:85–8.
37. Thivolet J, Nicolas JF. Skin aging and immune competence. Br J Dermatol. 1990;122:77–81.
38. Kos-Kudla B, Ostrowska Z, Marek B, Ciesielska-Kopacz N, Kajdaniuk D, Kudła M. Effects of hormone replacement therapy on endocrine and spirometric parameters in asthmatic postmenopausal women. Gynecol Endocrinol. 2001;15(4):304–11.
39. Sobel JD. Pathogenesis and epidemiology if vulvovaginal candidiasis. Ann N Y Acad Sci. 1988;544: 547–57.
40. Gonzalez-Intxaurraga MA, Stankovic R, Sorli R, Trevisan G. HPV and carcinogenesis. Acta Dermatolovenerol. 2002;11:1–8.
41. Harlow BL, Stewart EG. A population-based assessment of chronic unexplained vulvar pain: have we underestimated the prevalence of vulvodynia? J Am Med Womens Assoc. 2003;58(2):82–8.
42. Bachmann GA, Rosen R, Raymond A, Arnold LD. Chronic vulvar and other gynecologic pain: prev-

43. Robinson MK. Age and gender in influencing factors in skin sensitivity. In: Berardesca E, Fluhr JW, Maibach HI, editors. Sensitive skin syndrome. New York: Taylor & Francis; 2006. p. 169–80.
44. Farage M, Miller KW, Zolnoun D, Ledger WJ. Assessing sensory perception on the vulva and on extragenital sites. Open Womens Health J. 2012;6:6–18.
45. Farage M, Maibach H. Lifetime changes in the vulva and vagina. Arch Gynecol Obstet. 2005.
46. Elsner P, Wilhelm D, Maibach HI. Effect of low-concentration sodium lauryl sulfate on human vulvar and forearm skin. Age-related differences. J Reprod Med. 1991;36:77–81.

alence and characteristics in a self-reported survey. Obstet Gynecol Surv. 2006;61(5):313–4.

47. Sobel JD. Vaginal infections in adult women. Sex Transm Dis. 1990;74:1573–601.
48. Mao A, Paharkova-Vatchkova V, Hardy J, Miller MM, Kovats S. Estrogen selectively promotes the differentiation of dendritic cells with characteristics of langerhans cells. J Immunol. 2005;175:5148.
49. Mantyh PW, Koltzenberg M, Mandell LM, Tive L, Shelton DL. Antagonism of nerve growth factor-TrkA signaling and the relief of pain. Anesthesiology. 2011;115(1):189–204.
50. Di Marco E, Marchisio PC, Bondanza S, Franzi AT, Cancedda R, De Luca M. Growth-related synthesis and secretion of biologically active nerve growth factor by human keratinocytes. J Biol Chem. 1991;286(32):21718–22.

Vulval Disease in Postmenopausal Women

20

Allan B. MacLean and Maxine Chan

Contents

20.1	Structure of Normal Vulva	249
20.2	Vulval Changes Due to the Menopause or Estrogen Withdrawal	250
20.3	Vulval Infection	252
20.4	Vulval Patients	254
20.4.1	Classification (ISSVD 2006) of Vulval Dermatoses	255
20.5	Vulval Dermatitis/Eczema/Lichenification/Lichen Simplex Chronicus/Contact and Irritant Dermatitis	256
20.6	Lichen Sclerosus	257
20.6.1	The Relationship Between LS and Vulval Cancer	259
20.7	Lichen Planus	261
20.8	Vulval Intraepithelial Neoplasia	262
20.9	Paget's Disease of the Vulva	264
20.10	Vulval Cancer	265
20.10.1	Symptoms and Signs	265
20.10.2	Vulvodynia	267
20.11	Summary	270
References		270

A.B. MacLean, BMedSc, MD, FRCOG, FRCP Edin (✉)
Department of Obstetrics and Gynaecology,
Royal Free Campus, University College London,
Rowland Hill Street, London NW3 2PF, UK
e-mail: a.maclean@ucl.ac.uk

M. Chan, MB, BS, BSc
Department of Obstetrics and Gynaecology,
University College Hospital, London, UK
e-mail: maxine.chan@ucl.ac.uk

20.1 Structure of Normal Vulva

The vulva consists of the labia majora, labia minora, mons pubis, clitoris, perineum and the vestibule. From puberty the mons and lateral parts of the labia majora are covered in strong coarse hair and are distended with subcutaneous fat. In addition to hair follicles, they contain sebaceous, apocrine and eccrine (sweat) glands. The labia minora lie medially and are non-hair-bearing but contain multiple sebaceous glands. They extend from the frenulum of the clitoris to the perineum, varying considerably in shape and size but may become modified posteriorly with obstetric trauma or episiotomy scarring. Previous pregnancy may alter the course of vulval venous drainage, often in the interlabial sulcus between labia majora and minora, and the veins become tortuous in later life. The labia minora have a rich vascular supply such that in sexual response they become distended and engorged to pout apart to facilitate coital entry; when not distended they will fold together to protect the vestibule with urethral and vaginal orifices. The clitoris is attached to the pubo-ischial ramus and mostly covered by a prepuce such that only the tip or glans is visible.

The vulvovaginal vestibule is the cleft between the labia minora. It is covered by non-keratinised squamous epithelium extending down from the hymen or its remnants to the keratinised skin. The vestibule contains the entrance to the vagina, the urethral meatus and the ducts of the greater

(Bartholin's), lesser and paraurethral (Skene's) glands. Following childbirth (vaginal delivery) the vestibule and introitus may be altered in appearance, with scar tissue visible. Gaping of the introitus may be exaggerated with vaginal wall descent or prolapse.

The vagina, while a separate anatomical entity to the vulva, influences vulval function. It is lined by a stratified squamous epithelium that is rich in glycogen stores during the reproductive years, but not in prepubertal or postmenopausal women. The normal bacterial flora is usually dominated by lactobacilli, which alter the glycogen to lactic acid to maintain an acidic environment and reduce the proliferation of many organisms. Engorgement and transudation of the vagina are important components of normal sexual response; the loss of 'wetness' may become important after the menopause.

The normal histology and histopathology of skin lesions require an understanding that the vulval skin is an epidermis with different strata or layers (basal, parabasal, prickle cell, granular and cornified layers) and an underlying dermis with rete ridges or pegs at the epidermal–dermal interface compared with the mucosal epithelium and underlying stroma of the vagina.

20.2 Vulval Changes Due to the Menopause or Estrogen Withdrawal

It is widely known in gynaecology that the vagina 'suffers' atrophic changes due to estrogen absence or deficiency [1], but scientific understanding of what happens to vulval appearances and function in the perimenopause is limited [2]. Definitions of the 'perimenopause' are inconsistent, but broadly refer to the time of a woman's life when she is no longer producing estrogens in a regular, cyclical and physiological way. The periods are starting to become less regular or may be absent for 2–3 months at a time. There are vasomotor symptoms of night sweating and daytime flushes or flashes. In some publications, e.g. MacBride et al. [3], the changes are described as 'vulvovaginal atrophy', but almost all the descriptions are of vaginal changes, e.g. dryness, irritation, soreness, pain and bleeding with intercourse, change in pH and alteration of vaginal microbiological flora (microflora). Pallor, erythema, ecchymoses and architectural changes of labia minora and majora are more likely to represent some of the lesions described below and are unlikely to respond to replacement estrogens. Certainly that publication [3] includes a table of differential diagnoses for symptoms of vulvovaginal atrophy (lichen sclerosus, lichen planus, lichen simplex chronicus, contact dermatitis, vulval intraepithelial neoplasia, vulval cancer and extramammary Paget's disease), and all of these vulval conditions are discussed in the appropriate sections below.

The effects of estrogens are mediated via estrogen receptors. These have been demonstrated immunohistochemically in epidermal keratinocytes and dermal fibroblasts of hair-bearing and non-hair-bearing skin of the vulva and perineum, but at much lower frequency than in the vagina [4, 5]. More recent analysis has identified that ER (estrogen receptors) have alpha and beta configurations or isoforms and these are expressed in different structures, e.g. the nuclei of smooth muscle in the fibromuscular layer of the vulva express ERα but not ERβ [6]. That study included women with postmenopausal vaginal changes but concentrated on vulval lichen sclerosus (LS) and squamous hyperplasia. Nieves et al. [7] examined ER isoform expression in estrogen-deficient patients, but these were 2–9-year-old girls with labial fusion, and the findings may be different in women once they have been exposed to physiological levels of estrogens before they enter the menopause. The many body organs, tissues and cell types that contain estrogen receptors are listed in Table 1 of Farage et al. [8].

Changes in postmenopausal sexual function are often due to vaginal changes, such as reduced vaginal transudation, cervical mucus, stromal elasticity and epithelial thickness, which all follow estrogen deficiency some time after the menopause, i.e. not concurring with the last menstrual period but up to 4–5 years after the menopause [1]. Cumming et al. [9] describe postmenopausal sexual dysfunction and the factors that might cause low desire, low arousal and anorgasmia. Kao et al. [10] have reported the biopsychosocial factors associated with postmenopausal sexual difficulty and found hormone levels were not consistent predictors of pain severity.

Although the clitoris, labia minora, vestibule and lower vagina have awakened new interests in functional importance [11], there is still limited information about postmenopausal changes to innervation. Martin-Alguacil et al. [12] reviewed the role of vulva epithelium in sexual arousal, including how this is influenced by estrogen. Based mainly on animal studies, the authors relate this to changes in mechanical properties of the vulva, which can alter the way sensory nerve endings are stimulated; estrogen-receptor-mediated endothelial activity and the influence on central and peripheral neurotransmission. They cite experiments on rats [13, 14] in which estradiol was shown to widen touch receptor zones supplied by the pudendal nerve. In humans, Romanzi et al. [15] measured lower sensitivity to pressure and touch in women who were hypoestrogenic, had vulvovaginal atrophy or were postmenopausal, in particular those not on hormone replacement therapy. Connell et al. [16] found that increasing age and the menopause were associated with diminished vulval sensitivity, as represented by an increased threshold to vibratory sensation. It has also been demonstrated that topical estrogen replacement increases sensitivity of the vulval vestibule to mechanical stimuli [17]. Though the direct effect of estrogen on sensory receptors is unclear, the authors imply the indirect influence of improved blood flow and skin quality. Nevertheless, patients still respond to the pain of hypodermal needling and local anaesthetic infiltration. Post-operative pain still occurs as in any premenopausal patient. However, generalised unprovoked vulvodynia, with symptoms of burning, soreness, rawness and pain, occurs more frequently in postmenopausal women (see later).

Changes of the skin influenced by hormonal changes in postmenopausal women have been well reviewed. It is readily recognised that loss of estrogen in the menopausal years causes exposed skin to become thinner, dryer, less elastic and more wrinkled [18]. These changes can be reversed or improved, to a degree, with estrogen replacement [19]. However, there are few details or studies specific for vulval skin. Histologically, the epithelial and keratin layers of vulval skin are thickest during the reproductive years, when levels of circulating estrogen are highest, and become thinner after the menopause [20]. A series of studies found that vulval skin is intrinsically different in property to exposed skin [21, 22]. These studies described the use of bioengineering techniques to study water barrier function, skin hydration and friction coefficient in comparing vulval and forearm skin; the findings were that vulval skin is more capable of retaining water and has a higher friction coefficient. The differences between pre- and postmenopausal values were not significant, suggesting that vulval epithelium does not undergo the same age-related changes as the general skin. Farage [23] discusses how these factors cause vulval skin to react differently to irritants compared to skin elsewhere.

Some time after the last menstrual period, there is loss of subcutaneous fat from the labia majora and mons pubis so that the vulva becomes flatter and the introitus may gape. The loss of ligamentous support causes descent of the uterus and vaginal wall, with greater or lesser degrees of genital prolapse [24]. However, clinical observation is that the mons pubis may become more protuberant, either because of remodelling of the pubic symphysis or gradual descent of the fat of the lower abdominal wall. The inguinal nodes which are easily palpated in a younger woman are more difficult to define. The loss of labial bulk and skin tension means that surgical closure is more likely to be achieved without tension or need to reconstruct excised skin defects with advancement or rotational flaps.

There is reduction in hair density and colour but also hair coarseness, i.e. it becomes finer. Eventually it may become wispy and scanty, though there remains much variation (perhaps compounded by ethnic variations in the shape of the escutcheon).

It is suggested that there is a reduced number of capillaries and changes in the arteriolar wall of vessels after the menopause [25]. Estrogens promote blood flow to the skin. It does so in part

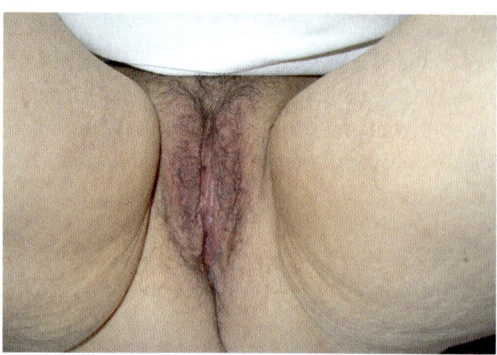

Fig. 20.1 Vulval angiomata

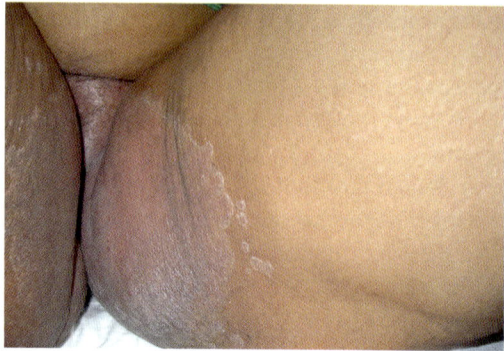

Fig. 20.2 Maceration due to *Candida albicans* in a poorly controlled diabetic

by acting on vascular endothelium to stimulate release of vasodilatory chemical mediators, such as nitric oxide and prostacyclin. Arora et al. [26] showed that cutaneous perfusion was increased during the high estrogen mid-cycle phase in premenopausal women, as well as in postmenopausal women on estrogen replacement. The increase in blood flow was both endothelium-mediated and endothelium-independent, suggesting the effect of estrogen on vascular smooth muscle. Increase in blood flow to the vulva leads to clitoral engorgement, which contributes importantly to sensitivity and sexual arousal [27]. Certainly the postmenopausal vulva is more likely to contain capillary angiomata (de Morgan's spots) (Fig. 20.1) and varicosities that require care when planning biopsies. Any reduction in blood supply may still cause wound complications with haematoma formation, but perhaps because of the wider use of aspirin in postmenopausal women. Surprisingly, wound closure with advancement or rotational flaps does not appear to be compromised with ischemic edges or corners, suggesting that skin vascularisation remains functionally adequate.

20.3 Vulval Infection

One of the more common reasons for women between puberty and the menopause to have vulval symptoms is infection and in particular due to the yeast *Candida albicans*. This occurs during pregnancy, while using oral contraceptives and following prolonged courses of broad-spectrum antibiotics.

It is commonly stated that the postmenopausal vulva is more vulnerable to infection, but on the basis of alterations within the vagina. Studies using swab and culture methods are now being replaced by molecular techniques for 'microbial communities', but little is available for description of what happens after the menopause [28].

It is most unlikely that postmenopausal women will have symptoms, e.g. chronic itch, vaginal discharge and dyspareunia due to vaginal yeasts, unless they are taking topical or systemic estrogen therapy [29] or are diabetic (Fig. 20.2). Before ascribing vulval symptoms in any postmenopausal women to yeasts, a low vaginal swab should be taken (by the woman when she is symptomatic or by her doctor) and examined for confirmation. Symptoms thought to be due to yeasts but associated with a negative swab require closer examination (as per the next section). Those women who have confirmed yeasts and are not on estrogen therapy should be screened/tested for diabetes mellitus.

The reasons for younger women being more susceptible to *Candida* species remain unclear, but include promotional changes in pH, direct effect of estrogens on adherence of yeasts to vaginal mucosa, effects of menstruation and tampon/menstrual pad use on vaginal microflora [30], an estrogen effect on vaginal immunity [31] and the availability of antifungal therapies as over-the-counter sales without an examination or prescription from their doctor [32].

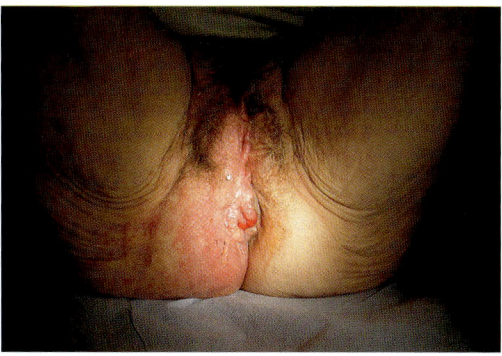

Fig. 20.3 Herpes zoster unilaterally involving the perineum and buttock

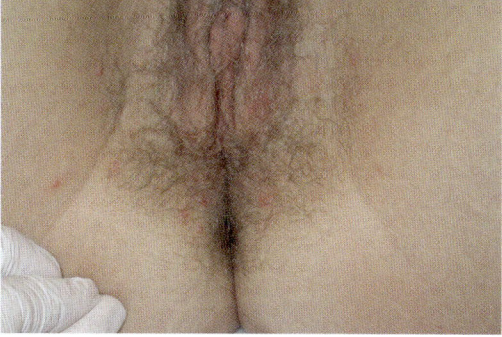

Fig. 20.4 Molluscum contagiosum

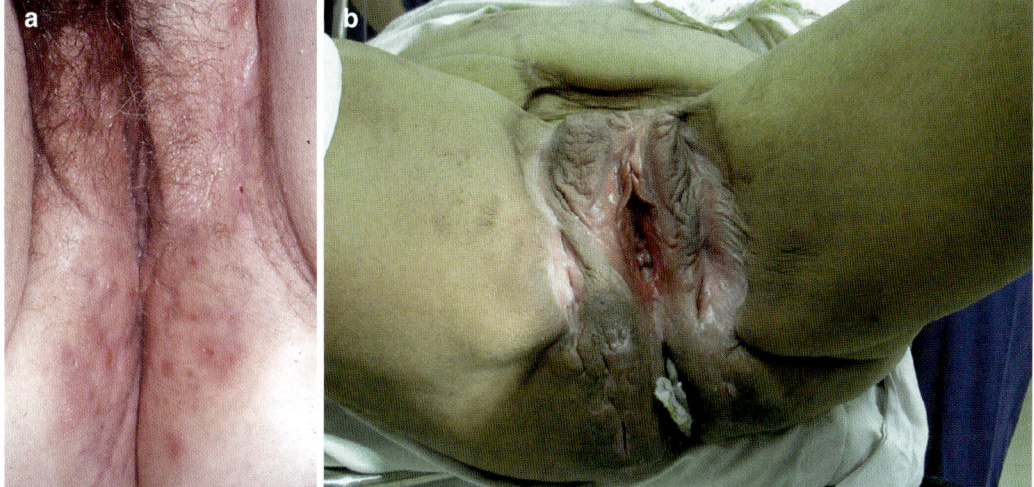

Fig. 20.5 Hidradenitis suppurativa. (**a**) Changes in the perianal area. (**b**) More extensive and with previous surgical changes

The impact of bacterial vaginosis and chlamydial or gonococcal bartholinitis is less likely in postmenopausal women. Viral changes associated with human papilloma virus will be discussed later. Herpes simplex lesions may still occur or reactivate in postmenopausal women. Rarely herpes zoster, due to varicella-zoster virus, can be seen involving part of the vulval area, i.e. unilateral involvement of thoracolumbar T12/L1 or sacral S2, S3 or S4 dermatomes (Fig. 20.3). *Molluscum contagiosum* has been seen in immune-competent postmenopausal women although more commonly seen in young adults (Fig. 20.4).

Superficial skin infections due to staphylococcal or streptococcal species are less frequently seen than in premenopausal women (partly associated with hair removal by waxing or shaving), but may follow skin damage from urinary or faecal incontinence (see section below on vulval dermatitis).

Deeper infections, e.g. *Hidradenitis suppurativa* (Fig. 20.5), do occur in perimenopausal women but usually settle after the menopause [33]. Skin infection complicating vulval surgery can complicate healing in any age group, particularly if obese, diabetic or immune-compromised. Necrotizing fasciitis or Fournier's gangrene is reported but extremely uncommon [34].

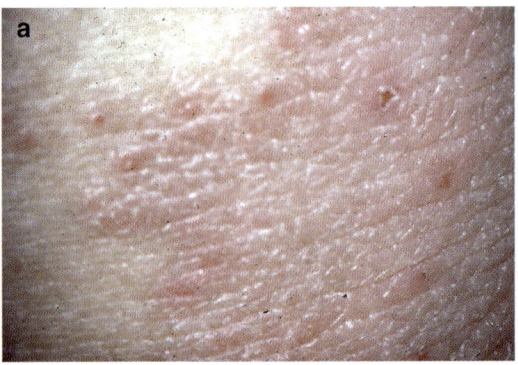 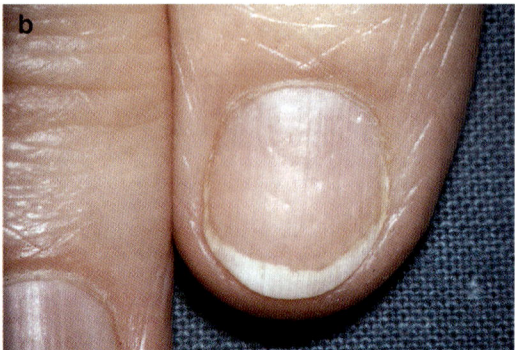

Fig. 20.6 (**a**) Vulval psoriasis and (**b**) nails showing pitting

20.4 Vulval Patients

The majority of patients who attend a gynaecology, dermatology or genitourinary clinic do so because they are symptomatic. For most, they will complain of itch or scratching (pruritus), while a minority will have pain, burning, soreness or rawness. Some will attend because of splitting, discomfort or sexual difficulty. However, some patients will be referred because abnormal, unusual or altered appearances will be noted when the patient attends for something else, e.g. to have a smear taken, or a gynaecological examination for other reasons.

While clinical appearances may allow the medical or nursing practitioner to make a diagnosis, more frequently it will require an appropriate history and to use correct examination techniques and biopsy procedures. History should include past history, e.g. flexural eczema or asthma, and family history, e.g. psoriasis and LS both having familial clustering. Other autoimmune disorders may be relevant. Careful documentation of all treatments previously used including topical applications is important to recognise that the appearances may have been modified, to avoid prescribing something that has not worked previously, and to identify possible contact allergens or irritants including soaps, perfumes, preservatives and components of sanitary pads.

Examination should include the fingernails (Fig. 20.6) and skin of the hands, wrists, elbows, scalp and face; the oral cavity (Fig. 20.7), gums and tongue; the trunk and the lower limbs. Examination of the vulva requires exposure of the pudendum from pubes and inguinal areas to the natal cleft and cannot be done easily with the patient lying flat on a couch; the dorsal position gives some viewing but the patient then needs turning on her side, sometimes with straightening of the upper leg, to get complete viewing. Adequate lighting is paramount. Colposcopy is not essential, but a colposcopy chair provides good positioning, and the associated light of the colposcope allows viewing without the examiner's head or hair obscuring the light source. Areas of colour change are noted and examined at higher magnification (a hand-held looking glass is an alternative to a colposcope and may now come with an in-built light source) for change in surface contour – exophytic or ulcerative. Red areas may represent altered capillary dilatation, but angiogenesis should be considered. White areas with abnormally thickened keratin may be the result of scratch damage but may represent more significant pathology.

Applications of 5 % acetic acid or 1 % toluidine blue solutions are not performed for every patient but certainly for anyone who has previously had an abnormal smear. Acetic acid penetrates mucosa quickly but not keratinised skin; it precipitates nucleoprotein so that neoplastic areas become visible (as for colposcopy of the cervix [35]), but it will take longer, the acetowhite epithelium may not be as obvious as on the cervix, and little information can be obtained if scratching has produced thickening of the keratin (hyperkeratosis or lichenification). Acetowhite epithelium

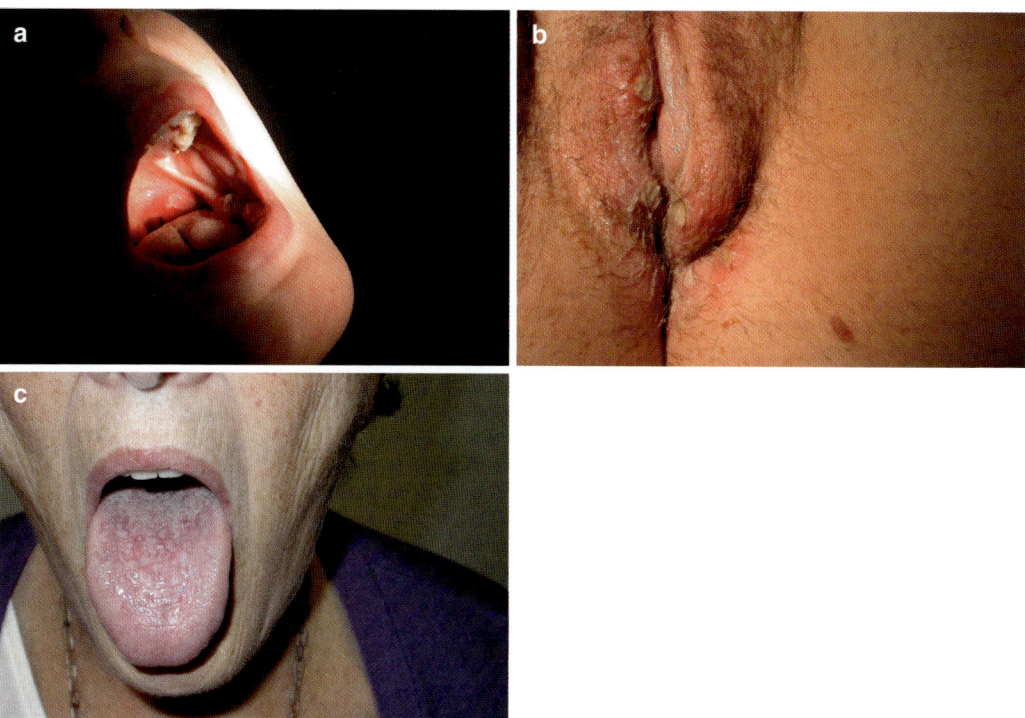

Fig. 20.7 (**a**) Pharyngeal and (**b**) vulval ulceration with Behcet's disease. (**c**) Appearance of tongue with oral lichen planus

does not equate to VIN or to HPV presence [36], and biopsy is required of the area. Toluidine blue stains the nuclei of cells (as haematoxylin does in histopathology). Surface squames consist mainly of cytoplasm with small pyknotic nuclei and therefore take up minimal blue staining. Where squamous differentiation and maturation is abnormal (as for VIN, usual type) the nuclei are larger, or if the surface cells have been scratched or scraped away, blue areas of staining will be defined, and these should be biopsied.

Biopsy is not necessary for every diagnosis. Some lesions, e.g. dermatitis/eczema, will be characteristic in their distribution, e.g. interlabial folds or perianal skin. Other lesions may have non-specific appearances as described above, and biopsy will be the only way to characterise the lesion (see classification below). Local anaesthesia, e.g. 2 % lignocaine with adrenaline as a vasoconstrictor, is infiltrated via a 27-gauge needle adjacent to but not into the lesion, and the biopsy is taken with a 4 mm biopsy (e.g. Stiefel) punch. Haemostasis is obtained with silver nitrate or Monsel's solution and pressure for a few minutes. If the patient is taking aspirin or warfarin, or multiple sites need to be biopsied to map out the extent of the lesion, e.g. Paget's or VIN, the biopsies are better taken in the theatre, often with a short general anaesthetic and the biopsy sites undersewn with sutures for haemostasis [37].

20.4.1 Classification (ISSVD 2006) of Vulval Dermatoses

- Spongiotic pattern: atopic dermatitis, allergic contact dermatitis, irritant contact dermatitis
- Acanthotic pattern (formerly squamous cell hyperplasia): psoriasis, lichen simplex chronicus, primary (idiopathic), secondary (superimposed on LS, lichen planus or other vulval disease)
- Lichenoid pattern: LS, lichen planus
- Dermal homogenisation/sclerosis pattern: LS
- Vesiculobullous pattern: pemphigoid (cicatricial type), linear immunoglobulin A disease

- Acantholytic pattern: Hailey–Hailey disease, Darier's disease, papular genitocrural acantholysis
- Granulomatous pattern: Crohn's disease, Melkersson–Rosenthal syndrome
- Vasculopathic pattern: aphthous ulcers, Behcet's disease, plasma cell vulvitis [38].

20.5 Vulval Dermatitis/Eczema/Lichenification/Lichen Simplex Chronicus/Contact and Irritant Dermatitis

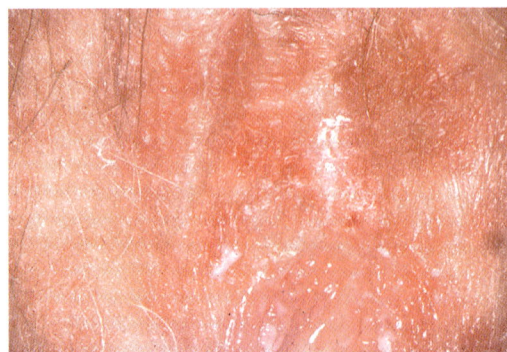

Fig. 20.8 Dermatitis caused by perfumed soap

Contact dermatitis occurs as an allergic response to various allergens including topical antibiotics, anaesthetic and antihistamine creams, deodorants and perfumes (e.g. Balsam of Peru as used in various haemorrhoid creams), lanolin, azodyes in nylons, biological washing powders, etc. An increasing number of referrals to vulval clinics are being seen because of the current trend to remove vulval hair. Some women have applied depilatory creams or waxes with subsequent irritant reaction, while others have inflicted skin damage by shaving.

An increasing challenge in the elderly is control of bladder and bowel function. Sometimes the vulval skin will be irritated by the constant wearing of pads or incontinence devices, but also by the effect of urine or faecal material in contact with the skin. Such events do not necessarily relate to the menopause, although researchers have highlighted the role estrogen plays in maintaining function of the lower urinary tract which in turn preserves urinary continence. As well as the genital tract, the urethra, bladder and pelvic floor also have estrogen receptors. Postmenopausal low levels of estrogen lead to urogenital atrophy and are associated with lower urinary tract symptoms, such as frequency, urgency, incontinence and nocturia [39]. The diminished action of estrogen reduces sensitivity of the urethral smooth muscle, which predisposes to incontinence. The prevalence of urge incontinence, in particular, increases with the menopause [40]. Elderly women have increased susceptibility to the so-termed incontinence dermatitis when the perineal skin is subject to urinary moisture under occlusion. The skin becomes inflamed and its barrier function is damaged by friction, rise in pH and faecal enzymes; this damage is perpetuated by chronic incontinence [41].

The clinical appearance of dermatitis (Fig. 20.8) is diffuse but sometimes focal erythema and oedema with superimposed infection or lichenification (Fig. 20.9). The terms 'lichen' and 'lichenification' cause confusion because of their similarity. Lichenification describes the patchwork covering of the rocks of the West of Scotland (and elsewhere) and is best illustrated by the appearance of the skin over the elbows and knuckles (metacarpophalangeal joints) where the shin is thickened and patterned unlike skin elsewhere. Biopsy is usually not required unless there is no response to treatment; then other diagnoses should be considered.

Patch testing may identify the allergen to allow removal or avoidance of the factor, and moisturising cream or mild steroids should provide local control. Haverhoek et al. [42] reported that 81 % of the patients that they saw with vulval pruritus had at least one contact allergen detected on patch `testing.

Some topical preparations will cause irritation over time (i.e. in a chronic fashion). The vulval appearances will be less obvious, with minimal erythema but with pallor or pigmentation and with dryness, thickening and cracking – lichenification or lichen simplex chronicus. Lichen simplex chronicus (previously known as

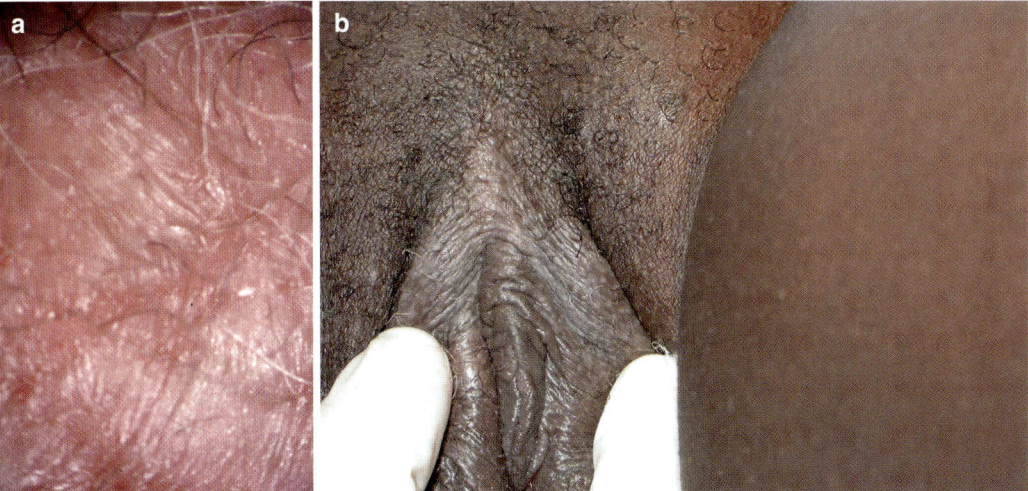

Fig. 20.9 (**a**, **b**) The appearance of lichenification

'neurodermatitis') occurs in normal skin which becomes thick and fissured in response to the trauma of constant scratching. These lesions are not usually symmetrical and occur in vulval areas accessible to scratching.

Treatment consists of the use of emollients or topical corticosteroids of low-to-moderate potency. Sometimes, sedation at night is useful to stop nocturnal scratching. Once control is gained, assessment for an underlying cause or lesion is often necessary.

20.6 Lichen Sclerosus

Lichen sclerosus represents approximately one quarter of the patients attending our vulval clinic, and the majority of them will be postmenopausal [43]. It is found once in every 800 prepubertal girls [44] and increases with age to be reported as frequent as 1 in 30 elderly women in residential care [45]. It is an inflammatory dermatosis and is frequently symptomatic, causing pruritus, sleeplessness, dyspareunia and constipation. It may produce major architectural changes and alterations in vulval appearance and function and has a small but important risk of cancer; in the UK 60–70 % of vulval squamous cell carcinomas occur against a background of LS [46].

Lichen sclerosus involves the pudendum either partially or completely as a 'figure of eight', encircling the vulva and anus and altering the clitoris and its prepuce, the labia minora and inner aspects of the labia majora and the fourchette and perineum. It is usually symmetrical, bilateral and central, but may involve more lateral structures including the genitofemoral creases and the natal cleft. It involves the skin, but does not involve the mucosa of the vestibule, vagina or anus (although 'overlap' with erosive lichen planus is recognised). The lesions consist of thin, pearly, ivory or porcelain white crinkly plaques. Sometimes there is shrinkage and absorption of the labia minora, but sometimes they coapt anteriorly to cause clitoral phimosis and narrowing of the introitus to make intercourse impossible and to impede micturition. Scratching may result in epidermal thickening (lichenification) but sometimes erosion and superficial ulceration (the previous term used by clinicians and endorsed by the ISSVD was 'lichen sclerosus et atrophicus'). Areas of ecchymoses and later haemosiderin pigmentation are common. LS may involve the trunk and limbs in up to 20 % of patients [47] (Fig. 20.10).

The histological features of LS include epidermal atrophy, dermal oedema, hyalinisation of the superficial dermal collagen and subdermal chronic inflammatory infiltrate. However,

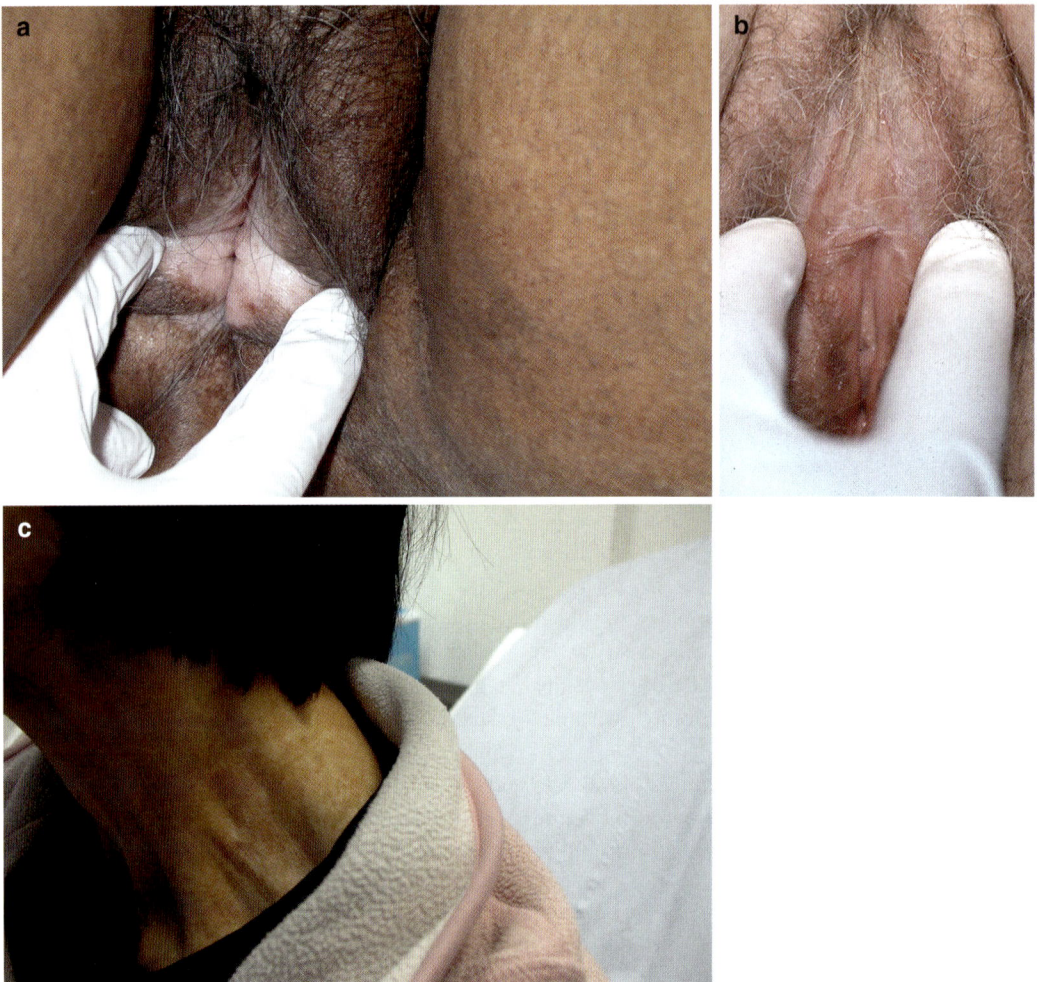

Fig. 20.10 (**a**) Lichen sclerosus. (**b**) Lichen sclerosus with phimosis. (**c**) Extragenital lichen sclerosus, involving the neck

occasionally the clinical features will resemble typical LS, and yet the biopsy shows minimal features. Sometimes the terms 'early' and 'late' are used to indicate the level of the inflammatory process, and these must not be misinterpreted as recent compared to longer duration.

The cause(s) of LS must consider the increased frequency in women (c.f., men) and with increasing age. It may show clustering within families, and a link with HLA DQ7 has been reported [48]. The association with autoimmunity has been widely reported. In the last decade Howard et al. [49] have found circulating basement membrane zone antibody in the serum of patients with LS, and Oyama et al. [50] describe an antibody to extracellular matrix protein 1. Farrell et al. [51] described the presence of interferon-gamma and other inflammatory cytokines within lesional epidermis, underlying dermis and within the inflammatory areas.

Explanation is required why LS is frequently seen in the UK, Europe, and especially Scandinavia, North and South America, Oceania and Southern Africa and yet is infrequent in Northern Africa, Arabia, Pakistan, India, Malaysia, Thailand, Singapore, Philippines and Hong Kong. The authors' observations are offset by data that a quarter of the women attending vulval clinic were born outside the UK, including countries within the areas listed above. It is rare to diagnose LS in women newly arrived in London, but prolonged domicile may be important. The authors are currently researching the possible role of vitamin D deficiency in causing LS. Vitamin D is generated from sun exposure to the head, arms and body and from oily fish and egg yolks within the diet. Data gathered to date include many older women do not leave the UK for holidays in the sun, and avoid sun exposure or use high factor sun block (some of the patients have developed skin cancers in exposed areas and have been warned by their dermatologists to keep out of the sun, plus our latitude of 56 north; pigmented skin in some patients and more protective clothing in some ethnic and religious groups reduce the effect of the sun in producing vitamin D in the skin); avoid eggs because of their concurrent cardiovascular morbidity and therapy to lower cholesterol levels; and have little enthusiasm for eating certain fish (or are vegetarian). A few women take cod liver oil or vitamin supplements, e.g. with calcium, to protect their bones as the current literature discourages the use of hormone replacement therapy. Serum levels of vitamin D are abnormally low in some of our patients, but we are comparing these with control patients because many older people in London, including those who arrive from other countries, may have chronically low vitamin D levels. Certainly vitamin D deficiency, with rickets and osteomalacia, is being reported from British studies. Vitamin D deficiency has been linked with autoimmune diseases and certain cancers. Dietary supplementation may become an easier option than sending every postmenopausal woman for a holiday in the sun.

The treatment of LS usually requires the super-potent topical corticosteroid clobetasol propionate and following the protocols described by the British Association of Dermatologists [52]. A fingertip or 'pea-sized' amount of clobetasol ointment (Dermovate) is applied at night for 4 weeks, alternate nights for 4 weeks and then twice a week for 4 weeks before review. The pharmacokinetics of clobetasol suggests one application per 24 h is adequate. Many patients require reassurance that the potent steroid will not damage their skin when used according to instructions and to use applications on a regular basis because stopping treatment will frequently cause a rebound of symptoms. A 30 g tube should last for at least 12 weeks, and most patients with ongoing symptoms require 30–60 g of clobetasol per year. Emollients are used during the day and a soap alternative while washing. Testosterone cream no longer has any role in treating women. Alternative treatment use must be done with careful vigilance because of the increased risk of malignancy in patients who do not respond to clobetasol.

20.6.1 The Relationship Between LS and Vulval Cancer

This relationship continues to be an area of debate, and the positive side of the argument has been presented elsewhere [46]. Several authors have reported a prevalence of carcinoma of 2.5–5 % in women who present with LS [47, 53, 54]. It is unlikely that the development of malignancy led to the appearance of LS, although many of these women denied having had symptoms for any duration.

Nevertheless, there are individual cases or series of cases that document carcinoma occurring some time after a clinical diagnosis of LS, in spite of the use of appropriate clobetasol therapy. Jones et al. [55] reported that women who develop cancer with LS are more likely to show clinical evidence of squamous hyperplasia and are more likely to have been symptomatic for 5 years or more [56]. Cooper et al. [57] reported that six women developed carcinoma in spite of treatment in their series. Renaud-Vilmer et al. [58] reported that among eight women who developed cancer, one had discontinued treatment 3 years earlier, and a second patient had used treatment irregularly.

In my own unpublished vulval clinic data up until 2010, there were 655 patients with a diagnosis of LS made at their first visit, and 19 of them had concurrent squamous cell carcinoma of the vulva (2.9 %) and 5 with recurrent carcinoma within residual areas of LS. In subsequent follow-up, five further patients developed carcinoma; the first after 2 years was probably inadequately applying her treatment, the second (and only premenopausal patient of these five) after 4 years was optimally treated but frequently was symptomatic, the third had her cancer recognised 8 years after starting treatment with steroid but then being changed to a calcineurin inhibitor (see below), the fourth after 10 years of good symptom control was changed to systemic steroid to manage her fibromyalgia and the fifth after 12 years of supervised treatment became symptomatic when the national supply of diflucortolone valerate (another super-potent steroid available in the UK) stopped temporarily.

There are concerns that certain treatments may increase the risk of cancer. There have been publications advocating the application of tacrolimus or pimecrolimus as alternatives to steroids, but following reports of apparently rapid progression to cancer, the US Food and Drug Administration released a warning advising caution with their use [59].

There is now increasing awareness of the appearance of histological changes within LS that seem to predispose to a risk of progression to carcinoma. Many authors have commented previously on the finding of basal cell atypia (e.g. Leibovitz et al. [60]), and the latest terminology for vulval intraepithelial neoplasia (VIN) includes differentiated VIN as the preferred term [61]. Initial response to this term was that it was only found with specimens of invasive cancer, but it is now an important biopsy finding for a patient who remains symptomatic without a diagnosis of cancer (see below).

Many vulval cancers which have LS in the adjacent skin have been studied for various molecular alterations including changes in tumour suppressor gene activity and increased expression of mutant p53 [62, 63] and allelic imbalance with loss of heterozygosity or allelic gain [64]. The authors' group has identified a mutation in codon 136 of exon 5 for p53 found in the areas of invasion and also in the adjacent LS [65]. Several patients with LS plus hyperplasia have progressed to carcinoma, and it is suggested that immunohistochemical staining of increased expression of p53 and Ki-67 may be a useful predictor of progression before invasion occurs [66].

Other factors that might place patients at increased risk of developing cancer include blood group; we found that 72 % of our patients with LS plus cancer were blood group A, compared with 38 % in a control population [67]. Similar associations with blood group A and the risk of gastric cancer suggest that the anti A antibody might be protective, or a link with particular polymorphisms increases susceptibility, e.g. to *Helicobacter* infection for gastric cancer [68]. After all this time of speculation, could another spirochaete, e.g. *Borrelia burgdorferi*, be linked with the risk of developing vulval cancer (Fig. 20.11)?

Recommendations for the specialist follow-up of women with LS:
1. Women in whom difficulty exists with symptom control. This includes women who require potent topical corticosteroid application three or more times a week or greater than 30 g of ointment per 6 months for symptom control.
2. Women previously treated for usual- or differentiated-type VIN and/or squamous cell carcinoma of the vulva. Differentiated VIN requires excision.
3. Women with clinical evidence of localised skin thickening/hyperkeratosis require biopsies. If the skin thickening contains carcinoma or precancerous changes, or the thickening is unresponsive to topical steroids, they should be referred.
4. Biopsies where the pathologist expresses 'concern' but cannot make a definite diagnosis of differentiated VIN should be referred. In this setting the clinician can choose between a limited period of intensive medical therapy with follow-up biopsies and excision at the outset [69].

The following mnemonic may be helpful when assessing LS:
L = labial changes (e.g. reduction or fusion)
I = introital changes (e.g. narrowing)
C = clitoral changes including phimosis
H = hyperkeratosis
E = elevated or eroded areas
N = neoplastic or suspicious area with hyperkeratosis or contour changes
S = symptom control

20 Vulval Disease in Postmenopausal Women

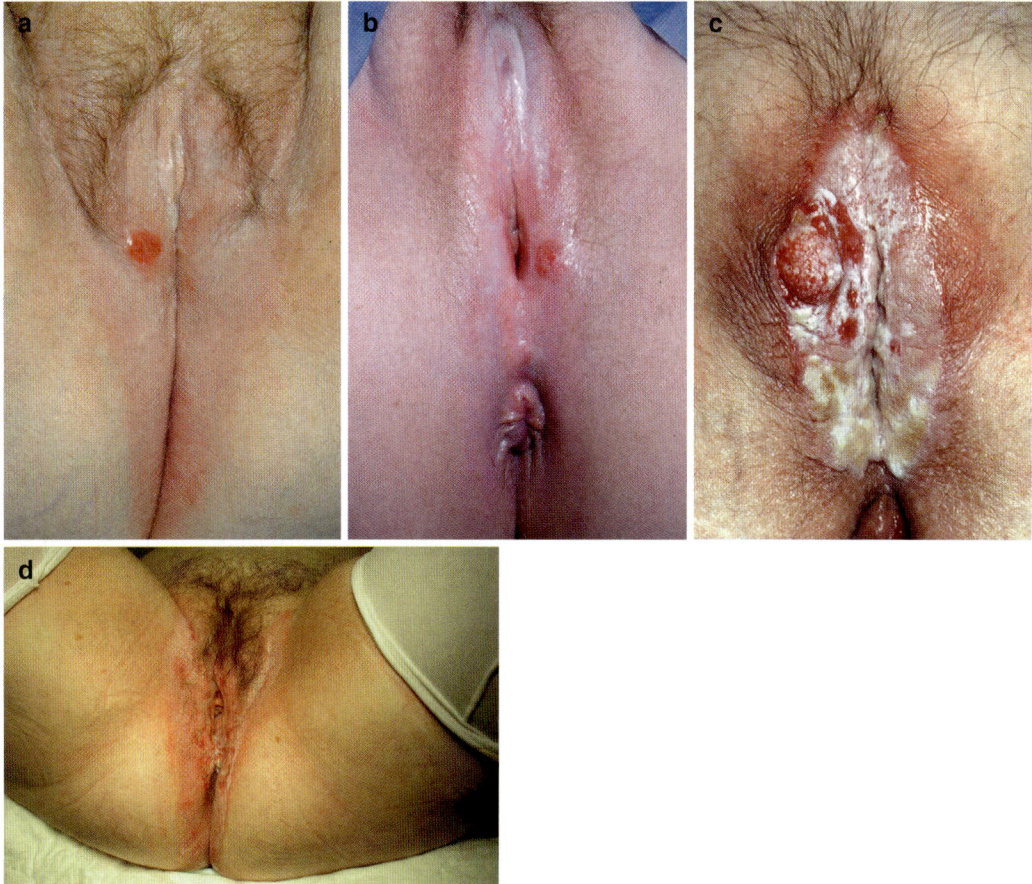

Fig. 20.11 (**a–d**) Examples of vulval cancer occurring in a background of lichen sclerosus

C = colour, usually with pallor but also ecchymoses and haemosiderin
L = localisation, usually central and symmetrical
E = extension posteriorly, causing anal symptoms and constipation
R = rest of the body; involvement elsewhere
O = other autoimmune conditions or associated symptoms
S = sexual difficulties
U = urinary difficulties
S = steroid use and misuse [70]

20.7 Lichen Planus

The lesions of lichen planus may be seen on mucous membranes or on cutaneous surfaces. Involvement of the vulva is usually with white patterned areas that are sometimes elevated and thickened (hypertrophic lichen planus) or may appear red and raw with features of erosion. Changes in the mouth are often seen. The vulval lesions may extend into the vagina where scarring, stenosis and adhesions make intercourse painful or impossible. In a small number of cases, 'crossover' from LS (involving the vulval skin) to lichen planus (involving the vestibule and vaginal mucosa) occurs (Fig. 20.12).

Histology will show liquefactive degeneration of the basal epidermal layer, long and pointed rete ridges, with parakeratosis, acanthosis and a dense dermal infiltrate of lymphocytes close to the dermal epidermal margin.

When the condition is severe, treatment can be difficult, requiring systemic steroids, azathioprine, hydroxychloroquine or other

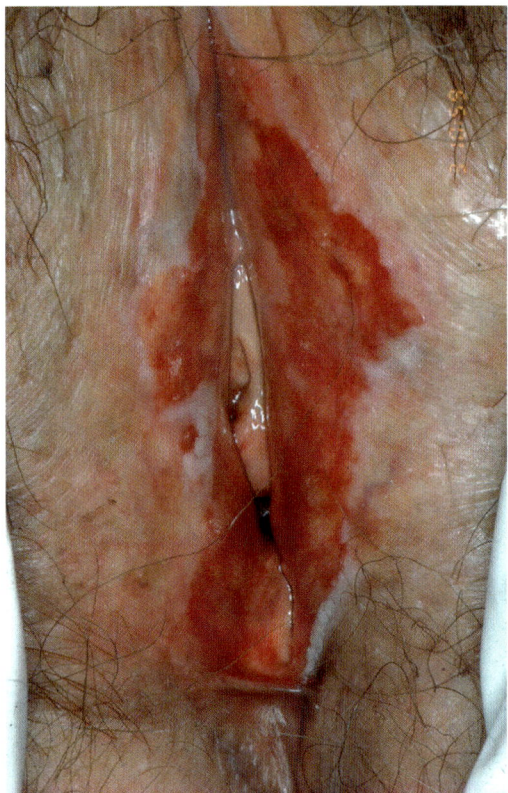

Fig. 20.12 Lichen planus with marked erosion of mucosal areas and loss of architecture

immune-modifying or chemotherapy agents such as methotrexate or mycophenolate mofetil. Lesser symptoms, particularly those externally on the vulva, can be managed with the application of topical corticosteroids; vaginal lesions can be managed with Colifoam (hydrocortisone) or Predfoam (prednisolone).

Rarely, vulval cancer will arise in association with hypertrophic lichen planus [71, 72].

20.8 Vulval Intraepithelial Neoplasia

Although this term sounds closely similar to cervical intraepithelial neoplasia, there are some striking differences. Cervical neoplasia occurs in the transformation zone in association with squamous and columnar epithelium. The cervix has an epithelium where depth of changes can be judged: the vulva is the skin (epidermis) and, in addition to a basal layer which may be convoluted with deep rete ridges, also has a spinous or prickle cell layer, a granular layer and a superficial cornified or keratinised layer. Thus, dividing VIN into VIN 1, VIN 2 and VIN 3 is not easy or reproducible. While CIN 1 is a common biopsy finding and is part of a spectrum with possible progression to CIN 3, VIN 1 is uncommon and does not appear to have neoplastic potential.

The ISSVD Vulval Oncology Subcommittee has made recommendations about the terminology of VIN [61]. They argue that intraepithelial neoplasia of the vulva should be divided into two types: the first, known as VIN of usual (sometimes classic) type, encompasses what was previously VIN 2 and VIN 3 and is almost always associated with oncogenic HPV. These lesions may be pigmented (brown), white (hyperkeratotic) or red in appearance, and the histological features are described as warty, basaloid or mixed – the distinction may not have any prognostic significance, and warty and basaloid features may be seen concurrently in multifocal disease or seen over different examinations. The second is called differentiated VIN, usually seen in older women with LS or squamous cell hyperplasia and not associated with HPV (see above in association with LS) (Fig. 20.13).

Patients with CIN are usually identified by abnormal cervical cytology, whereas women with VIN present with symptoms, including itching, irritation, discomfort or splitting with intercourse in more than 80 %.

We know that when loop excision of the cervix is performed to treat CIN, less than 1 % of specimens will be found with microinvasive carcinoma. However, the chances of finding invasive cancer within the lesions of usual-type VIN range between 15 and 22 %, as summarised by MacLean [54] from data from five publications. Nugent et al. [73] have reported that postmenopausal women with VIN were more likely than premenopausal women to have related carcinoma. The difficulty with recognising invasion is partly because keratinised lesions will not show colposcopically visible features of vessel atypia/

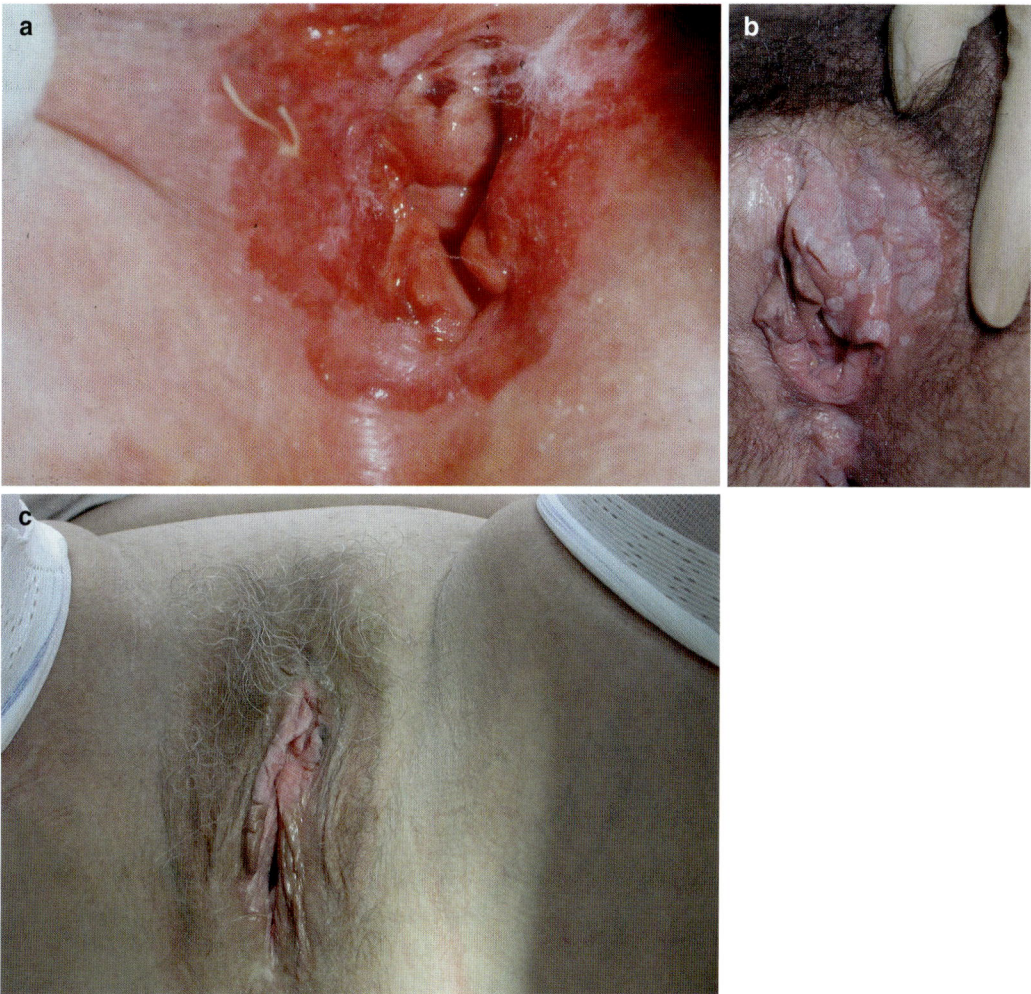

Fig. 20.13 (a–c) Examples of vulval intraepithelial neoplasia

abnormality (angiogenesis) as it does for the cervix. The significance of invasion, even as little as 1 mm below the epidermo-dermal junction of the nearest dermal junction of the nearest papilla, is the increased chance of lymph node metastases; this risk only becomes significant with measurements of more than 3–5 mm from the nearest basement membrane of CIN.

It has been difficult to recruit a large series of patients with VIN who have not been treated, because VIN is usually symptomatic (>80 %) and most patients will accept treatment to control itching, irritation, splitting with coitus, etc.

Jones and Rowan [74] recorded that of 105 women with VIN treated, four developed cancer. However, of eight women left untreated, seven developed cancer within 8 years.

van Seters et al. [75] reviewed data on 3,322 patients with VIN recorded in the published literature and could find 88 untreated patients, of whom 8 (9 %) progressed to invasive cancer. Jones and MacLean [76] have challenged this assumed low risk, partly because the vast majority of reported patients have been treated, partly because the follow-up interval is brief (mean = 33 months) and finally because if seven of the eight untreated patients came from Jones and Rowan [74], one further case of progression occurred in the other 80 untreated patients – this seems an underestimate. There is concern that nontreatment or undertreatment of VIN will pose a significant threat to those women who are older than 30 or who have other risk factors including smoking, multicentric disease, immunosuppression (transplant or HIV-positive patients) or have a lesion encroaching into the anal canal. We acknowledge that regression of VIN can occur in young women. Jones et al. [77] reported regression in 47 women, aged 15–45 (mean 24.6) years with 83 % 30 years or less. Twenty-seven were Polynesian; the lesions were small and papular and mainly multifocal. The median interval for regression was 9.5 months.

There is a growing number of reports that the diagnosis of VIN is increasing [78, 79] with trebling of the incidence reported in some countries. This is partly because of the spread of oncogenic HPV, but also because many young women have been or are still smokers. It is an increasing problem among immunosuppressed women, whether iatrogenic, e.g. with transplant patients, or the use of immunosuppressant therapy for other reasons, or among women infected with human immunodeficiency virus. We are seeing older patients who had treatment to their CIN 20–30 years ago presenting with vulval symptoms and having VIN. Perhaps all postmenopausal women coming for their smears (women in the UK over the age of 50 are offered 5 yearly screening until 65, unless recent smears have been abnormal when screening should continue) should be asked if they have any vulval symptoms; that would use the opportunity to examine without any additional embarrassment for the woman.

The treatment of VIN is complicated because the risk of underlying cancer, the risks of progression to cancer if untreated or undertreated and the associated symptoms must be balanced by every effort being made to preserve form and urinary, coital and anal functions. Several recent studies have warned of the implications of the diagnosis and treatment on the patients' psychosexual health, with increasing age being associated with worsening emotional health and sexual dysfunction [80]. Surgical excision (knife, Light Amplification for the Stimulated Emission of Radiation, diathermy) plus ablation remain the mainstay of treatment. Most patients express high levels of satisfaction following conservation surgery [81]. However, up to 50 % of patients will need at least one further treatment, and the risk of subsequent invasion is 4 % [77]. The immunomodifier imiquimod may have a role in shrinking the lesion's size to allow more complete excision with primary closure.

20.9 Paget's Disease of the Vulva

This is an uncommon lesion with uncertain malignant potential. Its appearance is of an eczematoid lesion with a scaly surface but vague margins, or it may be sharply bordered with a red and velvety texture, with areas or islands of hyperkeratosis. Histology classically shows large round atypical cells with oval nuclei and pale cytoplasm, singly or within clusters among the basal cells of the epidermis. These cells stain positively with cytokeratin 7, PAS and CEA and are regarded by many as carcinoma in situ. Their origin is uncertain; some believe they have migrated from deeper glandular structures, and others believe they are of Toker cell origin. Their similarity to Paget's cells seen in the nipple of the breast, usually with an underlying breast carcinoma, questions their association with cancers. Studies of a large number of vulval Paget's cases report that less than 10 % of cases will have an underlying adenocarcinoma of the vulva arising from an adnexal structure and another 20 % or more will have a carcinoma arising from adjacent viscera including the recto-colon, endocervix or endometrium, ovary, urinary tract or breast. Wilkinson and Brown [82] have proposed a classification that separates the lesions into those where Paget's lesion is in situ without any associated cancer, those with an underlying adenocarcinoma of a skin appendage or a subcutaneous gland and those that are secondary to an underlying anorectal adenocarcinoma, an urothelial cancer or an adenocarcinoma arising from elsewhere (this latter group may be suspected by finding cytokeratin 20 expression in Paget's lesion). A number of cases appear to progress from in situ to invasive adenocarcinomas if left un- or undertreated.

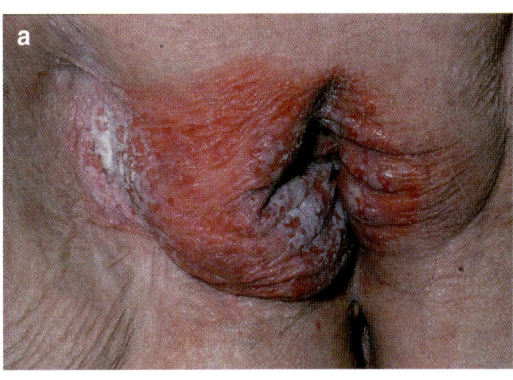
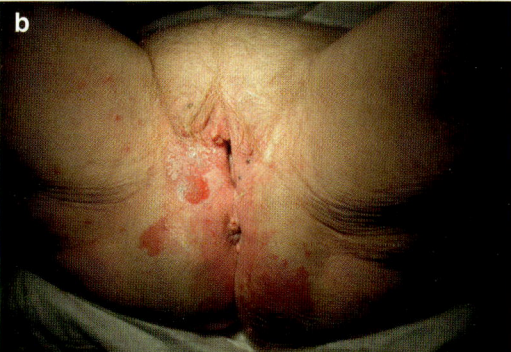

Fig. 20.14 (**a**, **b**) Two examples of Paget's disease of the vulva

Treatment by surgery is complicated with difficulty with primary closure, and plastic and reconstructive surgical techniques will be required. Achieving clear excision margins is difficult, and even when frozen section or definitive histology suggests clearance, recurrence in 50 % or more will occur. Currently there is some enthusiasm for using topical imiquimod, although series are small and follow-up is short [70, 83] (Fig. 20.14).

20.10 Vulval Cancer

As women get older there is an increasing risk of developing cancer and a variety of precancers, e.g. gynaecological cancers of the cervix, endometrium and ovary. In the UK vulval cancer is regarded as a rare cancer and is ranked 20th as the cause of cancer deaths in females (although it still causes more than one death each day), between cancers of the oral cavity (18th), bone and connective tissue (19th), mesothelioma (21st), gallbladder (22nd) and thyroid (23rd). In 2008 there were 1,157 new cases of vulval cancer diagnosed in the UK [84]. What is worrying is that vulval cancer rates are increasing, 20–25 % over the last 25 years. A similar upward trend, with an increasing incidence of vulval (vulvar) cancer of 2.4 % per year, is reported from the USA [85]. We now have one of the highest age-standardised incidences (2.5 per 100,000 female populations) in the world [84, 86]. There is little understanding why some populations with very high incidence of cervical cancer have reduced incidence of vulval cancer (some five- to tenfold variation in age-standardised incidence rates [86]), except it might reflect considerable variation in LS and its malignant potential.

These lesions are not unique to the menopause: vulval cancer in under 50 year olds was only 6 % in 1975, but accounted for 14 % in 2006–2008. However, much of the increase has been in postmenopausal women.

Delays in diagnosis continue to occur, due to patient embarrassment or reluctance to present, delays in referral from primary care and delays in taking an appropriate biopsy once the patient reaches the gynaecology department.

20.10.1 Symptoms and Signs

Cancer Research UK lists the symptoms and signs of vulval cancer as:

1. A lasting itch
2. Pain or soreness
3. Thickened, raised red, white or dark patches
4. An open sore or growth visible
5. Burning pain on passing urine
6. Vaginal discharge or bleeding
7. A spot that changes shape or colour
8. A lump or swelling

Unfortunately this list is not specific and includes symptoms and signs relevant to all (neoplastic and benign) vulval diseases and most gynaecological diseases in general. Among

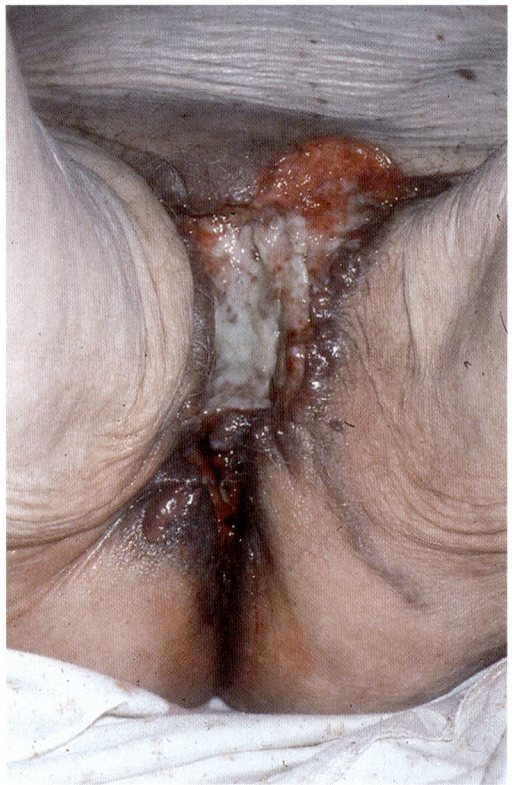

Fig. 20.15 An advanced vulval cancer and fungating inguinofemoral nodal areas diagnosed when patient transferred from a nursing home for transfusion and investigation of anaemia

1,000 women referred to a specialist vulval clinic with the above symptoms, only 26 had vulval cancer [43].

1. A lasting itch. The majority of women who come to vulval clinic have this symptom, although some will use this symptom to include irritation, soreness and rawness. Most women who attend vulval clinics have already used antifungals without benefit, hence a 'lasting itch'. There are many causes of itch or pruritus, and they have been discussed above.
2. Pain or soreness. Vulval cancer is not always painful. Figure 20.15 shows an example of an advanced cancer where the patient denied pain. Vulval pain/vulvodynia is described below.
3. Thickened, raised red, white or dark patches. The colour of vulval lesions does not always give a clue to their nature. However, vulval cancer arises in a background of LS, which is associated with white lesions, or vulval intraepithelial neoplasia, which may be white, red or pigmented. These lesions are described in greater detail above.

   Many vulval lesions will become thickened as the result of scratching (lichenification) and is seen with dermatitis/eczema, lichen simplex chronicus and psoriasis. However there are changes seen with LS and hypertrophic lichen planus with histological confirmation of hyperkeratosis and/or differentiated vulval intraepithelial neoplasia that have neoplastic potential.
4. An open sore or growth. When cancer develops the initial cellular growth is down into the dermis, initiating various events including angiogenic establishment of new vascular supply. As the tumour grows deeper and laterally, its volume increases until the contour of the epidermal surface is elevated and the lesion becomes exophytic. Later, when the tumour outgrows its vascular supply, the centre becomes necrotic and cavitation or ulceration is noted.

There are many benign reasons for epidermal 'growths' including condylomata acuminata, keratoacanthoma and basal cell papilloma, while the vulval contour may be altered by sebaceous cysts, inclusion cysts and soft tissue tumours including fibroepithelial stromal polyps, fibromas, lipomas, granular cell tumours, cellular angiofibromas, angiomyofibroblastomas and aggressive angiomyxomas [70, 87].

Cancer is not the only pathology that produces ulceration. Ulcers may occur commonly, as in the mouth, and are 'aphthae'; they may be seen with herpes simplex viral infection and syphilis, part of the linear or knifelike cuts seen with vulval Crohn's disease or the cavities associated with hidradenitis suppurativa and may be manifestations of Stevens–Johnson syndrome (Fig. 20.16) or Behcet's disease (Fig. 20.7) (include clinical photographs) or consequences of bullous eruptions.

The symptoms of burning with micturition, vaginal discharge or bleeding, a vulval spot that changes shape or colour or a lump or swelling are

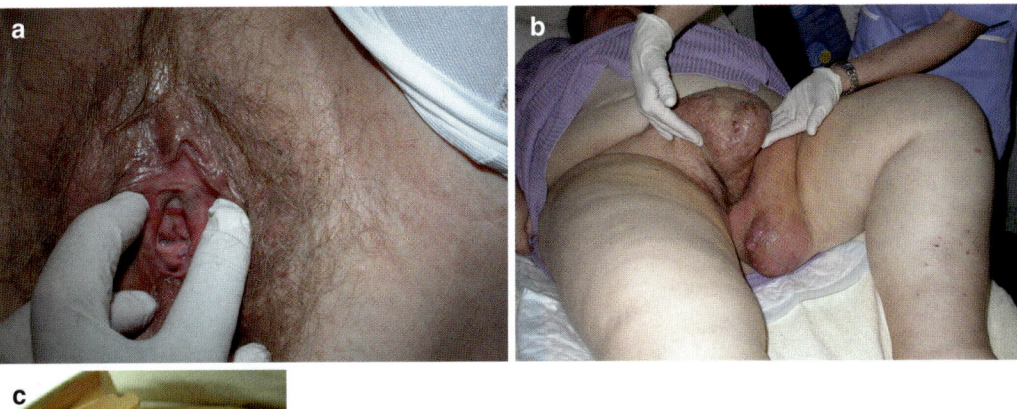
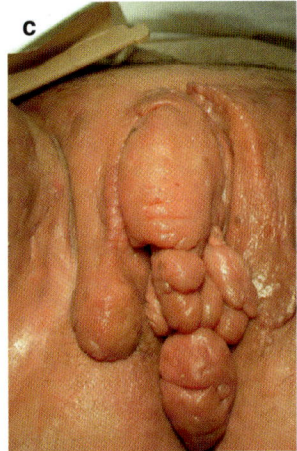

Fig. 20.16 Examples of lesions that might be confused with cancer. (**a**) Stevens–Johnson syndrome. (**b**) Hidradenitis. (**c**) Crohn's disease involving the vulva

even more non-specific. If urine is in contact with any vulval lesion or abraded vulval skin, discomfort can be expected. Vaginal discharge or bleeding may be manifestations of many genital tract pathologies or infections, but may be features of erosive lichen planus or desquamative inflammatory vaginitis. A spot that changes shape or colour might be a melanoma, but the vulval skin is normally hyperpigmented, and alteration (increase or decrease in pigment) may follow many conditions. A lump or swelling could range from a Bartholin's duct cyst or abscess, Gartner's duct cyst, encysted hydrocele of the canal of Nuck or any of the soft tissue swellings include above (Fig. 20.16).

Vulval cancer remains an uncommon cancer, but it should neither be forgotten nor ignored. There is no screening test to detect its precursors other than recognising LS, awareness of a past history of HPV and CIN and the importance of immune suppression. Careful examination and biopsy of suspicious lesions facilitate early diagnosis. However, women must be encouraged to present with and not ignore symptoms, and doctors must be willing to examine.

20.10.2 Vulvodynia

Vulval pain may be acute or chronic, defined as lasting for more than 3 months [88]. It is estimated that up to 16 % of women will have, or have had, vulval pain at some stage in their lifetime [89].

A task force of ISSVD members was formed in 1982 to survey the society's membership of their clinical, laboratory and therapeutic impressions of the 'burning vulva syndrome', and their report contained the following definitions [90]:

> Vulvodynia – chronic vulvar discomfort, especially that characterized by the patient's complaint of burning (and sometimes stinging, irritation or rawness). Vulvodynia should be differentiated from pruritus vulvae, which is associated with chronic itching. Vulvodynia can have multiple etiologies, and use of this term for a patient's problem should prompt a thorough diagnostic evaluation. Burning vulva syndrome (BVS) – vulvodynia of which no physical cause can be found or that persists despite appropriate treatment for associated physical findings. This diagnostic term implies an 'end-stage' condition, recalcitrant to a variety of treatments. Psychogenic factors have been strongly implicated but are not well defined.

Some of the differences between vulvodynia and pruritus vulvae were described in two articles by Marilynne McKay [91, 92], and the term 'essential vulvodynia' appears:

> typically occurs in elderly or postmenopausal patients who complain of diffuse and unremitting genital burning without evidence of vestibulitis or cutaneous changes. These patients describe pain patterns similar to post herpetic neuralgia (post zoster neuralgia) and 'glossodynia' (burning tongue) which suggests a problem with cutaneous perception either centrally or at the nerve root.

Thus, the terminology evolved, and the next report of the ISSVD committee on vulvodynia [93] used a division into subsets:
Vulval vestibulitis
Vestibular papillomatosis (thought to be caused by HPV changes but now recognised as normal microanatomy)
Cyclic vulvitis
Essential vulvodynia
Idiopathic vulvodynia

The most recent terminology and classification from ISSVD [94] is as follows:
(A) Vulval pain related to a specific disorder:
  1. Infectious: candidiasis, herpes infection, etc.
  2. Inflammatory: lichen planus, Crohn's disease, etc.
  3. Neoplastic: cancer, intraepithelial neoplasia, etc.
  4. Neurological: herpes neuralgia, spinal nerve compression, etc.

(B) Vulvodynia:
  1. Generalised:
     (a) Provoked: sexual, non-sexual or both
     (b) Unprovoked
     (c) Mixed: provoked and unprovoked
  2. Localised: vestibulodynia, clitorodynia, hemivulvodynia, etc.:
     (a) Provoked: sexual, non-sexual or both
     (b) Unprovoked
     (c) Mixed: provoked and unprovoked

This classification includes the following footnote:

> Vulvodynia is defined as vulval discomfort, most often described as burning pain, occurring in the absence of relevant visible findings or a specific, clinically identifiable neurological disorder. Specifically, a peripheral neuropathy (e.g., related to herpes zoster or simplex) should be excluded based on the list of associated symptoms, such as sphincter dysfunction, weakness in the lower limbs or sensory changes such as hypoaesthesia or anaesthesia involving the areas of discomfort. Vulvodynia is represented under the term vulval pain syndrome in the classification of the International Society for the Study of Pain. 'Relevant visible findings' takes into account the following considerations: 1. diffuse and periductal vestibular erythema (bilateral, usually symmetrical erythema localised around the openings of Bartholin's glands and minute epithelial depressions) is a normal finding and is therefore not responsible for vulval discomfort. 2. Such disorders as genital warts, naevi, cysts etc. may be present on the vulva but not be relevant (i.e., not necessarily responsible for vulval discomfort). 'Generalised' specifies involvement of the whole vulva, and 'localised' specifies involvement of a portion of the vulva such as the vestibule, clitoris, hemivulva etc. 'Unprovoked' means that the discomfort occurs spontaneously without a specific physical trigger; 'provoked' means that the discomfort is triggered by physical contact.

The latest ISSVD classification has attempted to differentiate those patients with pain due to infection, inflammation, neoplasia and neurological reasons and those with vulvodynia. It is therefore important that appropriate examination, and if necessary biopsy, is made to exclude other pathologies, e.g. lichen planus. Details of clinical findings are described in the relevant sections above [95].

Women with generalised vulvodynia usually have no clinical vulval findings.

Women with dysaesthesia vulvodynia were more likely to have altered tonic, phasic and endurance of pelvic floor muscle contractions when tested with pelvic floor electromyography compared with asymptomatic women [96, 97].

The cause of generalised unprovoked vulvodynia remains uncertain and elusive. It shows features of complex regional pain syndromes and neuropathy. It may tend to be unilateral and follow pudendal nerve distribution, and investigation with MRI will exclude neurological damage to nerve roots or of the nerve as it courses through the pelvis. Nerve damage may reduce the bulk of the pelvic floor muscles on the affected side. Some of these patients are unable to sit comfortably during consultation and pace around the room: presumably sitting increases stretching or stimulus of the pudendal nerve(s).

The nature of the symptoms, i.e. burning, soreness and rawness, shows similarity to postzoster neuralgia or trigeminal neuralgia. Terms such as dysaesthesia, allodynia and hyperaesthesia have been applied. Some patients will blame previous infection, believed to be inadequately treated, or gynaecological surgery for precipitating their problem. Some patients may be taking medication with peripheral neuropathy as a side effect, and several patients have commented that their symptoms were caused by ingestion of alcohol. Attempts to map out the neurological changes are often inconsistent, but may reward the patient in the thoroughness of an examination not usually performed in the gynaecology clinic.

Many of the patients who attend vulval clinics and are found to have 'vulvodynia' express dismay and frustration at the number of doctors they have seen before a diagnosis is offered, the many treatments attempted without apparent improvement and an inevitability of 'suffering pain' for always. It is not surprising that they exhibit psychological and psychosexual features, but it is uncertain as to whether this is the result or the cause of their vulvodynia.

Wylie et al. [98] reported that levels of psychological distress were significantly higher within the domains of somatisation; obsessive–compulsive, anxiety and phobic symptoms; interpersonal sensitivity; hostility; and paranoia among 82 British women with vulvodynia compared with 82 British women in a control group with general dermatology conditions. Women with vulvodynia are found to have worse levels of mental health-related quality of life. Schmidt et al. [99] examined 53 women with vulval dermatoses and vulval pain using quality of life, psychological profiles and general health rating scales including the Skindex questionnaire, Brief Symptom Inventory and a General Severity Index. On average, patients with dysaesthetic vulvodynia had higher scores on all quality of life scales than patients with vestibulitis and dermatoses. The authors commented that chronic pain in an intimate female organ is likely to affect a broad range of emotional functional dimensions of life. Sargeant and O'Callaghan [100] sent questionnaires to 51 women with vulval pain and 46 without and reported significantly worse levels of mental health-related quality of life among the women with pain. Masheb et al. [101] assessed 53 women with vulvodynia and found 9 (17 %) with current major depressive disorders (MDD) and 24 (45 %) with lifetime prevalence. Women with current major depressive disorder reported greater pain severity and worse functioning and quality of life. Among women with lifetime depressive disorder, the majority had their first episode before the onset of vulvodynia. Rates of current depression seemed lower than rates of depression in other women with chronic pain.

Management includes reassurance that more sinister causes of pain have been excluded and advice on bathing and the use of soap substitutes, emollients and sometimes local anaesthetic gel (a test patch applied and viewed on the flexor aspect of the wrist excludes stinging from a contact dermatitis or hypersensitivity). Assessment by a physiotherapist (physical therapist in the US) and the use of biofeedback will help a group of patients. Pain-modifying agents such as from the tricyclic group of antidepressants, e.g. amitriptyline, starting at 10 mg/night and gradually increasing to 50 mg, may reduce pain but sometimes at the expense of anticholinergic side effects, e.g. dry mouth, constipation and sleepiness. Better alternatives include gabapentin, starting at 300 mg per day and slowly and incrementally increasing to 2.7 g/day (more common side effects include altered proprioception, e.g. unable to walk to the toilet at night in the dark and palpitations due to heart block) or pregabalin which is currently more expensive but some claim to be more effective. There have been several patients who have had complete relief after psychosexual or cognitive behavioural therapies, but most patients benefit from a session(s) of listening by their clinician or psychologist (access to clinical psychologists are more difficult and yet for certain women will be hugely beneficial).

Reviews of treatments and results are provided by Nunns [102], Glazer and Ledger [103], Smart and MacLean [104], Bachmann et al. [105], Petersen et al. [106] and Danby and Margesson [88]. Unfortunately, there is no proven therapy that will be effective for all. The frequent requirement for combinations of therapy identifies the need for properly conducted clinical trials.

20.11 Summary

Women of all ages present with vulval symptoms. The menopause has a profound effect on the vagina but much less is known about changes in the vulva. However, it is no longer acceptable to treat a postmenopausal woman with itching for yeast infection or 'atrophy'. With increasing age the chance of significant pathology increases, and therefore all postmenopausal women must be examined. Lichen sclerosus is the most likely diagnosis among our population, but neoplasia must be considered. If the clinician is unable to examine or biopsy adequately, referral to a specialist clinic or consultant must be considered.

References

1. Nappi RE, Kokot-Kierepa M. Vaginal health: insights, views and attitudes (VIVA) – results from an international survey. Climacteric. 2012;15:36–44.
2. Farage MA, Maibach HI, Deliveliotou A, Creatsas G. Changes in the vulva and vagina throughout life. In: Farage MA, Maibach HI, editors. The vulva. New York: Informa Healthcare; 2006.
3. MacBride MB, Rhodes DJ, Shuster LT. Vulvovaginal atrophy. Mayo Clin Proc. 2010;85:87–94.
4. MacLean AB, Nicol LA, Hodgins MB. Immunohistochemical localisation of estrogen receptors in the vulva and vagina. J Reprod Med. 1990;35:1015–6.
5. Hodgins MB, Spike RC, Mackie RM, MacLean AB. An immunohistochemical study of androgen, estrogen and progesterone receptors in the vulva and vagina. Br J Obstet Gynaecol. 1998;105:216–22.
6. Taylor AH, Guzail M, Al-Azzawi F. Differential expression of estrogen receptor isoforms and androgen receptor in the normal vulva and vagina compared with vulval lichen sclerosus and chronic vaginitis. Dermatopathology. 2008;158:318–28.
7. Nieves M-A, Pfaff DW, Kow L-M, Schober JM. Estrogen receptors and their relation to neural receptive tissue of the labia minora. Sex Med. 2008;101:1401–6.
8. Farage MA, Neill S, MacLean AB. Physiological changes associated with the menstrual cycle. Obstet Gynecol Surv. 2009;64:58–72.
9. Cumming GP, Mauelshagen AE, Parrish MH. Postmenopausal sexual dysfunction. Obstet Gynaecol. 2010;12:1–6.
10. Kao A, Binik YM, Amsel R, Funaro D, Leroux N, Khalife S. Biopsychosocial predictors of postmenopausal dyspareunia: the role of steroid hormones, vulvovaginal atrophy, cognitive-emotional factors, and dyadic adjustment. J Sex Med. 2012;9:2066–76.
11. O'Connell HE, Eizenberg N, Rahman M, Cleave J. The anatomy of the distal vagina: towards unity. J Sex Med. 2008;5:1883–91.
12. Alguacil NM, Schober J, Kow L, Pfaff D. Arousing properties of the vulvar epithelium. J Urol. 2006;176:456–62.
13. Komisaruk BR, Adler NT, Hutchinson J. Genital sensory field: enlargement by estrogen treatment in female rats. Science. 1972;178:1295–8.
14. Kow LM, Pfaff DW. Effects of estrogen treatment on the size of receptive field and response threshold of pudendal nerve in the female rat. Neuroendocrinology. 1973;13:299–313.
15. Romanzi LJ, Groutz A, Feroz F, Blaivas JG. Evaluation of female external genitalia sensitivity to pressure/touch: a preliminary prospective study using Semmes-Weinstein monofilaments. Urology. 2001;57:1145–50.
16. Connell K, Guess MK, Bleustein CB, Powers K, Lazarou G, Mikhail M, Melman A. Effects of age, menopause, and comorbidities on neurological function of the female genitalia. Int J Impot Res. 2005;17:63–70.
17. Foster DC, Palmer M, Marks J. Effect of vulvovaginal estrogen on sensorimotor response of the lower genital tract: a randomised controlled trial. Obstet Gynecol. 1999;94:232–7.
18. Verdier-Sevrain S, Bonte F, Gilchrest B. Biology of estrogens in skin: implications for skin aging. Exp Dermatol. 2006;15:83–94.

19. Hall G, Phillips TJ. Estrogen and skin: the effects of estrogen, menopause, and hormone replacement therapy on the skin. J Am Acad Dermatol. 2005;53:555–68.
20. Jones ISC. A histological assessment of normal vulval skin. Clin Exp Dermatol. 1983;8:513–21.
21. Elsner P, Wilhelm D, Maibach HI. Frictional properties of human forearm and vulvar skin: influence of age and correlation with transepidermal water loss and capacitance. Dermatologica. 1990;181:88–91.
22. Elsner P, Wilhelm D, Maibach HI. Mechanical properties of human forearm and vulvar skin. Br J Dermatol. 1990;122:607–14.
23. Farage MA. Vulvar susceptibility to contact irritants and allergens: a review. Arch Gynecol Obstet. 2005;272:167–72.
24. Davey DA. The menopause and postmenopause. In: Dewhurst CJ, editor. Integrated obstetrics and gynecology for postgraduates. 2nd ed. Oxford: Blackwell; 1976.
25. Braude P, Hamilton-Fairley D. Hormonal changes during puberty, pregnancy and the menopause. In: Black M, Ambros-Rudolph C, Edwards L, Lynch P, editors. Obstetric and gynecologic dermatology. London: Mosby Elsevier; Oxford: 2008.
26. Arora S, Veves A, Caballaro E, Smakowski P, LoGerfo FW. Estrogen improves endothelial function. J Vasc Surg. 1998;27:1141–7.
27. Traish AM, Botchevar E, Kim NN. Biochemical factors modulating female genital sexual arousal physiology. J Sex Med. 2010;7:2925–46.
28. Berg RW, Davis CC. Microbial ecology of the vulva. In: Farage M, Maibach HI, editors. The vulva. New York: Informa Healthcare; 2006.
29. Fischer G. Chronic vulvovaginal candidiasis: what we know and what we have yet to learn. Aust J Dermatol. 2012;53:247–54.
30. Hickey RJ, Abdo Z, Zhou X, Nemeth K, Hansmann M, Osborn TW, et al. Effects of tampons and menses on the composition and diversity of vaginal microbial communities over time. BJOG. 2013;120:695–706.
31. Zhang Y, Leung DYM, Nordeen SK, Goleva E. Estrogen inhibits glucocorticoid action via protein phosphatase 5 (PP5) – mediated glucocorticoid receptor dephosphorylation. J Biol Chem. 2009;284:24542–52.
32. Sobel JD. Vulvovaginal candidosis. Lancet. 2007;369:1961–71.
33. Collier F, Smith RC, Morton CA. Diagnosis and management of hidradenitis suppurativa. BMJ. 2013;346:29–32.
34. Meltzer RM. Necrotizing fasciitis and progressive bacterial synergistic gangrene of the vulva. Obstet Gynecol. 1983;61:757–60.
35. MacLean AB. Acetowhite epithelium. Gynecol Oncol. 2004;95:691–4.
36. Van Beurden M, van der Vange N, de Craen AJ, Tjong-A-Hung SP, ten Kate FJ, ter Schegget J, et al. Normal findings in vulvar examination and vulvoscopy. Brit J Obstet Gynaecol. 1997;104:320–4.
37. Edwards L. Evaluation of vulvovaginal disease. In: Black M, Ambros-Rudolph C, Edwards L, Lynch P, editors. Obstetric and gynecologic dermatology. St. Louis: Mosby Elsevier; Oxford: 2008.
38. Lynch PJ, Moyal-Barracco M, Bogliatto F, Micheletti L, Scurry J. 2006 ISSVD classification of vulvar dermatoses: pathological subsets and their clinical correlates. J Reprod Med. 2007;52:3–9.
39. Robinson D, Cardozo L. Urogenital effects of hormone therapy. Best Pract Res Clin Endocrinol Metab. 2003;17:91–104.
40. Calleja-Agius J, Brincat MP. Urogenital atrophy. Climacteric. 2009;12:279–85.
41. Farage MA, Miller KW, Berardesca E, Maibach HI. Incontinence in the aged: contact dermatitis and other cutaneous consequences. Contact Dermatitis. 2007;57:211–7.
42. Haverhoek E, Reid C, Gordon L, Marshman G, Wood J, Selva-Nayagam P. Prospective study of patch testing in patients with vulval pruritus. Aust J Dermatol. 2008;49:80–5.
43. MacLean AB, Roberts DT, Reid WMR. Review of 1000 women seen at two specially designated vulval clinics. Curr Opin Obstet Gynaecol. 1998;8:159–62.
44. Powell J. Paediatric vulval disorders. J Obstet Gynecol. 2006;26:596–602.
45. Leibovitz A, Kaplun V, Saposhnicov N, Habot B. Vulvovaginal examinations in elderly nursing home women residents. Arch Gerontol Geriat. 2000;31:1–4.
46. MacLean AB. Are "non-neoplastic" disorders of the vulva premalignant? In: Luesley DM, editor. Cancer and pre-cancer of the vulva. London: Arnold; 2000.
47. Meyrick-Thomas RH, Ridley CM, MacGibbon DH, Black MM. Lichen sclerosus and autoimmunity—study of 350 women. Br J Derm. 1988;118:41–6.
48. Tasker GL, Wojnarowska F. Lichen sclerosus. Clin Exp Dermatol. 2003;28:128–33.
49. Howard A, Dean D, Cooper S, Kirtshig G, Wojnarowska F. Circulating basement membrane zone antibodies are found in lichen sclerosus of the vulva. Aust J Dermatol. 2004;45:12–5.
50. Oyama N, Chan I, Neill SM, South AP, Wojnarowska F, Kawakami Y, et al. Development of antigen-specific ELISA for circulating autoantibodies to extracellular matrix protein 1 in lichen sclerosus. J Clin Invest. 2004;113:1550–9.
51. Farrell A, Dean D, Millard PR, Charnock FM, Wojnarowska F. Cytokine alterations in lichen sclerosus: an immunohistochemical study. Br J Dermatol. 2006;155:931–40.
52. Neill SM, Lewis FM, Tatnall FM, Cox NH. British Association of Dermatologists' guidelines for the management of lichen sclerosus 2010. Br J Dermatol. 2010;163:672–82.
53. Friedrich EG. Vulvar dystrophy. Clin Obstet Gynecol. 1985;28:178–87.
54. MacLean AB. Vulval cancer: prevention and screening. Best Pract Res Clin Obstet Gynecol. 2006;20:379–95.
55. Jones RW, Sadler L, Grant S, Whineray J, Exeter M, Rowan D. Clinically identifying women with vulvar

lichen sclerosus at increased risk of squamous cell carcinoma: a case control study. J Reprod Med. 2004;49:808–11.
56. Jones RW, Joura EA. Analyzing prior clinical events at presentation in 102 women with vulvar carcinoma: evidence of diagnostic delays. J Reprod Med. 1999;44:766–8.
57. Cooper SM, Gao XH, Powell JJ, Wojnarowska F. Does treatment of vulvar lichen sclerosus influence its prognosis? Arch Dermatol. 2004;140:702–6.
58. Renaud-Vilmer C, Cavelier-Balloy B, Porcher R, Dubertret L. Vulvar lichen sclerosus—effect of long-term application of a potent steroid on the course of the disease. Arch Dermatol. 2004;140:709–12.
59. Edwards L. Lichen sclerosus. In: Black MM, Ambros-Rudolph C, Edwards L, Lynch P, editors. Obstetric and gynecologic dermatology. London: Mosby-Elsevier; Oxford: 2008.
60. Leibowitch M, Neill S, Pelisse M, Moyal-Barracco M. The epithelial changes associated with squamous cell carcinoma of the vulva: a review of the clinical, histological and viral findings in 78 women. Br J Obstet Gynaecol. 1990;97:1135–9.
61. Sideri M, Jones RW, Wilkinson EJ, Preti M, Heller DS, Scurry J, et al. Squamous vulvar intraepithelial neoplasia: 2004 modified terminology, ISSVD Vulvar Oncology Subcommittee. J Reprod Med. 2005;30:807–10.
62. Kagie MJ, Kenter GG, Tollenaar RAE, Hermans J, Trimbos JB, Fleuren GJ. p53 protein overexpression, a frequent observation in squamous cell carcinoma of the vulva and in various synchronous vulva epithelia, has no value as a prognostic parameter. Int J Gynecol Pathol. 1997;16:124–30.
63. Kohlberger PD, Kainz CH, Breitenecker G, Gitsch G, Sliutz G, Kölbl H, et al. Prognostic value of immunohistochemically detected p53 expression in vulvar carcinoma. Cancer. 1995;76:1786–9.
64. Pinto AP, Lin MC, Sheers, Muto MG, Sun D, Crum CP. Allelic imbalance in lichen sclerosus, hyperplasia and intraepithelial neoplasia of the vulva. Gynecol Oncol. 2000;77:171–6.
65. Rolfe KJ, MacLean AB, Crow JC, Benjamin E, Reid WMN, Perrett CW. TP53 mutations in vulval lichen sclerosus adjacent to squamous cell carcinoma of the vulva. Br J Cancer. 2003;89:2249–53.
66. Rolfe KJ, Eva LJ, MacLean AB, Crow JC, Perrett CW, Reid WM. Cell cycle proteins as molecular markers of malignant change in lichen sclerosus. Int J Gynecol Cancer. 2001;11:113–8.
67. Rolfe KJ, Nieto JJ, Reid WM, Perrett CW, MacLean AB. Is there a link between vulval cancer and blood group. Eur J Gynaecol Oncol. 2002;23:111–2.
68. Oba-Shinjo SM, Uno M, Ito LS, Shinjo SK, Marie SK, Hamajima N. Association of Lerwis and Secretor gene polymorphisms and *Helicobacter pylori* seropositivity among Japanese-Brazilians. J Gastroenterol. 2004;39:717–23.
69. Jones RW, Scurry J, Neill S, MacLean AB. Guidelines for the follow-up of women with vulvar lichen sclerosus in specialist clinics. Am J Obstet Gynecol. 2008;198:496.e1.
70. MacLean AB, Reid WMR. Benign disease of the vulva and the vagina. In: Shaw RW, Luesley D, Monga A, editors. Gynecology. 4th ed. London: Churchill Livingstone; 2011.
71. Dwyer CM, Kerr RE, Millan DW. Squamous cell carcinoma following lichen planus of the vulva. Clin Exp Dermtol. 1995;20:171–2.
72. Zaki I, Dalziel KL, Solomonsz FA, Stevens A. The under reporting of skin disease in association with squamous cell carcinoma of the vulva. Clin Exp Dermtol. 1996;21:334–7.
73. Nugent EK, Brooks RA, Barr CD, Case AS, Mutch DG, Massad LS. Clinical and pathologic features of vulvar intraepithelial neoplasia in premenopausal and postmenopausal women. J Low Gen Tract Dis. 2011;15:15–9.
74. Jones RW, Rowan DM. Vulvar intraepithelial neoplasia III: a clinical study of the outcome in 113 cases with relation to the later development of invasive vulvar carcinoma. Obstet Gynecol. 1994;84:741–5.
75. van Seters M, van Beurden M, de Craen AJM. Is the assumed natural history of vulvar intraepithelial neoplasia III based on enough evidence? A systematic review of 3322 published patients. Gynecol Oncol. 2005;97:645–51.
76. Jones RW, MacLean AB. Re: is the assumed natural history of vulvar intraepithelial neoplasia III based on enough evidence? A systematic review of 3322 published patients. Gynecol Oncol. 2006;101:371–2.
77. Jones RW, Rowan DM, Stewart AW. Vulvar intraepithelial neoplasia: aspects of the natural history and outcome in 405 women. Obstet Gynecol. 2005;106: 1319–26.
78. Jones RW, Baranyai J, Stables S. Trends in squamous cell carcinoma of the vulva: the influence of vulvar intraepithelial neoplasia. Obstet Gynecol. 1997;90: 448–52.
79. Joura EA, Losch A, Haider-Angeler MG, et al. Trends in vulvar neoplasia. Increasing incidence of vulvar intraepithelial neoplasia and squamous cell carcinoma of the vulva in young women. J Reprod Med. 2000;45:613–5.
80. Shylasree TS, Karanjgaokar V, Tristram A, Wilkes AR, MacLean AB, Fiander AN. Contribution of demographic, psychological and disease-related factors to quality of life in women with high-grade vulval intraepithelial neoplasia. Gynecol Oncol. 2008;110:185–9.
81. Fong KL, Jones RW, Rowan DM. Women's perception of the outcome of the surgical management of vulvar intraepithelial neoplasia. J Reprod Med. 2008;53:952–4.
82. Wilkinson EJ, Brown H. Vulvar Paget disease of urothelial origin: a report of 3 cases and a proposed classification of vulvar Paget disease. Hum Pathol. 2002;33:549–54.
83. Sanderson P, Innamaa A, Palmer J, Tidy J. Imiquimod therapy for extramammary Paget's disease of the

vulva: a viable non-surgical alternative. J Obstet Gynaecol. 2013;33:479–83.
84. Cancer Research UK website: Vulval cancer incidence statistics. 2010.
85. Howe HL, Wingo PA, Thun MJ, Ries LA, Rosenberg HM, Feigal EG, et al. Annual report to the nation on the status of cancer (1973 through 1998), featuring cancers with increasing trends. J Nat Cancer Inst. 2001;93:824–42.
86. Sankaranarayanan R, Ferlay J. Worldwide burden of gynaecological cancer: the size of the problem. Best Pract Res Clin Obstet Gynaecol. 2006;20:207–25.
87. McCluggage WG. Recent developments in vulvovaginal pathology. Histopathology. 2009;54:156–73.
88. Danby CS, Margesson LJ. Approach to the diagnosis and treatment of vulvar pain. Dermatol Ther. 2010;23: 485–504.
89. Harlow BL, Stewart EG. A population based assessment of chronic unexplained vulvar pain: have we underestimated the prevalence of vulvodynia? J Am Med Womens Assoc. 2003;58:82–8.
90. McKay M. Burning vulva syndrome: report of the ISSVD Task Force. J Reprod Med. 1984;29:457.
91. McKay M. Vulvodynia versus pruritus vulvae. Clin Obstet Gynecol. 1985;28:123–33.
92. McKay M. Vulvitis and vulvovaginitis: cutaneous considerations. Am J Obstet Gynecol. 1991;165:1176–82.
93. McKay M, Frankman O, Horowitz BJ, Lecart C, Micheletti L, Ridley CM, et al. Vulvar vestibulitis and vestibular papillomatosis. Report of the ISSVD Committee on Vulvodynia. J Reprod Med. 1991;36: 413–5.
94. Moyal-Barracco M, Lynch PJ. 2003 ISSVD terminology and classification of vulvodynia: a historical perspective. J Reprod Med. 2004;49:772–7.
95. MacLean AB, Siddiqui G. Terminology and diagnosis of vulval pain. J Obstet Gynaecol. 2013;33:651–4.
96. Glazer HI, Jantos M, Hartmann EH, Swencionis C. Electromyographic comparisons of the pelvic floor in women with dysesthetic vulvodynia and asymptomatic women. J Reprod Med. 1998;43: 959–62.
97. Glazer HI. Dysesthetic vulvodynia. Long-term follow-up after treatment with surface electromyography-assisted pelvic floor muscle rehabilitation. J Reprod Med. 2000;45:798–802.
98. Wylie K, Hallam-Jones R, Harrington C. Psychological difficulties within a group of patients with vulvodynia. J Psychosom Obstet Gynaecol. 2004;25:257–65.
99. Schmidts S, Bauer A, Grief C, Merker A, Elsner P, Strauss B. Vulvar pain. Psychological profiles and treatment responses. J Reprod Med. 2001;46: 377–84.
100. Sargeant HA, O'Callaghan F. Predictors of psychological well-being in a sample of women with vulval pain. J Reprod Med. 2009;54:109–16.
101. Masheb RM, Wang E, Lozano C, Kerns RD. Prevalence and correlates of depression in treatment-seeking women with vulvodynia. J Obstet Gynaecol. 2005;25:786–91.
102. Nunns D. Vulval pain syndromes. Br J Obstet Gynecol. 2000;107:1185–93.
103. Glazer HI, Ledger WJ. Clinical management of vulvodynia. Rev Gynaecol Pract. 2002;2:83–90.
104. Smart OC, MacLean AB. Vulvodynia. Curr Opin Obstet Gynecol. 2003;15:497–500.
105. Bachmann GA, Rosen R, Pinn VW, Utian WH, Ayers C, Basson R, et al. Vulvodynia: a state-of-the-art consensus on definitions, diagnosis and management. J Reprod Med. 2006;51:447–56.
106. Petersen CD, Lundvall L, Kristensen E, Giraldi A. Vulvodynia. Definition, diagnosis and treatment. Acta Obstet Gynecol. 2008;87:893–901.

Vulvodynia in Menopause

Miranda A. Farage, Kenneth W. Miller,
Nancy Phillips, Micheline Moyal-Barracco,
and William J. Ledger

Contents

21.1	**Introduction**	275
21.2	**Definition**	276
21.3	**Epidemiology**	276
21.4	**Vulvodynia and Menopause: Physiological Considerations**	277
21.5	**Diagnosis**	278
21.6	**Treatment**	279
21.6.1	Vulvar Care Measures	279
21.6.2	Topical Medications	280
21.6.3	Oral Medications	280
21.6.4	Botox	281
21.6.5	Physical Therapy	281
21.6.6	Counseling	281
21.6.7	Additional Treatment Options	281
21.7	**Surgery**	282
21.8	**Special Consideration of the Menopausal Woman**	282
21.9	**Summary**	282
References		282

M.A. Farage, MSc, PhD (✉)
Clinical Innovative Sciences, The Procter
and Gamble Company, 6110 Center Hill Avenue,
Cincinnati, OH 45224, USA
e-mail: Farage.m@pg.com

K.W. Miller, PhD
Global Product Stewardship, The Procter
and Gamble Company, Cincinnati, OH, USA
e-mail: Miller.kw.1@pg.com

21.1 Introduction

Vulvodynia is a chronic pain condition impacting women's psychosexual well-being, self-esteem, and quality of life. Vulvodynia is frequently underdiagnosed and therefore inadequately managed. Despite research efforts, the pathophysiology remains unclear, and there are no evidence-based treatment guidelines. A multifaceted treatment of vulvodynia is therefore advocated, including pharmacological, physical, and psychosocial measures. Even less information is available for vulvodynia in menopausal women, who have considerable physiologic, anatomic, and functional differences compared to premenopausal women. This chapter will review vulvodynia with special consideration for the menopausal population.

N. Phillips, MD
Department of Obstetrics, Gynecology
and Reproductive Science, Rutgers-Robert
Wood Johnson Medical School,
125 Paterson Street, New Brunswick, NJ 08901, USA
e-mail: phillina@rwjms.rutgers.edu

M. Moyal-Barracco, MD
Department of Dermatology,
Hôpital Tarnier Cochin, Paris, France
e-mail: micheline@barracco.net

W.J. Ledger, MD
Department of Obstetrics and Gynecology,
Weill Medical College,
New York, NY, USA
e-mail: wjledger@med.cornell.edu

Table 21.1 Classification of vulvodynia

Definition		Generalized[a]	Localized[b]
Provoked	Present only with contact, sexual or nonsexual	✓	✓
Unprovoked	Present without contact	✓	✓
Mixed	Provoked & unprovoked	✓	✓

[a]Involvement of the entire vulva
[b]Involvement of a portion of the vulva, such as the vestibule
Adapted from Moyal-Barracco and Lynch [1]

21.2 Definition

The International Society for the Study of Vulvovaginal Disease (ISSVD) defines *vulvodynia* as vulvar discomfort, most often described as burning pain, occurring in the absence of relevant visible findings (either infectious, inflammatory, or neoplastic) or of a specific clinically identifiable neurologic disorder. The pain is chronic, and women often see many health-care providers prior to proper diagnosis and the initiation of appropriate treatment.

Vulvodynia is classified as (1) localized or generalized and (2) provoked, unprovoked, or both (Table 21.1) [1, 2]. In localized vulvodynia, the pain occurs in a specific location on the vulva, most frequently the vestibule, at the entrance to the vagina (vestibulodynia). More rarely, the pain is confined to the clitoris or to other parts of the vulva such as labia majora or minora. In generalized vulvodynia, the pain affects the entire vulvar region. The discomfort of both localized and generalized vulvodynia is further subdivided as either provoked, unprovoked, or both [1, 3]. Provoked pain is caused by contact with the affected area (e.g., sexual intercourse, tampon insertion, tight clothing), whereas unprovoked pain is present commonly without any direct contact. Provoked *vestibulodynia* is the most common subset of vulvodynia. Generalized unprovoked vulvodynia and other subsets are less frequently encountered [4].

While the earliest accounts describing symptoms of vulvodynia were found even in the first century [5], the term "vulvodynia" was suggested by Tovell and Young in 1978 [6]. Later in 1987, Dr. Edward Friedrich coined the term "vulvar vestibulitis" along with the diagnostic criteria known as Friedrich's criteria. These criteria include (1) severe pain in the vulvar vestibule upon touch or attempted vaginal entry, (2) tenderness to pressure localized within the vulvar vestibule, and (3) vulvar erythema of various degrees [7]. From 1987 to 2003, different definitions and classifications of vulvodynia were discussed, including vulvar dermatoses, vulvitis (cyclic candidiasis), vulvar papillomatosis, essential vulvodynia, dysesthetic vulvodynia, and vulvar vestibulitis syndrome (VVS) [8]. The confusion was the result of disagreement as to whether vulvodynia was a symptom (secondary to infection, inflammation, neoplasm, etc.) or a primary disorder. The 17th Congress of the ISSVD established the current definition and classification system of vulvodynia 2003, published in 2004 [1]. This classification separated chronic vulvar pain into two categories: (1) vulvar pain due to identifiable medical causes and (2) vulvar pain in the absence of any known medical cause.

21.3 Epidemiology

Estimates of the prevalence of vulvodynia range from 4 to 16 % over a woman's lifetime [9, 10]. In response to a self-administered questionnaire sent to ethnically diverse women in Boston, 16 % of respondents reported a history of burning vulvar pain for at least 3 months, and 7 % had the pain at the time of the survey [9]. A population-based survey in southeastern Michigan reported that 8.5 % of women over the age of 18 years were currently suffering with vulvodynia [10], and a New Jersey study found a 9.9 % lifetime prevalence with 3.8 % of respondents reporting current pain [11].

The occurrence of vulvodynia may be underestimated because of frequent misdiagnosis. Both physicians and affected women are frequently not aware of this condition; they either persistently or even desperately look for an organic cause to the symptoms or dismiss it as a psychological "all in the head" issue. In the Boston survey, 40 % of symptomatic women chose to not seek treatment, and those who did often saw three or four physicians without a correct diagnosis [9].

Vulvodynia affects both reproductive and nonreproductive-aged women; however, statistics of vulvodynia in postmenopausal women are lacking. In a large population-based sample ($N=12,435$), Harlow showed that 64 % of patients with vulvodynia were aged between 18 and 35, 22 % between 45 and 54, and 14 % between 55 and 64 [12]. Most of the patients with provoked vestibulodynia (the most frequent pattern of vulvodynia) are premenopausal, the mean age being 27.8 years old in a recent study [13]. Unprovoked vulvodynia is more likely to occur in postmenopausal women; in a series of 159 patients with unprovoked, most frequently generalized, vulvodynia, the mean age was 56 (Moyal-Barracco M, unpublished data).

Menopausal women with chronic vulvar pain are frequently diagnosed with vulvovaginal atrophy (VVA). A 2013 Internet-based survey of postmenopausal women designed to assess the effects of VVA found 44 % of respondents experienced dyspareunia and 37 % experienced vulvar irritation ($N=3046$). Although the most common symptom was vaginal dryness (55 %), the study suggests a definite need for evaluation and treatment of postmenopausal women with vulvovaginal symptoms [14]. Genital atrophy due to loss of estrogen is not the only cause of vulvar discomfort in menopausal women, and likely evaluation of women with these complaints will also uncover other etiologies such as vulvodynia. Though the onset of vulvodynia is usually during reproductive years, it may persist or even start in the postmenopausal years. Postmenopausal women complaining of persisting discomfort in the absence of visible findings, despite treatment with hormonal replacement therapy either local or systemic or both, should be considered to possibly suffer from vulvodynia [15].

21.4 Vulvodynia and Menopause: Physiological Considerations

The age-related morphological and physiological changes of the vulva and vagina over a lifetime are well established, as is the hormonal mediation of these events [16]. At birth, the vulva and vagina exhibit the effects of residual maternal estrogens which dissipate by the fourth postnatal week [17, 18]. During puberty, adrenal and gonadal steroid hormones induce maturation of these tissues [19], which continue to undergo changes during the reproductive years, linked to the menstrual cycle and pregnancy [20]. At menopause, there is a dramatic loss of estrogen, which leads to vulvar and vaginal atrophy. Pubic hair becomes sparse, the labia majora loses subcutaneous fat, and the skin of the vulva thins. The vaginal mucosa loses glycogen, with a subsequent rise in the vaginal pH and decrease of vaginal secretions. Decreased vaginal blood flow and pelvic floor muscle tone also occurs [21–23]. Symptoms are variable among women, but may include dyspareunia, irritation, burning, or itching [24]. As such, the symptoms of VVA may mimic those of vulvodynia.

Perimenopause, the transition period to menopause, usually begins at the median age of 45 years and lasts for about 4 years. Perimenopause is characterized by menstrual cycle irregularity, with an increase in the number of anovulatory cycles. The symptoms vary and include cramps, bloating, and breast tenderness as well as hot flashes, migraine, and vaginal dryness [25]. Menopause is established 1 year after the last menstrual period [26].

Estrogens also affect many levels of the pain pathway, including the tissue inflammatory response, sensory neurons and dorsal root ganglia, spinal cord, supraspinal centers such as opioidergic/

serotonergic pain modulation systems, limbic circuits for affective states, and stress responses [27]. Estrogen receptors present in the central and peripheral nervous systems are known to influence all aspects of neural activity from membrane permeability to gene regulation. The transition into menopause, with the accompanying change in systemic estrogen concentration, may therefore affect chronic pain [22].

21.5 Diagnosis

The evaluation of postmenopausal women with vulvar pain includes a detailed history and a targeted physical exam. Vulvodynia should always be considered in the differential diagnosis. The history should document the nature of the pain, onset, severity, and effect on everyday life and/or sexual function. In addition to dyspareunia and pain provoked by any local contact, women with provoked vulvodynia may report constant or intermittent spontaneous discomfort such burning, aching, rawness, or irritation [28]. Vaginal symptoms including discharge, bleeding, should be sought. Nongenital menopausal symptoms, all medications, and all vulvar contacts (soaps, detergents, over-the-counter products) should be reviewed. Recent research has shown increasing evidence for comorbidity of vulvodynia and other chronic pain conditions such as fibromyalgia, interstitial cystitis, temporomandibular joint and muscle disorder (TMD), and irritable bowel syndrome [29] (Figs. 21.1 and 21.2). As such, patients with vulvar pain should be asked about symptoms related to these pain disorders as their presence may heighten the concern for vulvodynia.

A careful inspection of the vulva and vagina should be undertaken aiming at ruling out an inflammatory, infectious, or neoplastic cause of the pain and to sustain the diagnosis of provoked vulvodynia through the cotton swab test. For instance, the pain of provoked vestibulodynia is elicited by lightly touching the vestibule with a moistened cotton swab.

The presence of vulvar lesions does not exclude the diagnosis of vulvodynia. For example, the presence of psoriasis or warts on one labium majus cannot be held responsible for a spontaneous diffuse chronic burning vulvar pain or for an introital dyspareunia. Indeed vulvodynia may be associated with other nonrelevant conditions. In addition, anatomic variants such as vestibular papillae, Fordyce's granules, or vestibular erythema should not be misinterpreted as causes of vulvar pain. As opposed to abnormal vestibular erythemas, physiological vestibular erythemas are macular (not raised), focal (posterior part of the vestibule, particularly around the openings of the Bartholin's gland), symmetrical, and have ill-defined borders.

Pelvic exams should include palpation of the levator muscles to assess muscle spasm, bladder, and urethra for tenderness and bimanual exam

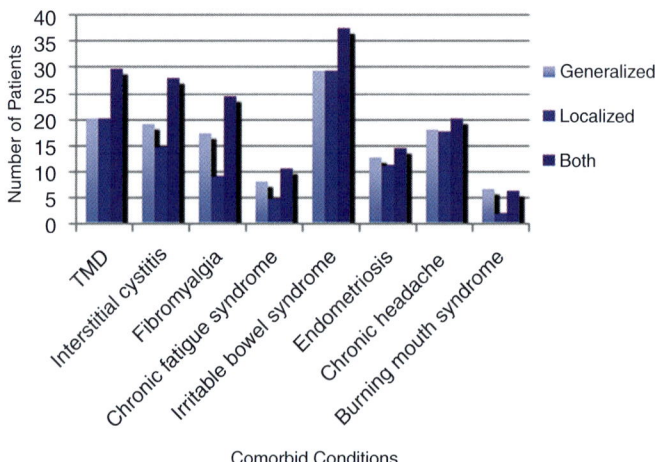

Fig. 21.1 Distribution of the eight comorbid conditions in each of the three types of vulvodynia (generalized, local, and both) in 1,457 women with self-reported vulvodynia. *TMD* temporomandibular joint, and muscle disorder (Source of data is Ref. [29])

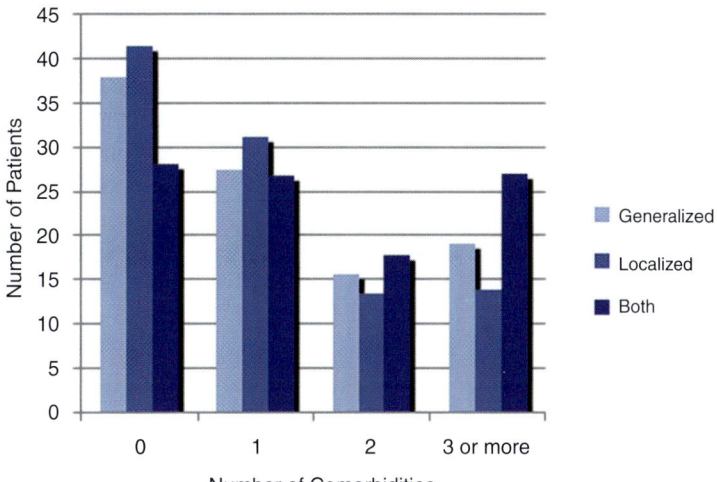

Fig. 21.2 Number of comorbidities in women with the three types of vulvodynia. Based on comorbidities in Fig. 21.1 (Source of data is Ref. [29])

to exclude pelvic pathology. Neurologic exam includes a search for sphincter disturbances (urinary, anal) by history taking and search for objective neurologic abnormalities such as anesthesia or hypoesthesia and perineal reflex abolition such as the "anal wink;" that is, scratching the perianal area gently with the sharp end of a cotton swab and observing the contracture of the external anal sphincter.

In the absence of any visible vulvar lesions or skin changes, a biopsy is not indicated and would not aid in the diagnosis of vulvodynia. In a menopausal woman, vulvovaginal atrophy is one of the possible causes of provoked vulvar pain, and signs such as loss of pubic hair, labial flattening or fusion, loss of vaginal rugae, or an elevated pH should be documented. In VVA, a vaginal wet prep would show an increase in vaginal parabasal cells and white blood cells without evidence of any pathogens such as yeast or bacterial vaginosis. Addition of a drop of Wright's stain to the wet prep will more clearly define the presence of parabasal cells. Vaginal cultures should be sent if evidence of infection is present. Vaginal specimens should be systematically taken to look for infection either responsible for or associated with the pain.

In menopausal women complaining from dyspareunia, a trial of topical estrogen (in the absence of contraindications) should be the first-line treatment especially if there is evidence of VVA on exam. If symptoms do not resolve with these measures, treatments for vulvodynia should be initiated. Spontaneous diffuse vulvar burning is not a manifestation of VVA and, in the absence of relevant findings, is more likely related to vulvodynia.

21.6 Treatment

There is no "one size fits all" treatment of vulvodynia. Experts agree that a multifaceted treatment is the best approach to this condition [30, 31]. Choices will depend on the patient, her partner, the local health-care system, and the costs. Vulvar care measures, pharmacological treatments (both topical and oral); physical therapy; and personal, couple, or sexual counseling, are all possible components of successful treatment.

The National Vulvodynia Association (NVA) is an excellent source for educational materials which actively promotes support for these patients (www.nva.org).

21.6.1 Vulvar Care Measures

Gentle genital hygiene is important to prevent irritation which may aggravate vulvodynia. The vulva should be washed with plain warm water only or with a gentle, unscented soap and then patted dry. Vulvar irritants such as bath salts or

Table 21.2 Treatment guidelines for vulvodynia in menopause

Comorbidity	Vulvovaginal atrophy should be adequately treated prior to and during vulvodynia treatment
Multiple treatments	Only one treatment should be introduced at a time
Dosage	Medications should be started at the lowest dose and titrated upwards slowly. In older women, a longer interval between advancing doses can be considered
Documentation	Patient pain diaries and examinations with specific pain location and severity recorded in the patients chart will help document response and guide treatment
Adjunct therapy	Physical therapy is a helpful adjunct to medical therapy
Counseling options	Counseling should be offered (individual, couple, sexual) as appropriate
Surgery	Surgery should be reserved for localized vestibulodynia only after failure of medical therapy and careful evaluation of risks and benefits

Adapted from Phillips and Bachman [28]

over-the-counter feminine hygiene products, such as douches, sprays, and scented wipes, should be avoided. Ice packs (easily made by freezing water in a 16 oz. plastic soda or water bottle) can be applied through clothing for temporary relief. Adequate lubrication during intercourse and vaginal moisturizers for noncoital lubrication should be encouraged [33] (Table 21.2).

21.6.2 Topical Medications

Lidocaine anesthetic ointment can be used both for symptomatic relief and to reduce coital pain in women with localized vestibulodynia. Lidocaine gel 5 % applied externally 10–20 min prior to intercourse aids in reducing pain with penetration with minimal effect on overall sexual sensation in many women. Direct application to the clitoris should be avoided. One study showed that daily applications of topical lidocaine were equally effective as biofeedback in relieving symptoms at 12 months [34], whereas in another double-blind, placebo-controlled study, lidocaine failed to improve vulvodynia symptoms more than placebo when applied four times a day for 12 weeks [35]. Many topical medications have been used anecdotally or shown to be effective in small studies or case series. These include 2–6 % gabapentin formulation [36], compounded topical estradiol 0.03 % with testosterone 0.1 % [37], capsaicin [38], amitriptyline 2 % cream (sometimes combined with baclofen 2 %) [39], or nifedipine cream [40]. None of these treatments are evidence based, and all of these treatments are off-label for the treatment of vulvodynia.

Intolerance to topical treatments is common. Although contact dermatitis has been documented [41], discomfort (mostly burning) following topical applications is related neither to an allergy nor to an irritation. Diluting topical preparations with tolerated substances, such as lubricating gels, estrogen creams, and mineral or vegetable oils, may be helpful.

21.6.3 Oral Medications

Oral medications for vulvodynia are aimed at the treatment of neurogenic pain. The most frequently prescribed treatment is the tricyclic antidepressants, amitriptyline, desipramine, or nortriptyline. The latter two have a more favorable side effect profile with less sedation and anticholinergic effects. Documentation of a normal electrocardiogram (ECG) is recommended by some in patients over the age of 50. Dosage is started low, usually at 10 mg at night and slowly titrated upward by 10 mg every 1–2 weeks until relief is achieved. Generally, if there is no relief at a dosage of 75 mg, then treatment is discontinued. Patients must not stop tricyclics abruptly.

Gabapentin has been shown in small studies to provide relief for vulvodynia with fewer side effects than the tricyclic antidepressants. Gabapentin 100 mg at bedtime increased by 100 mg every 2–7 days to a maximum of 3,600 mg/day in divided doses is one treatment regimen. Side effects include nausea and sedation. Gabapentin was put on the Food and Drug Administration (FDA) MedWatch list for rare reports of rhabdomyolysis (2011) [42]. Patients should be informed to call with any muscle aches or pains or new-onset dark urine for evaluation. A randomized controlled trial is currently ongoing [43].

Other medications used in the treatment of vulvodynia include pregabalin (titrated slowly to a maximal dose of 600 mg daily in divided doses), venlafaxine (37.5 mg initially to a maximum daily dose of 375 mg), and duloxetine (20–60 mg daily). None of these treatments have an evidence-based efficacy [44], and a high and potentially serious side effect profile limits their use.

21.6.4 Botox

Botulinum neurotoxin type A (Botox) injections into the vestibule seems to be a safe and effective treatment of provoked vestibulodynia [45, 46]. This treatment has been used in small numbers of women in two randomized trials. Botox is postulated to relieve both the muscular hyperactivity of the perineum and to reduce the pain through a blockage of the release of neuropeptides and neurotransmitters. Cost may prove to be a limiting factor of this treatment.

21.6.5 Physical Therapy

Patients with provoked vestibulodynia, compared to non-affected women, have pelvic floor muscle hypertonicity (i.e., increased tension) [47], which may exacerbate or propagate the condition. Pelvic floor physical therapy has been shown to provide vulvovaginal pain relief and improve sexual functioning. Patients report a physical, emotional, and sexual improvement with physical therapy, especially if it is part of a multifaceted treatment approach [48–50]. Pelvic floor physiotherapists utilize internal and external soft tissue mobilization and massage, release of trigger points, biofeedback, and postural exercises. Patients are provided with at-home exercises which help shorten the course of treatment. Medical professionals can provide instructional exams for patients, demonstrating muscle relaxation and contraction and/or advice vaginal dilators for women in addition to physical therapy or for those women who cannot or choose not to use physical therapy. No study has been carried out to evaluate the efficacy of physiotherapy in unprovoked vulvodynia. Spinal cord stimulation and transcutaneous electrical nerve stimulation are less frequently used to treat vulvodynia [51, 52].

21.6.6 Counseling

Psychological, sexual, and relationship disturbances are frequently encountered in patients with vulvodynia. Often these conditions are secondary to the ongoing pain, and therapy is part of the multifaceted management of vulvodynia, either provoked or unprovoked [30–32]. Cognitive behavioral therapy that involves learning and practice of specific pain-relevant coping and self-management skills was shown to yield better outcomes and greater patient satisfaction in patients with vulvodynia than a less directive approach [53, 54]. Additionally, cognitive behavioral therapy (CBT) was shown to result in similar outcomes as electromyographic biofeedback and vestibulectomy), including significantly reduced pain and improved psychological adjustment and sexual function [55]. Individual, couple, or sexual counseling should be recommended as appropriate. Again, the National Vulvodynia Association (NVA) is an excellent source for educational materials for these patients (www.nva.org).

21.6.7 Additional Treatment Options

The effect of acupuncture and other alternative therapies on pain and psychosexual adjustment requires further investigation [56]. Local or regional nerve blocks have been shown in small studies to be effective in the treatment of vulvodynia [57]. Combinations of anesthetics (lidocaine, bupivacaine) and steroids (triamcinolone acetonide, methylprednisolone) are infiltrated locally, via a pudendal nerve block or via caudal epidural injections. Repetitive treatments may be necessary.

21.7 Surgery

Surgical management of vulvodynia has been advocated only for provoked vestibulodynia, and all experts agree that surgery should never be the first-line treatment [58]. Many experts however do not recommend this treatment at all. Although a wide variety of surgical procedures have been advocated [59–64], randomized trials with appropriate short- and long-term outcome measures are lacking. Complete improvement of dyspareunia occurred globally in 60 % of the published studies with rates varying from 0 to 100 % [65]. A recent meta-analysis of surgical outcomes for vestibulodynia estimated a 31–100 % effect rate with a median of 79 % who reported partial to complete relief [66]. There is no data looking at surgical outcomes in postmenopausal women.

21.8 Special Consideration of the Menopausal Woman

All treatments for vulvodynia are off-label. In older women, there are potentially more risks in treatment than in their younger counterparts. Older patients are more likely to have chronic medical conditions, to be on one or more medications, or to be more affected by side effects such as sedation or dry mouth or eyes. Slower upward titrations of medications or more frequent monitoring may be necessary. Primary care or specialist consultation should be sought as needed, especially prior to initiation of medications.

Vulvovaginal atrophy is a condition secondary to the lack of estrogen, present in a large percentage of postmenopausal women. Local estrogen or nonhormonal moisturizers should be used to correct the vulvovaginal atrophy which could be the only cause of introital dyspareunia or an aggravating factor in a patient suffering from provoked vestibulodynia. Estrogen therapy should be continued throughout vulvodynia treatment. Estrogen topical creams, vaginal inserts, or rings can be used.

21.9 Summary

Vulvodynia is a chronic and potentially debilitating pain condition. Though vulvodynia is more common during the reproductive years, there is clear evidence that this condition may affect menopausal women. The etiology of vulvodynia remains unknown, and evidence-based treatment options are not available. Little data exists on vulvodynia in menopausal women; however, evidence suggests that menopausal changes may have an effect on chronic pain conditions. The management of vulvodynia in menopause should include a multifaceted approach with special attention to the correction of estrogen deficiency and to the specific psychosexual and social context of menopause.

References

1. Moyal-Barracco M, Lynch PJ. 2003 ISSVD terminology and classification of vulvodynia: a historical perspective. J Reprod Med. 2004;49(10):772–7.
2. Danby CS, Margesson LJ. Approach to the diagnosis and treatment of vulvar pain. Dermatol Ther. 2010;23(5):485–504.
3. Haefner HK, Collins ME, Davis GD, Edwards L, Foster DC, Hartmann EDH, et al. The vulvodynia guideline. J Low Genit Tract Dis. 2005;9(1):40–51.
4. Edwards L. Subsets of vulvodynia: overlapping characteristics. J Reprod Med. 2004;49(11):883–7.
5. McElhiney J, Kelly S, Rosen R, Bachmann G. Satyriasis: the antiquity term for vulvodynia? J Sex Med. 2006;3(1):161–3.
6. Tovell HM, Young AWJ. Classification of vulvar diseases. Clin Obstet Gynecol. 1978;21(4):955–61.
7. Friedrich EGJ. Vulvar vestibulitis syndrome. J Reprod Med. 1987;32(2):110–4.
8. Masheb RM, Nash JM, Brondolo E, Kerns RD. Vulvodynia: an introduction and critical review of a chronic pain condition. Pain. 2000;86(1–2):3–10.

9. Harlow BL, Stewart EG. A population-based assessment of chronic unexplained vulvar pain: have we underestimated the prevalence of vulvodynia? J Am Med Womens Assoc. 2003;58(2):82–8.
10. Reed BD, Harlow SD, Sen A, Legocki LJ, Edwards RM, Arato N, et al. Prevalence and demographic characteristics of vulvodynia in a population-based sample. Am J Obstet Gynecol. 2012;206((2):170.e1–9.
11. Arnold LD, Bachmann GA, Rosen R, Rhoads GG. Assessment of vulvodynia symptoms in a sample of US women: a prevalence survey with a nested case control study. Am J Obstet Gynecol. 2007;196(2):128. e1–6.
12. Harlow BL, Vazquez G, MacLehose RF, Erickson DJ, Oakes JM, Duval SJ. Self-reported vulvar pain characteristics and their association with clinically confirmed vestibulodynia. J Womens Health (Larchmt). 2009;18(9):1333–40.
13. Bois K, Bergeron S, Rosen NO, McDuff P, Grégoire C. Sexual and relationship intimacy among women with provoked vestibulodynia and their partners: associations with sexual satisfaction, sexual function, and pain self-efficacy. J Sex Med. 2013;10(8):2024–35.
14. Kingsberg SA, Wysocki S, Magnus L, Krychman ML. Vulvar and vaginal atrophy in post-menopausal women: findings from the REVIVE (REal Women's VIews of Treatment Options for Menopausal Vaginal ChangEs) survey. J Sex Med. 2013;10(7):1790–9.
15. Bachmann G, Rosen RC. Vulvodynia and Menopause. Menopause Manag. 2006;15(2):14–21.
16. Farage M, Maibach H. Lifetime changes in the vulva and vagina. Arch Gynecol Obstet. 2006;273(4):195–202.
17. Altchek A. Vulvovaginitis, vulvar skin disease, and pelvic inflammatory disease. Pediatr Clin N Am. 1981;28(2):397–432.
18. Elvik SL. Vaginal discharge in the prepubertal girl. J Pediatr Health Care. 1990;4(4):181–5.
19. Marshall WA, Tanner JM. Variations in pattern of pubertal changes in girls. Arch Dis Child. 1969;44(235):291–303.
20. Wagner G, Ottesen B. Vaginal physiology during menstruation. Ann Intern Med. 1982;96(6 Pt 2):921–3.
21. Burger HG. The menopausal transition. Baillieres Clin Obstet Gynaecol. 1996;10(3):347–59.
22. Griebling TL, Liao Z, Smith PG. Systemic and topical hormone therapies reduce vaginal innervation density in post-menopausal women. Menopause. 2012;19(6):630–5.
23. Notelovitz M, Mattox JH. Suppression of vasomotor and vulvovaginal symptoms with continuous oral 17beta-estradiol. Menopause. 2000;7(5):310–7.
24. Kao A, Binik YM, Kapuscinski A, Khalife S. Dyspareunia in post-menopausal women: a critical review. Pain Res Manag. 2008;13(3):243–54.
25. Erickson KL, Montagna W. New observations on the anatomical features of the female genitalia. J Am Med Womens Assoc. 1972;27(11):573–81.
26. Ginsberg J. What determines the age at the menopause? BMJ. 1991;302(6788):1288–9.
27. Craft RM, Mogil JS, Aloisi AM. Sex differences in pain and analgesia: the role of gonadal hormones. Eur J Pain. 2004;8(5):397–411.
28. Phillips N, Bachman G. Vulvodynia: an often-overlooked cause of dyspareunia in the menopausal population. Menopausal Med. 2010;18(2):S1. S3–S5.
29. Nguyen RH, Veasley C, Smolenski D. Latent class analysis of comorbidity patterns among women with generalized and localized vulvodynia: preliminary findings. J Pain Res. 2013;6:303–9.
30. Nunns D, Mandal D, Byrne M, McLelland J, Rani R, Cullimore J, et al. Guidelines for the management of vulvodynia. Br J Dermatol. 2010;162(6):1180–5.
31. Backman H, Widenbrant M, Bohm-Starke N, Dahlof L. Combined physical and psychosexual therapy for provoked vestibulodynia-an evaluation of a multidisciplinary treatment model. J Sex Res. 2008;45(4):378–85.
32. Spoelstra SK, Dijkstra JR, van Driel MF, Weijmar Schultz WCM. Long-term results of an individualized, multifaceted, and multidisciplinary therapeutic approach to provoked vestibulodynia. J Sex Med. 2011;8(2):489–96.
33. O'Hare PM, Sherertz EF. Vulvodynia: a dermatologist's perspective with emphasis on an irritant contact dermatitis component. J Womens Health Gend Based Med. 2000;9(5):565–9.
34. Danielsson I, Torstensson T, Brodda-Jansen G, Bohm-Starke N. EMG biofeedback versus topical lidocaine gel: a randomized study for the treatment of women with vulvar vestibulitis. Acta Obstet Gynecol Scand. 2006;85(11):1360–7.
35. Foster DC, Kotok MB, Huang L, Watts A, Oakes D, Howard FM, et al. Oral desipramine and topical lidocaine for vulvodynia: a randomized controlled trial. Obstet Gynecol. 2010;116(3):583–93.
36. Boardman LA, Cooper AS, Blais LR, Raker CA. Topical gabapentin in the treatment of localized and generalized vulvodynia. Obstet Gynecol. 2008;112(3):579–85.
37. Goldstein AT, Burrows L. Vulvodynia. J Sex Med. 2008;5(1):5–14. Quiz 15.
38. Steinberg AC, Oyama IA, Rejba AE, Kellogg-Spadt S, Whitmore KE. Capsaicin for the treatment of vulvar vestibulitis. Am J Obstet Gynecol. 2005;192(5):1549–53.
39. Pagano R, Wong S. Use of amitriptyline cream in the management of entry dyspareunia due to provoked vestibulodynia. J Low Genit Tract Dis. 2012;16(4):394–7.
40. Bornstein J, Tuma R, Farajun Y, Azran A, Zarfati D. Topical nifedipine for the treatment of localized provoked vulvodynia: a placebo-controlled study. J Pain. 2010;11(12):1403–9.
41. Margesson LJ. Contact dermatitis of the vulva. Dermatol Ther. 2004;17(1):20–7.
42. Potential Signals of Serious Risks/New Safety Information Identified by the Adverse Event

43. Reporting System (AERS) between October–December 2011. http://www.fda.gov/Drugs/GuidanceCompliance RegulatoryInformation/Surveillance/AdverseDrugEffects/ucm295585.htm.
43. Brown CS, Foster DC, Wan JY, Rawlinson LA, Bachmann GA. Rationale and design of a multicenter randomized clinical trial of extended release gabapentin in provoked vestibulodynia and biological correlates of response. Contemp Clin Trials. 2013;36(1):154–65.
44. Leo RJ, Dewani S. A systematic review of the utility of antidepressant pharmacotherapy in the treatment of vulvodynia pain. J Sex Med. 2013;10(10):2497–505.
45. Bertolasi L, Frasson E, Cappelletti JY, Vicentini S, Bordignon M, Graziottin A. Botulinum neurotoxin type A injections for vaginismus secondary to vulvar vestibulitis syndrome. Obstet Gynecol. 2009;114(5):1008–16.
46. Pelletier F, Parratte B, Penz S, Moreno J, Aubin F, Humbert P. Efficacy of high doses of botulinum toxin A for treating provoked vestibulodynia. Br J Dermatol. 2011;164(3):617–22.
47. Reissing ED, Brown C, Lord MJ, Binik YM, Khalifé S. Pelvic floor muscle functioning in women with vulvar vestibulitis syndrome. J Psychosom Obstet Gynaecol. 2005;26(2):107–13.
48. Bergeron S, Brown C, Lord M, Oala M, Binik YM, Khalifé S. Physical therapy for vulvar vestibulitis syndrome: a retrospective study. J Sex Marital Ther. 2002;28(3):183–92.
49. Goldfinger C, Pukall CF, Gentilcore-Saulnier E, McLean L, Chamberlain S. A prospective study of pelvic floor physical therapy: pain and psychosexual outcomes in provoked vestibulodynia. J Sex Med. 2009;6(7):1955–68.
50. Gentilcore-Saulnier E, McLean L, Goldfinger C, Pukall CF, Chamberlain S. Pelvic floor muscle assessment outcomes in women with and without provoked vestibulodynia and the impact of a physical therapy program. J Sex Med. 2010;7(2 Pt 2):1003–22.
51. Murina F, Bianco V, Radici G, Felice R, Di Martino M, Nicolini U. Transcutaneous electrical nerve stimulation to treat vestibulodynia: a randomised controlled trial. BJOG. 2008;115(9):1165–70.
52. Nair AR, Klapper A, Kushnerik V, Margulis I, Del Priore G. Spinal cord stimulator for the treatment of a woman with vulvovaginal burning and deep pelvic pain. Obstet Gynecol. 2008;111(2 Pt 2):545–7.
53. Masheb RM, Kerns RD, Lozano C, Minkin MJ, Richman S. A randomized clinical trial for women with vulvodynia: cognitive-behavioral therapy vs. supportive psychotherapy. Pain. 2009;141(1–2):31–40.
54. Reese JB. Results from an RCT testing a psychosocial treatment for vulvodynia: methodological strengths and future directions. Pain. 2009;141(1–2):8–9.
55. Bergeron S, Binik YM, Khalifé S, Pagidas K, Glazer HI, Meana M, et al. A randomized comparison of group cognitive–behavioral therapy, surface electromyographic biofeedback, and vestibulectomy in the treatment of dyspareunia resulting from vulvar vestibulitis. Pain. 2001;91(3):297–306.
56. Curran S, Brotto LA, Fisher H, Knudson G, Cohen T. The ACTIV study: acupuncture treatment in provoked vestibulodynia. J Sex Med. 2010;7(2 Pt 2):981–95.
57. Murina F, Tassan P, Roberti P, Bianco V. Treatment of vulvar vestibulitis with submucous infiltrations of methylprednisolone and lidocaine. An alternative approach. J Reprod Med. 2001;46(8):713–6.
58. Landry T, Bergeron S, Dupuis M, Desrochers G. The treatment of provoked vestibulodynia: a critical review. Clin J Pain. 2008;24(2):155–71.
59. Woodruff JD, Genadry R, Poliakoff S. Treatment of dyspareunia and vaginal outlet distortions by perineoplasty. Obstet Gynecol. 1981;57(6):750–4.
60. Bornstein J, Zarfati D, Goldik Z, Abramovici H. Perineoplasty compared with vestibuloplasty for severe vulvar vestibulitis. Br J Obstet Gynaecol. 1995;102(8):652–5.
61. Bergeron S, Bouchard C, Fortier M, Binik YM, Khalifé S. The surgical treatment of vulvar vestibulitis syndrome: a follow-up study. J Sex Marital Ther. 1997;23(4):317–25.
62. Eva LJ, Narain S, Orakwue CO, Luesley DM. Is modified vestibulectomy for localized provoked vulvodynia an effective long-term treatment? A follow-up study. J Reprod Med. 2008;53(6):435–40.
63. Goetsch MF. Simplified surgical revision of the vulvar vestibule for vulvar vestibulitis. Am J Obstet Gynecol. 1996;174(6):1701–5. Discussion 1705–7.
64. Goldstein AT, Klingman D, Christopher K, Johnson C, Marinoff SC. Surgical treatment of vulvar vestibulitis syndrome: outcome assessment derived from a postoperative questionnaire. J Sex Med. 2006;3(5):923–31.
65. Tommola P, Unkila-Kallio L, Paavonen J. Surgical treatment of vulvar vestibulitis: a review. Acta Obstet Gynecol Scand. 2010;89(11):1385–95.
66. Andrews JC. Vulvodynia interventions–systematic review and evidence grading. Obstet Gynecol Surv. 2011;66(5):299–315.

Dermatologic Conditions of the Vulva During Menopause

22

Caroline D. Lynch and Nancy Phillips

Contents

22.1	Introduction	285
22.2	The Role of the Women's Health Provider	286
22.3	Vulvar Skin Screening	286
22.4	ISSD Classification of Disorders	287
22.5	Clinical History	287
22.6	Physical Exam	288
22.7	The Dermatoses	289
22.7.1	Lichen Sclerosus	289
22.7.2	Lichen Simplex Chronicus	290
22.7.3	Other Dermatoses	291
22.8	Systemic Diseases	293
22.9	Summary	294
References		294

C.D. Lynch, MD • N. Phillips, MD (✉)
Department of Obstetrics, Gynecology, and Reproductive Science, Rutgers-Robert Wood Johnson Medical School, 125 Paterson Street, New Brunswick, NJ 08907, USA
e-mail: Cdl81@rwjms.rutgers.edu; phillna@rwjms.rutgers.edu

22.1 Introduction

The aim of this chapter is to provide an overview of the vulvar skin conditions commonly found in the aging female. These disorders are underreported and may be undertreated. These conditions most commonly present with pruritus or pain [1]. Other symptoms include difficulty urinating, defecating, walking, and/or interrupted, painful relations. Skin discoloration or rash can be present. Diagnosis may be delayed due to the woman's embarrassment in presenting for gynecological care of these lesions and/or discussing the symptoms with her clinician. Many may accept these distressing symptoms as signs of aging to be expected with menopause.

Vulvar skin disorders present the practitioner with a diagnostic challenge. Although biopsy is not always required to make a diagnosis, it should be performed when lesions are present that cannot be adequately characterized. If conservative management is elected, biopsy should be performed if initial treatment fails. Treatment should also include education regarding vulvar hygiene, with removal of contact irritants when identified and topical steroid creams. Despite treatment, symptoms are often chronic and persistent, interfering with sexuality, activity level, and overall quality of life and may involve continuous active management to achieve partial relief of distress for the aging woman. Our objective is to provide the practitioner with a simple diagnostic framework and treatment plan for vulvar skin dysplasias.

22.2 The Role of the Women's Health Provider

Women may not report symptoms of vulvar itching and pain at their annual visit. Many find the complaint embarrassing. Practitioners are often more comfortable discussing chronic medical conditions rather than sexual health complaints. Thus, the health-care provider with a focus or interest in women's health plays an important role in diagnosis and treatment of vulvar dysplasias. This includes gynecologists, mid-level providers in women's health, and primary care providers; although dermatologists and gynecologic oncologists have a key referral role when there is a refractory case, a lesion suspicious for and/or a biopsy-confirmed malignancy.

The American Cancer Society recommends that women have a full-body skin examination annually beginning at age 40 [2, 3]. In a survey of 201 female veterans, 68.7 % reported that they did not regularly undergo full-body skin exam (FBSE) [4]. Primary care physicians (PCP) are often the gatekeepers, responsible for referral within managed care organizations, and trusted with the initial medical opinion in many conditions. Those who work in the field of obstetrics and gynecology play a key role in a woman's primary health care. A cross-sectional survey of patients from primary care and dermatology clinics found that patients have a high level of confidence in their PCP's ability to treat their skin conditions [5]. Although previous reviews found primary care providers not as likely to do be as thorough as dermatologists in the diagnosis of lesions, electronic age offers the ability to bridge the diagnostic gap that may be created by lack of access to specialists. With electronic medical records, digital images may be inserted to document the lesion. In remote areas without access to specialists, telemedicine offers the ability to guide diagnostic and treatment options for dermatologic conditions.

22.3 Vulvar Skin Screening

The role of the women's health-care provider in screening for vulvar skin disorders is not limited to skin cancer screening.

The majority of vulvar skin disorders diagnosed either on exam, or when a woman presents with vulvar pruritus or pain, are not malignant. See Table 22.1 for common differential diagnoses of vulvar pruritus or pain.

As a woman ages, and particularly after menopause and its resultant hypo-estrogenism, vulvar skin and vaginal mucosa undergo progressive physical changes. Estrogen plays a key role in cellular remodeling, angiogenesis, and response to oxidative stressors [6]; therefore, decreasing estrogen levels affect the macro- and microstructure of the perineum. Estrogen receptors are located in the vagina, the vulva (to a lesser degree), and the urethra [7]. Withdrawal of estrogen leads to decreased cell turnover, blood supply, and vaginal mucosal and vulvar sebaceous gland secretions. The vaginal mucosa atrophies and becomes more alkaline. The vulvar skin thins and pigmentation decreases uniformly. The labia become less full, reflecting a loss of both fat and collagen. Turgor decreases as a result of decreased glycosaminoglycan [8]. The result is vulvovaginal atrophy, also called atrophic vaginitis, as it is believed to account for vulvovaginal pain and dryness in up to 50 % of postmenopausal women. Bothersome local symptoms may be present even in 10–25 % of women using systemic hormone therapy [1, 9].

Vulvovaginal atrophy affects both the structure and function of the vulvar skin. Thinning,

Table 22.1 Differential diagnosis of vulvar pruritus or pain

Acute
Bacterial or fungal infections
Contact dermatitis
Chronic
Dermatoses
Lichen sclerosus
Lichen simplex chronicus/squamous cell hyperplasia
Other dermatoses
Vulvovaginal atrophy
Neoplasia or preneoplastic lesions
Vulvodynia
Infection
Human papillomavirus infection
Vulvar manifestations of systemic illnesses
Crohn's disease, Bechet's

more friable skin, with the loss of the hair barrier and increased vulvar permeability, becomes more susceptible to damage from local irritants. Microvasculature changes contribute to dysfunctional response to infection. Increased vaginal pH can result in colonization with pathologic organisms.

Immune function is also a contributing factor to the development of vulvar dermatoses. In recent years, research has focused on the estrogen effects of the immune system. Aging skin has been noted to show a decrease in Toll-like receptors, which serve a primary role in cutaneous host defense [10]. Proinflammatory cytokines contribute to decreasing collagen and inflammation [11]. Thus, not only does the hypo-estrogenic vulva have a diminished barrier, but it also has a limited ability to protect against infectious microorganisms and topical irritants. Furthermore, it has a decreased response to healing after insult.

22.4 ISSD Classification of Disorders

Many nonmalignant vulvar skin disorders present with the same symptoms as premalignant or malignant vulvar conditions. A skin biopsy will result in a definitive diagnosis via histopathology; however, it requires technical skill and may result in scarring. The original classification system of nonneoplastic dermatologic conditions of the vulva by the International Society for the Study of Vulvovaginal Disease (ISSVD) was based on gross description and histopathology (Table 22.2). However, in 2011, the ISSVD presented a stepwise diagnostic approach that aims to help providers make a diagnosis based on clinical presentation. The classification was based on pathophysiology, etiology, and commonalities among clinical presentation. The goal of the ISSVD was to simplify the terminology in order to arrive at a differential diagnosis. In contrast to the original classification of vulvovaginal skin diseases, the most recent classification aims to diagnose without a biopsy. However, if a biopsy is necessary, it should be performed by a healthcare provider trained in the procedure and ideally interpreted by a dermatopathologist (pathologist with specialty training in dermatological disorders) whenever possible.

The classification of vulvar disorders is shown in Table 22.2.

Table 22.2 Nomenclature for vulvar disease

1. Nonneoplastic epithelial disorders of skin and mucosa
   (a) Lichen sclerosis
   (b) Squamous hyperplasia, not otherwise specified (formerly "hyperplastic dystrophy without atypia")
   (c) Other dermatoses
2. Mixed nonneoplastic and neoplastic epithelial disorders
3. Intraepithelial neoplasia
   (a) Squamous intraepithelial neoplasia (formerly "dystrophies with atypia")
   (b) VIN, usual type
   (c) VIN, differentiated type
   (d) Nonsquamous intraepithelial neoplasia
   (e) Paget's disease
   (f) Tumors of melanocytes, noninvasive
4. Invasive tumors
   (a) VIN, Vulvar intraepithelial neoplasia
   (b) Paget disease

Adapted from Lynch et al. [12]

22.5 Clinical History

All women, especially postmenopausal women, should be asked about symptoms related to vulvovaginal atrophy and vulvar skin conditions. These symptoms include vulvar itching, burning, bleeding, changes in pigmentation, sores, lumps, ulcers, or pain with intercourse. When present, symptom duration, intensity, and modifying factors should be assessed. All vulvovaginal contacts should be reviewed, including over-the-counter remedies, soaps, shampoos, and sanitary products. These topical irritants should be eliminated. See Table 22.3 for a list of common irritants and possible suggestions for their removal.

For intermittent symptoms, contact/symptom diaries can be recommended. Skin conditions elsewhere, such as oral lesions or eczema should be documented. Systemic disease and all medications should be reviewed.

22.6 Physical Exam

The ISVVD 2012 publication's diagnostic approach to vulvar disorders represents a philosophical return to the physical exam. Table 22.4 offers descriptive terms useful for universal documentation of vulvar lesions and clear communication with specialists.

Physical exam of the vulva begins with visual inspection. Optimal patient positioning is in dorsal lithotomy position in gynecological stirrups, although a frog-legged position on a non-gyn examination table also may be used. Lighting should be adequate. A magnifying glass can aid visualization, but is not always necessary. Acetic acid application is not recommended because its accuracy in enhancing vulvar lesions has not been validated.

Visual inspection should include assessment of aging changes in the vulvovaginal area. Loss of hair, thinning skin, increase or loss of pigmentation should be noted. Ulcerations, excoriations, or any lesions should be noted and documented as specifically as possible in the patient chart. Localization, symmetry, and number and distribution of abnormal areas should be recorded. Border asymmetry, color, and size are also key elements to note. A cotton swab can be used to diagnose provoked vestibulodynia (through elicitation of pain with point contact through the vestibule).

The surface appearance of a lesion provides clinically helpful information. If the surface is rough, it may be due to either a crust or a scale. A crust commonly appears yellow or hemosiderin colored, and its presence implies a lesion that has involved excoriation, erosion, or any type of disruption of

Table 22.3 Tips for removing common vulvar skin irritants

Avoid scented bath products, detergents, lotions, or powders
Wear natural-fiber undergarments without dyes
At night, consider going without undergarments
Avoid tightly fitting leggings, pants or nylons
Do not scrub the vulvar area during bathing; avoid all soap to the area
Avoid activities that put tremendous pressure on the perineal area, such as biking or spin class

Table 22.4 Descriptive terminology useful for describing vulvar lesions

Blister	A compartmentalized fluid-filled elevation of the skin or mucosa
Bulla (pl. bullae)	A large (>0.5 cm) fluid-filled blister; the fluid is clear
Cyst	A closed cavity lined by epithelium that contains fluid or semisolid material
Edema	A poorly marginated area of swelling due to the abnormal accumulation of fluid in the dermis and/or subcutaneous tissue; edema may be skin colored, pink, or red
Erosion	Shallow defect in the skin surface; absence of some, or all, of the epidermis down to the basement membrane; the dermis is intact
Excoriation	An erosion or ulcer caused by scratching; excoriations are often linear or angular in configuration
Fissure	A thin linear erosion of the skin surface
Lesion	A visible or palpable abnormality
Macule	A *macule* is a flat, distinct, colored area of skin that is less than 1 cm in diameter
Nodule	A large (>1.0 cm) papule; often hemispherical or poorly marginated; it may be located on the surface, within or below the skin; nodules may be cystic or solid
Papule	A *papule* is a circumscribed, solid elevation of skin with no visible fluid, varying in size from a pinhead to 1 cm
Patch	Large (>1.0 cm) area of color change; no elevation and no substance on palpation
Plaque	Large (>1.0 cm) elevated, palpable, and flat-topped lesion
Pustule	Pus-filled blister; the fluid is white or yellow
Rash	Numerous or diffuse abnormalities (it is preferable to describe the specific abnormalities using the other terms in this list)
Ulcer	Deeper defect; absence of the epidermis and some, or all, of the dermis
Vesicle	Small blister beneath the skin

Adapted from Lynch et al. [13]

the epithelial layer. A scale is characterized by reactive keratinization, such as in eczema.

Lichenification refers to the process of cutaneous thickening that occurs secondary to chronic itching or rubbing contact. As a dermatological description, it lacks specificity for the naked eye or magnifying glass. The skin may be erythematous (red), white, or skin colored. It may or may not have excoriations. Histologically, lichenification appears as a thickened epidermal layer.

Properties that may indicate an allergic reaction include red plaques and evidence of itching, such as excoriations. A clinical history of sensitive skin, seasonal allergies, and/or asthma suggests a person with "atopy." Atopic or contact dermatitis may be causing or contributing to the chronic itching.

Inflammation typically includes the appearance of excoriations and erythema (representing reactive microvasculature). Eczematous conditions are related to atopic dermatitis but typically occur without contact irritants.

Differentiating a premalignant condition from vulvar carcinoma is difficult based on appearance alone. A biopsy is recommended in cases of non-healing erosions, ulcerative lesions, hyperpigmented lesions, or any vulvar lesion demonstrating lack of response to treatment.

A trained health-care provider can perform a vulvar punch biopsy in the office. The site is prepped with an antibacterial solution, and 1 or 2 % lidocaine is injected subcutaneously. A punch biopsy instrument is pressed against the skin in a circular fashion to penetrate the dermis. The biopsy site should include the most abnormal appearing skin lesion as well as an adjacent potion of normal appearing skin (the very edge of the lesion). Multiple biopsy sites may be needed. Forceps and scissors are used to remove the sample. Direct pressure, Monsel solution, silver nitrate, or suture may be utilized for hemostasis. Post-biopsy care includes keeping the area clean and dry, although a topical antibiotic ointment may be prescribed.

General principles of therapy include the removal of topical irritants, focus on skin hygiene, and anti-inflammatory therapy, usually in the form of topical steroid cream. Systemic treatment for vulvar dysplasias or dermatoses is prescribed for severe, recurrent or resistant disease, or in an immunocompromised individual.

Additionally, in a patient with concomitant vulvovaginal atrophy, the addition of local estrogen therapy, in the absence of contraindications, should be considered as an adjunct to any specific therapies. Vaginal creams, rings, or tablets may be used. If VIN or cancer is present on biopsy, referral to a gynecologic oncologist is recommended.

22.7 The Dermatoses

Nonneoplastic epithelial lesions fall into one of the following three categories: (1) lichen sclerosis, (2) squamous cell hyperplasia/lichen simplex chronicus, and (3) other dermatoses.

22.7.1 Lichen Sclerosus

Lichen sclerosus has many synonyms. Pathologists may still use "lichen sclerosus et atrophicus" or "lichen albus," which refer to atrophy and whitened appearance. However, the ISSVD promotes use of the term lichen sclerosus to describe a histologically confirmed condition that typically presents with the patient complaining of pruritus in the anogenital area.

The exact incidence of lichen sclerosus is not objectively known, largely because it is believed to be underreported. In a gynecology clinic, rates are estimated to be 1.7 % [14, 15]. Patients are most often postmenopausal and Caucasian.

Lichen sclerosis likely has a multitude of mechanisms. Investigators have found a 30 % correlation between lichen sclerosus and autoimmune diseases [16]. A genetic cause has been suggested, but not confirmed [17]. The tendency of patients to be postmenopausal at presentation suggests a contribution of biological skin aging. The etiology is likely multifactorial, with changes in aging skin being critical.

Although lichen sclerosis may be asymptomatic, most women report dyspareunia, chronic itching, discomfort, or dysuria. It is thought that the inflammation affects terminal nerve fibers leading to chronic itching [15].

As the Latin alternative name, lichen albus, suggests, the skin typically has a whitish appearance. It forms a porcelain-white plaque in a figure-of-eight pattern around the clitoris and anus. Excoriations and skin thickening from chronic itching may be present. Initially, there is a loss of vulvar skin structure. Over time, the architecture is disturbed leading to retraction of the clitoris, labial adhesions, and narrowing of the introitus. This loss of architecture is a key differing feature from vitiligo, which is also characterized by depigmentation. Secondary complications due to the stenotic introitus include urethral obstruction, chronic or recurrent UTIs, and anorgasmia. The genital mucosa and cervix are spared. Diagnosis is based on histopathology to exclude premalignant or malignant lesions.

Lichen sclerosis has a controversial association with squamous cell carcinoma of the vulva. Vulvar cancer affects 4 % of women per year. Vulvar cancer in older women is typically not related to HPV, as it is in younger women [18]. Frequent surveillance for squamous cell carcinoma is recommended in all women with lichen sclerosis, with biopsy recommended for new or indeterminate lesions.

Histopathology demonstrates thickened epidermis and lymphocytic infiltrate. Nuclear abnormalities on histology may be present, representing a possible continuum from lichen sclerosus to squamous cell carcinoma [19].

Ultra-potent topical corticosteroids are the primary intervention for lichen sclerosis. Clobetasol propionate 0.05 % is most often prescribed. Clobetasol is available as a cream, gel, and ointment. Ointments are formulated to provide a barrier, are typically less irritating, and provide longer medication exposure following application. Recommended dosing is 0.05 % clobetasol propionate once nightly for 4 weeks, every other night for 4 weeks then by twice a week for 4 weeks [20]. The dosage regimen should be titrated to response. There is no agreement on the frequency of clobetasol application for maintenance. Switching to less potent corticosteroids such as hydrocortisone 1 % for maintenance is recommended.

Skin atrophy, as has been demonstrated in other parts of the body after prolonged topical steroid use, is rare in the vulvar. Although short-term overuse of potent topical corticosteroids may induce local atrophy, long-term atrophic changes have not been demonstrated. The modified mucous membranes of the labia and clitoris are relatively resistant to these changes [21, 22]. Risks of developing Cushing syndrome from prolonged topical steroid use are largely theoretical.

Testosterone and progesterone topical preparations are not recommended as multiple studies have found clobetasol propionate superior to both [23]. Studies evaluating tacrolimus, photodynamic therapy, topical retinoids, and local injection of corticosteroids were largely underpowered to determine efficacy [14, 20].

Once an adequate treatment regimen is established, reexamination is necessary every 4–6 months. These exams are intended to both monitor response and to observe for skin changes that may suggest progression to squamous cell carcinoma.

22.7.2 Lichen Simplex Chronicus

Lichen simplex chronicus (squamous cell hyperplasia) is a chronic eczematous condition characterized by a repetitive "itch-scratch" cycle. Lichen simplex chronicus can occur in any age group, including children, but is most common in older women. Women with lichen simplex chronicus experience intense itching, often with disruption of both daily activity and sleep. Clinically, the skin is erythematous and thickened (lichenified) with excoriations. The affected vulvar area may appear reddened, grayish, or whitish. There may be moderate inflammation. The affected skin area is typically symmetric.

The cornerstone of treatment for lichen sclerosis is to break the "itch-scratch" cycle. Identifying and removing chemical or environmental irritants achieve this goal. This includes evaluation for underlying yeast vulvovaginitis, with treatment if present. Mid- to high-potency topical steroids prescribed for daily use will decrease inflammation. Antihistamines will aid in reduction of the intense pruritus. Antihistamines with sedating properties, such as hydroxyzine or doxepin, will decrease nocturnal scratching and improve disrupted sleep patterns, whereas those with nonsedating properties can be used during the day. Topical steroids should be weaned as the condition improves. A biopsy is recommended initially, if the diagnosis is uncertain or if there is a poor response to treatment. Histologically, the lesions will show irregular thickening of the epidermis with a prominent nucleated keratin layer. Rete ridges, downward projections of epidermis into the dermis, will be thickened. Although biopsy results may be nonspecific, the absence of malignant or premalignant changes is documented. In refractory, biopsy-confirmed cases, systemic steroids may be used.

Table 22.5 Differentiating allergic and irritant contact dermatitis

Condition	Allergic contact dermatitis	Irritant contact dermatitis
Signs/symptoms	Delayed-onset pruritus, edema, vesicles or bullae	Immediate burning and stinging
Diagnosis	Patch testing by allergist	History of irritant use
Treatment	Remove offending agent(s), topical hydrocortisone, sitz baths	Remove offending agent(s), topical hydrocortisone, sitz baths

22.7.3 Other Dermatoses

According to the 2006 ISSVD Classification, the "other dermatoses" include (1) inflammatory dermatoses, (2) bullous dermatoses, and (3) ulcerative dermatoses. There are similarities within the subdivisions, suggesting a continuum of illness.

22.7.3.1 Inflammatory Dermatoses: Allergic

Allergic dermatitis is diagnosed in up to 54 % of patients presenting with vulvar pruritus [24]. Allergic dermatitis may be exogenous, attributed to irritants, which causes immediate symptoms, or endogenous, an underlying atopy/allergic reaction which is typically more gradual in onset. See Table 22.5 for tips differentiating the two conditions. Clinically, the two are difficult to differentiate, although evaluation and treatment are similar. These inflammatory dermatoses may be the vulvar manifestation of eczema and appear as poorly defined, patchy, erythematous lesions.

Allergic dermatitis can be diagnosed by eliciting a history of atopy or allergies or identification of an offending allergen or irritant. Patients may have extra-genital manifestations of eczema. Vulvovaginal candidiasis must be ruled out. Biopsy is generally not required, but if performed will show nonspecific changes, such as inflammation, spongiosis, or parakeratosis. Treatment is a multifaceted and includes removal of irritants, skin hydration with emollients, and the application of mid-high-potency topical corticosteroids. In refractory cases, systemic steroids or immune modulators may be required.

Inflammatory dermatoses may represent vulvar manifestation of psoriasis. Similar to atopic eczema, psoriasis is defined by the presence of specific lesions and usually a history of nongenital psoriasis. Psoriatic lesions are thick erythematous plaques with silvery scales Successful treatment of psoriasis may require systemic therapy with one of the several FDA-approved immunomodulating biologic agents such as infliximab, adalimumab, etanercept, alefacept, and ustekinumab [25]. For local relief, high-potency corticosteroids are often prescribed. Referral to a dermatologist or healthcare professional with experience in treating psoriasis is recommended.

Intertrigo is an inflammatory condition commonly associated with obesity. Intertrigo is characterized by an erythematous rash that often presents in the genitocrural folds. Candida (yeast) is the most common organism that presents in conjunction with intertrigo. Treatment is aimed at keeping skin folds clean and dry. Antifungal powder has both a moisture-wicking quality and antifungal properties. If inflammation is present, a topical corticosteroid may be used, although treatment of the fungal infection is first-line treatment. Diaper rash creams can also be useful as a protective barrier.

22.7.3.2 Inflammatory Disorders: Lichen Planus

Lichen planus is a mucocutaneous inflammatory disorder thought to be caused by a disturbance in the cell-mediated immune system. A genetic component of the genital form has been postulated. Lichen planus commonly presents in women aged 50–60 and can affect the hair, nails, mouth, and/or genital area. The exact incidence of lichen planus is not clearly documented. Lichen planus has three genital manifestations – erosive, papulosquamous, and hypertrophic. The erosive type is the most common form.

The appearance of erosive lichen planus is variable, including white epithelium or red or purple papules. The classic presentation found on mucous membranes is of white, lacy, or fern-like striae, called "Wickham's striae." In the erosive form, vaginal ulcerations may be present. Commonly, the six Ps (planar [flat], purple, polygonal, pruritic, papules, plaques) are cited as common signs [26]. Unlike lichen sclerosis or lichen simplex chronicus, itching is not the most common presenting symptom. More commonly, patients present with burning and dyspareunia.

Vulvovaginal-gingival syndrome occurs when lichen planus also involves the oral mucosa. Typically, the vulva is spared in lichen planus, whereas, lichen sclerosus involves the labia majors but does not include the vagina. In long-standing disease, vulvar and vaginal architecture may be disrupted. Vaginal discharge is a common complaint in addition to burning and dyspareunia, due to the desquamation of surface (parabasal) cells. Lichen planus is especially difficult to treat in the menopausal woman as the skin changes that are typically seen with menopause may be associated with decreased immune response as well as delayed healing.

Despite the potential of delayed healing, a biopsy is recommended for diagnosis of lichen planus. Histologically a band-like lymphocytic infiltrate and colloid bodies in the basal layer of the epidermis will be seen [27].

Papulosquamous and hypertrophic lichen sclerosis are less common than erosive lichen planus. Papulosquamous lichen sclerosis is characterized by pruritic papules. Thickened (hypertrophic) plaques are common in the hypertrophic form, which may appear similar to squamous cell carcinoma.

Once diagnosis is established, treatment focuses on symptom control. Initial treatment is with high-potency steroids topically, although systemic steroids may be needed. Vaginal suppositories of 25 mg of hydrocortisone are usually effective for vaginal manifestations. They are dosed in a tapering fashion starting at twice a day over several months. Vaginal stenosis or other architectural changes from long-standing disease cannot be reversed. Oral pharmacotherapy with immunomodulators or biologic agents is initiated in persistent or refractory cases. Lichen planus is a chronic condition for which management rather than cure is the goal of treatment.

22.7.3.3 Inflammatory Disorders: Other Conditions

Other conditions that can have both oral and genital manifestations, like lichen planus, include aphthous ulcers and Bechet's disease.

Aphthous ulcers, or "canker sores," are more common in women than men. These ulcers are likely related to immunodeficiency, although no direct cause has been identified. Nutritional deficiencies have been associated with their development, namely, B12, iron, thiamine, and zinc [28]. However, vitamin supplementation is not successful in prevention or treatment of vaginal aphthous ulcers. Recurrent or severe apthous ulcers have been associated with CMV, HIV, mycoplasma, EBV, or inflammatory bowel disease. A short course of oral or topical corticosteroids can be effective, but colchicine, dapsone, cyclosporine, or thalidomide may be required in difficult to treat cases [29].

Bechet's disease may present with aphthous – appearing ulcers in the genital, oral, and ocular mucosa. Typically presenting in Asian or Middle Eastern females in the third or fourth decade of life, this systemic illness may be persistent and progressive. Bechet's disease involves systemic vasculitis that affects the GI tract, brain, joints, lungs, and large vessels as well as microvasculature. Topical steroids are recommended for treatment of vaginal lesions. Control of systemic symptoms is necessary to prevent further erosion. If Bechet's disease is suspected, a rheumatologist referral is recommended.

Hidradenitis suppurativa is a chronic condition affecting apocrine glands. The glands become blocked, an inflammatory process ensues and superinfection leads to abscess formation. The process is recurrent and leads to scarring and formation of sinus tracts. The most commonly affected sites are the axillae, inguinal, perianal, perineal, inframammary, and retro-auricular regions.

Both genetic and environmental factors are thought to play a role in the pathophysiology of hidradenitis. A hormonal cause is postulated, likely in relation to androgens, as disease is generally from puberty until age 40. Other factors for disease development include obesity, diabetes and a likely familial predisposition. Population studies in postmenopausal women are scarce, but since androgen levels decrease in this population, the incidence of hidradenitis may be lower than in younger women.

Diagnosis is by history and physical exam. Treatment is challenging and aimed at prevention. Incision and drainage is useful for symptom relief, but frequent recurrence necessitates wide local excision of most severely affected areas. Topical clindamycin or intralesional triamcinolone is effective for treatment of local infection [30].

Medical treatments options include systemic steroids, antibiotics, antiandrogens, cyclosporine, or infliximab. Antiandrogens are largely not looked favorably upon as treatment in the aging female as testosterone levels are low in this population.

22.7.3.4 Pigmented and Depigmented Lesions

Vitiligo is a rare skin condition. The exact prevalence is unknown, but is thought to be 0.38 % in the USA [31]. Vitiligo is characterized by depigmented skin, which, histopathologically, is due to a loss of melanocytes in the epidermis. The perineal and perianal skin may be affected, with a generally symmetric distribution.

The pathophysiology of vitiligo is unknown. Familial patterns of vitiligo suggest a genetic contribution [32]. There may also be an association with autoimmune disorders. Unlike lichen sclerosis, vitiligo has no risk of progression to squamous cell carcinoma and does not cause progressive scarring. Vitiligo may however, co-exist with lichen sclerosis. Vitiligo has equal prevalence among different ethnicities. It is, however, more noticeable and possibly more disfiguring in individuals of darker skin tone.

Treatment, when desired by the patient, includes UVB phototherapy and topical immunomodulators. The most important aspect of treatment may be ruling out other conditions such a lichen sclerosis, which can produce a depigmentation but with loss of vulvar architecture. Vitiligo is not associated with pruritus or dyspareunia.

Hyperpigmentation of vulva is commonly associated with nevi. Common names include moles or skin tags. In the vulvar area, nevi should be closely monitored for progression, just as they should in any part of the body. Melanoma is the second most common vulvar malignancy after squamous cell carcinoma although both are rare primary vulvar diseases.

As with skin lesions, the ABCDs should be closely monitored on an annual basis at the minimum:
A. Asymmetry
B. Border (irregular)
C. Color (a change in color or blackish/bluish appearance)
D. Diameter (greater than 6 mm)

With electronic medical records, the feasibility of including a digital image of the lesion is increased and recommended. When a lesion changes appearance, has bleeding, pruritus, or surface skin breaks, a biopsy is recommended. The biopsy follows the same technique as previously described if it is a flat lesion. A raised lesion can be excised in the office after infiltration of local anesthetic. A dermatopathologist is optimal when available, as they usually offer the highest level of interpretation. After excision and healing of a benign lesion, there is no exact recommendation of ongoing surveillance. Yearly clinical exams are warranted, but may be biyearly in a high-risk patient, such as one with a history of a melanoma in a nonperineal location.

22.8 Systemic Diseases

Anogenital involvement in Crohn's disease is common, affecting up to 80 % of patients with bowel disease, depending on the definition of perianal involvement [33]. Although t he disease is usually diagnosed in younger women, 80 % of cases are diagnosed before age 40 [3]. External lesions secondary to Crohn's are typically ulcers, so called "knife-cut" ulcers that appear to be stab wounds. The interlabial and genitocrural folds are especially prone to external manifestations of Crohn's. Fistulas may develop over time, which require surgical management. Treatment of the lesions is with topical corticosteroids. Control of the primary illness is paramount.

Acanthosis nigricans is a skin manifestation of hyperinsulinemia. The development of skin lesions is believed to be secondary to insulin-like growth factor stimulation of keratinocytes and dermal fibroblasts. Lesions are raised plaques with irregular contour, typically occurring in groups, most commonly located on the neck, axillae, and genitocrural folds. Patients diagnosed with acanthosis nigricans should be screened for insulin resistance and diabetes, if not previously diagnosed. Typically, the lesions regress when glucose levels are well controlled.

22.9 Summary

The aging or postmenopausal female is prone to the development of vulvar dystrophies and dermatoses. In addition to primary conditions, systemic illness also may have genital manifestations. Benign and premalignant or malignant lesions may present with similar symptoms or clinical appearance. A biopsy is not always required but is strongly recommended, especially if the lesion cannot be characterized or is not responsive to treatment. Common treatment of vulvar dystrophies and dermatoses includes high-potency topical steroids and removal of environmental irritants. Local estrogen therapy, in appropriate women without contraindications to its use, should be considered as an adjunct to other therapies. Frequent follow-up is recommended to monitor progress with treatment, and referral should be initiated as warranted.

References

1. Boardman L. Diagnosis and management of vulvar skin disorders. ACOG practice bulletin: clinical management guidelines. May 2008 (Number 93).
2. Robinson JK, Ramos-e-Silva M. Women's dermatologic diseases, health care delivery, and socioeconomic barriers. Arch Dermatol. 2006;142(3):362–4. Epub 22 Mar 2006.
3. LeBlanc WG, Vidal L, Kirsner RS, Lee DJ, Caban-Martinez AJ, McCollister KE, et al. Reported skin cancer screening of US adult workers. J Am Acad Dermatol. 2008;59(1):55–63. Epub 26 Apr 2008.
4. Federman DG, Kravetz JD, Haskell SG, Ma F, Kirsner RS. Full-body skin examinations and the female veteran: prevalence and perspective. Arch Dermatol. 2006;142(3):312–6. Epub 22 Mar 2006.
5. Federman DG, Reid M, Feldman SR, Greenhoe J, Kirsner RS. The primary care provider and the care of skin disease: the patient's perspective. Arch Dermatol. 2001;137(1):25–9. Epub 15 Feb 2001.
6. Thornton M. Estrogens and aging skin. Dermatoendocrinology. 2013;5(2):264–70.
7. Calleja-Agius J, Brincat MP. Urogenital atrophy. Climacteric. 2009;12(4):279–85. Epub 24 Apr 2009.
8. Raine-Fenning NJ, Brincat MP, Muscat-Baron Y. Skin aging and menopause: implications for treatment. Am J Clin Dermatol. 2003;4(5):371–8.
9. Willhite LA, O'Connell MB. Urogenital atrophy: prevention and treatment. Pharmacotherapy. 2001;21:464–80.
10. Iram N, Mildner M, Prior M, Petzelbauer P, Fiala C, Hacker S, et al. Age-related changes in expression and function of Toll-like receptors in human skin. Development. 2012;139(22):4210–9. Epub 5 Oct 2012.
11. Borg M, Brincat S, Camilleri G, Schembri-Wismayer P, Brincat M, Calleja-Agius J. The role of cytokines in skin aging. Climacteric. 2013;16(5):514–21. Epub 11 May 2013.
12. Lynch PJ, Moyal-Barroco M, Bogliatto F, Micheletti L, Scurry J. 2006 ISSVD classification of vulvar dermatoses: pathologic subsets and their clinical correlates. J Reprod Med. 2007;52(11):20A.
13. Lynch PJ, Moyal-Barroco M, Scurry J, Stockdale C. 2011 ISSVD terminology and classification of vulvar dermatological disorders: an approach to clinical diagnosis. J Low Genit Tract Dis. 2012;16(4):339–44.
14. Goldstein AT, Marinoff SC, Christopher K, Srodon M. Prevalence of vulvar lichen sclerosis in a general gynecology practice. J Reprod Med. 2005;50(7):477.
15. Wang JB, Yan H, Yang HY, Si JY, Jia LP, Li K, Yu J. Histological and ultrastructural changes of lichen sclerosis et atrophicus. Chin Med. 1991;104(10):868–71.
16. Cooper SM, Ali I, Baldo M, Wojnarowska F. The association of lichen sclerosus and erosive lichen planus of the vulva with autoimmune disease: a case-control study. Arch Dermatol. 2008;144(11):1432–5.
17. Sherman V, McPherson T, Baldo M, Salim A, Gao XH, Wojnarowska F. The high rate of familial lichen sclerosus suggests a genetic contribution: an observational cohort study. J Eur Acad Dermatol Venereol. 2010;24(9):1031–4. Epub 6 Mar 2010.
18. Berek JS, Hacker NF. Gynecologic oncology. Philadelphia: Lippincott Williams & Wilkins; 2010.
19. Scurry J, Whitehead J, Healey M. Histology of lichen sclerosus varies according to site and proximity to carcinoma. Am J Dermatopathol. 2001;23(5):413–8.

20. Chi CC, Kirtschig G, Baldo M, Brackenbury F, Lewis F, Wojnarowska F. Topical interventions for genital lichen sclerosus. Cochrane Database Syst Rev. 2011;7(12):CD008240. Epub Dec 7.
21. Dalziel KL, Woinarowska F. Long term control of vulval lichen sclerosis after treatment with a potent topical steroid cream. J Reprod Med. 1993;38(1):25.
22. Stewart EG. Vulvar lichen sclerosis. UpToDate 2014. Wolters Kluwer Health. Available from: http://www.uptodate.com/contents/vulvar-lichen-planus.
23. Bracco GL, Carli P, Sonni L, Maestrini G, De Marco A, Taddei GL, et al. Clinical and histologic effects of topical treatments of vulval lichen sclerosus. A critical evaluation. J Reprod Med. 1993;38(1):37–40. Epub 1 Jan 1993.
24. Fisher AA, Rietschel RL, Fowler JF. Fisher's contact dermatitis. 6th ed. Hamilton: Decker; 2008.
25. Smith CH, Anstey AV, Barker JN, Burden AD, Chalmers RJ, Chandler DA. British association of dermatologists' guidelines for biologic interventions for psoriasis 2009. Br J Dermatol. 2009;161:987–1019.
26. Usatine RP, Tinitigan M. Diagnosis and treatment of lichen planus. Am Fam Physician. 2011;84(1):53–60. Epub 20 Jul 2011.
27. Ramer MA, Altchek A, Deligdisch L, Phelps R, Montazem A, Buonocore PM. Lichen planus and the vulvovaginal-gingival syndrome. J Periodontol. 2003;74(9):1385–93. Epub 31 Oct 2003.
28. Volkov I, Rudoy I, Abu-Rabia U, Masalha T, Masalha R. Case report: recurrent aphthous stomatitis responds to vitamin B12 treatment. Can Fam Physician Med Fam Can. 2005;51(51):844–5. Epub 1 Jul 2005.
29. Letsinger JA, McCarty MA, Jorizzo JL. Complex aphthosis: a large case series with evaluation algorithm and therapeutic ladder from topicals to thalidomide. J Am Acad Dermatol. 2005;52(3 Pt 1):500–8.
30. Jemec GB, Wendelboe P. Topical clindamycin versus systemic tetracycline in the treatment of hidradenitis suppurativa. J Am Acad Dermatol. 1998;39(6):971–4. Epub 8 Dec 1998.
31. Chen JJ, Huang W, Gui JP, Yang S, Zhou FS, Xiong QG, et al. A novel linkage to generalized vitiligo on 4q13-q21 identified in a genomewide linkage analysis of Chinese families. Am J Hum Genet. 2005;76(6):1057–65. Epub 6 Apr 2005.
32. Spritz RA. The genetics of generalized vitiligo and associated autoimmune disease. Pigment Cell Res. 2007;20(4):271–8.
33. Safar B, Sands D. Perianal Crohn's disease. Clin Colon Rectal Surg. 2007;20(4):282–93. Epub 1 Nov 2007.

Part IV

Menopause and Autoimmune Disease

The Effects of Menopause on Autoimmune Diseases

23

Miranda A. Farage, Kenneth W. Miller, and Howard I. Maibach

Contents

23.1	Introduction	299
23.2	Immunosenescence: How the Immune System Ages	300
23.3	Gender and Immunity	303
23.4	Aging and the Development of Autoimmunity	305
23.5	Specific Effects of Estrogen on Autoimmunity	307
23.6	What Is Known About the Estrogen Deficiency of Menopause and Specific Autoimmune Diseases	308
23.6.1	Systemic Lupus Erythematosus	308
23.6.2	Rheumatoid Arthritis	310
23.6.3	Scleroderma	311
23.6.4	Sjögren's Syndrome	311
23.6.5	Multiple Sclerosis	311
23.6.6	Autoimmune Hepatitis	311
23.7	Summary	312
23.8	Expert Commentary	313
23.9	Five-Year View	313
23.10	Key Issues	313
	References	314

M.A. Farage, MSc, PhD (✉)
Clinical Innovative Sciences, The Procter and Gamble Company, 6110 Center Hill Avenue, Cincinnati, OH 45224, USA
e-mail: Farage.m@pg.com

K.W. Miller, PhD
Global Product Stewardship, The Procter & Gamble Company, Cincinnati, OH, USA
e-mail: Miller.kw.1@pg.com

H.I. Maibach, MD
Department of Dermatology, University of California, School of Medicine, San Francisco, CA, USA
e-mail: MaibachH@derm.ucsf.edu

23.1 Introduction

Life expectancy in human beings has increased dramatically in the last century [1] and is expected to continue to increase, hitting 100 years in the United States and other industrialized countries by about 2040 [2]. In the United States, life expectancy has increased 10 % since 1970 from an average of 70.8 years to an average of 78.3 years [3]. Women, on average, currently live nearly 3 years longer than men [2].

The dramatic gains in life expectancy achieved have allowed for concomitant gains in an understanding of immune system aging, termed *immunosenescence*. Recent analyses of immune system aging have revealed that individual longevity is closely tied to the preservation of healthy immune function [4].

The immunosenescence that occurs as humans age is therefore of increasing interest in medicine and deserving of research effort as life expectancy, particularly in developed countries, is increasing at a more rapid rate than concomitant improvements in meeting the medical needs of the elderly [5]. This is particularly true in women, who at current life expectancies will spend more than a third of their lifetimes in menopause.

Menopause, a period of time defined by the cessation of menstruation, is an experience common to all aging females. Cessation of menses

---

Adapted with permission from *Expert Rev Obs Gyn* 7(6), 557–571 (2012) with permission of Expert Reviews Ltd.

results from a gradual deterioration in ovarian function, with declining production of follicles and falling levels of numerous endogenous hormones. Estrogen produced in postmenopausal females, furthermore, is of a different form than that which is predominant during the reproductive years. Levels of the ovarian-derived 17β estradiol (E2), as ovarian follicles cease production, plunge as menopause nears, and estrogen in the form of estrone (E1) becomes the predominant form. Estrone is produced by secretion of androstenedione by the ovarian stroma and the adrenal gland and is aromatized to estrone in the peripheral circulation. Conversion to estrone occurs primarily in adipose tissue, but also in the muscle, liver, bone, bone marrow, fibroblasts, and hair roots [6]. Postmenopausal deficits in estrogen and progesterone, and the replacement of E2, the primary estrogen of the reproductive years, to E1 carry impact far beyond the immune system.

Estrogen, with receptors in nearly every tissue of the body, is a principal regulator of homeostasis in the female body, with the hormonal tides characteristic of a woman's reproductive years having demonstrable effects on nearly every body system. The sudden and dramatic removal of estrogen from the female body, particularly in the form of estradiol, is a veritable tsunami with significant and largely negative effects on many body tissues, including a loss of skin integrity and tone, poorer muscle tone (affecting heart, vasculature, eye, and bladder function; declining brain function; and deterioration in bone strength). Estrogen levels, and particularly the estrogen withdrawal of menopause, undeniably impact autoimmunity in women as well.

Autoimmune disease as a category affects an estimated 50 million Americans [7] and is the top cause of morbidity in women in the United States [7]. The annual cost of only seven of the 100+ known autoimmune diseases (Crohn's disease, ulcerative colitis, systemic lupus erythematosus [SLE], multiple sclerosis [MS], rheumatoid arthritis [RA], psoriasis, and scleroderma) is estimated, through epidemiological studies, to total as much as $70 billion annually [7].

The development of autoimmunity clearly involves genetic and environmental contributions to existing levels of endogenous estrogen, and the precise contributions of each are not fully understood. Additional research, to focus on how autoimmune disease is impacted by the plummeting estrogen levels associated with menopause, is needed.

23.2 Immunosenescence: How the Immune System Ages

The immune system undergoes constant physiological changes over the human life span [8]. The infant has no immunity of its own at birth; immune function develops quickly over the first few years and then builds to a complete maturation by puberty [9]. In fertile women, immunity fluctuates cyclically in sync with the menstrual cycle, dramatic changes occur during pregnancy, and as well as the postpartum period [9].

Throughout life, homeostasis is preserved in all systems through tightly regulated interactions between numerous interdependent body tissues [8] (Fig. 23.1). Driven by inalterable genetic factors; environmental insults, such as ultraviolet (UV) light; and lifestyle factors like nutrition and nicotine use [10], body tissues, with age, experience a progressive deterioration of cellular and tissue functions, largely due to genetic decay and the by-products of metabolism [10]. The study of aging in the immune system has revealed that immunosenescence represents a substantial remodeling of major immune functions [8].

Immunosenescence in both genders impacts cellular, humoral, and innate immunity [11]. Significant consequences of aging include atrophy of the thymus, changes in both the total numbers and subsets of lymphocytes, changes in the function of both B and T cells, changes in the patterns of secretion of cytokines and growth factors, disruption of intracellular signaling, changes in the patterns of antibody production, loss of antibody repertoire, loss of response to antigens and mitogens, and disruption of immunological tolerance (Table 23.1). Gender-specific increases in some aspects of immunosenescence have been observed and will be discussed below.

Although aging affects many immune cell types, the cumulative effects of aging on T-cell

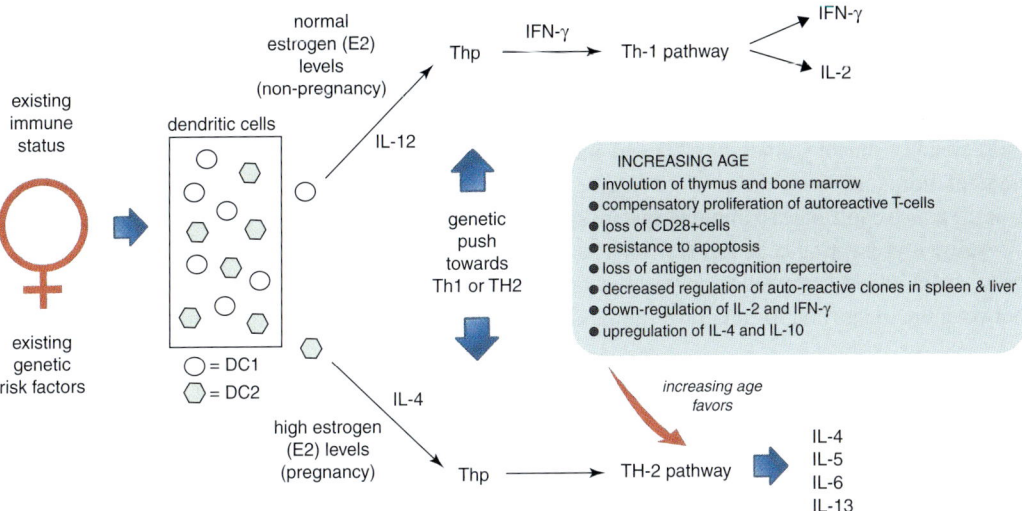

Fig. 23.1 Interaction between genetic factors, estrogen, and aging in the development of Th1/TH2 differentiation and subsequent autoimmune diseases in aging women (Reprinted with permission from *Expert Rev Obs Gyn* 7(6), 557–571 (2012) with permission of Expert Reviews Ltd)

function are the most consistently observed and most extensive [12]. The human thymus decreases in both size and cellularity in a process called thymic involution; thymus tissue is replaced with fat [13]. By age sixty, thymus-derived hormones are absent from the circulation.

Involution of the thymus in humans occurs in concert with a depletion of naïve T cells and a shift in the T cell population towards memory CD4+ cells [14]. In young adulthood, the CD4+ subset is characterized by roughly equivalent numbers of memory and naïve CD4+ cells but in older adults becomes predominantly memory CD4+ [15], a shift which reduces the potential antigenic repertoire [16]. The shift towards memory T cells with age is largely a consequence of the imbalance in T-cell maturation produced by thymus involution [17] paired with an age-related impairment of T-cell proliferation [18] in concert with clonal expansion of T cells activated by specific antigens [16]. The shift towards memory cells in the T-cell compartment affects cytokine production as well, with less interleukin (IL)-2 produced (primarily a product of naïve T cells) but more IL-4 (primarily a product of memory T cells) [19].

The cumulative loss of T helper (Th) cells with age plays a profound role in immunosenescence, ultimately affecting both cellular and humoral immunity. Disruption of T-cell helper cells and alterations of cytokine levels which control B-cell functions compromise humoral immunity substantially, with decreased production of long-term immunoglobulin (Ig)-producing B cells as well as a reduction of Ig diversity [5]. Although B-cell numbers do not change significantly, there is a significant impairment of B-cell response to primary antigenic stimulation [16]; specific immunoglobulins produced become more random, and those produced have decreased affinity for their specific antigen [16]. With age, therefore, the B-cell repertoire poised to respond to new antigenic challenge is limited, and the predominance of memory T cells seen with thymic involution is mirrored in the B-cell compartment [20]. IL-15, particularly, stimulates proliferation of memory T cells; IL-15 levels are nearly double in healthy adults 95 or older (3.05 pg/mL as compared to both older adults [aged 60–89] 1.94 pg/mL and midlife adults [aged 30–59] 1.73 pg/mL) [21].

Immunosenescence is compounded by the presence in the aged of a chronic low-grade inflammation characterized by increased proinflammatory cytokines such as Il-6 and tumor necrosis factor alpha (TNF-α), compounds that create oxidative stress and decrease cellular antioxidant capacity [11]. These proinflammatory cytokines are positively associated with stress as well as salivary cortisol levels and may play a significant role in creating the degenerative changes associated with aging [18]. Other body processes, most notably innate immunity [22] and interactions of immunity with the neuroendocrine system [23], also contribute to immune system aging.

Antigen-presenting cells (APCs) such as dendritic cells and macrophages serve as a bridge between the innate and the adaptive immune systems. APCs interact with foreign molecules and release pathogen-specific cytokines that drive the activation of naïve CD4 helper cells into either Th1 or T helper 2 (Th2) effector cells [24].

Production of IL-12 and interferon gamma (IFN-γ) drives commitment of naïve T cells to the Th1 lineage. Th1 cells produce cytokines which favor a cell-mediated response (IL-2, lymphotoxin, IFN-γ, tumor necrosis factor beta [TNFβ]), warding off intracellular pathogens, mounting

Table 23.1 Changes in immune function with age (both men and women)

Immune function	Change	Reference
B cell	Reduction in early progenitor B cells in the bone marrow	[110]
	Increase in polyclonal response against diverse mitogens	[8]
	Decrease of specific antigen response	[8]
	Production of antibodies independent of T-cell activation	[5]
	Oligoclonal expansion of B cells	[5]
	Increase in B1 cell fraction of B cells	[49]
	Maturation of B cells blocked (believed to be inability to rearrange Ig genes because of decrease in expression of RAG-1 and RAG-2 recombinases	[111]
	Reduced output of naïve B cells	[110]
	Accumulation of oligoclonally expanded, functionally incompetent memory lymphocytes	[110]
	Decreased numbers of circulating B cells	[112]
	CD20+ B cells decrease	[15]
	Reduced antigen-recognition repertoire of B cells	[113]
	Class switch alterations in immunoglobulins produced	[114]
	Stimulated B cells show significant alterations in cellular structures with role in signal transduction	[115]
	Increase of IgA and several IgG subclasses	[116]
Lymphocytes	Reduction in total numbers	[59]
Molecular	Alterations in cell surface receptors (e.g., loss of co-stimulatory receptor CD28 expression in CD8+ cells)	[117]
	Alterations in cytokine and cytokine receptor alterations in T cells	[118]
	Alterations in effector molecules	[119,120]
	Interleukin 6 levels increase	[121]
	Alterations in transcriptional regulators	[119]
	Diminished RAG expression as result of defective bone marrow microenvironment	[5]
	Reduced activity of transcription factors like E2A and Pax-5	[5]
Systemic	Decline in humoral immunity	[119]
	Increased levels of circulating proinflammatory cytokines IL-6 and TNF-α	[122]
	Decreased microbicidal activity against *C. albicans* and *E. coli* with reduced reactive oxygen species produced during the respiratory burst	[123]
	Decreased response of activated neutrophils to cytokines that suppress apoptosis	[124]
	Frequency of monoclonal gammopathies increases with age (doubles from 2 % at age 50 to 4 % at age 70)	[125]
NK cells	Total cell numbers increase	[15]
	NK cytotoxic function impaired	[5]

Table 23.1 (continued)

Immune function	Change	Reference
T-cell functions	Reduced diversity of T-cell repertoire	[119]
	Decrease of T-helper (Th) cells	[8]
	Decrease of T-suppressor cells	[8]
	Decrease in expression of lymphocyte growth factors	[8]
	Decrease in expression of specific lymphocyte receptors	[8]
	Disruption of intracellular signaling	[126]
	Reduced diversity of antigen recognition repertoire (about 10^8 in young adults to 10^6 in elderly)	[127]
	Impaired proliferation in response to antigenic stimulation	[128]
	Changes in cytokine profiles	[119]
	Atrophy of the thymus with reduction of thymic production of T cells	[129]
	Substantial reduction in numbers of naïve lymphocytes	[129]
	Impaired helper function of naïve CD4+ T cells	[130]
	Decline in CD3+ and CD5 +populations	[15]
	Accumulation of CD 28- CD8+ circulating T cells	[119]
	Loss of CD28 which abrogates normal T-cell elimination	[131]
	Decrease in total numbers of CD4+ and CD8+ cells	[15]
	Decrease in suppressor-inducer naïve T cells (CD4+CD45RA+) decrease	[15]
	Increase in helper-inducer T cells (CD4CD29+)	[15]
	Increase in CD4+/CD8+ ratio	[15]
	Clonal expansion of CD8+ T cells	[132]
	Impaired response of CD44^{hi}CD8+ cells to IL-15	[133]
	Impaired maturation of naïve CD4+ cells into Th1 or Th2 cells	[134]
	Decreased postactivation of Il-2	[135]
	Alterations in several components of signaling complex in both memory and naïve T cells in aged mice	[126]
	Naïve T cells defective, production of lower levels of Il-2, increased levels of Il-4, reduced proliferative capability, reduced capability of differentiation into effecter cells (much driven by Il-2 deficit)	[16]

CD cluster of differentiation, *E2A* estradiol, *Ig* immunoglobulin, *IL* interleukin, *NK* natural killer, *RAG* recombinase-activating gene, *Th* T-helper, *TNF* tumor necrosis factor

delayed-type hypersensitivity responses to viral and bacterial antigens, and eliminating tumor cells [16].

Production of IL-4 and IL-10 drives commitment to the Th2 subtypes [24]. Th2 cells release cytokines which produce an environment favoring humoral immunity (IL-4, IL-5, IL-6, IL-10, and IL-13) by stimulating Th2-cell proliferation, differentiation, and participation in humoral immunity [16].

In the aged, however, naïve cells are less likely to become effectors; in those that do, there is a documented shift towards a Th2 cytokine response [16].

The molecular and cellular changes associated with aging have substantial clinical ramifications. The elderly have impaired ability to achieve immunization but much higher levels of circulating autoantibodies (due to the lack of naïve effectors), impaired response to viral infections, increased risk of bacterial infections, and increased risk of both neoplastic and autoimmune disease [8].

23.3 Gender and Immunity

Immunosenescence does not affect men and women equally [12]. The dysregulation in T-cell function, for example, that is associated with aging, occurs much more dramatically in women than in men [25,26].

Gender-specific differences in immunosenescence are at least partly attributable to sex hormones, evidenced by the fact that men and postmenopausal women have reduced T-cell immunity as compared to premenopausal women [27]. The fact that men live shorter lives, on average, than women is also partially attributed to the thymic involution produced by higher circulating levels of androgens in men [28], and a recent study has documented greater age-associated decline of less differentiated lymphocytes and increase of highly differentiated T cells in females [29].

Much is known about the influence of sex hormones on immunity in general. Androgens, estrogen, and progesterone all influence immune functions; estrogen in the form of 17β estradiol has been particularly associated with profound influences on the immune system (Table 23.2).

Females, in general, have superior immune vigilance as compared to males, with both humoral and cell-mediated arms mounting more vigorous responses to immune stimulation [30]. Women maintain higher antibody levels than men, as well as higher levels of circulating IL-1, IL-4, and INF-γ [31]. Females reject grafts faster [32]. A general pattern is observed in which estrogen enhances humoral immunity, while androgens as well as progesterone tend to suppress it [33]. Women respond to antigenic stimulation with a predominantly Th2 response, with increased antibody production [34]. Estrogen stimulates the Th2 response by stimulating Th lymphocytes to secrete type 2 cytokines which promote the synthesis of antibodies [35]. High estrogen levels associated with pregnancy also produce a shift towards Th2 response [36].

Conversely, men respond to antigenic stimulation primarily with a Th1 response [34]. Androgens stimulate Th cells to produce type 1 cytokines, which suppress Th2 activity and stimulate CD8

Table 23.2 Biological functions of estrogen

Immune function	Immune characteristic	Reference
B cell	Induction of antibody production	[38]
	Produces higher overall immunoglobulin levels	[31]
	Promotes antibody response to foreign antigens	[31]
	Increases IgG and IgM levels	[35]
	Produces polyclonal induction of B cells in vitro	[136]
Cytokines and effector molecules	Stimulates proinflammatory serum markers	[137]
	Downregulates soluble cell adhesion molecules in women	[138]
	Inhibits expression of monocyte chemoattractant protein-1	[139]
	Stimulates interleukin production (IL-1, IL-4, IL-6, IL-10 in macrophages; IL-4, IL-5,IL-6; and 1-0 in Th2 cells	[38]
	Stimulates cellular response to cytokines	[31]
	Stimulates secretion of IL-4, IFN-γ, and IL-1	[31]
	Stimulates production of anti-apoptosis protein Bcl-2	[140]
	Inhibits IL-1-induced expression of cell adhesion molecules	[139]
	Inhibits of TNF-α expression	[141]
	Downregulates soluble TNF-α	[142]
T cell	Downregulates number of immature T lymphocytes	[143]
Systemic	Stimulates resistance to certain infections	[31]
	Downregulates induction of tolerance	[31]
	Stimulates graft rejection	[31]
T cell	Stimulates involution of the thymus	[143]
	Stimulates production of regulatory T cells (Tregs)	[53]
	Downregulates CD4 T cells	[31]
	Stimulates an increase CD4/CD8 ratios	[31]

CD cluster of differentiation, *IFN-γ* interferon gamma, *Ig* immunoglobulin, *IL* interleukin, *Th* T helper, *TNF-α* tumor necrosis factor alpha cells [37], a process that produces inflammation as the predominant immune response [34].

The fact that estrogen favors a stronger overall immune response, particularly with regard to antibody response in women, is a mixed blessing. Although it produces a superior resistance to infection as compared to men, it also increases the risk in women of autoimmune disease [38].

23.4 Aging and the Development of Autoimmunity

There are at least 70 documented autoimmune diseases [38], and the prevalence of autoimmune disease is rapidly rising worldwide, for reasons not completely understood [39]. Although the disorders share a pathogenic immunity against the body's own tissues that is the product of a progressive disorganization of immune function, the precise etiology is unknown. Autoimmunity appears to be a multifactorial process in which genetic, environmental, and biochemical processes all participate.

A genetic or familial predisposition to autoimmunity clearly plays a role. Pairwise analyses examined discordant familiar risks for seven common autoimmune diseases using a large national databank that included the records of 172,242 patients. Records examined demonstrated a genetic pattern of inheritance for RA, SLE, type I diabetes, ankylosing spondylitis, Crohn's disease, celiac disease, and ulcerative colitis. Incidence of each of the seven autoimmune diseases analyzed was associated additionally with at least three of the others [40].

Environmental factors such as pollution or occupational exposures or contact with viral, bacterial, or parasitic pathogens may trigger autoimmunity. Lifestyle differences like nutritional choices, sleep patterns, medications, and stress may also trigger illness [38].

Endogenous factors also play a role; for example, sex hormones are a major influence [31]. The most striking gender-based difference in immune system function is the remarkable female predominance of autoimmune diseases [41]. An estimated 78 % of those affected by autoimmune disease are women [34].

Gender-specific patterns in the development of autoimmune diseases suggest a strong role of sex hormones, as predominance in the female sex changes with age at disease diagnosis, lending strong support [42]. Autoimmunity in males shows less age-dependent variation. Autoimmune diseases prevalent in males typically present before the sixth decade with the appearance of autoantibodies, acute inflammation, and increase in the proinflammatory cytokines characteristic of a Th1 response.

Those that manifest primarily in females are more complicated. Autoimmune diseases that manifest early in life in females generally have a clear antibody-mediated pathology. Those with increased incidence in females that appear after the age of 50 (in menopause) tend to be characterized by a more chronic disease course and fibrotic Th-mediated pathology.

A central role for sex hormones in autoimmune disease in women is also evidenced by the dramatic differences in prevalence during the different reproductive periods of a woman's life, which are themselves driven by profound modulation of circulating levels of sex steroids, particularly estrogen [31]. Many autoimmune diseases in which women predominate are exacerbated by the higher levels of female sex steroids in pregnancy (a period that is also characterized by a shift towards Th2 response), primarily estrogen, which worsens disease, while androgens produce beneficial effect.

Strict correlation of autoimmunity with estrogen levels, however, is not observed. Other female-predominant autoimmune diseases, such as multiple sclerosis and rheumatoid arthritis, worsen during pregnancy [43] and improve in the postmenopausal period [44] (Table 23.3).

The influence on autoimmune disease of the decreasing levels of estrogen associated with aging in women is essentially unascertained. The declining efficacy of the immune system with age, in both genders, is accompanied by a characteristic increase in both the variety and level of circulating autoantibodies [8]. Antinuclear antibody (ANA) levels remain constant until about age 60 and then rise. About 5 % of healthy individuals of that age have high ANA titers (1:160), compared to 37 % of those over 70 years of age [45].

Table 23.3 Preponderance of females afflicted with autoimmune diseases

Autoimmune disease	Target of autoantibodies	Percent female	F/M differential	Peak of prevalence	Pathway	Effect of menopause
Hashimoto's thyroiditis	Thyroid gland	95 %[a]	37:1[b]	40s in women, 50s in men	Th2	Associated with early menopause
Sjögren's syndrome	Mucous membranes and salivary glands	94 %[a]	14:1[b]	30–40s	Th2	Worsens
SLE	DNA (primarily double stranded)	89 %[a]	11:1[b]	Late 20s, early 30s	Th2	Improves
Grave's disease	Thyroid	88 %[a]	6:1[b]	Late 40s to early 60s	Th2	Can precipitate premature menopause
Scleroderma	Connective tissue	92 %[a]	3.5:1[b]	40s	Th2	Little affect
Diabetes mellitus	Pancreas	48 %[a]	5:1[b]	20s	Th1	Worsens
Rheumatoid arthritis	Synovial joints	75 %[a]	2.5:1[b]	60s	Th1	Worsens
Multiple sclerosis	Central nervous system	64 %[a]	Unknown	Late 20s	Th1	Worsens
Myasthenia gravis	Muscle tissue	73 %[a]	2.5:1[b]	Early 30s	Unknown	Unknown

DNA deoxyribonucleic acid, *F/M* female/male, *NA* not applicable, *SLE* systemic lupus erythematosus
[a]Source reference: Ackerman [144]
[b]Source reference: Papenfuss [30]

Although autoantibodies, found in the blood of all healthy humans, serve a useful function in a healthy adult, acting to clear away cellular debris produced by routine injury and inflammation [46], the number of different circulating autoantibodies has proven to be a good predictor of autoimmune disease. The risk of developing childhood diabetes within 5 years, for example, is only 10 % with the presence of one autoantibody specificity, but increases to as much as 80 % if there are three [34]. Autoantibody levels are normally kept in check by immune tolerance processes, but can (through age or overt disease) reach clinically significant levels, at which point the binding of self-antigens activates the complement cascade and results in cytotoxicity or other immune pathology [34]. Rising levels of antibodies, apart from the number of different specificities, are also associated with a generally increased risk of autoimmunity in old age [8].

What specifically causes the documented increase in both autoantibodies and autoimmunity in older adults is a matter of debate. With age, the normally tight orchestration of interdependent immune functions begins to decay, with progressive perturbation of immune function that can eventually lead to autoimmune disease [8]. Increased autoimmunity appears to be primarily the result of the combined effects of the reduction in naïve T cells (produced by thymus involution) in concert with an activation of self-reactive memory B cells.

B-cell activation may result from a variety of antigenic stimuli [47]. Exposure to an infectious agent with molecular mimicry of a self-antigen may prompt a memory response [16]. Cumulative exposure to a variety of antibody specificities, in the presence of chronic infections, for example, may also produce hyperstimulation of B cells. In a study of the elderly in Cameroon (where multiple chronic infections are not uncommon), the pattern of autoantibodies observed in the elderly subjects was markedly different from that in industrialized countries, suggesting a role for long-term multiple antigen exposures [48]. Normal aging can also reduce the efficiency of normal physical immune barriers, resulting in increased pathogen intrusion [49]. Innate immunity also deteriorates with age, which can contribute to chronic immune stimulation. The persistence of high antigen levels can also make co-stimulatory T cells less susceptible to downregulation [49].

Other sources of B-cell memory activation are neoantigens which are revealed by a progressive loss of tissue integrity and increased inflammation as individuals age [50]. Inappropriate activation of lymphocytes can also result from defective clearance of cellular debris, resulting in prolonged exposure to autoantigens [49]. Self-antigens may also acquire alterations that increase immunogenicity. For example, posttranslational modification of proteins increases in immunosenescence; particular modifications, such as isoaspartyl formation, can trigger an autoimmune response [49].

Improper self-antigen recognition by dendritic cells (DC) and T cells initiates, through release of specific cytokines (as described above), destructive Th1 or Th2 responses. Rheumatoid arthritis, for example, is characterized by an exaggerated Th1 self-reactive immunity, SLE by an excessive Th2 [24]. Estrogens are known to drive physiological selection of Th1 or Th2 pathways.

A perturbation in immune receptor signaling may underlie the increase in autoimmune phenomena in the elderly, particularly those that contribute to the regulation of immune tolerance. Optimal immune function necessitates a tight balance of the signaling pathways in both T- and B-cell compartments; these pathways are altered in both compartments in SLE and other autoimmune diseases [51].

Other aspects of aging can increase immune dysfunction as well: stress, with associated increased cortisol levels; sleep dysregulation and associated effects on immunity; decrease in physical activity and negative effects on immunocompetence; and nutritional deficiencies common in old age with a negative impact on immunocompetence [4].

23.5 Specific Effects of Estrogen on Autoimmunity

In women, the cumulative physiological degeneration associated with normal aging is augmented by a dramatic and systemic estrogen deprivation. Estrogens generally favor immune processes involving CD4+ Th2 cells and B cells [52], thereby promoting B-cell-mediated autoimmune diseases. Physiological levels of estrogen, however, also stimulate the expansion of CD4+CD25+regulatory T cells (Treg cells), which help maintain tolerance to self-antigens and therefore ameliorate autoimmune disease, as well as the expression of the FOXP3 gene, a marker for Treg cell function [53]. Follicular helper T cells (Tfh cells), in contrast, appear to drive autoantibody production in the germinal center and are associated with the development of systemic autoimmunity [54].

Androgens, on the other hand, encourage processes involving CD4+Th1 cells and CD8+ cells, acting to suppress or ameliorate B-cell-mediated autoimmune diseases [31]. The influence of these hormones on the immune system, therefore, produces more autoimmune pathology in women in autoimmune disease mediated by Th2-dominant processes and more in men when Th1 processes are involved (see Table 23.3).

Hormonal manipulations can alter immune reactivity and modulate disease expression [41]. Estrogens provoke involution of the thymus [38]; treatment of castrated animals with exogenous sex hormones causes massive atrophy of the thymus [55]. Thymus regeneration occurs following ovariectomy [5], and thymus involution occurs during pregnancy, which reverts after lactation ceases [56].

Estrogen-induced involution of the thymus is associated with a reduction in numbers of immature T lymphocytes [38]. Estrogen affects T-cell subset composition, as well as T-cell function and activation [12]. Oral estrogen replacement therapy has been shown to restore T-cell function [57].

Estrogen drastically reduces not only the size of the thymus but also of the bone marrow cavity as well, the sites where most deletion of autoreactive cells occurs. B cells developing at alternative sites (liver and spleen), where less stringent selection occurs, may escape normal controls [31].

Estrogens, in fact, stimulate lymphopoiesis outside of the bone marrow [58]. Mice treated with exogenous estrogen develop impressive hemopoietic centers in the liver and spleens filled with antibody-producing cells [31].

Estrogen depletion in women, characteristic of postmenopausal women, has been specifically associated with reductions in B cells and T cells [59] and Th-derived cytokines [60] as well as an impaired immune response to viral infections [61]. In vitro, estrogen stimulates Th1 cytokine production by T cells [47].

Estrogens diminish the number of monocytes, through apoptosis, as well as through a modulation of the cell cycle which delays mitosis [62]. Autoreactive B-cell apoptosis, particularly, is inhibited [63]. Estrogen however simultaneously induces a rapid maturation of B lymphocytes [38] and stimulates Th lymphocytes to secrete type 2 cytokines that promote antibody production [35,37].

23.6 What Is Known About the Estrogen Deficiency of Menopause and Specific Autoimmune Diseases

It is known that many natural, pathological, and therapeutic conditions can change serum estrogen levels, including the menstrual cycle, pregnancy, menopause, use of oral contraceptives, use of hormonal replacement treatment, and disease. The estrogen withdrawal of menopause, however, is a significant hormonal transition and one with numerous physiological ramifications. The interrelationship of menopause and autoimmune diseases is complex and not yet fully understood. Recent literature has noted that autoimmune disease and/or autoimmune disease treatments can play a role in causing premature ovarian failure (POF) resulting in early menopause [64,65]. In addition, some symptoms and effects of autoimmune disease (e.g., increased cardiovascular risk, increased fracture risk, cognitive decline, urinary incontinence/irritable bladder, etc.) can be similar to those of normal aging, which increases the challenge of distinguishing the expected effects of menopause and aging from those of autoimmune disease [64,66]. These aspects of the relationship between menopause and autoimmune disease will not be discussed in this chapter, which shall rather concentrate on effects of menopause on selected autoimmune diseases.

The normal immunosenescence evidenced in both sexes may be modulated in some degree by changing levels and forms of endogenous estrogen. The production of cytokines Il-6, Il-1, and TNF-α increases after menopause, as does the physiological response to those cytokines [11]. There is a postmenopausal decrease in CD4 T and B lymphocytes, as well as decrease in the cytotoxic activity of natural killer (NK) cells [33].

In vitro analysis of three different T-cell signaling proteins (Janus kinase 2 [JAK2], Janus kinase 3 [JAK3], and CD3-zeta) found that postmenopausal levels were substantially reduced as compared to premenopausal levels [12]. In addition, Jurkat T cells exposed to premenopausal levels of E2 also formed significantly more IL-2 producing colonies as compared to those exposed to postmenopausal levels (75.3 ± 2.2 vs 55.7 ± 2.1 [$P<0.0001$]) [12]. Studies suggest a normalization of cellular response after hormone replacement therapy (HRT) [11].

23.6.1 Systemic Lupus Erythematosus

Systemic lupus erythematosus (SLE) is an autoimmune disorder characterized by the production of pathogenic autoantibodies, primarily to nuclear antigens, as well as dysregulation of both T and B cells [67]. B cells display accelerated maturity [68]. SLE patients exhibit monocyte-derived dendritic cells (DCs) which display an activated, proinflammatory phenotype [68].

SLE has a female preponderance of 9:1. Although there are X-chromosome abnormalities associated with SLE [69], estrogen itself is strongly implicated in SLE autoimmunity [11]. SLE is associated with a disrupted sex hormone balance characterized by lower amounts of androgens and dramatically higher levels of the estrogen metabolite, 16-hydroxyestrone [70]. Pregnancy worsens the disease [24]; incidence of SLE diminishes after menopause [38,44,71]. Administration of an estrogen receptor blocker (fulvestrant) to human female SLE patients produces clinical improvement [72] as does treatment with testosterone [73], and long-term remission has been seen following abrupt medication-induced menopause [74].

Increased risk has been associated with higher lifetime levels of estrogen exposure. In a cohort of 238,308 adult women evaluated prospectively over 27 years, the 262 women diagnosed with SLE over the course of the study were analyzed for relative risk factors. Increased risk was associated with early menarche (aged less than 10) (relative risk [RR] 2.1, 95 % confidence interval [CI] 1.4–3.2) and oral contraceptive use (RR 1.5, 95 % CI 1.1–2.1) [75]. Menstrual irregularity increased risk of SLE diagnosis in a Japanese case-control study [76]. Menstrual cycles of abnormal length (either long or short) increased risk as well [77]. Estradiol treatment of mouse lupus-prone strains produces disease onset, increases autoantibody production, and increases risk of mortality [24].

Hormonal fluctuations also appear to influence the course of SLE. Dual studies evaluated the course of disease in early-onset SLE patients versus late-onset patients; later-onset patients (after the age of 50) had lower incidences of renal disease, arthritis, malar rash, and photosensitivity as compared to patients who were younger at diagnosis [78]. Younger patients had a more aggressive disease course as well, with time from symptom onset to diagnosis being 3 years as compared to 5 years in older patients [78]. Similar results were observed in a study of 125 Chinese SLE patients [79]. A pooled analysis which compared 714 late-onset patients with 4,700 early-onset patients confirmed earlier results, finding also a lower incidence of purpura, alopecia, and Raynaud's in the late-onset group. The late-onset group, however, had a higher prevalence of rheumatoid factor, with antibodies to ribonucleoprotein (RNP) and sphingomyelin (SM) less frequently [80].

SLE patients have also been evaluated for effect of previous hysterectomy (with and without concomitant oophorectomy). SLE patients ($N=3,389$) who had undergone hysterectomy were less likely to develop nephritis or positive anti-double-stranded deoxyribonucleic acid (dsDNA) antibodies than age-matched SLE patients who had not (Odds ratio 6.66 [95 % CI=3.09–14.38] in European patients and 2.74 [95 % CI=1.43–5.25] in African-American patients). SLE patients with hysterectomy before disease onset had later onset of disease ($P=0.0001$) [67].

The role of estrogen, rather than age alone, was investigated by studies which utilized younger SLE patients who underwent ovarian failure produced by cyclophosphamide. Significantly fewer flares were observed in the group with ovarian failure as compared to normally menstruating SLE women [81]. The cyclophosphamide group, however, was significantly older than the control group (37.9 years as compared to 25.5 years). Other research, however, followed two groups of SLE patients, one early onset and one late, and concluded that the decrease in disease activity after menopause could not conclusively be determined to be related to hormonal status [82].

Hormone replacement therapy (HRT) has documented benefits for women with regard to some aspects of aging and in some cases may be medically necessary [83]. Postmenopausal osteoporosis, for example, directly tied to estrogen deficiency, may require hormonal intervention, shown to reduce the risk of hip fractures as much as 30 % [84]. HRT, however, in patients with SLE, which is induced or exacerbated by oral contraceptives, has the potential to produce disease flares.

Examination of the effects of HRT in postmenopausal women found that in 351 postmenopausal SLE patients, combined estrogen/progesterone hormone replacement (0.625 mg conjugated estrogen daily, plus 5 mg medroxyprogesterone for 12 days/month) given for 12 months produced only a small increase in the risk of disease flares (0.64 probability in HRT patients vs 0.51 in placebo controls, with most flares mild or moderate [$p=0.01$]). HRT use did not significantly increase the risk of severe flares [83].

An overall assessment of the consequences of SLE in postmenopausal patients looked at damage accrual in SLE as part of the LUMINA (Lupus in Minorities: Nature vs Nurture) study and found that despite the drop in disease activity in the postmenopausal period (with a reduction in the risk of renal disease), overall damage scores were higher due to an increase in cardiovascular disease. Whether higher damage accrual is related to the changing hormones of menopause or due simply to longer disease duration is as yet undetermined [85]. It is known that estrogen promotes SLE through estrogen receptor-α (ER-α) by inducing IFN-γ [86]. Testosterone is most likely protective in SLE patients by driving the Th1 immune pathway [11].

Although no differences are observed in SLE patients as compared to normal controls with regard to circulating estrogen levels (17β-estradiol), number of estrogen receptors, or binding affinities of estrogen receptor to estrogen, and blocking of the estrogen receptors using fulvestrant in patients with moderately active SLE produced a significant decrease in disease activity (as measured by the SLE disease activity index [SLEDAI] score) [72].

Female SLE patients have abnormal metabolism of sex hormones, with an increase in the production of 16-hydroxyestrone and metabolites that may produce a chronic state of excessive estrogen [87]. Elevated aromatase activity (an enzyme found in all organ system and integral to sexual reproduction that converts androgens into estrogens) is also observed in SLE patients [38].

The molecular mechanism leading to a gender preponderance in SLE appears to be demethylation of CD40 ligand on CD40+ T cells [88], which, appearing on an inactive X chromosome, results in overexpression of CD40 ligand on CD4+ cells [89]. SLE patients are typically characterized by high titers of autoantibodies directed against nuclear antigens, antibodies which have been demonstrated to potentially arise from germline-coded polyreactive antibodies induced to class switch to IgG by a proinflammatory milieu [90].

23.6.2 Rheumatoid Arthritis

Rheumatoid arthritis (RA) is an autoimmune disease in which multiple components of the immune system produce tissue damage and contribute to systemic inflammation. T cells, B cells, and macrophages infiltrate into the inflamed synovial membrane whose resident cells proliferate and differentiate; macrophages and other activated tissue-resident cells begin to produce cytokines which induce B- and T-cell responses that act in concert to erode bone and cause destruction of cartilage. RA is associated with an altered sex hormone balance characterized by lower amounts of androgens and higher estrogens [70]. RA incidence increases with postmenopause, suggesting that decreased E2 levels are involved in disease onset. The incidence of RA incidence peaks in the seventh decade [91]. Pregnancy ameliorates disease activity [92]; however, the postpartum period is a time of high risk for new-onset RA [93]. Aromatase inhibitor, a compound that interferes with estrogen production, triggers onset of rheumatoid arthritis or produces arthritis flares in both premenopausal and postmenopausal women [94].

Rheumatoid arthritis is characterized by a profile of generalized immunosenescence typical with age. Early-onset RA may represent premature immunosenescence [95], loss of T-cell diversity and T-cell reactivity, slide towards proliferative arrest, and significant production of inflammatory cytokines. Levels of autoantibodies increase as well [91]. In addition, RA patients carry large, clonally expanded populations of CD4+ and CD8+ cells; C4+ clones are consistently autoreactive [91].

Menopause is associated with an increased risk of disease onset. In a cohort of nearly 32,000 women in Iowa, those who reached menopause before age 45 had a higher risk of RA than women who reached menopause after age 51 [96]. Similar results were obtained in a study that evaluated 18,326 Swedish women and compared those who entered menopause before 45 to those who reached menopause after 45 years of age [97]. Menopause before age 45 has also been shown to be associated with milder RA severity. A study of 134 postmenopausal female RA patients with menopause before age 45 was significantly more likely to experience mild/moderate rheumatoid factor-negative (RF-negative) RA, rather than severe RA or mild/moderate RF-positive RA [98]. The same study found no major difference in RA severity associated with oral contraceptive use or a history of breastfeeding.

Another author followed RA patients over a 6-year period; the 209 female patients evaluated were divided into premenopausal and postmenopausal groups. Postmenopausal subjects had greater joint damage as measured radiographically as well as by health assessment questionnaires. In addition, comparison with both premenopausal women and men determined that estrogen deprivation of menopause was a significant factor in the disparity of damage between men and women [99]. Although the use of HRT does not appear to influence the risk of developing RA [100], HRT improves both symptoms and progression of disease [101].

23.6.3 Scleroderma

Scleroderma is an autoimmune disease of the connective tissues characterized by a buildup of collagen in body tissues. Typically involving primarily the skin on the hands and face, scleroderma can affect many organ systems, including the heart, lungs, and kidneys. Scleroderma affects mostly women, with onset typically around the same time as menopause; early menopause increases risk [102]. Scleroderma involves significant vasculopathy which is accentuated by menopause-related loss of estrogen. A prospective Italian study found that the estrogen removal of the postmenopausal period was a risk factor for the development of pulmonary arterial hypertension (PAH) in scleroderma patients, with relative risk due to postmenopausal state of 5.2 ($p=0.000$) [103]. Twenty-three postmenopausal scleroderma patients were subsequently treated with HRT for a mean follow-up of 7.5 years. None of the HRT scleroderma patients developed PAH as compared to 19.5 % of those not on HRT [104].

23.6.4 Sjögren's Syndrome

Sjögren's syndrome (SS) is an autoimmune disorder that affects mucous membranes as well as tear ducts and salivary glands but may also impact other organs such as the kidneys, stomach, intestines, vasculature, lungs, liver, pancreas, and central nervous system. The large majority of SS patients are women, with onset after the age of 40. SS is associated with a T-cell infiltration of the exocrine glands with associated autoantibodies [105]. Estrogen suppresses disease development, while ovariectomy leads to an SS-like condition with increased epithelial cell apoptosis [24]. Estrogen-deficient mice develop an autoimmune exocrinopathy resembling SS [106]. It is believed that estrogen deficiency may influence autoantigen cleavage in such a way that it results in autoimmune exocrinopathy in postmenopausal women [106].

23.6.5 Multiple Sclerosis

Multiple sclerosis (MS) is an episodic autoimmune disease in which autoantibodies attack the central nervous system (CNS), particularly the myelin sheath; symptoms vary with the location of the attack. MS is typically diagnosed in young adulthood. As the target tissue of MS is the central nervous system, MS has debilitating and systemic effects. More women than men suffer from MS; estrogen influence is also suggested by the fact that MS symptoms improve during pregnancy but worsen postpartum. MS pathogenesis is largely driven by antigen-specific CD4+ Th1 cells, specific for the central nervous system, which secrete proinflammatory cytokines such as IFN-γ, TNF-α, and IL-12. Active disease is well correlated with T-cell production of proinflammatory cytokines [24]. Most (54 %) MS patients reported a worsening of symptoms after menopause; 75 % of those who had used HRT (at all stages of menopause) reported improvement [107].

23.6.6 Autoimmune Hepatitis

Autoimmune hepatitis (AIH) is an autoantibody-induced inflammation of the liver, although a variety of autoantibodies (directed against specific liver antigens as well as nuclear DNA, mitochondrial antigens, and smooth muscle antigens) are involved. AIH also affects predominantly females, most often with onset in childhood but also postmenopause [47], although men may be affected more often than women in old age. Autoantibodies are directed against hepatocytes, the putative result of an insidious progressive destruction of the hepatic parenchyma [47]. AIH often ameliorates during pregnancy; many cases, however, are diagnosed in the postpartum period [108,109].

23.7 Summary

Immunosenescence is a complex phenomenon, involving cellular, humoral, and innate immunity in a downward spiral of dysregulation of the tightly interdependent responses characteristic of young adulthood, with multiple effects on hematopoiesis, immune cell proliferation and differentiation, and immune cell function. The eventual result is an immune system that is hyperactivated but defective, which sets the stage for a rise in autoantibodies and thus autoimmunity.

Unraveling the respective roles of genes, hormones, lifestyle factors, and environment in autoimmunity in general and in postmenopausal women in particular has yet to be accomplished. Although the general understanding that estrogen skews immune responses towards Th2 pathways while androgens drive the Th1 pathway explains many of the gender discrepancies and age-related peaks of disease observed, it does not explain all. There are discrepancies, and it proves difficult to attach hormones to specific mechanisms.

Obviously other factors are at play. Genetic and epigenetic components need further investigation. The major autoimmune diseases of the connective tissue all have a strong predominance in women, and tissue specificity for Th1 or Th2 responses may be a factor as well.

The specificity of Ig subclass may influence autoimmunity as autoimmunity is characterized by a marked increase of IgM levels produced by B cells. The role of sex hormones in autoimmunity and in the menopausal period is unmistakable but not easily understood. Estrogen, progesterone, and testosterone share the same precursor: cholesterol, as well as common intermediate metabolites that are known to interact with the immune system. Levels of both estrogen and progesterone decline rapidly as menopause nears; progesterone levels drop more steeply than estrogen. Progesterone (Pg) may substantially impact autoimmune development, as Pg receptors are ubiquitous in immune organs, tissues, and cells. Progesterone has different immunomodulatory effects from estrogen but shares interdependent signaling pathways.

The profound female predisposition to autoimmunity as well as the fact that significant immune derangement occurs during the estrogen-infused months of pregnancy suggests the likelihood that, in general, lower physiological amounts of estrogen stimulate Th1 effects, whereas higher doses stimulate Th2.

The presence of at least two different types of estrogen receptors also allows for multiple levels of control, as does the fact that at menopause, the predominant circulating form of estrogen changes. In addition, the X chromosome, apart from female hormones, may contribute to the female predominance in autoimmune diseases. Racial differences have yet to be seriously explored; other factors implicated in autoimmunity have lacked significant research effort as well. For example, geographical differences in autoimmune disease prevalence have been noted, as has level of industrialization. Increased parity has also been associated with an increased risk in autoimmunity.

With steadily expanding life expectancy, immunosenescence in general, and autoimmunity in old age in particular, should be given increased medical focus. The role of menopause, with its attendant depletion of estrogen, in autoimmune disease should be an important part of that research effort, given the drastic dichotomy in incidence of autoimmune disease in women and men and the longer expected female life span. A better understanding of the interplay between genetic, hormonal, and environmental factors that lead to autoimmunity in menopause is necessary to provide appropriate prevention and/or treatment options for older patients, preserving health into old age and providing an increased quality of life throughout those additional years.

23.8 Expert Commentary

Estrogen rules a women's body. With estrogen receptors in every organ system and nearly every tissue and organ, estrogen's actions continue to be catalogued, but a comprehensive understanding of its dominion over the physiology of the female has yet to be attained. Estrogen maintains female health, protecting a women's cardiovascular system, maintaining bone health, and preserving neural health and brain function. It ferries her from childhood to motherhood yet eventually brings the curtain down on her fertility. Estrogen can also betray her, promoting cancers in the reproductive organs (breast, ovary, and uterus) and causing both mood swings and migraines. It also plays a role in autoimmune disease.

The dramatic preponderance of autoimmune disease in females makes a leading role for estrogen in autoimmune disease nearly certain. The specific contributions that estrogen makes to autoimmunity, however, have been difficult to tease out, due largely to the magnitude of estrogen's influence in female physiology, with seemingly infinite possible actions in multiple biochemical processes. The fact that estrogen, over the life span of the human female, shapeshifts also complicates the picture. Estradiol (E2), the predominant form during the reproductive years, is complemented by estriol (E3) during pregnancy and replaced as the dominant form by estrone (E1) after menopause. Another complicating factor is the existence of dual forms of receptors which act to modulate how estrogen is expressed. Variations in the circulating level of the different forms of estrogen also modulate immune processes, particularly with regard to whether immune response is driven towards cellular (Th1 pathway) or humoral (Th2 pathway) immune responses. A better understanding of the role of estrogen in immune processes is critical for elucidating the role that aging (and its associated estrogen withdrawal in women) plays in both the development and the course of autoimmune disease.

23.9 Five-Year View

This review revealed a disturbing absence of data on the influence of menopause on autoimmune disease given its predominance in women and the fact that autoimmunity increases with age, an absence possibly related to an existing deficit in the understanding of the physiological basis for autoimmune disease in general. A meaningful understanding of the physiology is a challenging goal because autoimmunity clearly has multifactorial origins: a genetic component clearly provides a foundation, estrogen plays a documented role, and prevalence shows a clear correlation with age. The influence of heredity on autoimmunity is being rapidly unveiled now and will no doubt contribute greatly to the elucidation of the relative additional contributions of (1) epigenetic processes, (2) changes in hormone levels, and (3) immunosenescence on immune function. A better understanding of the processes by which molecular events, hormonal shifts, and immunosenescence impact a healthy immune system will provide a physiological basis for better ways to treat both immunosenescence and autoimmunity, a critical goal as the world population, particularly in the developed world, continues to age.

23.10 Key Issues

- Life expectation worldwide continues to rise, as does the prevalence of autoimmune disease.
- Autoimmune diseases affect predominantly women.
- Data on the experience of autoimmunity in postmenopausal women are lacking.
- A genetic foundation for autoimmune risk clearly exists, with both numerous specific genes (including X linked) associated with autoimmunity as well as epigenetic processes that contribute to the development of disease.
- A progressive decay of immune system integrity remodels immune function at a basic level.

Thymic atrophy, which substantially affects T-cell-dependent immune function, shifts immune response towards a humoral response.
- Estrogen has multiple actions in the immune system, creating clear gender-related differences in immune response in men and women.
- Estrogen clearly plays a role in the preponderance of autoimmunity in females and acts to promote humoral immunity in females.
- Autoimmunity appears to be a multifactorial process in which genetic, environmental, and internal physiological effectors like estrogen participate.
- Estrogen's specific effects on autoimmune disease are little understood.
- Autoimmunity appears to be a multifactorial process in which genetic, environmental, and biochemical processes all participate. As both autoimmunity and average life expectancy are on the rise, how these components specifically influence both the development and course of autoimmunity is critical to understand.

References

1. Bulati M, Pellicanò M, Vasto S, Colonna-Romano G. Understanding ageing: biomedical and bioengineering approaches, the immunologic view. Immun Ageing. 2008;5:9.
2. Oeppen J, Vaupel JW. Demography. Broken limits to life expectancy. Science. 2002;296(5570):1029–31.
3. Kochanek KD, Xu JQ, Murphy SLEA. Deaths: preliminary data for 2009. National vital statistics reports; vol 59, no 4. Hyattsville: National Center for Health Statistics; 2011.
4. Larbi A, Franceschi C, Mazzatti D, Solana R, Wikby A, Pawelec G. Aging of the immune system as a prognostic factor for human longevity. Physiology (Bethesda). 2008;23:64–74.
5. Aw D, Silva AB, Palmer DB. Immunosenescence: emerging challenges for an ageing population. Immunology. 2007;120(4):435–46.
6. Menopause. http://emedicine.medscape.com/article/264088-overview.
7. Tobias L. A briefing report on autoimmune diseases and AARDA: past, present, and future. Eastpointe: American Autoimmune Related Diseases Association (AARDA); 2010.
8. Ramos-Casals M, García-Carrasco M, Brito MP, López-Soto A, Font J. Autoimmunity and geriatrics: clinical significance of autoimmune manifestations in the elderly. Lupus. 2003;12(5):341–55.
9. Mund E. Gender differences in immunity over human lifespan. Eur Respir Mon. 2003;25:26–38.
10. Farage MA, Miller KW, Elsner P, Maibach HI. Functional and physiological characteristics of the aging skin. Aging Clin Exp Res. 2008;20(3):195–200.
11. Gameiro CM, Romão F, Castelo-Branco C. Menopause and aging: changes in the immune system–a review. Maturitas. 2010;67(4):316–20.
12. Ku LT, Gercel-Taylor C, Nakajima ST, Taylor DD. Alterations of T cell activation signalling and cytokine production by postmenopausal estrogen levels. Immun Ageing. 2009;6:1.
13. Mello Coelho VD, Bunbury A, Rangel LB, Giri B, Weeraratna A, Morin PJ, et al. Fat-storing multilocular cells expressing CCR5 increase in the thymus with advancing age: potential role for CCR5 ligands on the differentiation and migration of preadipocytes. Int J Med Sci. 2009;7(1):1–14.
14. Crétel E, Veen I, Pierres A, Binan Y, Robert P, Loundou A, et al. Immune profile of elderly patients admitted in a geriatric short care unit. Rev Med Interne. 2011;32(5):275–82.
15. Utsuyama M, Hirokawa K, Kurashima C, Fukayama M, Inamatsu T, Suzuki K, et al. Differential age-change in the numbers of CD4+CD45RA1+ and CD4+ CD29+ T cell subsets in human peripheral blood. Mech Ageing Dev. 1992;63(1):57–68.
16. Stacy S, Krolick KA, Infante AJ, Kraig E. Immunological memory and late onset autoimmunity. Mech Ageing Dev. 2002;123(8):975–85.
17. Aspinall R, Andrew D. Thymic involution in aging. J Clin Immunol. 2000;20(4):250–6.
18. Luz C, Collaziol D, Preissler T, da Cruz IM, Glock L, Bauer ME. Healthy aging is associated with unaltered production of immunoreactive growth hormone but impaired neuroimmunomodulation. Neuroimmunomodulation. 2006;13(3):160–9.
19. Kurashima C, Utsuyama M. Age-related changes of cytokine production by murine helper T cell subpopulations. Pathobiology. 1997;65(3):155–62.
20. Listì F, Candore G, Modica MA, Russo M, Di Lorenzo G, Esposito-Pellitteri M, et al. A study of serum immunoglobulin levels in elderly persons that provides new insights into B cell immunosenescence. Ann N Y Acad Sci. 2006;1089:487–95.
21. Gangemi S, Basile G, Monti D, Merendino RA, Di Pasquale G, Bisignano U, et al. Age-related modifications in circulating IL-15 levels in humans. Mediators Inflamm. 2005;2005(4):245–7.
22. Solana R, Pawelec G, Tarazona R. Aging and innate immunity. Immunity. 2006;24(5):491–4.
23. Glaser R, Kiecolt-Glaser JK. Stress-induced immune dysfunction: implications for health. Nat Rev Immunol. 2005;5(3):243–51.
24. Nalbandian G, Kovats S. Estrogen, immunity & autoimmune disease. Curr Med Chem Immun Endo Metab Agents. 2005;5:85–91.
25. Dolomie-Fagour L, Gatta B, Nguyen TDT, Corcuff J. Bioavailable estradiol in man: relationship with

25. age and testosterone. Clin Chim Acta. 2008;398(1–2): 145–7.
26. Vermeulen A, Kaufman JM, Goemaere S, van Pottelberg I. Estradiol in elderly men. Aging Male. 2002;5(2):98–102.
27. Pietschmann P, Gollob E, Brosch S, Hahn P, Kudlacek S, Willheim M, et al. The effect of age and gender on cytokine production by human peripheral blood mononuclear cells and markers of bone metabolism. Exp Gerontol. 2003;38(10):1119–27.
28. Ongrádi J, Kövesdi V. Factors that may impact on immunosenescence: an appraisal. Immun Ageing. 2010;7:7.
29. García Verdecia B, Saavedra Hernández D, Lorenzo-Luaces P, de Jesús Badía Alvarez T, Leonard Rupalé I, Mazorra Herrera Z, et al. Immunosenescence and gender: a study in healthy Cubans. Immun Ageing. 2013;10(1):16.
30. Papenfuss TL, Whitacre CC. Sex hormones, pregnancy, and immune function. In: Pfaff DW, Arnold AP, Etgen AM, Fahrbach SE, Rubin RT, editors. Hormones, brain, and behavior. San Diego: Academic; 2009. p. 367–76.
31. Ahmed SA, Hissong BD, Verthelyi D, Donner K, Becker K, Karpuzoglu-Sahin E. Gender and risk of autoimmune diseases: possible role of estrogenic compounds. Environ Health Perspect. 1999;107 Suppl 5:681–6.
32. Ansar Ahmed S, Penhale WJ, Talal N. Sex hormones, immune responses, and autoimmune diseases. Mechanisms of sex hormone action. Am J Pathol. 1985;121(3):531–51.
33. Gameiro C, Romao F. Changes in the immune system during menopause and aging. Front Biosci (Elite Ed). 2010;2:1299–303.
34. Fairweather D, Frisancho-Kiss S, Rose NR. Sex differences in autoimmune disease from a pathological perspective. Am J Pathol. 2008;173(3):600–9.
35. Beagley KW, Gockel CM. Regulation of innate and adaptive immunity by the female sex hormones oestradiol and progesterone. FEMS Immunol Med Microbiol. 2003;38(1):13–22.
36. Marzi M, Vigano A, Trabattoni D, Villa ML, Salvaggio A, Clerici E, et al. Characterization of type 1 and type 2 cytokine production profile in physiologic and pathologic human pregnancy. Clin Exp Immunol. 1996;106(1):127–33.
37. Grimaldi CM, Cleary J, Dagtas AS, Moussai D, Diamond B. Estrogen alters thresholds for B cell apoptosis and activation. J Clin Invest. 2002;109(12):1625–33.
38. González DA, Díaz BB, Rodríguez Pérez MDC, Hernández AG, Chico BND, de León AC. Sex hormones and autoimmunity. Immunol Lett. 2010;133(1):6–13.
39. Shapira Y, Agmon-Levin N, Shoenfeld Y. Defining and analyzing geoepidemiology and human autoimmunity. J Autoimmun. 2010;34(3):J168–77.
40. Hemminki K, Li X, Sundquist K, Sundquist J. Shared familial aggregation of susceptibility to autoimmune diseases. Arthritis Rheum. 2009;60(9):2845–7.
41. Olsen NJ, Kovacs WJ. Effects of androgens on T and B lymphocyte development. Immunol Res. 2001;23(2–3):281–8.
42. Selmi C, Brunetta E, Raimondo MG, Meroni PL. The X chromosome and the sex ratio of autoimmunity. Autoimmun Rev. 2012;11:A531–7.
43. Buyon JP. The effects of pregnancy on autoimmune diseases. J Leukoc Biol. 1998;63(3):281–7.
44. Sánchez-Guerrero J, Villegas A, Mendoza-Fuentes A, Romero-Díaz J, Moreno-Coutiño G, Cravioto MC. Disease activity during the premenopausal and postmenopausal periods in women with systemic lupus erythematosus. Am J Med. 2001;111(6):464–8.
45. Shoenfeld Y, Isenberg DA. The mosaic of autoimmunity. Immunol Today. 1989;10(4):123–6.
46. Tiller T, Tsuiji M, Yurasov S, Velinzon K, Nussenzweig MC, Wardemann H. Autoreactivity in human IgG+ memory B cells. Immunity. 2007;26(2):205–13.
47. Béland K, Lapierre P, Alvarez F. Influence of genes, sex, age and environment on the onset of autoimmune hepatitis. World J Gastroenterol. 2009;15(9):1025–34.
48. Njemini R, Meyers I, Demanet C, Smitz J, Sosso M, Mets T. The prevalence of autoantibodies in an elderly sub-Saharan African population. Clin Exp Immunol. 2002;127(1):99–106.
49. Hasler P, Zouali M. Immune receptor signaling, aging, and autoimmunity. Cell Immunol. 2005;233(2):102–8.
50. Boren E, Gershwin ME. Inflamm-aging: autoimmunity, and the immune-risk phenotype. Autoimmun Rev. 2004;3(5):401–6.
51. Fülöp TJ, Larbi A, Dupuis G, Pawelec G. Ageing, autoimmunity and arthritis: perturbations of TCR signal transduction pathways with ageing – a biochemical paradigm for the ageing immune system. Arthritis Res Ther. 2003;5(6):290–302.
52. Cai Y, Zhou J, Webb DC. Estrogen stimulates Th2 cytokine production and regulates the compartmentalisation of eosinophils during allergen challenge in a mouse model of asthma. Int Arch Allergy Immunol. 2012;158(3):252–60.
53. Tai P, Wang J, Jin H, Song X, Yan J, Kang Y, et al. Induction of regulatory T cells by physiological level estrogen. J Cell Physiol. 2008;214(2):456–64.
54. Linterman MA, Rigby RJ, Wong RK, Yu D, Brink R, Cannons JL, et al. Follicular helper T cells are required for systemic autoimmunity. J Exp Med. 2009;206(3):561–76.
55. Bodey B, Siegel SE, Kaiser HE. Involution of the mammalian thymus and its role in the aging process. In: Immunological aspects of neoplasia – the role of the thymus. Dordrecht: Kluwer Academic Publishers; 2004. p. 147–66.
56. Bodey B, Bodey BJ, Siegel SE, Kaiser HE. Involution of the mammalian thymus, one of the leading regulators of aging. In Vivo. 1997;11(5):421–40.
57. Porter VR, Greendale GA, Schocken M, Zhu X, Effros RB. Immune effects of hormone replacement therapy in post-menopausal women. Exp Gerontol. 2001;36(2):311–26.

58. Grimaldi CM, Michael DJ, Diamond B. Cutting edge: expansion and activation of a population of autoreactive marginal zone B cells in a model of estrogen-induced lupus. J Immunol. 2001;167(4):1886–90.
59. Giglio T, Imro MA, Filaci G, Scudeletti M, Puppo F, De Cecco L, et al. Immune cell circulating subsets are affected by gonadal function. Life Sci. 1994;54(18):1305–12.
60. Kumru S, Godekmerdan A, Yilmaz B. Immune effects of surgical menopause and estrogen replacement therapy in peri-menopausal women. J Reprod Immunol. 2004;63(1):31–8.
61. Chakravarti B, Abraham GN. Aging and T-cell-mediated immunity. Mech Ageing Dev. 1999;108(3):183–206.
62. Thongngarm T, Jenkins JK, Ndebele K, McMurray RW. Estrogen and progesterone modulate monocyte cell cycle progression and apoptosis. Am J Reprod Immunol. 2003;49(3):129–38.
63. Medina KL, Strasser A, Kincade PW. Estrogen influences the differentiation, proliferation, and survival of early B-lineage precursors. Blood. 2000;95(6):2059–67.
64. Sammaritano LR. Menopause in patients with autoimmune diseases. Autoimmun Rev. 2012;11(6–7):A430–6.
65. Lobo R. Primary and secondary amenorrhea and precocious puberty: etiology, diagnostic evaluation, management. In: Katz VL, Lentz GM, Lobo RA, Gershenson DM, editors. Comprehensive gynecology. Philadelphia: Mosby Elsevier; 2007. p. 933–61.
66. Bultink IEM, Lems WF, Kostense PJ, Dijkmans BAC, Voskuyl AE. Prevalence of and risk factors for low bone mineral density and vertebral fractures in patients with systemic lupus erythematosus. Arthritis Rheum. 2005;52(7):2044–50.
67. Namjou B, Scofield RH, Kelly JA, Goodmon EL, Aberle T, Bruner GR, et al. The effects of previous hysterectomy on lupus. Lupus. 2009;18(11):1000–5.
68. Vallin H, Blomberg S, Alm GV, Cederblad B, Rönnblom L. Patients with systemic lupus erythematosus (SLE) have a circulating inducer of interferon-alpha (IFN-alpha) production acting on leucocytes resembling immature dendritic cells. Clin Exp Immunol. 1999;115(1):196–202.
69. Zandman-Goddard G, Peeva E, Shoenfeld Y. Gender and autoimmunity. Autoimmun Rev. 2007;6(6):366–72.
70. Cutolo M. Estrogen metabolites: increasing evidence for their role in rheumatoid arthritis and systemic lupus erythematosus. J Rheumatol. 2004;31(3):419–21.
71. Mok CC, Lau CS, Ho CT, Wong RW. Do flares of systemic lupus erythematosus decline after menopause? Scand J Rheumatol. 1999;28(6):357–62.
72. Abdou NI, Rider V, Greenwell C, Li X, Kimler BF. Fulvestrant (Faslodex), an estrogen selective receptor downregulator, in therapy of women with systemic lupus erythematosus. Clinical, serologic, bone density, and T cell activation marker studies: a double-blind placebo-controlled trial. J Rheumatol. 2008;35(5):797.
73. Dinesh RK, Hahn BH, Singh RP. PD-1, gender, and autoimmunity. Autoimmun Rev. 2010;9(8):583–7.
74. Catania G, Rossi E, Marmont A. Familial SLE: sustained drug-free remission in a mother successfully treated for anal cancer, but development of SLE in a 16-year old daughter. Lupus. 2012;21(6):672–4.
75. Costenbader KH, Feskanich D, Stampfer MJ, Karlson EW. Reproductive and menopausal factors and risk of systemic lupus erythematosus in women. Arthritis Rheum. 2007;56(4):1251–62.
76. Minami Y, Sasaki T, Komatsu S, Nishikori M, Fukao A, Yoshinaga K, et al. Female systemic lupus erythematosus in Miyagi Prefecture, Japan: a case-control study of dietary and reproductive factors. Tohoku J Exp Med. 1993;169(3):245–52.
77. Cooper GS, Dooley MA, Treadwell EL, St Clair EW, Gilkeson GS. Hormonal and reproductive risk factors for development of systemic lupus erythematosus: results of a population-based, case-control study. Arthritis Rheum. 2002;46(7):1830–9.
78. Font J, Pallarés L, Cervera R, López-Soto A, Navarro M, Bosch X, et al. Systemic lupus erythematosus in the elderly: clinical and immunological characteristics. Ann Rheum Dis. 1991;50(10):702–5.
79. Ho CT, Mok CC, Lau CS, Wong RW. Late onset systemic lupus erythematosus in southern Chinese. Ann Rheum Dis. 1998;57(7):437–40.
80. Boddaert J, Huong DLT, Amoura Z, Wechsler B, Godeau P, Piette J. Late-onset systemic lupus erythematosus: a personal series of 47 patients and pooled analysis of 714 cases in the literature. Medicine (Baltimore). 2004;83(6):348–59.
81. Mok CC, Wong RW, Lau CS. Ovarian failure and flares of systemic lupus erythematosus. Arthritis Rheum. 1999;42(6):1274–80.
82. Urowitz MB, Ibañez D, Jerome D, Gladman DD. The effect of menopause on disease activity in systemic lupus erythematosus. J Rheumatol. 2006;33(11):2192–8.
83. Buyon JP, Petri MA, Kim MY, Kalunian KC, Grossman J, Hahn BH, et al. The effect of combined estrogen and progesterone hormone replacement therapy on disease activity in systemic lupus erythematosus: a randomized trial. Ann Intern Med. 2005;142(12 Pt 1):953–62.
84. Askanase AD. Estrogen therapy in systemic lupus erythematosus. Treat Endocrinol. 2004;3(1):19–26.
85. González LA, Pons-Estel GJ, Zhang JS, McGwin GJ, Roseman J, Reveille JD, et al. Effect of age, menopause and cyclophosphamide use on damage accrual in systemic lupus erythematosus patients from LUMINA, a multiethnic US cohort (LUMINA LXIII). Lupus. 2009;18(2):184–6.
86. Bynoté KK, Hackenberg JM, Korach KS, Lubahn DB, Lane PH, Gould KA. Estrogen receptor-alpha deficiency attenuates autoimmune disease in (NZB x NZW)F1 mice. Genes Immun. 2008;9(2):137–52.

87. Cutolo M, Sulli A, Capellino S, Villaggio B, Montagna P, Seriolo B, et al. Sex hormones influence on the immune system: basic and clinical aspects in autoimmunity. Lupus. 2004;13(9):635–8.
88. Lu Q, Wu A, Tesmer L, Ray D, Yousif N, Richardson B. Demethylation of CD40LG on the inactive X in T cells from women with lupus. J Immunol. 2007;179(9):6352–8.
89. Rider V, Jones S, Evans M, Bassiri H, Afsar Z, Abdou NI. Estrogen increases CD40 ligand expression in T cells from women with systemic lupus erythematosus. J Rheumatol. 2001;28(12):2644–9.
90. Zhang J, Jacobi AM, Wang T, Berlin R, Volpe BT, Diamond B. Polyreactive autoantibodies in systemic lupus erythematosus have pathogenic potential. J Autoimmun. 2009;33(3–4):270–4.
91. Weyand CM, Fulbright JW, Goronzy JJ. Immunosenescence, autoimmunity, and rheumatoid arthritis. Exp Gerontol. 2003;38(8):833–41.
92. Olsen NJ, Kovacs WJ. Hormones, pregnancy, and rheumatoid arthritis. J Gend Specif Med. 2002;5(4):28–37.
93. Silman A, Kay A, Brennan P. Timing of pregnancy in relation to the onset of rheumatoid arthritis. Arthritis Rheum. 1992;35(2):152–5.
94. Abdou NI, Rider V. Gender differences in autoimmune diseases: immune mechanisms and clinical applications. In: Lagato M, editor. Principles of gender-specific medicine. London: Academic; 2010. p. 585–91.
95. Lindstrom TM, Robinson WH. Rheumatoid arthritis: a role for immunosenescence? J Am Geriatr Soc. 2010;58(8):1565–75.
96. Merlino LA, Cerhan JR, Criswell LA, Mikuls TR, Saag KG. Estrogen and other female reproductive risk factors are not strongly associated with the development of rheumatoid arthritis in elderly women. Semin Arthritis Rheum. 2003;33(2):72–82.
97. Pikwer M, Bergström U, Nilsson J, Jacobsson L, Turesson C. Early menopause is an independent predictor of rheumatoid arthritis. Ann Rheum Dis. 2012;71(3):378–81.
98. Pikwer M, Nilsson J, Bergström U, Jacobsson LT, Turesson C. Early menopause and severity of rheumatoid arthritis in women older than 45 years. Arthritis Res Ther. 2012;14(4):R190.
99. Kuiper S, van Gestel AM, Swinkels HL, de Boo TM, da Silva JA, van Riel PL. Influence of sex, age, and menopausal state on the course of early rheumatoid arthritis. J Rheumatol. 2001;28(8):1809–16.
100. Doran MF, Crowson CS, O'Fallon WM, Gabriel SE. The effect of oral contraceptives and estrogen replacement therapy on the risk of rheumatoid arthritis: a population based study. J Rheumatol. 2004;31(2):207–13.
101. Holroyd CR, Edwards CJ. The effects of hormone replacement therapy on autoimmune disease: rheumatoid arthritis and systemic lupus erythematosus. Climacteric. 2009;12(5):378–86.
102. Bhadauria S, Moser DK, Clements PJ, Singh RR, Lachenbruch PA, Pitkin RM, et al. Genital tract abnormalities and female sexual function impairment in systemic sclerosis. Am J Obstet Gynecol. 1995;172(2 Pt 1):580–7.
103. Scorza R, Caronni M, Bazzi S, Nador F, Beretta L, Antonioli R, et al. Post-menopause is the main risk factor for developing isolated pulmonary hypertension in systemic sclerosis. Ann N Y Acad Sci. 2002;966:238–46.
104. Beretta L, Caronni M, Origgi L, Ponti A, Santaniello A, Scorza R. Hormone replacement therapy may prevent the development of isolated pulmonary hypertension in patients with systemic sclerosis and limited cutaneous involvement. Scand J Rheumatol. 2006;35(6):468–71.
105. Hayashi Y, Arakaki R, Ishimaru N. Apoptosis and estrogen deficiency in primary Sjögren syndrome. Curr Opin Rheumatol. 2004;16(5):522–6.
106. Ishimaru N, Arakaki R, Watanabe M, Kobayashi M, Miyazaki K, Hayashi Y. Development of autoimmune exocrinopathy resembling Sjögren's syndrome in estrogen-deficient mice of healthy background. Am J Pathol. 2003;163(4):1481–90.
107. Smith R, Studd JW. A pilot study of the effect upon multiple sclerosis of the menopause, hormone replacement therapy and the menstrual cycle. J R Soc Med. 1992;85(10):612–3.
108. Buchel E, Van Steenbergen W, Nevens F, Fevery J. Improvement of autoimmune hepatitis during pregnancy followed by flare-up after delivery. Am J Gastroenterol. 2002;97(12):3160–5.
109. Samuel D, Riordan S, Strasser S, Kurtovic J, Singh-Grewel I, Koorey D. Severe autoimmune hepatitis first presenting in the early post partum period. Clin Gastroenterol Hepatol. 2004;2(7):622–4.
110. Allman D, Miller JP. B cell development and receptor diversity during aging. Curr Opin Immunol. 2005;17(5):463–7.
111. Huppert FA, Solomou W, O'Connor S, Morgan K, Sussams P, Brayne C. Aging and lymphocyte subpopulations: whole-blood analysis of immune markers in a large population sample of healthy elderly individuals. Exp Gerontol. 1998;33(6):593–600.
112. Franceschi C, Cossarizza A. Introduction: the reshaping of the immune system with age. Int Rev Immunol. 1995;12(1):1–4.
113. Johnson SA, Cambier JC. Ageing, autoimmunity and arthritis: senescence of the B cell compartment – implications for humoral immunity. Arthritis Res Ther. 2004;6(4):131–9.
114. Frasca D, Riley RL, Blomberg BB. Humoral immune response and B-cell functions including immunoglobulin class switch are downregulated in aged mice and humans. Semin Immunol. 2005;17(5):378–84.
115. Whisler RL, Liu BQ, Newhouse YG, Walters JD, Breckenridge MB, Grants IS. Signal transduction in human B cells during aging: alterations in stimulus-induced phosphorylations of tyrosine and serine/threonine substrates and in cytosolic calcium responsiveness. Lymphokine Cytokine Res. 1991;10(6):463–73.

116. Paganelli R, Quinti I, Fagiolo U, Cossarizza A, Ortolani C, Guerra E, et al. Changes in circulating B cells and immunoglobulin classes and subclasses in a healthy aged population. Clin Exp Immunol. 1992;90(2):351–4.
117. Fann M, Chiu WK, Wood 3rd WH, Levine BL, Becker KG, Weng N. Gene expression characteristics of CD28 null memory phenotype CD8+ T cells and its implication in T-cell aging. Immunol Rev. 2005;205:190–206.
118. Mo R, Chen J, Han Y, Bueno-Cannizares C, Misek DE, Lescure PA, et al. T cell chemokine receptor expression in aging. J Immunol. 2003;170(2):895–904.
119. Weng N. Aging of the immune system: how much can the adaptive immune system adapt? Immunity. 2006;24(5):495–9.
120. Tarazona R, DelaRosa O, Alonso C, Ostos B, Espejo J, Peña J, et al. Increased expression of NK cell markers on T lymphocytes in aging and chronic activation of the immune system reflects the accumulation of effector/senescent T cells. Mech Ageing Dev. 2000;121(1–3):77–88.
121. Ershler WB, Sun WH, Binkley N, Gravenstein S, Volk MJ, Kamoske G, et al. Interleukin-6 and aging: blood levels and mononuclear cell production increase with advancing age and in vitro production is modifiable by dietary restriction. Lymphokine Cytokine Res. 1993;12(4):225–30.
122. Brüünsgaard H, Pedersen BK. Age-related inflammatory cytokines and disease. Immunol Allergy Clin N Am. 2003;23(1):15–39.
123. Niwa Y, Kasama T, Kawai S, Komura J, Sakane T, Kanoh T, et al. The effect of aging on cutaneous lipid peroxide levels and superoxide dismutase activity in guinea pigs and patients with burns. Life Sci. 1988;42(4):351–6.
124. Tortorella C, Piazzolla G, Spaccavento F, Pece S, Jirillo E, Antonaci S. Spontaneous and Fas-induced apoptotic cell death in aged neutrophils. J Clin Immunol. 1998;18(5):321–9.
125. Mattila PS, Tarkkanen J. Age-associated changes in the cellular composition of the human adenoid. Scand J Immunol. 1997;45(4):423–7.
126. Miller RA, Garcia G, Kirk CJ, Witkowski JM. Early activation defects in T lymphocytes from aged mice. Immunol Rev. 1997;160:79–90.
127. Naylor K, Li G, Vallejo AN, Lee W, Koetz K, Bryl E, et al. The influence of age on T cell generation and TCR diversity. J Immunol. 2005;174(11):7446–52.
128. Quadri RA, Plastre O, Phelouzat MA, Arbogast A, Proust JJ. Age-related tyrosine-specific protein phosphorylation defect in human T lymphocytes activated through CD3, CD4, CD8 or the IL-2 receptor. Mech Ageing Dev. 1996;88(3):125–38.
129. Linton PJ, Dorshkind K. Age-related changes in lymphocyte development and function. Nat Immunol. 2004;5(2):133–9.
130. Swain S, Clise-Dwyer K, Haynes L. Homeostasis and the age-associated defect of CD4 T cells. Semin Immunol. 2005;17(5):370–7.
131. Vallejo AN, Weyand CM, Goronzy JJ. Functional disruption of the CD28 gene transcriptional initiator in senescent T cells. J Biol Chem. 2001;276(4):2565–70.
132. Messaoudi I, Lemaoult J, Guevara-Patino JA, Metzner BM, Nikolich-Zugich J. Age-related CD8 T cell clonal expansions constrict CD8 T cell repertoire and have the potential to impair immune defense. J Exp Med. 2004;200(10):1347–58.
133. Goronzy JJ, Weyand CM. Aging, autoimmunity and arthritis: T-cell senescence and contraction of T-cell repertoire diversity – catalysts of autoimmunity and chronic inflammation. Arthritis Res Ther. 2003;5(5):225–34.
134. Kiecolt-Glaser JK, Preacher KJ, MacCallum RC, Atkinson C, Malarkey WB, Glaser R. Chronic stress and age-related increases in the proinflammatory cytokine IL-6. Proc Natl Acad Sci U S A. 2003; 100(15):9090–5.
135. Whisler RL, Beiqing L, Chen M. Age-related decreases in IL-2 production by human T cells are associated with impaired activation of nuclear transcriptional factors AP-1 and NF-AT. Cell Immunol. 1996;169(2):185–95.
136. Kanda N, Tamaki K. Estrogen enhances immunoglobulin production by human PBMCs. J Allergy Clin Immunol. 1999;103(2 Pt 1):282–8.
137. O'Connor M, Motivala SJ, Valladares EM, Olmstead R, Irwin MR. Sex differences in monocyte expression of IL-6: role of autonomic mechanisms. Am J Physiol Regul Integr Comp Physiol. 2007;293(1): R145–51.
138. Lamon-Fava S, Posfai B, Schaefer EJ. Effect of hormonal replacement therapy on C-reactive protein and cell-adhesion molecules in postmenopausal women. Am J Cardiol. 2003;91(2):252–4.
139. Miller AP, Feng W, Xing D, Weathington NM, Blalock JE, Chen Y, et al. Estrogen modulates inflammatory mediator expression and neutrophil chemotaxis in injured arteries. Circulation. 2004;110(12):1664–9.
140. Bynoe MS, Grimaldi CM, Diamond B. Estrogen up-regulates Bcl-2 and blocks tolerance induction of naive B cells. Proc Natl Acad Sci U S A. 2000; 97(6):2703–8.
141. Srivastava S, Weitzmann MN, Cenci S, Ross FP, Adler S, Pacifici R. Estrogen decreases TNF gene expression by blocking JNK activity and the resulting production of c-Jun and JunD. J Clin Invest. 1999;104(4):503–13.
142. Koh KK, Ahn JY, Jin DK, Yoon B, Kim HS, Kim DS, et al. Effects of continuous combined hormone replacement therapy on inflammation in hypertensive and/or overweight postmenopausal women. Arterioscler Thromb Vasc Biol. 2002;22(9): 1459–64.
143. Tanriverdi F, Silveira LFG, MacColl GS, Bouloux PMG. The hypothalamic-pituitary-gonadal axis: immune function and autoimmunity. J Endocrinol. 2003;176(3):293–304.
144. Ackerman LS. Sex hormones and the genesis of autoimmunity. Arch Dermatol. 2006;142(3):371–6.

24. Genes, Hormones, Immunosenescence, and Environmental Agents: Toward an Integrated View of the Genesis of Autoimmune Disease

Miranda A. Farage, Kenneth W. Miller, and Robert G. Lahita

Contents

24.1	Introduction	319
24.2	The Genetic Underpinnings of Autoimmune Disease	322
24.3	Contributions of Gender to Autoimmune Disease	324
24.3.1	Estrogen	324
24.3.2	Estrogen Receptors	326
24.3.3	Microchimerism	327
24.3.4	X Chromosome	327
24.4	The Contribution of Environmental Agents in Autoimmune Disease	328
24.5	Immunosenescence and Autoimmune Disease	329
24.6	Genes, Estrogen, Environment, and Aging: Hints of a Nexus in SLE	331
24.6.1	The Genetic Foundation of SLE	331
24.6.2	The Contribution of Estrogen to SLE	331
24.6.3	The Role of Environment in SLE	332
24.6.4	The Contribution of Immunosenescence to SLE	332
24.7	NF-KB: Insights from One Protein's Role in Gene Regulation	332
24.7.1	NF-Kβ and the Genetic Predilection for Autoimmune Disease	334
24.7.2	NF-Kβ and Sex Hormones	334
24.7.3	NF-Kβ and Environment and Aging	334
24.8	Epigenetics: The Missing Link in an Integrated Theory of Autoimmune Disease	335
24.8.1	Mechanisms of Epigenetic Change	336
24.8.2	Epigenetic Contributions to Autoimmunity and Gender	336
24.9	Summary	338
	References	338

M.A. Farage, MSc, PhD (✉)
Clinical Innovative Sciences, The Procter and Gamble Company, 6110 Center Hill Avenue, Cincinnati, OH 45224, USA
e-mail: Farage.m@pg.com

K.W. Miller, PhD
Global Product Stewardship, The Procter and Gamble Company, Cincinnati, OH, USA
e-mail: Miller.kw.1@pg.com

R.G. Lahita, MD, PhD
Department of Medicine, Newark Beth Israel Medical Center, Newark, NJ, USA
e-mail: r.lahita@att.net

24.1 Introduction

The immune system prevents an immune response to the body's own tissues, generating immune tolerance with regard to self-antigens during T-cell generation in the thymus and B-cell generation in the bone marrow. Mechanisms of tolerance to sequestered or otherwise aberrant self-antigens exist in the periphery as well [1].

Autoimmune disease (AID), nonetheless, exists and is increasing in prevalence worldwide [2]. A group of at least 80 distinct syndromes, these are mostly of relatively rare complaints that together comprise a wide range of genetically complex diseases that afflict as much as 10 % of the population [3]. Autoimmune disorders are defined by a dysregulation of immune function that potentiates a breakdown in immune tolerance. The breakdown in immune tolerance in turn permits an overexpression of autoantibodies and autoreactive T cells [3] that will, unchecked, eventually result in inflammation and tissue destruction [4]. Autoimmune diseases target a variety of tissue types but share certain characteristics, foremost being the fact that they affect far more women than men (Tables 24.1a, Part 1 and 24.1b Part 2).

Table 24.1a Part 1: selected gender influences implied or positively associated with specific autoimmune diseases

Autoimmune disease	Percent female patients (highest estimate)	X chromosome	MHC/HLA association (selected)	Non-MHC gene associations
Autoimmune hepatitis	Type I 9:1 Type II: 3:1 [5]	NA	A1-88 DRB* 0301 DRB* 0401 DRB* 0404 [5]	IgA [5]
Crohn's disease[a]	58 % [6]	NA	HLA-DRB1*07 [7]	IL23R, NOD2 CARD9 IL18RAP, CUL2, C1orf106, PTPN22, and MUC19 [8]
Hyperthyroidism/Graves' disease	95 % [9]	(Skewed) inactivation [10]	DR3 DRB108 [12]	CTLA4 [11]
Multiple sclerosis	60 % [13]	NA	DR2 DR3 DRA DRB1 [9]	CTLA4 [14]
Primary biliary cirrhosis	88 % [15]	NA [16]	DRB1*0801 [17]	IL12A and IL12RB2, CTLA4 [17]
Psoriasis	38 % [18]	NA	HLA-C [19]	IL12B IL23A [19]
Rheumatoid arthritis	72 % [15]	Yes [20]	DRB1-0101, DRB1-0102, DRB1-0404, others [12]	PTPN22, STAT4 [21],
Scleroderma	84 % [15]	Yes [22]	HLA-DRB1*01 and HLA-DRB1*11 [23]	BANK1, C8orf13-BLK, IL-23R, IRF5, STAT4, TBX21, and TNFSF4 [24]
Sjögren's syndrome	95 % [5]	Gene dosage [25]	–[26]	–
Systemic lupus erythematosus	90 % [13]	[27]	DR3, DR8, DR15 [12]	STAT4, IRF5, ITGAM [28]
Type I diabetes	50 % [9]	NA	DR3 DR4 [12]	Lymphoid tyrosine phosphatase (PTPN22) and the cytotoxic T lymphocyte-associated antigen-4 (CTLA-4) gene [29]
Ulcerative colitis	50 % [5]	NA	B27[b] [30]	ECM1, CDH1, HNF4a, and laminin B1 [30]

HLA human leukocyte antigen, IgA immunoglobulin, IL interleukin, MHC major histocompatibility complex, NA not available
[a]Occupational exposures
[b]Common HLA associations selected from typically multiple possible examples; HLA displays ethnic variation

Table 24.1b Part 2: selected gender influences implied or positively associated with specific autoimmune diseases

Autoimmune disease	MZ/DZ	Geo-epidemiology prevalence/100,000	Associated environmental exposures
Autoimmune hepatitis	NA	NA	Acne drug minocycline associated [31] statins particularly in patients genetically predisposed by HLA [32]
Crohn's disease[a]	NA	Highest: North America (201) [9] Lowest: Israel 2[b] [34]	Tobacco smoke [33]
Hyperthyroidism/Graves' disease	31/4.7 % [35]	Highest: N. Europe, China (1200) [9] Lowest: Africa (<10) [9]	Tobacco smoke [33] Radiation [36]
Multiple sclerosis	31 %/5 % [35]	Highest: N. Europe (200) Lowest: South and Central America and the Caribbean (<20) [9]	Tobacco smoke [33] UV [37], EBV [38]
Primary biliary cirrhosis	62.5 %/0 [39]	NA	Tobacco smoke [33]
Psoriasis	67 %/15 % [35]	Highest: France (3058) Lowest: indigenous S. American: 0 [9]	Periodontal disease [40]
Rheumatoid arthritis	15/3.5 % [35]	–	Tobacco smoke [33]
Scleroderma	–	–	Tobacco smoke [33]
Systemic lupus erythematosus	33 %/2 % [35]	–	EBV, silica, nail polish[a], hair dye[a] [36]; tobacco smoke [33]
Type I diabetes	70/13 % [35]	Highest: N. Europe (700) Lowest: Central America (<20) [9]	–
Ulcerative colitis	18.7/3 % [35]	Highest: North America (300) Lowest: Central and South America (<3) [9]	–

DZ dizygotic, *EBV* Epstein-Barr virus, *HLA* human leukocyte antigen, *MZ* monozygotic, *NA* not available
[a]Occupational exposures
[b]Common HLA associations selected from typically multiple possible examples; HLA displays ethnic variation

The mechanisms which underlie this diverse group of diseases are still poorly understood. Many autoimmune diseases display both genetic predisposition and familial associations, firmly establishing a genetic foundation for their eventual development [2,41].

Most also have obvious environmental triggers as well; a wide variety of environmental insults including infectious agents, pharmaceuticals, dietary factors, smoking, chemicals, and pollutants are shown to increase the risk [2,41].

In addition, since autoimmune disease affects predominantly women (80 % of autoimmune disease sufferers are female) [13], with the activity of disease fluctuating in parallel with estrogen levels, sex steroids are widely proposed as a key component of autoimmune pathology [42].

Finally, as both the levels of circulating of autoantibodies (in association with a general dysregulation of immune function) and the risk of autoimmune disease are observed to increase as humans age [43], it is probable that immunosenescence also plays a role.

Although the precise pathways through which a genetic predisposition to autoimmune disease becomes a full-blown autoimmune disease (through the influence of endogenous hormones, environmental insults, and the natural decay of the aging immune system) are still unknown [3], progress suggests that lifelong epigenetic changes to deoxyribonucleic acid (DNA) are a primary means to gene regulation. Because of this, autoimmune diseases, potentially devastating conditions with complex etiology and paradoxical nature, are better understood.

24.2 The Genetic Underpinnings of Autoimmune Disease

The existence of a genetic platform that confers susceptibility to or protection against autoimmune disease has been long suspected. Only a handful of these diseases display strict Mendelian inheritance [44]. Certain autoimmune diseases, nonetheless, consistently occur at statistically improbable levels in certain families [45].

Apart from Mendelian inheritance, familial aggregation is modest [44]. For example, despite the fact that a family history of systemic lupus erythematosus (SLE) increases the risk 25-fold, only 2 % of an AID patient's close relatives actually develop the disease [46]. Thus, the manner in which the genome confers protection or susceptibility through modulation of immune tolerance is not solidly identified, and patients in which a genetic profile has been firmly linked to the development of disease are a substantial minority [47]. This situation arises because many of the identified genetic associations have odds ratios (typically 1.1–1.5) that are too small to meaningfully increase individual risk [44].

The genetic contribution to autoimmunity is "extraordinarily complex" [44]. Refinements in methodologies in molecular biology, however, are beginning to unlock the genetic basis of autoimmunity. Culpable genes in the pathogenesis of autoimmune diseases were first pursued through candidate gene association studies, then by linkage analysis in affected families, and then through genome-wide association scans [44] (Table 24.2). Genome-wide association studies, built on the completion of the Human Genome and the haplotype map (HapMap) projects, have particularly accelerated solid associations between disease and specific genes, courtesy of their ability to scan the entire genome for polymorphisms implicated in disease [44].

More than 200 genetic loci have now been documented as contributing to various autoimmune diseases [4]. Some genetic variants, that is, human leukocyte antigens (HLAs), have been reliably associated with several different autoimmune diseases, including type I diabetes mellitus (T1DM), rheumatoid arthritis (RA), and SLE [3]; the signal transducer and activator of transcription 4 (STAT4) (a transcription factor gene) haplotype is associated with an increased risk of both RA and SLE [21]. Through these genetic techniques, multiple potential pathways for the origin of autoimmunity have emerged. These are primarily related to innate immunity, cytokine signaling, or lymphocyte activation [3], and include molecules like intracellular tyrosine phosphatases, tumor necrosis factor(s), intracellular pattern recognition receptors, nuclear factor kappa-light-chain-enhancer (NF-Kβ) and other transcription factors, cytokines (and their receptors), cell-surface receptors, signaling molecules, enzymes, autoantigens, and major histocompatibility complex (MHC) profiles [44].

Table 24.2 Ability to establish genetic foundation spurred by ongoing innovations in molecular methodology

Technique	Strength	Weakness	Approximate year of innovation	References
Linkage analysis	Solid identification of AID with Mendelian inheritance	AIDs with strict Mendelian inheritance make up a small fraction of known AID	1953	[44]
Candidate gene studies	Useful for identifying gene associations in disease with more complex, non-Mendelian inheritance	Requires large sample sizes as well as an existing understanding of disease mechanisms with implied plausibility of specific gene. Also requires case/control matching	1986	[44]
Genome-wide association scans	Does not require prior plausibility for specific genes	Requires huge databases (Human Genome Project and HapMap project made those available)	2005	[44]

AID autoimmune disease, *HapMap* haplotype map

Intriguingly, the loci identified are often shown to be common to a number of autoimmune diseases [4], and the presence of an autoimmune disease in one individual increases the risk in close family members to a variety of others. For example, analysis of variants of the protein tyrosine phosphatase (PTPN) gene in Swedish patients with autoimmune diseases such as RA, T1DM, or Crohn's disease ($N = 172,242$) found that the relative risk of several autoimmune diseases increased in offspring when the parent suffered from an existing autoimmune disease [45] (Table 24.3). Pairwise analyses demonstrated a shared familial risk for RA, SLE, T1DM, ankylosing spondylitis (AS), Crohn's disease, celiac disease, and ulcerative colitis (UC) (see Table 24.3).

A genome-wide association study looked at single-nucleotide polymorphisms (SNPs) outside the MHC and identified a total of 107 SNPs that were associated with an increased risk for at least one of seven individual autoimmune diseases: celiac disease, Crohn's disease, multiple sclerosis (MS), psoriasis, RA, SLE, and T1DM. Again, a substantial proportion (44 %) of the SNPs identified were also implicated in more than one disease [48]. The implicated SNPs clustered near deoxyribonucleic acid (DNA) sequences that encoded proteins also implicated in the same subsets of diseases [49].

Such proteins, with genes located in proximity to genes implicated in the increased risk for multiple autoimmune diseases, may represent an underlying shared mechanism that constitutes the physiological basis for disease risk. This is a theory supported by the observation that autoimmune patients frequently suffer from more than one autoimmune disorder at a time or from different autoimmune diseases during different stages of their lives [3].

Genome-wide association studies ostensibly reveal a set of genes common to many autoimmune diseases which represent little increased risk on their own [44]. Multiple polymorphisms, however, each carry a slight risk on their own, but together create a lower threshold for the development of an autoimmune event [3]. It is also possible that in rare instances, copy number [44] or somatic mutations de novo can create a genetic platform for autoimmune disease [50, 51]. It is reported that somatic mutation can, in adults, generate B cells with autoreactive antigen receptors [52].

Concordance rates among monozygotic (MZ) twins, although consistently higher than those in dizygotic (DZ) twins, are low (see Table 24.1b, Part 2). This observation and the observation that in animal studies the gender bias characteristic of autoimmune disease was revealed to be strain specific suggest an interaction between sex chromosomes and the background genes [36]. It makes it clear that AID requires more than just a genetic foundation. Despite the fact that genome-wide association studies have identified multiple significant associations with specific genetic loci, concordance rates for MZ twins are still below 50 % (with a few exceptions), a statistic that suggests additional complementary mechanisms in the genesis of AID [47].

Table 24.3 Familial clustering associated with high-risk gene variants in autoimmune disease (selected associations)

Disease diagnosed in parent	Relative risk (as standardized incidence ratio [SIR]) of disease in offspring						
	AS	CD	CE	RA	SLE	T1DM	UC
Ankylosing spondylitis	–	NIR	NIR	1.41	NIR	NIR	NIR
Celiac disease	NIR	1.61	–	1.31	2.72	1.91	1.27
Crohn's disease	1.86	–	NIR	1.14	NIR	NIR	NIR
Systemic lupus erythematosus	NIR	NIR	NIR	1.77	–	NIR	NIR
Type I diabetes mellitus	1.44	NIR	NIR	1.72	1.87	–	NIR
Ulcerative colitis	1.72	2.55	NIR	1.15	NIR	1.29	–

The source of the data is Hemminki et al. [45]
AS ankylosing spondylitis, *CD* Crohn's disease, *CE* celiac disease, *NIR* no increased risk, *RA* rheumatoid arthritis, *SIR* standardized incidence ratio, *SLE* systemic lupus erythematosus, *T1DM* type I diabetes mellitus, *UC* ulcerative colitis

24.3 Contributions of Gender to Autoimmune Disease

The most striking feature in the diverse group of disorders that make up AID, arguably, is their definitive predominance for females [53] (see Tables 24.1a, Part 1 and 24.1b Part 2). Autoimmune disease is one of the top ten causes of death in women under the age of 65 [54], the second highest cause of chronic illness, and the top cause of morbidity in women in the United States [55]. Suspicion with regard to the physiological basis for the dramatic surfeit of female AID patients has rested primarily on the female sex hormone estrogen [56], with lots of evidence to support it [46]. The role of estrogen in immune function as well as autoimmune disease is supported by a substantial body of evidence [42].

24.3.1 Estrogen

The immune response is heightened in women as compared to men [57]. Both cellular and humoral immune responses are more vigorous in women than men, making women more resistant to infection, but also more subject to autoimmune diseases [41]. Women typically respond to infection (natural and by vaccination) as well as trauma with the increased antibody production characteristic of a T-helper 2 cell (Th2) immune response, while men respond with a T-helper 1 cell (Th1) response, characterized predominantly by inflammation [58]. Estrogen's effect on T-helper cells appears to be estrogen dependent. Low doses of estrogen stimulate Th1 response and higher doses, Th2 [59], a phenomenon also driven by increasing levels of circulating estrogen of pregnancy. Such a shift is also observed during pregnancy [60]. The Th2 response, wherein estrogen stimulates Th lymphocytes to secrete type II cytokines, thereby promotes synthesis of antibodies [61].

Estrogen drastically reduces the size of the bone marrow cavity and induces significant atrophy of the thymus, sites where deletions of autoreactive cells occur. Estrogens are known to stimulate lymphopoiesis outside of marrow (promoting auto reactivity by bypassing the normal selection process) [62], so B cells may develop at alternative sites (liver and spleen) where less stringent selection is occurring. Mice treated with endogenous estrogen have extensive hemopoietic centers in the liver and spleen with B-cell activation including autoantibody-rousing cells in the spleen and liver [42].

Estrogen, a principal regulator of proinflammatory molecules [52], is known to exert numerous effects on individual immune parameters (Table 24.4).

Numerous intrinsic (e.g., pregnancy, menopause, disease states) and extrinsic (e.g., oral contraceptives, hormone replacement therapy [HRT]) factors influence serum estrogen levels. The course of autoimmune diseases typically fluctuates in parallel to changes in estrogen levels [46]; the role that sex hormones play is clearly evidenced by dramatic differences in prevalence related to circulating levels of estrogen over the female life span [42].

Autoimmune hepatitis (AIH), for example, often ameliorates during pregnancy, with an increase in first-time diagnoses in the postpartum period [75,76]. The severity of MS as well as RA decreases during pregnancy, particularly in the third trimester when hormone levels are highest [46].

SLE varies over the course of the menstrual cycle, with flares much more likely during peak estrogen periods such as the high estrogen levels of pregnancy [52]. Similarly, in vitro fertilization procedures and drugs that induce ovulation also induce SLE flares or the onset of SLE symptoms [52]. New diagnoses and flares of existing SLE are rare in the postmenopausal period [52].

Treatment of human peripheral blood mononuclear cells (PBMCs) from SLE patients enhanced total immunoglobulin G (IgG) production as well as anti-double-stranded DNA (dsDNA) autoantibody levels; PBMCs from healthy individuals, however, did not; the disparity proved to be interleukin (IL)-10 dependent

Table 24.4 Biological functions of estrogen in the immune system

Immune function	Immune characteristic	References
B cell	Induction of antibody production	[41]
	Produces higher overall immunoglobulin levels	[42]
	Promotes antibody response to foreign antigens	[42]
	Increases IgG and IgM levels	[61]
	Produces polyclonal induction of B cells in vitro	[63]
	Alters existing thresholds for B-cell apoptosis as well as B-cell activation	[64]
	Induces rapid maturation of B lymphocytes	[41]
T cell	Downregulates the number of immature T lymphocytes	[65]
	Stimulates involution of thymus	[65]
	Stimulates production of regulatory T cells (Tregs)	[66]
	Downregulates CD4 T cells	[42]
	Stimulates an increase CD4/CD8 ratios	[42]
	Stimulates T-cell activation markers	[52]
	Stimulates proliferation of T cells	[52]
Other cell types	Stimulate proliferation of macrophages	[52]
	Decrease the number of monocytes	[67]
Cytokines and effector molecules	Stimulate proinflammatory serum markers	[68]
	Downregulate soluble cell adhesion molecules in women	[69]
	Inhibit expression of monocyte chemoattractant protein-1	[70]
	Stimulate interleukin production (IL-1, IL-4, IL-6, and IL-10 in macrophages; IL-4, IL-5, IL-6, and 1-0 in Th2 cells	[41]
	Stimulate cellular response to cytokines	[42]
	Stimulate secretion of IL-4, IFN-γ and IL-1	[42]
	Stimulate production of antiapoptosis protein Bcl-2	[71]
	Inhibit IL-1-induced expression of cell adhesion molecules	[70]
	Inhibit of TNF-α expression.	[72]
	Downregulate soluble TNF-α	[73]
	Suppress IL-2 secretion by T cells as well as receptor expression in activated peripheral blood T cells	[5]
	Induce Th2 pathway cytokines, downregulate Th1	[52]
	Inflammatory chemokines (MCP-1, MCP-5 as well as NO synthase [iNOS4] and cyclooxygenase-2)	[74]
Systemic	Stimulates resistance to certain infections	[42]
	Increases antibody-secreting cells (IgG and IgA)	[46]
	Downregulates induction of tolerance	[42]
	Stimulates graft rejection	[42]
	Suppresses apoptosis	[52]

CD cluster of differentiation, *IFN-γ* interferon gamma, *Ig* immunoglobulin, *IL* interleukin, *iNOS* inducible nitric oxide synthase, *MCP* monocyte chemoattractant protein, *Th* T helper, *TNF-α* tumor necrosis factor alpha

[77]. Testosterone significantly inhibited IgM and IgG production by PBMC [78].

Similar estrogen effects were observed in animal models [46]. Animal studies confirm that hormonal manipulations can influence disease expression [53]. In a murine lupus model of experimental autoimmune encephalomyelitis (EAE) in which male mice were castrated, castration produced SLE with disease parameters very similar to that in female mice, while ovariectomized females produced disease parameters similar to male mice of the same strain (NZBxNZW) F1 [46]. Estradiol protected the female mice from EAE.

In other animal studies, five different genes, all regulated by either estradiol or dihydrotestosterone, contributed to autoimmunity (in vivo mouse model with lupus) [79].

The importance of the hormonal component in autoimmunity was illuminated by an experiment in mice, which isolated the chromosomal from the hormonal component by moving the testis-determining gene SRY from the Y chromosome to an autosomal chromosome [80]. This approach revealed that although the XY genotype alone stimulated autoantibody proliferation, androgens exerted an overriding suppressive effect [81]. Male sex hormones appear to mask the otherwise immunostimulatory influence of the XY genotype.

In contrast, however, estradiol increases susceptibility to experimental myasthenia gravis, experimental autoimmune uveoretinitis, and lupus [5]. The effects of estrogen on female-predominant AIDs, however, are not generalizable—some are abrogated by testosterone and some are amplified [82]. Gender differences in autoimmunity are at least partially mediated by regulation at the level of the estrogen receptor.

24.3.2 Estrogen Receptors

Nuclear receptors are factors that bind to DNA and act to regulate gene expression at the transcription level (thus known also as transcription factors) and include receptors for estrogens and androgens [52]. Estrogen (17-β estradiol), which is the principal estrogen in circulation during the reproductive years, acts as a ligand for two different nuclear receptor proteins, thus forming two functionally distinct estrogen receptors, estrogen receptor alpha (ERα) and estrogen receptor beta (ERβ), which exist in both homo- and heterodimers.

Estrogen receptors translocate to the nucleus where they bind to estrogen-responsive elements (EREs) in gene promoters and thus act as an on/off switch for gene transcription. The estrogen/estrogen-receptor (E/ER) complex may also interact with other transcription factors such as NF-Kβ, which is capable of binding to non-ERE sites in other promoters [83].

Both types of estrogen receptors are found all over the body, including the ovary, womb, breast, bone, and immune cells, T and B cells, dendritic cells, neutrophils, macrophages, natural killer (NK) cells, thymic stroma cells, bone marrow, and endothelial cells [83].

Although both ERα and ERβ both act to modulate gene expression of estrogen-responsive genes, they modulate that expression in very different ways [52]. ERα deficiency in a murine model of lupus, for example, resulted in disease abrogation and prolonged survival, while ERβ deficiency had minimal effect [84].

Estrogen receptors also occur in two places, with distinctive purposes. Membrane-associated ERs amplify signal transduction cascades, where nuclear ones induce gene transcription. Mature lymphocytes express membrane-associated ERs which are activated by estrogen to invoke increased calcium flex in antigen-activated cells [83].

The effects of estrogen-receptor regulation of immunity and their implications for autoimmunity are many. In one study, estrogen-receptor blockers blocked estrogen-receptor activation in lupus T cells but not in healthy controls [85]. Decreased ERα in macrophages resulted in the stimulation of a cluster of differentiation 4 (CD4) cells [82]. Estradiol (E2), acting via ERα, increased proinflammatory cytokine expression, enhanced proliferative and interferon alpha (INF-α) production by CD4+T cells [82], and differential expression of ER-α and ER-β observed in SLE and RA [83].

The presence of two ERs, occurring in two different places, adds another layer to hormonal regulation of immune processes since the same estrogen produces different effects at one receptor versus another [41], giving the body the ability to fine-tune immune response.

Estrogen, then, is believed to be involved in the regulation of a wide variety of immune cells and a key player in the dysregulation of immunity that leads to both autoimmune and autoinflammatory diseases. Paradoxically, however, comparisons of estrogen levels in female patients with different autoimmune diseases (including AID patients) showed no difference between patients and healthy controls, an indication that estrogen is just part of a more complex etiology [78,86]. In fact, estrogen is not the only component of female gender with the potential to contribute to autoimmunity.

24.3.3 Microchimerism

Fetomaternal microchimerism is the presence, after pregnancy and delivery, of foreign fetal cells in the mother. These include hemapoietic progenitor cells with the capacity to induce autoimmunity and which have been implicated in autoimmune disease, in particular, Graves' disease [87]. It is known that fetal cells are found in peripheral blood of nearly all women during pregnancy, including hematopoietic progenitor cells with the potential to become both effectors and targets of immune processes, and that maternal DNA can be detected by polymerase chain reaction (PCR) in a majority of cord blood samples [87].

Female subjects with autoimmune thyroid disease (Graves and Hashimoto's) are often shown to have microchimeric fetal cells in their thyroid glands [87]. In addition, women with autoimmune thyroid disease with sons had higher prevalence of male cells in their thyroid than women with sons but healthy thyroids [87].

Sixty percent of women with Graves' disease with onset during reproductive years developed the disease in the postpartum period [87]. Also supporting microchimerism as the etiological basis of Graves' disease is a large study that found a significant increase in thyroid peroxidase autoantibody (TPO) associated with increase in parity [88].

24.3.4 X Chromosome

Interestingly, in a murine model in which the authors artificially produced XX, XY mice without alteration of actual gonads, the XX genotype was associated with greater severity of EAE and pristane-induced lupus than XY [46], demonstrating that the sex chromosomes beyond the influence of the sex hormones themselves, contribute to autoimmunity.

The X chromosome itself is implicated in the genesis of autoimmunity, with the presence of two copies of the X chromosome in women held responsible for the observed female predominance in AID. Aberrant, congenital X-chromosome doses, as in Klinefelter's syndrome (XXY) in men, which greatly increases the risk for female-predominant autoimmune disease, underlines the X chromosome's importance [15]. Gene expression in X and Y, however, is not well understood. The fact that the X chromosome itself contains 1,000 unique genes, including genes associated with systemic sclerosis, autoimmune thyroid disease, and SLE [89], in and of itself infers a substantial role of the X chromosome in the regulation of autoimmunity.

In women, one X chromosome is habitually but randomly inactivated to preserve equal gene expression in men and women. However, the inactivated X is not completely inactivated, meaning that some X-associated genes are overexpressed in women [46] as compared to males. Partial inactivation of X, then, may contribute to gender disparity in AID. The mouse strain BXSB, with a translocation mutation in which part of the X chromosome has been transferred to the Y, develops lupus-like syndrome with high frequency in males, shown to involve overexpression of Toll-like receptors (TLR)-7, shown to be a key player in lupus development [46].

In addition, although the choice of which X chromosome to inactivate is random, certain cell types are preferentially inactivated or maintained, resulting in "skewed inactivation" that acts to modulate gene expression. A high percentage of women with systemic sclerosis display skewed X inactivation [46]; skewed X-chromosome inactivation is also implicated in scleroderma in association with reduced regulatory T cell (T_{reg}) activity [83].

Finally, there is sometimes spontaneous loss of the X chromosome with age, observed in increasing frequency with age in blood cells of patients with systemic sclerosis and autoimmune thyroid disease [46]. The origin and the effect of this spontaneous loss are unclear.

Beyond issues of gender created by the gene complement of sex chromosomes and hormones that the complement stimulates, environmental interactions contribute to autoimmunity as well.

24.4 The Contribution of Environmental Agents in Autoimmune Disease

The fact that monozygotic pairs of female twins (with identical genetic and hormonal constitutions) can attribute only 20 % of their phenotypic variance to their shared genetic polymorphisms implicates environmental exposures in the development of autoimmune disease [3]. These exposures are numerous and contribute to a variety of autoimmune diseases. Geographic clusterings of specific diseases are observed, with wide disparities in prevalence in different parts of the world. Even in the confines of the US, multiple sclerosis has dramatic geographical specificity, with a prevalence of 61/100,000 in the West, compared to only 3/100,000 in the South [33].

Autoimmunity is associated with seemingly improbable environmental factors like season of birth or weather patterns [3].

Many environmental factors, both intrinsic and extrinsic, are associated with the development of autoimmune disorders (Table 24.5). The internal biological environment (e.g., endogenous hormones and aging) obviously contributes to autoimmune disease; extrinsic insults, including environmental agents like ultraviolet (UV) light, chemical or other occupational exposures, pollutants, or health habits like smoking or alcohol consumption, are now recognized as important components of autoimmune disease as well. Environmental factors may initiate immunity through nonspecific activation of resting T cells, modification or release of previously sequestered proteins, cross-reactivity between virus and self-protein (molecular mimicry), and modulation of gene expression [5]. Viruses and other infectious agents are also potential environmental inducers of AID as well, although, since viral infection can occur years before the actual onset of a particular AID, definitive associations are difficult to establish [5].

Table 24.5 Environmental triggers for autoimmune disease and their epigenetic effects

Environmental exposures	Action	References
Methionine, S-adenosylmethionine	Cofactor involved in DNA methylation	[90]
Folic acid	Cofactor involved in DNA methylation	[91]
Choline	Source of methyl group in DNA methylation	[92]
Betaine	Methyl donor in DNA methylation	[92]
Resveratrol	Inhibits HDAC	[93]
Dietary fat	DNA methylation	[94]
Nickel	Inhibits DNA methyltransferase	[80]
Vinclozolin (fungicide)	DNA methylation in germ line	[95]
Methoxychlor (pesticide)	DNA methylation in germ line	[95]
Pollutants	DNA methylation	[96]
Asbestos	Increases methylation	[80]
Alcohol consumption	Hypermethylation of promoter for HERP gene	[80]
Tobacco	Hypermethylation of tumor-suppressor gene in lungs, methylation of other tissues	[80]
Marijuana	NA	[80, 97]
Stress (mice)	Increase methylation in brain-derived neurotrophic factor gene in hippocampus	[98]

DNA deoxyribonucleic acid, *HDAC* histone deacetylase, *HERP* homocysteine-induced endoplasmic reticulum protein, *NA* not available

Potential contributions to autoimmunity from the environment are virtually endless and differ widely with occupation, place of residence, hobbies, and medical history. Environmental interactions, like diet, occupation, exposure to environmental chemicals, radiation, UV light, pathogenic organisms, and medications, can also differ by gender [36] and contribute to gender disparities in AID prevalence [99]. Interestingly, the lupus-like syndrome produced by the drug procainamide has a male to female ratio of 2:1, while in asymptomatic patients, the ratio is 5:1, implying an as yet unresolved interaction between gender determinants and susceptibility to an environmental exposure, procainamide, in the development of lupus [36].

Environmental insults may increase with age, including cortisol levels, sleep dysregulation, decrease in physical activity, increase in oxidative stress, or nutritional deficiencies [100].

24.5 Immunosenescence and Autoimmune Disease

The immune system undergoes extensive remodeling as humans age, characterized by a progressive deterioration in the ability to mount an effective immune response. However, an unexplained paradox is a simultaneous increase in autoantibody production [43]. The clinical consequences of this remodeling include a risk of neoplasia and infectious disease, as well as autoimmune disease [43]. Immunosenescence is a subject of increasing interest in medicine, as life expectancy, especially in developed countries, increases without a parallel improvement in health in old age [101].

The immune system, a complex and exquisitely regulated collection of interdependent molecular pathways of both innate and adaptive defense, begins to undergo dysregulation of cell homeostasis. This causes multiple changes in immune function which increase susceptibility to the development of autoimmune diseases [43] (Table 24.6). Old age is characterized by the rising incidence of autoimmunity [103] and an associated increase in both levels of circulating antibodies and numbers of specific antibodies in circulation. Persistent high antigen levels activate memory cells, and costimulatory T cells become less susceptible to downregulation [117].

Although immunosenescence affects all cell types and results in deterioration of both humoral and cellular immunity and multiple cell types, age-associated cumulative effects on T-cell function are the most dramatic and most detrimental [118]. With age, there is a decrease in thymic epithelial space and thymic cellularity, called thymic involution; in humans, the increase in perivascular thymic space is replaced progressively with fat [101]. Humoral immunity as well is severely compromised in the aged as a result of decreased production of long-term Ig-producing B cells and the loss of immunoglobulin diversity and affinities [101].

Although B-cell numbers do not change significantly, B cells do exhibit a decreased response to primary antigenic stimulation [119]. B-cell response (immunoglobulins produced) becomes more random [119] with decreased affinity of IgG produced for a given antigen [119], and IL-15 stimulates proliferation of memory T cells. IL-15 levels nearly double in healthy adults 95 years or older (3.05 pg/mL) as compared to both older adults (60–89, 1.94 pg/mL) and midlife adults (30–59, 1.73 pg/mL) [120]. With an increasing number of memory B cells, the number of autoantibodies also increases with age [121].

Antinuclear antibody (ANA) levels remain constant until age 60 and then increase rapidly. Over the age of 70, more than a third of otherwise healthy senior citizens exhibit high levels of circulating antibody.

Autoantibodies rise because the efficiency of physical barriers is reduced, with higher exposure to pathogens and novel exposure to previously sequestered self-antigens [117]. Infections can trigger immune-mediated inflammatory disease, either by cross-reactivity or by interfering with signaling processes regulating immune response [122]. Increasing autoantibodies in old age may also be the result of reactivation of self-reactive memory B cells originally generated in childhood but reactivated [119].

Table 24.6 Changes in immune function with age (both men and women)

Immune function	Change	References
B cell	Reduction in early progenitor B cells in bone marrow	[102]
	Increase in polyclonal response against diverse mitogens	[43]
	Decrease of specific-antigen response	[43]
	Production of antibodies independent of T-cell activation	[101]
	Oligoclonal expansion of B cells	[101]
	Increase in B1 cell fraction of B cells	[103]
	Maturation of B cells blocked (believed to have inability to rearrange Ig genes because of the decrease in expression of RAG-1 and RAG-2 recombinases)	[104]
	Reduced output of naïve B cells	[102]
	Accumulation of oligoclonally expanded, functionally incompetent memory lymphocytes	[102]
	Decreased numbers of circulating B cells	[105]
	CD20+ B cells decrease	[106]
	Reduced antigen-recognition repertoire of B cells	[107]
	Class switch alterations in immunoglobulins produced	[108]
	Stimulated B cells show significant alterations in cellular structures with a role in signal transduction	[109]
	Increase of IgA and several IgG subclasses	[110]
Lymphocytes	Reduction in total numbers	[111]
Molecular	Alterations in cell-surface receptors (e.g., loss of costimulatory receptor CD28 expression in CD8+ cells)	[112]
	Alterations in cytokine and cytokine receptor alterations in T cells	[113]
	Alterations in effector molecules	[114, 115]
	Interleukin 6 levels increase	[116]
	Alterations in transcriptional regulators	[114]

CD cluster of differentiation, *Ig* immunoglobulin, *RAG* recombinase-activating gene

Defective clearance of cellular debris can also result in prolonged exposure to autoantigens in higher concentrations than normal with subsequent activation of lymphocytes [103]. An increased basal level of inflammatory activity may result from increased production of proinflammatory cytokines such as IL6, tumor necrosis factor (TNF) alpha, and free radicals [123].

A large percentage of older people have relatively high titers of autoantibodies due to higher exposure to exogenous factors such as polypharmia or multiple infections, with cumulative exposure to antibody specificities, supported by a study in Cameroonians 60 years and older [124]. Autoantibodies (AABs) were observed at a rate similar to US averages (49 %) but with a markedly different pattern which implied a strong contribution from extrinsic factors, putatively the widespread presence of chronic infection [124]. In a US study which evaluated Medicare files for the prevalence of AIDs, the risk increased 41 % with a prior infection-related medical visit and by 90 % with a prior (pathogen-free) transfusion [125].

Immunosenescence does not affect men and women equally. Men (and postmenopausal women), for example, have reduced T-cell immunity as compared to premenopausal women [126]. Furthermore, different forms of estrogen are produced at different points of the female life span. During the reproductive years, the primary circulating form of estrogen is estradiol (E2), produced in the ovaries; after menopause, it is estrone (E1), which is produced primarily by adipose tissues. Estrone is the primary form of circulating estrogen in men at all ages. Estradiol binds both estrogen receptors (α and β) at equal affinity. Estrone however, has a fivefold higher affinity for ERα than for ERβ [127].

24.6 Genes, Estrogen, Environment, and Aging: Hints of a Nexus in SLE

Human lupus is a systemic autoimmune disease which primarily affects women, characterized by the formation of autoantibodies to nuclear antigens like DNA, with varied pathogenicity, for example, deposition of immune complexes in the kidneys or in the skin [128].

SLE, one of the more common autoimmune diseases and therefore one of the most studied, is nonetheless a disease whose pathogenesis is still somewhat murky. Dysregulation of immune function seems to be global, as multiple genes appear to more or less simultaneously escape control [52]. In a study which analyzed SLE sera, 30 disparate proteins (cytokines, chemokines, growth factors, and soluble receptors) were observed to be outside the range observed in normal controls [52], highlighting the multifactorial etiology of AIDs like SLE, a complexity that has made definitive etiologies elusive. Over the last several years, however, the multidisciplinary profile of SLE has come together that moves toward integration of the disparate influences on SLE for a more comprehensive understanding.

24.6.1 The Genetic Foundation of SLE

SLE has solid evidence of a genetic foundation. Multiple genetic loci are identified with risk [128]; HLA variant HLA DR3-DQ2.5-C4AQ0 is strongly associated with SLE (odds ratio [OR] 2.8, 95 % confidence interval [CI] 1.7–4.5) [129]. No single gene or group of structural gene defects, however, has emerged as a defining genetic factor [74]. In addition, there is minimal concordance between MZ twins, implying an existence for other complementary components as well [128].

24.6.2 The Contribution of Estrogen to SLE

Estrogen is abnormally metabolized in SLE, with an increase in the production of 16-hydroxyestrone and estriol metabolites which putatively lead to a chronic hyperestrogenic state [41]. Estrogen is clearly an important component of disease course, which fluctuates in close parallel to estrogen levels [130].

In addition, when a cohort of 238,308 women was evaluated prospectively, risk factors for SLE showed a strongly positive association with cumulative estrogen exposure. Menarche earlier than age 10 (relative risk [RR] 2.1, 95 % CI 1.4–3.2), the use of oral contraceptives (RR 1.5, 95 % CI 1.1–2.1), and the use of HRT (RR 1.9, 95 % CI 1.2–3.1) in menopause all raise the risk significantly [131].

Several etiological pathways have been implicated in estrogen's effects. One strong candidate is the strong association of SLE with an observed demethylation of CD40 ligand on CD40+T cells [132]. This demethylation, when present on the inactive X chromosome, results in the overexpression of CD40 ligand on CD4+ cells, which in turn induces the production of autoantibodies [85].

SLE is characterized by the largest number of detectable autoantibody specificities among the autoimmune diseases, which could result from T-cell escape from normal regulation [52]; autoantibody secretion could result from abnormal T-cell regulation. Estrogen-dependent T-cell stimulation, therefore, provides a specific pathway between hormone activation of the T cell, increased T-cell interactions with B cells, and the subsequent overexpression of autoantibodies characteristic of SLE [52].

Expression of the T-cell activator calcineurin is increased when estrogen is cultured with SLE T cells but not with T cells from normal women. This is an upregulation of T-cell function that appears to be estrogen driven since estradiol, bound to the ER, evokes a direct increase in calcineurin expression in T cells from female lupus patients. This does not happen in males, implying a disease-related alteration of the ER specific to women [133]. Estrogen stimulation of calcineurin expression is dose dependent [130]. Thus, estrogen stimulation of calcineurin expression may be what upregulates T-cell regulation, adding to the existing genetic-, environmental-, and immunosenescence-burdened threshold for disease.

ERα also plays a role in SLE disease activity. ERα promotes lupus by inducing interferon (IFN) and cytokines [134]. A deficit in ERα attenuates lupus in NZB/NZW mice disruption of ERα in female NZB/NZW, delays onset of glomerulonephritis, increases survival, and delays the production of autoantibodies; ERα deficiency in male mice increases survival and decreases anti-DNA antibodies [134].

A decrease in SLE disease activity also correlates with abrogation of interferon alpha/beta (INF-αβ) signaling, implicating INF receptors in SLE pathogenesis [135]. Increased levels of estradiol could seemingly be assumed to cause dose-dependent effects across the immune system. Estrogen levels in autoimmune diseases like SLE, however, do not differ dramatically from normal controls. Clearly, then, estrogen does not act in a vacuum.

24.6.3 The Role of Environment in SLE

SLE, in addition to strong evidence for both genetic and sex-hormone components to the disease state, is the autoimmune disease most strongly associated with a specific environmental component. Numerous lupus-like syndromes are widely recognized to result from exposure to over 100 different pharmaceuticals (most commonly procainamide and hydralazine). Drug-induced lupus syndromes, in fact, permitted the use of mouse models in targeted investigation into pathogenic mechanisms, for example, the realization that 5-azacytidine (known to inhibit DNA methylation) causes CD4+T cells to become autoreactive with the ability to respond to antigen-presenting cells (APCs) directly (without exposure to antigen). Intriguingly, the effects were reversible when the drug was removed [128]. Bacterial and viral infections are also believed to be environmental triggers [136]. Ultraviolet light is also known to cause lupus flares [128].

24.6.4 The Contribution of Immunosenescence to SLE

Defects in apoptosis mechanism as well as impaired clearance of apoptotic cells have also been implicated in SLE pathogenesis. Impaired clearance creates a progressive accumulation of autoantigens with an increasing likelihood of an autoimmune response [137]. Regulation of apoptosis is also deranged with increased age, with impaired clearance of cellular debris [138], a factor which could augment effects produced by estrogen.

As the pathogenic basis for SLE is further revealed, we begin to glimpse a variety of known, implicated, and potential mechanisms, from disparate influences but which have plausible interdependent actions with plausible ability to create a genesis of autoimmunity. The genetic platform of susceptibility is built upon, brick by brick, by the multiple potential influences of the immune dysregulation characteristic of increasing age, the chromosomal and hormonal contributions of gender, and a lifetime of environmental insults. Combined, they push the immune system gradually toward immunodysregulation until the threshold is crossed to overt SLE [139]. The question is how that happens.

24.7 NF-KB: Insights from One Protein's Role in Gene Regulation

NF-Kβ is a family of transcription factors ubiquitous in the cytoplasm of immune cells, which clearly plays a fundamental role in immunoregulation (Table 24.7). NF-Kβ proteins occur as dimers and its distribution can differ between tissues. Nuclear factor-Kβ1 (aka p50) and RelA (aka p65) heterodimers are expressed ubiquitously; nuclear factor-Kβ2 (aka p52), RelB, and

Table 24.7 NF-Kβ family of proteins

NF-Kβ protein	Responsible gene	Protein also known as
NF-κβ1	NF κβ1	p50
NF-κβ2	NF κβ2	p52
RelA	RELA	p65
RelB	RELB	–
c-Rel	REL	–

NF-κβ nuclear factor kappa-light-chain-enhancer, also sometimes NF-kappa B

c-Rel are expressed only in lymphoid cells and tissues. The intercellular balance between different nuclear factor-Kβ dimers determines which complex will bind target DNA sequences. NF-Kβ is activated by specific factors like lipopolysaccharide (LPS), TNF-α, and IL-1 as well as by nonspecific factors like UV radiation or oxidative stress, which leads to dissociation of nuclear factor-Kβ from a binding protein inhibitory Kβ (IKβ), allowing NF-Kβ to enter the nucleus [1]. In some normal cells, such as B cells, some T cells, Sertoli cells, and some neurons, NF-Kβ is constitutively located in the nucleus [140].

Nearly countless genes, many of which are implicated in pathways to AID (e.g., inflammatory molecules, apoptosis inhibitors, growth factors, proteins for viral replication, and self-regulatory proteins for NF-Kβ actions) appear to either alter NF-Kβ regulation or to be altered by NF-Kβ (Table 24.8). Not surprisingly, NF-Kβ is often proposed as an agent in the pathogenesis of autoimmune disease.

NF-Kβ appears to encourage autoimmune disease in several ways. It increases tolerance to self-antigens by acting on APCs and thymocytes in such a way that negative selection is deranged, causing increased survival of autoreactive T cells in the peripheral circulation and an enhanced susceptibility to environmental insults with the potential to trigger autoimmune disease [1].

NF-Kβ also initiates the inflammatory response when activated by bacterial or viral interaction with TLRs on macrophages, dendritic cells, and other cells that effect innate immunity [1]. NF-Kβ, in turn, activates transcription for genes encoding inflammation-related cytokines, chemokines, and other molecules required for the migration of inflammatory and phagocytic cells into areas of infection or injury [1]. TLRs in the endoplasmic reticulum, endosomes, and lysosomes also recognize bacterial and nuclear DNA and, through

Table 24.8 NF-Kβ pathways to autoimmunity: inducers of NF-Kβ, its target genes, and associated diseases

Inducers	Bacteria and their products
	Chemicals
	Disease
	Environmental agents
	Fungi and their products
	Growth factors
	Hormones
	Mediators of apoptosis
	Mitogens
	Pharmaceuticals
	Physiological stress
	Proinflammatory cytokines
	Radiation
	Viruses and their products
Target genes	Acute-phase proteins
	Antigen presentation proteins
	Apoptosis regulation proteins
	Cell adhesion molecules
	Cell-surface receptors
	Chemokines
	Cytokines
	Early response genes
	Enzymes
	Growth factors
	Immune receptors
	Stress response genes
	Transcription factors
	Virus particles
Associated immune diseases	Burkett's lymphoma and Epstein-Barr virus (EBV) [141]
	Cancer of the vulva [142]
	Cervical cancer [143]
	Crohn's disease [144]
	Hodgkin's lymphoma [145]
	Inflammatory bowel disease (IBD) [146]
	Multiple myeloma [147]
	Multiple sclerosis (MS) [148]
	Ovarian cancer [149]
	Rheumatoid arthritis (RA) [150]
	Systemic lupus erythematosus (SLE) [151]
	Type I diabetes [152]

NF-Kβ, induce autoimmune reactions [153]. Inflammation, in turn, causes tissue breakdown and the erosion of peripheral tolerance [1].

NF-Kβ also promotes stimulation of an immune response in the absence of antigen due to dysregulation of apoptosis, as many of NF-Kβ target genes are also NF-Kβ inducers, creating a continual feedback loop that can drive an inflammatory response explosively even in the dearth or absence of antigenic stimuli [1]. Reduction of NF-Kβ activity, in fact, promotes the survival of a hyperactivated autoreactive T cells [13].

Functional control of apoptosis is integral for both the development and selection of both T and B cells. NF-Kβ regulates apoptosis in many cell types; whether apoptosis is induced or suppressed depends on the specific type of cell, the specific inducer, and the relative level of intracellular levels of subunits [1].

24.7.1 NF-Kβ and the Genetic Predilection for Autoimmune Disease

NF-Kβ builds upon genetically conferred risk by acting to inappropriately induce gene products. NF-Kβ, once activated, is able to enter the nucleus. There, it binds rapidly to DNA, stimulating the expression of target genes, including many cytokines, chemokines, and other factors involved in immune-cell signaling (see Table 24.8). Monocytes and B cells appear to produce express active NF-Kβ; T cells, however, require proteasome-dependent activation [13].

24.7.2 NF-Kβ and Sex Hormones

Estrogens, interestingly, are known to regulate NF-Kβ activity. 17-β estradiol raises NF-Kβ levels as well as the levels of TNF-α that it induces in a dose-dependent fashion, causing enough overexpression of relevant cytokines to potentially cause autoimmune disease in the physiological context [13]. High concentrations of E2 modulates NF-KB signaling and affects T-cell survival [82]; estrogen regulates inflammation [154]. Estrogen acts to regulate inflammation through posttranslational modification of STAT-1 and NF-Kβ proteins [74].

NF-Kβ interacts directly with estrogen, binding to both ERs, and forming both homo- and heterodimers. When bound, ERs translocate to the nucleus where they bind to EREs in gene promoters, thereby directly controlling gene transcription. The E/ER complex may also interact with other transcription factors such as additional NF-Kβ, capable of binding to transcription factors that are not estrogen related.

Estrogen interactions with NF-Kβ intriguingly also appear to drive gender specificity of autoimmune disease. A recent report revealed that peroxisome proliferator-activated receptor (PPARα) mediates inflammatory responses by activating NF-Kβ and thus inducing production of INF-γ and TNF downregulation of Th2 cytokines. Men are less prone to develop some autoimmune diseases because CD4+T cells express higher levels of PPARα [155].

24.7.3 NF-Kβ and Environment and Aging

Cigarette smoke, an environmental factor associated with numerous autoimmune diseases, is known to induce the release of TNF, TNF alpha receptors, IL-1, IL-6, IL-8, and granulocyte macrophage colony-stimulating factors (GM-CSF) and decrease IL-10 and IFN-gamma [33]. Many of these cytokines and other factors are inducers of the NF-Kβ pathway. Numerous other chemical agents and environmental threats are implicated in the modulation of the actions (see Table 24.8).

The NF-Kβ functions are implicated in the processes of immunosenescence itself [156]. In another positive feedback loop, the progressive deterioration of immune functions regulated by multiple cytokines and other regulatory factors that are known inducers are targets of NF-Kβ actions, it is probable that immunosenescence augments NF-Kβ contributions to autoimmune disease. Suppression of NF-Kβ activity is a common denominator in at least T1DM, SLE, MS, Crohn's disease, and RA.

Table 24.9 Role of NF-Kβ in various autoimmune diseases

Disease	Affected genes	Effect on NF-Kβ	References
Crohn's disease	NOD2	Decreased cell signaling	[13]
	TNF	Suppresses activation	[157]
Diabetes mellitus type I (mouse)	LMP2	Prevents activation, which also suppresses LMP2	[158]
Diabetes mellitus type I (human)	SUMO4	Over ubiquitination prevents activation	[159]
Inflammatory bowel disease	TNF	Suppresses (TNF suppressed also)	[160]
Multiple sclerosis	NF-Kβ family	Undefined, possibly related to NF-Kβ inhibitory protein I Kβ	[161]
Rheumatoid arthritis	NF-Kβ	Increased HDCA activity, promoter demethylation	[162]
Sjögren's syndrome	LMP2	Suppresses activity, which also suppresses LMP2	[163]
Systemic lupus erythematosus	NF-Kβ	Decreased activity	[164]

LMP latent membrane protein, *NF-Kβ* nuclear factor kappa-light-chain-enhancer, *NOD* nucleotide-binding oligomerization domain, *TNF* tumor necrosis factor, *SUMO* small ubiquitin-related modifier

NF-Kβ, then, provides an example of a transcription factor, one of many that provide a link between the genetic background of the individual and the influences of aging, estrogen, and environmental interactions on that genetic predisposition, driving genetic risk toward the onset of autoimmune disease [1] (Table 24.9).

24.8 Epigenetics: The Missing Link in an Integrated Theory of Autoimmune Disease

Epigenetic actions are cell specific, and these actions represent stable changes to DNA that act to regulate gene expression, but do not cause mutation. Epigenetic changes do not alter DNA sequence, but instead control gene expression [47]. These epigenetic changes effect real-time control of homeostasis in the body and maintain the normal function of every cell and its metabolism.

Epigenetic mechanisms confer "phenotypic plasticity" to the genotypic platform by giving the body, at the cellular level, an ability to respond to both internal and external environmental cues [165]. Cells, for example, monitor inventories of necessary compounds and are able to modulate transcription of appropriate genes through epigenetic mechanisms [166]. Epigenetic modifications of DNA are abundant in every cell, changes which are stable because they are heritable during cell division [165].

Epigenetic changes are involved in normal development as well as in disease. Epigenetic variation over time depends on genotype, environment, sex hormone interactions, and undoubtedly other undetermined stochastic factors [80]. Such epigenetic changes provide a ready explanation for discordance in MZ twins with regard to epigenetic diseases that clearly have a strong genetic foundation [94], literally serving as the physiological link between the genome and the genesis of disease. Phenotypic differences in identical twins, caused by epigenetic changes, increase steadily with age ("epigenetic drift"), driven by regular environmental insult [47].

Epigenetic changes are effected by three primary mechanisms as follows: (1) methylation or demethylation of DNA, particularly in promoter sequences of genes; (2) histone modifications, which effect steric changes to chromatin that act to regulate gene transcription; and (3) micro ribonucleic acid (miRNA) particles, typically 22 nucleotides in length, which bind to and degrade complementary messenger RNA (mRNA) after transcription, therefore preventing translation [47] (Table 24.10). Monozygotic twins, with age, show increasing variance in total DNA methylation as well as in acetylation of histone H3K9, with older sets of twins acquiring significantly more epigenetic variance than younger sets [165].

Table 24.10 Epigenetic mechanisms

Effector	Chemical action	Effect
Histone modification	N-terminal histone tails are acetylated, deacetylated, methylated, or demethylated	Modifies steric accessibility to target genes
DNA methylation	Methyl group added to cytosine residues in cytosine-rich promoter regions	Generally silences affected gene
MicroRNA	Binds and degrades complementary miRNA	Blocks translation of target genes

DNA deoxyribonucleic acid, *miRNA* microRNA, *RNA* ribonucleic acid

24.8.1 Mechanisms of Epigenetic Change

24.8.1.1 DNA Methylation

Inherited patterns of DNA methylation are largely wiped away shortly after an embryo is fertilized, with a rapid eradication of the paternal genome patterns but only partial demethylation of maternal DNA. Genome-wide remethylation occurs in the blastocyst stage and tissue-specific remethylation follows later [80]. DNA methylation enzymes DNMT1, DNMT3a, and DNMT3b enact these changes during fetal development; they reproduce epigenetic markings after cell division as well as maintain or copy methylation marks after DNA replication that remethylate in the blastocyte stage [80].

DNA methylation occurs mainly in DNA sequences in which cytosine residues precede guanine residues to yield 5-methylcytosine (5-meC). This resulting dinucleotide is called C-phosphate-G (CpG). Many areas of the human genome are rich in CpGs; CpG-rich areas are known as CpG islands. CpG islands typically occur in gene promoter regions and are usually unmethylated in normal cells [80].

24.8.1.2 Histone Modifications

Chromatin is made up of four core histones, wrapped in 147 base pairs (bp) of DNA. Four epigenetic modifications to DNA in conjunction with histones (typically what is called the "histone tail," a stretch of DNA that protrudes from the histone) are commonly observed: acetylation, methylation, phosphorylation, and ubiquitination [80]. Histone methylation is controlled by histone methyltransferases and demethylases [166].

DNA methylation and histone modification are coupled through both DNA methyltransferases (DNMTs) and different families of methylated DNA binding proteins that associate with histone-modifying enzymes in multiprotein complexes; both regulate transcription in the nucleus and affect nuclear architecture that also acts to regulate gene expression, therefore producing multiple levels of regulation of gene expression [137].

The third more recent epigenetic effectors are miRNAs, typically 22-nucleotide noncoding RNAs that control gene expression at the post-transcriptional level by binding (through partial sequence homology) to the three prime untranslated region (3′UTR) of RNAs, producing translation inhibition or degradation of miRNAs [74].

MicroRNA acting posttranslationally provides a mechanism for quantitative regulation of genes (rather than off/on signals at the genome level) and acts to fine-tune cellular responses to environmental influences [167], thereby regulating immune-cell development as well as maintaining immune homeostasis and immune tolerance [74].

24.8.2 Epigenetic Contributions to Autoimmunity and Gender

ER function is regulated by epigenetic mechanisms. ER occurs in nearly every immune-cell type and is distributed at the cellular membrane, cytoplasm, nucleus, and mitochondria [168].

ER-α is epigenetically regulated; T cells from SLE patients have decreased total genomic methylation compared with age-matched controls [52].

Nuclear ERs provide DNA-dependent regulation of gene expression mediated through the histone-acetylation enzyme histone acetyltransferase (HAT). The binding of HATs to the ER produces acetylation of local histones, which in turn cause steric changes that facilitate gene transcription by permitting transcription factor binding with promoter regions of estrogen-responsive genes.

Dysregulated mRNA expression has also been observed to be estrogen driven in association with autoimmune disease [169].

DNA methylation is also involved in genomic imprinting (the preferential gender-specific silencing of genetic material, for example, the paternal X chromosome in mammals) and X-chromosome inactivation [80].

It is also reported that differentiation of T-helper cells in the direction of either the Th1 or Th2 pathways is epigenetically regulated—Th1 cells have a demethylated IFN-γ promoter, with repressive epigenetic histone modifications at the IL-4 to IL-13 locus, while Th2 cells carry the opposite profile [170].

24.8.2.1 Aging

Global DNA methylation decreases with age [80], simultaneously coupled with hypermethylation specific to CpG island gene promoters or ribosomal DNA clusters [80], changes that almost certainly contribute to immunosenescence [80].

Several papers have reported age-associated changes in global and specific histone profiles, as well as in several histone-modifying enzymes [171].

The biological basis of aging is a progressive decline in the ability to adapt to the environment due to loss of normal gene regulation precipitated by changes in gene promoters or gene silencing regions [165]. Age-associated changes to DNA methylation patterns or histones and their regulatory enzymes certainly increase the risk for dysregulation of gene expression, including the myriad of genes related to immunoregulatory molecules.

24.8.2.2 Environment

An expansive list of environmental factors are now known to directly or indirectly induce epigenetic changes that, through changes in gene expression, modulate immune-cell function. Epigenetics then provides molecular mechanisms that explain the environmental effects on the development of autoimmune disorders [3]. The fact that many autoimmune disease are striking greater numbers of individuals, in populations whose background of genetic, gender, and aging can be assumed to be relatively stable, is an indication of the importance of environmental interactions in autoimmune disease. Genetically identical laboratory animals raised under identical conditions similarly evidence environmental importance and also evidence epigenetic drift [80].

One of the first and most interesting examples of the power of epigenetics was the Dutch Hunger Winter. A severe famine at the end of World War II affecting a specific area of the Netherlands suggests that famine exposure at a critical period in utero can lead to adverse phenotypes. In this group, there was an increased risk of coronary artery disease (CAD) specific for exposure to famine early in gestation. A similar influence of the environment has been shown in agouti mice, in which epigenetic changes related to diet determine coat color; foods rich in methyl donors change the coat color in offspring, a modification produced by altered DNA methylation [47,172].

Many other environmental interactions effect epigenetic changes that contribute to disease (see Table 24.5).

24.8.2.3 Systemic Lupus Erythematosus

Lupus, one of the most investigated of autoimmune diseases, is arguably also the most well characterized in terms of epigenetic etiology [128]. DNA methylation patterns have been associated with immune dysregulation in SLE. A study which looked at genome-wide DNA methylation patterns in a cohort of MZ twins discordant for SLE found DNA methylation differences in genes relevant to SLE pathogenesis, with a decrease in total methylation content [173]. Human SLE patients have reduced total deoxymethylcytosine content and decreased levels of DNMT1, an enzyme which drives the methylation of cytosine residues; demethylated T cells stimulated antibody production by autologous B cells [47]. Drug-induced lupus is predictably induced by procainamide and hydralazine (methylation inhibitors) [47] and is the mechanism found with other drugs as well.

Global acetylation of H3 and H4 histones was observed in active SLE CD4+ cells, a change negatively correlated with disease activity.

Estrogen and the female chromosome complement are known to contribute to female predisposition to lupus (in a mouse model) through both hormonal influence and epigenetic effects on the X chromosome [174].

Epigenetic processes contribute to dysregulation of both B- and T-cell function [47,165,175]. Numerous associations of lupus with miRNA changes have been observed. In human patients, PBMC displayed abnormal miRNA expression patterns in PBMC as compared to controls [74], although the association of these abnormal patterns with overt dysregulation was not consistent, a conundrum which may involve sex-hormone levels or other environmental influences [167]. Specific miRNAs have recently been identified to influence T-cell sensitivity and selection [167] as well as the IFN-gamma pathway; the underexpression of miR-146a in lupus patients effects alterations in type I IFN pathways via key signaling proteins. Models have also observed disrupted miRNA patterns in lupus-affected mice [74].

Epigenetic changes are now being identified as the root of nearly every autoimmune disease. The accumulation of epigenetic changes that disrupt immune function and contribute to a breakdown in immune tolerance through DNA methylation, histone modification, and miRNA binding creates autoimmune disease through aberrant regulation of gene expression.

Epigenetics is then the missing link in the chain of events that produces autoimmune disease from the starting point of modest genetic risk. That risk, acted on by a lifetime of hormone changes, environmental interactions, and inexorable aging, eventually results in a full-blown autoimmune disease. Epigenetics, reversible but acting at the DNA level, defines mechanisms that can explain the environmental effects on the development of autoimmune disorders [3].

24.9 Summary

Although autoimmunity is affected largely by autoantibodies, the development of autoimmune disease requires an aberrant yet sophisticated interplay of a multitude of immunoactive genes, resulting after years of random boosts in risk from genes, estrogen, environmental insults, and the inexorable process of aging, in a point at which immune tolerance and the onset of autoimmune disease occurs. Up until the last few years, the manner in which the process unfolds within the body, in which both set internal parameters and variable external risks act in concert to bring about disease, has been somewhat mysterious.

Epigenetics is a new frontier in understanding the etiology of complex disease, providing a firm footing for etiology theories by defining mechanisms by which environmental conditions, both internal and external, are acted upon to create disease. Moreover, since epigenetic changes are reversible, they provide great potential for therapies in autoimmune diseases. Further research will provide better understanding of epigenetic processes. With targeted intervention, a cure for autoimmune disease may be on the horizon.

References

1. Kuryłowicz A, Nauman J. The role of nuclear factor-kappaB in the development of autoimmune diseases: a link between genes and environment. Acta Biochim Pol. 2008;55(4):629–47.
2. The Autoimmune Diseases Coordinating Committee. Progress in autoimmune disease research. Report to Congress. NIH publication 05-5140. 2005.
3. Javierre BM, Hernando H, Ballestar E. Environmental triggers and epigenetic deregulation in autoimmune disease. Discov Med. 2011;12(67):535–45.
4. Cho JH, Gregersen PK. Genomics and the multifactorial nature of human autoimmune disease. N Engl J Med. 2011;365(17):1612–23.
5. Béland K, Lapierre P, Alvarez F. Influence of genes, sex, age and environment on the onset of autoimmune hepatitis. World J Gastroenterol. 2009;15(9):1025–34.
6. Kurata JH, Kantor-Fish S, Frankl H, Godby P, Vadheim CM. Crohn's disease among ethnic groups in a large health maintenance organization. Gastroenterology. 1992;102(6):1940–8.
7. Reinshagen M, Loeliger C, Kuehnl P, Weiss U, Manfras BJ, Adler G, et al. HLA class II gene frequencies in Crohn's disease: a population based analysis in Germany. Gut. 1996;38(4):538–42.
8. Rivas MA, Beaudoin M, Gardet A, Stevens C, Sharma Y, Zhang CK, et al. Deep resequencing of GWAS loci identifies independent rare variants associated with inflammatory bowel disease. Nat Genet. 2011;43(11):1066–73.

9. Shapira Y, Agmon-Levin N, Shoenfeld Y. Defining and analyzing geoepidemiology and human autoimmunity. J Autoimmun. 2010;34(3):J168–77.
10. Brix TH, Knudsen GPS, Kristiansen M, Kyvik KO, Orstavik KH, Hegedüs L. High frequency of skewed X-chromosome inactivation in females with autoimmune thyroid disease: a possible explanation for the female predisposition to thyroid autoimmunity. J Clin Endocrinol Metab. 2005;90(11):5949–53.
11. Djilali-Saiah I, Larger E, Harfouch-Hammoud E, Timsit J, Clerc J, Bertin E, et al. No major role for the CTLA-4 gene in the association of autoimmune thyroid disease with IDDM. Diabetes. 1998;47(1):125–7.
12. Gough SCL, Simmonds MJ. The HLA region and autoimmune disease: associations and mechanisms of action. Curr Genomics. 2007;8(7):453–65.
13. Dale E, Davis M, Faustman DL. A role for transcription factor NF-kappaB in autoimmunity: possible interactions of genes, sex, and the immune response. Adv Physiol Educ. 2006;30(4):152–8.
14. Fukazawa T, Yanagawa T, Kikuchi S, Yabe I, Sasaki H, Hamada T, et al. CTLA-4 gene polymorphism may modulate disease in Japanese multiple sclerosis patients. J Neurol Sci. 1999;171(1):49–55.
15. Invernizzi P, Pasini S, Selmi C, Gershwin ME, Podda M. Female predominance and X chromosome defects in autoimmune diseases. J Autoimmun. 2009;33(1):12–6.
16. Miozzo M, Selmi C, Gentilin B, Grati FR, Sirchia S, Oertelt S, et al. Preferential X chromosome loss but random inactivation characterize primary biliary cirrhosis. Hepatology. 2007;46(2):456–62.
17. Hirschfield GM, Liu X, Xu C, Lu Y, Xie G, Lu Y, et al. Primary biliary cirrhosis associated with HLA, IL12A, and IL12RB2 variants. N Engl J Med. 2009; 360(24):2544–55.
18. Nigam P, Singh D, Matreja VS, Saxena HN. Psoriatic arthritis: a clinico-radiological study. J Dermatol. 1980;7(1):55–9.
19. Chandran V, Raychaudhuri SP. Geoepidemiology and environmental factors of psoriasis and psoriatic arthritis. J Autoimmun. 2010;34(3):J314–21.
20. Chabchoub G, Uz E, Maalej A, Mustafa CA, Rebai A, Mnif M, et al. Analysis of skewed X-chromosome inactivation in females with rheumatoid arthritis and autoimmune thyroid diseases. Arthritis Res Ther. 2009;11(4):R106.
21. Remmers EF, Plenge RM, Lee AT, Graham RR, Hom G, Behrens TW, et al. STAT4 and the risk of rheumatoid arthritis and systemic lupus erythematosus. N Engl J Med. 2007;357(10):977–86.
22. Ozbalkan Z, Bagişlar S, Kiraz S, Akyerli CB, Ozer HTE, Yavuz S, et al. Skewed X chromosome inactivation in blood cells of women with scleroderma. Arthritis Rheum. 2005;52(5):1564–70.
23. Gladman DD, Kung TN, Siannis F, Pellett F, Farewell VT, Lee P. HLA markers for susceptibility and expression in scleroderma. J Rheumatol. 2005;32(8):1481–7.
24. Agarwal SK, Reveille JD. The genetics of scleroderma (systemic sclerosis). Curr Opin Rheumatol. 2010;22(2):133–8.
25. Bizzarro A, Valentini G, Di Martino G, DaPonte A, De Bellis A, Iacono G. Influence of testosterone therapy on clinical and immunological features of autoimmune diseases associated with Klinefelter's syndrome. J Clin Endocrinol Metab. 1987;64(1):32–6.
26. Harley JB, Reichlin M, Arnett FC, Alexander EL, Bias WB, Provost TT. Gene interaction at HLA-DQ enhances autoantibody production in primary Sjögren's syndrome. Science. 1986;232(4754):1145–7.
27. Desai-Mehta A, Lu L, Ramsey-Goldman R, Datta SK. Hyperexpression of CD40 ligand by B and T cells in human lupus and its role in pathogenic autoantibody production. J Clin Invest. 1996;97(9):2063–73.
28. Chung SA, Taylor KE, Graham RR, Nititham J, Lee AT, Ortmann WA, et al. Differential genetic associations for systemic lupus erythematosus based on anti-dsDNA autoantibody production. PLoS Genet. 2011; 7(3):e1001323.
29. Barker JM. Clinical review: type 1 diabetes-associated autoimmunity: natural history, genetic associations, and screening. J Clin Endocrinol Metab. 2006; 91(4):1210–7.
30. Thompson AI, Lees CW. Genetics of ulcerative colitis. Inflamm Bowel Dis. 2011;17(3):831–48.
31. Teitelbaum JE, Perez-Atayde AR, Cohen M, Bousvaros A, Jonas MM. Minocycline-related autoimmune hepatitis: case series and literature review. Arch Pediatr Adolesc Med. 1998;152(11):1132–6.
32. Alla V, Abraham J, Siddiqui J, Raina D, Wu GY, Chalasani NP, et al. Autoimmune hepatitis triggered by statins. J Clin Gastroenterol. 2006;40(8): 757–61.
33. Arnson Y, Shoenfeld Y, Amital H. Effects of tobacco smoke on immunity, inflammation and autoimmunity. J Autoimmun. 2010;34(3):J258–65.
34. Kappelman MD, Rifas-Shiman SL, Kleinman K, Ollendorf D, Bousvaros A, Grand RJ, et al. The prevalence and geographic distribution of Crohn's disease and ulcerative colitis in the United States. Clin Gastroenterol Hepatol. 2007;5(12):1424–9.
35. Brooks WH, Le Dantec C, Pers J, Youinou P, Renaudineau Y. Epigenetics and autoimmunity. J Autoimmun. 2010;34(3):J207–19.
36. Pollard KM. Gender differences in autoimmunity associated with exposure to environmental factors. J Autoimmun. 2012;38(2–3):J177–86.
37. Orton S, Wald L, Confavreux C, Vukusic S, Krohn JP, Ramagopalan SV, et al. Association of UV radiation with multiple sclerosis prevalence and sex ratio in France. Neurology. 2011;76(5):425–31.
38. Ascherio A, Munch M. Epstein-Barr virus and multiple sclerosis. Epidemiology. 2000;11(2):220–4.
39. Selmi C, Mayo MJ, Bach N, Ishibashi H, Invernizzi P, Gish RG, et al. Primary biliary cirrhosis in monozygotic and dizygotic twins: genetics, epigenetics, and environment. Gastroenterology. 2004;127(2):485–92.
40. Ogrendik M. Does periodontopathic bacterial infection contribute to the etiopathogenesis of the autoimmune disease rheumatoid arthritis? Discov Med. 2012;13(72):349–55.

41. González DA, Díaz BB, Rodríguez Pérez MDC, Hernández AG, Chico BND, de León AC. Sex hormones and autoimmunity. Immunol Lett. 2010;133(1):6–13.
42. Ahmed SA, Hissong BD, Verthelyi D, Donner K, Becker K, Karpuzoglu-Sahin E. Gender and risk of autoimmune diseases: possible role of estrogenic compounds. Environ Health Perspect. 1999;107 Suppl 5:681–6.
43. Ramos-Casals M, García-Carrasco M, Brito MP, López-Soto A, Font J. Autoimmunity and geriatrics: clinical significance of autoimmune manifestations in the elderly. Lupus. 2003;12(5):341–55.
44. Gregersen PK, Olsson LM. Recent advances in the genetics of autoimmune disease. Annu Rev Immunol. 2009;27:363–91.
45. Hemminki K, Li X, Sundquist K, Sundquist J. Shared familial aggregation of susceptibility to autoimmune diseases. Arthritis Rheum. 2009;60(9):2845–7.
46. Rubtsov AV, Rubtsova K, Kappler JW, Marrack P. Genetic and hormonal factors in female-biased autoimmunity. Autoimmun Rev. 2010;9(7):494–8.
47. Meda F, Folci M, Baccarelli A, Selmi C. The epigenetics of autoimmunity. Cell Mol Immunol. 2011;8(3):226–36.
48. Cotsapas C, Voight BF, Rossin E, Lage K, Neale BM, Wallace C, et al. Pervasive sharing of genetic effects in autoimmune disease. PLoS Genet. 2011;7(8): e1002254.
49. Gervin K, Vigeland MD, Mattingsdal M, Hammerø M, Nygård H, Olsen AO, et al. DNA methylation and gene expression changes in monozygotic twins discordant for psoriasis: identification of epigenetically dysregulated genes. PLoS Genet. 2012;8(1): e1002454.
50. Manheimer-Lory AJ, Zandman-Goddard G, Davidson A, Aranow C, Diamond B. Lupus-specific antibodies reveal an altered pattern of somatic mutation. J Clin Invest. 1997;100(10):2538–46.
51. Davidson A, Manheimer-Lory A, Aranow C, Peterson R, Hannigan N, Diamond B. Molecular characterization of a somatically mutated anti-DNA antibody bearing two systemic lupus erythematosus-related idiotypes. J Clin Invest. 1990;85(5):1401–9.
52. Rider V, Abdou NI. Hormones: epigenetic contributors to gender-based autoimmunity. In: Zouali M, editor. The epigenetics of autoimmune diseases. Chichester: Wiley; 2009. p. 309–26.
53. Olsen NJ, Kovacs WJ. Effects of androgens on T and B lymphocyte development. Immunol Res. 2001;23(2–3):281–8.
54. Walsh SJ, Rau LM. Autoimmune diseases: a leading cause of death among young and middle-aged women in the United States. Am J Public Health. 2000;90(9):1463–6.
55. IOM (Institute of Medicine). Women's health research: progress, pitfalls, and promise. Washington, DC: The National Academies Press; 2010.
56. Gameiro C, Romao F. Changes in the immune system during menopause and aging. Front Biosci (Elite Ed). 2010;2:1299–303.
57. Papenfuss TL, Whitacre CC. Sex hormones, pregnancy, and immune function. In: Pfaff DW, Arnold AP, Etgen AM, Fahrbach SE, Rubin RT, editors. Hormones, brain, and behavior. San Diego: Academic; 2009. p. 367–76.
58. Fairweather D, Frisancho-Kiss S, Rose NR. Sex differences in autoimmune disease from a pathological perspective. Am J Pathol. 2008;173(3):600–9.
59. Delpy L, Douin-Echinard V, Garidou L, Bruand C, Saoudi A, Guéry J. Estrogen enhances susceptibility to experimental autoimmune myasthenia gravis by promoting type 1-polarized immune responses. J Immunol. 2005;175(8):5050–7.
60. Marzi M, Vigano A, Trabattoni D, Villa ML, Salvaggio A, Clerici E, et al. Characterization of type 1 and type 2 cytokine production profile in physiologic and pathologic human pregnancy. Clin Exp Immunol. 1996;106(1):127–33.
61. Beagley KW, Gockel CM. Regulation of innate and adaptive immunity by the female sex hormones oestradiol and progesterone. FEMS Immunol Med Microbiol. 2003;38(1):13–22.
62. Grimaldi CM, Michael DJ, Diamond B. Cutting edge: expansion and activation of a population of autoreactive marginal zone B cells in a model of estrogen-induced lupus. J Immunol. 2001;167(4):1886–90.
63. Kanda N, Tamaki K. Estrogen enhances immunoglobulin production by human PBMCs. J Allergy Clin Immunol. 1999;103(2 Pt 1):282–8.
64. Nalbandian G, Kovats S. Estrogen, immunity & autoimmune disease. Curr Med Chem Immun Endoc Metab Agents. 2005;5:85–91.
65. Tanriverdi F, Silveira LFG, MacColl GS, Bouloux PMG. The hypothalamic-pituitary-gonadal axis: immune function and autoimmunity. J Endocrinol. 2003;176(3):293–304.
66. Tai P, Wang J, Jin H, Song X, Yan J, Kang Y, et al. Induction of regulatory T cells by physiological level estrogen. J Cell Physiol. 2008;214(2):456–64.
67. Thongngarm T, Jenkins JK, Ndebele K, McMurray RW. Estrogen and progesterone modulate monocyte cell cycle progression and apoptosis. Am J Reprod Immunol. 2003;49(3):129–38.
68. O'Connor M, Motivala SJ, Valladares EM, Olmstead R, Irwin MR. Sex differences in monocyte expression of IL-6: role of autonomic mechanisms. Am J Physiol Regul Integr Comp Physiol. 2007;293(1):R145–51.
69. Lamon-Fava S, Posfai B, Schaefer EJ. Effect of hormonal replacement therapy on C-reactive protein and cell-adhesion molecules in postmenopausal women. Am J Cardiol. 2003;91(2):252–4.
70. Miller AP, Feng W, Xing D, Weathington NM, Blalock JE, Chen Y, et al. Estrogen modulates inflammatory mediator expression and neutrophil chemotaxis in injured arteries. Circulation. 2004;110(12):1664–9.

71. Bynoe MS, Grimaldi CM, Diamond B. Estrogen up-regulates Bcl-2 and blocks tolerance induction of naive B cells. Proc Natl Acad Sci U S A. 2000;97(6):2703–8.
72. Srivastava S, Weitzmann MN, Cenci S, Ross FP, Adler S, Pacifici R. Estrogen decreases TNF gene expression by blocking JNK activity and the resulting production of c-Jun and JunD. J Clin Invest. 1999;104(4):503–13.
73. Koh KK, Ahn JY, Jin DK, Yoon B, Kim HS, Kim DS, et al. Effects of continuous combined hormone replacement therapy on inflammation in hypertensive and/or overweight postmenopausal women. Arterioscler Thromb Vasc Biol. 2002;22(9):1459–64.
74. Dai R, Zhang Y, Khan D, Heid B, Caudell D, Crasta O, et al. Identification of a common lupus disease-associated microRNA expression pattern in three different murine models of lupus. PLoS One. 2010;5(12):e14302.
75. Buchel E, Van Steenbergen W, Nevens F, Fevery J. Improvement of autoimmune hepatitis during pregnancy followed by flare-up after delivery. Am J Gastroenterol. 2002;97(12):3160–5.
76. Samuel D, Riordan S, Strasser S, Kurtovic J, Singh-Grewel I, Koorey D. Severe autoimmune hepatitis first presenting in the early post partum period. Clin Gastroenterol Hepatol. 2004;2(7):622–4.
77. Kanda N, Tsuchida T, Tamaki K. Estrogen enhancement of anti-double-stranded DNA antibody and immunoglobulin G production in peripheral blood mononuclear cells from patients with systemic lupus erythematosus. Arthritis Rheum. 1999;42(2):328–37.
78. Kanda N, Tsuchida T, Tamaki K. Testosterone inhibits immunoglobulin production by human peripheral blood mononuclear cells. Clin Exp Immunol. 1996;106(2):410–5.
79. Gubbels Bupp MR, Jørgensen TN, Kotzin BL. Identification of candidate genes that influence sex hormone-dependent disease phenotypes in mouse lupus. Genes Immun. 2008;9(1):47–56.
80. Aguilera O, Fernández AF, Muñoz A, Fraga MF. Epigenetics and environment: a complex relationship. J Appl Physiol. 2010;109(1):243–51.
81. Palaszynski KM, Smith DL, Kamrava S, Burgoyne PS, Arnold AP, Voskuhl RR. A yin-yang effect between sex chromosome complement and sex hormones on the immune response. Endocrinology. 2005;146(8):3280–5.
82. Abdou N, Rider V. Gender differences in autoimmune diseases: immune mechanisms and clinical applications. In: Legato MJ, editor. Principles of gender-specific medicine. London: Academic; 2009. p. 585–91.
83. Pennell LM, Galligan CL, Fish EN. Sex affects immunity. J Autoimmun. 2012;38(2–3):J282–91.
84. Cunningham M, Gilkeson G. Estrogen receptors in immunity and autoimmunity. Clin Rev Allergy Immunol. 2011;40(1):66–73.
85. Rider V, Jones S, Evans M, Bassiri H, Afsar Z, Abdou NI. Estrogen increases CD40 ligand expression in T cells from women with systemic lupus erythematosus. J Rheumatol. 2001;28(12):2644–9.
86. Abdou NI, Rider V, Greenwell C, Li X, Kimler BF. Fulvestrant (Faslodex), an estrogen selective receptor downregulator, in therapy of women with systemic lupus erythematosus. Clinical, serologic, bone density, and T cell activation marker studies: a double-blind placebo-controlled trial. J Rheumatol. 2008;35(5):797.
87. Galofré JC. Microchimerism in Graves' disease. J Thyroid Res. 2012;2012:724382.
88. Greer LG, Casey BM, Halvorson LM, Spong CY, McIntire DD, Cunningham FG. Antithyroid antibodies and parity: further evidence for microchimerism in autoimmune thyroid disease. Am J Obstet Gynecol. 2011;205(5):471.e1–4.
89. Zandman-Goddard G, Peeva E, Shoenfeld Y. Gender and autoimmunity. Autoimmun Rev. 2007;6(6):366–72.
90. Tremolizzo L, Carboni G, Ruzicka WB, Mitchell CP, Sugaya I, Tueting P, et al. An epigenetic mouse model for molecular and behavioral neuropathologies related to schizophrenia vulnerability. Proc Natl Acad Sci U S A. 2002;99(26):17095–100.
91. Kim K, Friso S, Choi S. DNA methylation, an epigenetic mechanism connecting folate to healthy embryonic development and aging. J Nutr Biochem. 2009;20(12):917–26.
92. Shaw GM, Carmichael SL, Yang W, Selvin S, Schaffer DM. Periconceptional dietary intake of choline and betaine and neural tube defects in offspring. Am J Epidemiol. 2004;160(2):102–9.
93. Choi S, Friso S. Epigenetics: a new bridge between nutrition and health. Adv Nutr. 2010;1(1):8–16.
94. MacFarlane AJ, Strom A, Scott FW. Epigenetics: deciphering how environmental factors may modify autoimmune type 1 diabetes. Mamm Genome. 2009;20(9–10):624–32.
95. Anway MD, Cupp AS, Uzumcu M, Skinner MK. Epigenetic transgenerational actions of endocrine disruptors and male fertility. Science. 2005;308(5727):1466–9.
96. Baccarelli A, Wright RO, Bollati V, Tarantini L, Litonjua AA, Suh HH, et al. Rapid DNA methylation changes after exposure to traffic particles. Am J Respir Crit Care Med. 2009;179(7):572–8.
97. Fernández-Ruiz J, Gómez M, Hernández M, de Miguel R, Ramos JA. Cannabinoids and gene expression during brain development. Neurotox Res. 2004;6(5):389–401.
98. Roth TL, Zoladz PR, Sweatt JD, Diamond DM. Epigenetic modification of hippocampal Bdnf DNA in adult rats in an animal model of post-traumatic stress disorder. J Psychiatr Res. 2011;45(7):919–26.
99. Borchers AT, Gershwin ME. Sociological differences between women and men: implications for autoimmunity. Autoimmun Rev. 2012;11(6–7):A413–21.

100. Larbi A, Franceschi C, Mazzatti D, Solana R, Wikby A, Pawelec G. Aging of the immune system as a prognostic factor for human longevity. Physiology (Bethesda). 2008;23:64–74.
101. Aw D, Silva AB, Palmer DB. Immunosenescence: emerging challenges for an ageing population. Immunology. 2007;120(4):435–46.
102. Allman D, Miller JP. B cell development and receptor diversity during aging. Curr Opin Immunol. 2005;17(5):463–7.
103. Hasler P, Zouali M. Immune receptor signaling, aging, and autoimmunity. Cell Immunol. 2005; 233(2):102–8.
104. Huppert FA, Solomou W, O'Connor S, Morgan K, Sussams P, Brayne C. Aging and lymphocyte subpopulations: whole-blood analysis of immune markers in a large population sample of healthy elderly individuals. Exp Gerontol. 1998;33(6):593–600.
105. Franceschi C, Cossarizza A. Introduction: the reshaping of the immune system with age. Int Rev Immunol. 1995;12(1):1–4.
106. Utsuyama M, Hirokawa K, Kurashima C, Fukayama M, Inamatsu T, Suzuki K, et al. Differential age-change in the numbers of CD4+CD45RA+ and CD4+CD29+ T cell subsets in human peripheral blood. Mech Ageing Dev. 1992;63(1):57–68.
107. Johnson SA, Cambier JC. Ageing, autoimmunity and arthritis: senescence of the B cell compartment—implications for humoral immunity. Arthritis Res Ther. 2004;6(4):131–9.
108. Frasca D, Riley RL, Blomberg BB. Humoral immune response and B-cell functions including immunoglobulin class switch are downregulated in aged mice and humans. Semin Immunol. 2005;17(5):378–84.
109. Whisler RL, Liu BQ, Newhouse YG, Walters JD, Breckenridge MB, Grants IS. Signal transduction in human B cells during aging: alterations in stimulus-induced phosphorylations of tyrosine and serine/threonine substrates and in cytosolic calcium responsiveness. Lymphokine Cytokine Res. 1991;10(6):463–73.
110. Paganelli R, Quinti I, Fagiolo U, Cossarizza A, Ortolani C, Guerra E, et al. Changes in circulating B cells and immunoglobulin classes and subclasses in a healthy aged population. Clin Exp Immunol. 1992;90(2):351–4.
111. Giglio T, Imro MA, Filaci G, Scudeletti M, Puppo F, De Cecco L, et al. Immune cell circulating subsets are affected by gonadal function. Life Sci. 1994;54(18):1305–12.
112. Fann M, Chiu WK, Wood 3rd WH, Levine BL, Becker KG, Weng N. Gene expression characteristics of CD28null memory phenotype CD8+ T cells and its implication in T-cell aging. Immunol Rev. 2005;205:190–206.
113. Mo R, Chen J, Han Y, Bueno-Cannizares C, Misek DE, Lescure PA, et al. T cell chemokine receptor expression in aging. J Immunol. 2003;170(2):895–904.
114. Weng N. Aging of the immune system: how much can the adaptive immune system adapt? Immunity. 2006;24(5):495–9.
115. Tarazona R, DelaRosa O, Alonso C, Ostos B, Espejo J, Peña J, et al. Increased expression of NK cell markers on T lymphocytes in aging and chronic activation of the immune system reflects the accumulation of effector/senescent T cells. Mech Ageing Dev. 2000;121(1–3):77–88.
116. Ershler WB, Sun WH, Binkley N, Gravenstein S, Volk MJ, Kamoske G, et al. Interleukin-6 and aging: blood levels and mononuclear cell production increase with advancing age and in vitro production is modifiable by dietary restriction. Lymphokine Cytokine Res. 1993;12(4):225–30.
117. Farage MA, Miller KW, Maibach HI. The effects of menopause on autoimmune diseases. Expert Rev Obstet Gynecol. 2012;7(6):557–71.
118. Ku LT, Gercel-Taylor C, Nakajima ST, Taylor DD. Alterations of T cell activation signalling and cytokine production by postmenopausal estrogen levels. Immun Ageing. 2009;6:1.
119. Stacy S, Krolick KA, Infante AJ, Kraig E. Immunological memory and late onset autoimmunity. Mech Ageing Dev. 2002;123(8):975–85.
120. Gangemi S, Basile G, Monti D, Merendino RA, Di Pasquale G, Bisignano U, et al. Age-related modifications in circulating IL-15 levels in humans. Mediators Inflamm. 2005;2005(4):245–7.
121. Fairweather D, Rose N. Immunopathogenesis of autoimmune diseases. In: Luebke R, House RV, Kimber I, editors. Immunotoxicology and immunopharmacology. Boca Raton: CRC Press; 2007. p. 423–36.
122. Hasler P, Zouali M. Subversion of B lymphocyte signaling by infectious agents. Genes Immun. 2003;4(2):95–103.
123. Gameiro CM, Romão F, Castelo-Branco C. Menopause and aging: changes in the immune system–a review. Maturitas. 2010;67(4):316–20.
124. Njemini R, Meyers I, Demanet C, Smitz J, Sosso M, Mets T. The prevalence of autoantibodies in an elderly sub-Saharan African population. Clin Exp Immunol. 2002;127(1):99–106.
125. Rogers MAM, Levine DA, Blumberg N, Fisher GG, Kabeto M, Langa KM. Antigenic challenge in the etiology of autoimmune disease in women. J Autoimmun. 2012;38(2–3):J97–102.
126. Pietschmann P, Gollob E, Brosch S, Hahn P, Kudlacek S, Willheim M, et al. The effect of age and gender on cytokine production by human peripheral blood mononuclear cells and markers of bone metabolism. Exp Gerontol. 2003;38(10):1119–27.
127. Zhu BT, Han G, Shim J, Wen Y, Jiang X. Quantitative structure-activity relationship of various endogenous estrogen metabolites for human estrogen receptor alpha and beta subtypes: Insights into the structural determinants favoring a differential subtype binding. Endocrinology. 2006;147(9):4132–50.

128. Strickland FM, Richardson BC. Epigenetics in human autoimmunity. Epigenetics in autoimmunity—DNA methylation in systemic lupus erythematosus and beyond. Autoimmunity. 2008;41(4):278–86.
129. Jönsen A, Bengtsson AA, Sturfelt G, Truedsson L. Analysis of HLA DR, HLA DQ, C4A, FcgammaRIIa, FcgammaRIIIa, MBL, and IL-1Ra allelic variants in Caucasian systemic lupus erythematosus patients suggests an effect of the combined FcgammaRIIa R/R and IL-1Ra 2/2 genotypes on disease susceptibility. Arthritis Res Ther. 2004;6(6):R557–62.
130. Rider V, Foster RT, Evans M, Suenaga R, Abdou NI. Gender differences in autoimmune diseases: estrogen increases calcineurin expression in systemic lupus erythematosus. Clin Immunol Immunopathol. 1998;89(2):171–80.
131. Costenbader KH, Feskanich D, Stampfer MJ, Karlson EW. Reproductive and menopausal factors and risk of systemic lupus erythematosus in women. Arthritis Rheum. 2007;56(4):1251–62.
132. Lu Q, Wu A, Tesmer L, Ray D, Yousif N, Richardson B. Demethylation of CD40LG on the inactive X in T cells from women with lupus. J Immunol. 2007;179(9):6352–8.
133. Rider V, Jones SR, Evans M, Abdou NI. Molecular mechanisms involved in the estrogen-dependent regulation of calcineurin in systemic lupus erythematosus T cells. Clin Immunol. 2000;95(2):124–34.
134. Bynoté KK, Hackenberg JM, Korach KS, Lubahn DB, Lane PH, Gould KA. Estrogen receptor-alpha deficiency attenuates autoimmune disease in (NZB x NZW)F1 mice. Genes Immun. 2008;9(2):137–52.
135. Jørgensen TN, Roper E, Thurman JM, Marrack P, Kotzin BL. Type I interferon signaling is involved in the spontaneous development of lupus-like disease in B6.Nba2 and (B6.Nba2 x NZW)F(1) mice. Genes Immun. 2007;8(8):653–62.
136. New discoveries on environmental triggers of lupus. http://lupusresearchinstitute.org/news/discoveries/080528.
137. Ballestar E, Esteller M, Richardson BC. The epigenetic face of systemic lupus erythematosus. J Immunol. 2006;176(12):7143–7.
138. Aprahamian T, Takemura Y, Goukassian D, Walsh K. Ageing is associated with diminished apoptotic cell clearance in vivo. Clin Exp Immunol. 2008;152(3):448–55.
139. Grimaldi CM, Hill L, Xu X, Peeva E, Diamond B. Hormonal modulation of B cell development and repertoire selection. Mol Immunol. 2005;42(7):811–20.
140. Gilmore T. NK-kB Transcription factors. http://www.bu.edu/nf-kb/.
141. Knecht H, Berger C, Rothenberger S, Odermatt BF, Brousset P. The role of Epstein-Barr virus in neoplastic transformation. Oncology. 2001;60(4):289–302.
142. Seppänen M, Vihko KK. Activation of transcription factor NF-kappaB by growth inhibitory cytokines in vulvar carcinoma cells. Immunol Lett. 2000;74(2):103–9.
143. Ramdass B, Maliekal TT, Lakshmi S, Rehman M, Rema P, Nair P, et al. Coexpression of Notch1 and NF-kappaB signaling pathway components in human cervical cancer progression. Gynecol Oncol. 2007;104(2):352–61.
144. Peña AS, Peñate M. Genetic susceptibility and regulation of inflammation in Crohn's disease. Relationship with the innate immune system. Rev Esp Enferm Dig. 2002;94(6):351–60.
145. Staudt LM. The molecular and cellular origins of Hodgkin's disease. J Exp Med. 2000;191(2):207–12.
146. Atreya I, Atreya R, Neurath MF. NF-kappaB in inflammatory bowel disease. J Intern Med. 2008;263(6):591–6.
147. Gilmore TD. Multiple myeloma: lusting for NF-kappaB. Cancer Cell. 2007;12(2):95–7.
148. Satoh J, Illes Z, Peterfalvi A, Tabunoki H, Rozsa C, Yamamura T. Aberrant transcriptional regulatory network in T cells of multiple sclerosis. Neurosci Lett. 2007;422(1):30–3.
149. Huang S, Robinson JB, Deguzman A, Bucana CD, Fidler IJ. Blockade of nuclear factor-kappaB signaling inhibits angiogenesis and tumorigenicity of human ovarian cancer cells by suppressing expression of vascular endothelial growth factor and interleukin 8. Cancer Res. 2000;60(19):5334–9.
150. Greetham D, Ellis CD, Mewar D, Fearon U, Ultaigh SN, Veale DJ, et al. Functional characterization of NF-kappaB inhibitor-like protein 1 (NFkappaBIL1), a candidate susceptibility gene for rheumatoid arthritis. Hum Mol Genet. 2007;16(24):3027–36.
151. Oikonomidou O, Vlachoyiannopoulos PG, Kominakis A, Kalofoutis A, Moutsopoulos HM, Moutsatsou P. Glucocorticoid receptor, nuclear factor kappaB, activator protein-1 and C-jun N-terminal kinase in systemic lupus erythematosus patients. Neuroimmunomodulation. 2006;13(4):194–204.
152. Eldor R, Yeffet A, Baum K, Doviner V, Amar D, Ben-Neriah Y, et al. Conditional and specific NF-kappaB blockade protects pancreatic beta cells from diabetogenic agents. Proc Natl Acad Sci U S A. 2006;103(13):5072–7.
153. Hurst J, von Landenberg P. Toll-like receptors and autoimmunity. Autoimmun Rev. 2008;7(3):204–8.
154. Dai R, Phillips RA, Karpuzoglu E, Khan D, Ahmed SA. Estrogen regulates transcription factors STAT-1 and NF-kappaB to promote inducible nitric oxide synthase and inflammatory responses. J Immunol. 2009;183(11):6998–7005.
155. Dunn SE, Ousman SS, Sobel RA, Zuniga L, Baranzini SE, Youssef S, et al. Peroxisome proliferator-activated receptor (PPAR)alpha expression in T cells mediates gender differences in development of T cell-mediated autoimmunity. J Exp Med. 2007;204(2):321–30.

156. Csiszar A, Wang M, Lakatta EG, Ungvari Z. Inflammation and endothelial dysfunction during aging: role of NF-kappaB. J Appl Physiol. 2008; 105(4):1333–41.
157. Levine A, Shamir R, Wine E, Weiss B, Karban A, Shaoul RR, et al. TNF promoter polymorphisms and modulation of growth retardation and disease severity in pediatric Crohn's disease. Am J Gastroenterol. 2005;100(7):1598–604.
158. Hayashi T, Faustman D. NOD mice are defective in proteasome production and activation of NF-kappaB. Mol Cell Biol. 1999;19(12):8646–59.
159. Gale EA, Gillespie KM. Diabetes and gender. Diabetologia. 2001;44(1):3–15.
160. van Heel DA, Udalova IA, De Silva AP, McGovern DP, Kinouchi Y, Hull J, et al. Inflammatory bowel disease is associated with a TNF polymorphism that affects an interaction between the OCT1 and NF(-kappa)B transcription factors. Hum Mol Genet. 2002;11(11):1281–9.
161. Miterski B, Böhringer S, Klein W, Sindern E, Haupts M, Schimrigk S, et al. Inhibitors in the NFkappaB cascade comprise prime candidate genes predisposing to multiple sclerosis, especially in selected combinations. Genes Immun. 2002;3(4):211–9.
162. Okamoto T, Tsuchiya A. NF-kappaB as a therapeutic target of rheumatoid arthritis. Nihon Rinsho Meneki Gakkai Kaishi. 2007;30(5):383–9. Japanese.
163. Krause S, Kuckelkorn U, Dörner T, Burmester G, Feist E, Kloetzel P. Immunoproteasome subunit LMP2 expression is deregulated in Sjogren's syndrome but not in other autoimmune disorders. Ann Rheum Dis. 2006;65(8):1021–7.
164. Kammer GM, Tsokos GC. Abnormal T lymphocyte signal transduction in systemic lupus erythematosus. Curr Dir Autoimmun. 2002;5:131–50.
165. Feinberg AP. Phenotypic plasticity and the epigenetics of human disease. Nature. 2007;447(7143): 433–40.
166. Luo J, Kuo MH. Linking nutrient metabolism to epigenetics. Cell Sci Rev. 2009;6:49–54.
167. Tang Y, Luo X, Cui H, Ni X, Yuan M, Guo Y, et al. MicroRNA-146A contributes to abnormal activation of the type I interferon pathway in human lupus by targeting the key signaling proteins. Arthritis Rheum. 2009;60(4):1065–75.
168. Leader JE, Wang C, Popov VM, Fu M, Pestell RG. Epigenetics and the estrogen receptor. Ann N Y Acad Sci. 2006;1089:73–87.
169. Dai R, Ahmed SA. MicroRNA, a new paradigm for understanding immunoregulation, inflammation, and autoimmune diseases. Transl Res. 2011;157(4): 163–79.
170. Baguet A, Bix M. Chromatin landscape dynamics of the Il4-Il13 locus during T helper 1 and 2 development. Proc Natl Acad Sci U S A. 2004;101(31): 11410–5.
171. Calvanese V, Lara E, Kahn A, Fraga MF. The role of epigenetics in aging and age-related diseases. Ageing Res Rev. 2009;8(4):268–76.
172. Wolff GL, Kodell RL, Moore SR, Cooney CA. Maternal epigenetics and methyl supplements affect agouti gene expression in Avy/a mice. FASEB J. 1998;12(11):949–57.
173. Javierre BM, Fernandez AF, Richter J, Al-Shahrour F, Martin-Subero JI, Rodriguez-Ubreva J, et al. Changes in the pattern of DNA methylation associate with twin discordance in systemic lupus erythematosus. Genome Res. 2010;20(2):170–9.
174. Strickland FM, Hewagama A, Lu Q, Wu A, Hinderer R, Webb R, et al. Environmental exposure, estrogen and two X chromosomes are required for disease development in an epigenetic model of lupus. J Autoimmun. 2012;38(2–3):J135–43.
175. Korganow A, Knapp A, Nehme-Schuster H, Soulas-Sprauel P, Poindron V, Pasquali J, et al. Peripheral B cell abnormalities in patients with systemic lupus erythematosus in quiescent phase: decreased memory B cells and membrane CD19 expression. J Autoimmun. 2010;34(4):426–34.

Menopause and Aging Skin in the Elderly

25

Camil Castelo-Branco and Jhery Davila

Contents

25.1	Introduction	345
25.2	**Morphological Alterations**	346
25.2.1	Epidermis	346
25.2.2	Dermis	346
25.3	**Function Alterations**	347
25.4	**Aging, Menopause, and Changes in the Skin and Appendages**	347
25.5	**Estrogen and Skin**	347
25.5.1	Effects on Nails	348
25.5.2	Effects on Pilosebaceous Follicles	348
25.5.3	Effects on Eccrine Sweat Glands and Apocrine Glands	349
25.6	**Physiology of Aging**	349
25.7	**Aging Pathophysiology**	350
25.8	**Intrinsic Factors**	350
25.8.1	Epidermis	350
25.8.2	Dermis	351
25.8.3	Changes in Hair	352
25.8.4	Cutaneous Nerves and Glands	352
25.9	**Extrinsic Factors**	352
25.9.1	Sun Exposure	352
25.9.2	Tobacco	353
25.9.3	Free Radicals	353
25.10	**Skin Diseases and Aging**	353
25.11	**Psychological Impact**	355
References		356

C. Castelo-Branco, MD, PhD (✉)
J. Davila, MD
Faculty of Medicine, Clinic Institute of Gynecology, Obstetrics and Neonatology, Hospital Clinic-Institut D'Investigacions Biomèdiques August Pi Sunyer, University of Barcelona,
Villarroel #170, Barcelona 08036, Spain
e-mail: castelobranco@ub.edu;
dr_jdavila@outlook.com

25.1 Introduction

The aging body, and therefore the aging skin, is a constant concern in all civilizations. The most developed society has higher prevalence of diseases associated with senescence. In industrialized countries, birth rate decreases, and life expectancy increases making an aging society. Moreover, in modern societies, the worship given to physical appearance makes aging a transcendent topic. Skin aging is defined as a series of changes occurring with age and that are determined by intrinsic and extrinsic factors. Chronological or intrinsic aging is a set of clinical, physiological, biochemical, and histological changes, involving epidermal cell turnover, dermal substance clearance, thickness and cellularity of the dermis, ability of thermoregulation, immune response, sensory perception, secretion of sebaceous and sweat glands, and vitamin D synthesis. Extrinsic factors not only accelerate the chronological process of skin aging but also may exaggerate and introduce qualitative changes in it. Among the extrinsic factors, the most important is ultraviolet radiation (UV) exposure. The sun exposure is responsible for most of the cosmetic trouble (atrophy, spots, and wrinkles) and clinical complaints (telangiectasia, basal and squamous cell carcinoma, and melanoma) affecting elderly people. Other well-defined extrinsic factor is pollution. All these factors act on the skin, causing changes at the morphological and functional level; therefore, the prevention or delay of its effects may preserve the skin improving the quality of life. For all these reasons, identifying biomarkers of aging in the skin is currently a topic of great interest.

25.2 Morphological Alterations

25.2.1 Epidermis

The gradual thinning of the skin and atrophy are changes that occur with aging. These phenomena, which start at 30 and intensify between 40 and 50, coinciding with menopause, are more pronounced in areas exposed to sunlight. At the microscopic level, this is described as a lack of basal-granular-squamous cell differentiation and loss of the architectural polarity.

25.2.2 Dermis

The dermis is the physical support of a multitude of anatomical structures (capillaries, veins, receptors and nerve endings, glands). In aged skin, a decreased cellular thickness of the dermis and a flattening and widening of the dermal papillae are detected.

The main components of the dermis are collagen, elastin, and fibroblasts. Collagen represents about 80 % dry weight of adult skin, having a high tensile strength that prevents the skin tear by elongation. Elastin, which represents nearly 5 % of the dermis, is an elastic protein that maintains skin tension. Finally, the fibroblast is the cell that synthesizes all matrix components – collagen, elastin, and ground substance.

There are at least eight different types of collagen, and they are all composed of three polypeptide chains. The most abundant collagen is type I, which is the only type identified in the bone and the predominating form in adult skin [1]. Type III is also common in the skin but in a lower concentration than type I. Type IV is the major structural component of basement membranes and is responsible for their mechanical elasticity.

The hair and nails are constituted largely by keratin, which is hard and insoluble, whereas skin is almost pure collagen. The collagen's fibrous protein has a high tensile strength capable of withstanding mechanical stresses. Collagen is found in the connective tissue of the skin, tendons, cartilage, bone matrix, and eye cornea [2, 3]. The genesis of human collagen type I requires the presence of fibroblasts. These cells synthesized procollagen I, which is subsequently transformed into collagen in the extracellular space. Successively, the collagen fibril must undergo a series of changes in the extracellular space to improve its stability and tensile strength, becoming less soluble and more stable. Collagen has different catabolism in the diverse tissues with a higher renewal rate in the bone and muscle and lower turnover in the skin and tendons. Differences between tissues are due to the disparity in the solubility and cross-links of the different collagens [4]. The glycosylation of the collagen may be involved in the age-related formation cross-links of collagen. This is a key process for understanding skin aging.

Collagen synthesis and enzymes involved in posttranslational processing of the collagen in the skin are impaired in the process of aging [5]. Collagen stability increases with age because a majority of cross-links between collagen molecules becomes non-reductible [6].

Morphological and histochemical changes occurring in the collagen at the sunlight-exposed skin are similar to those that occur later and less sharply in unexposed skin during aging. Besides an age-related decrease in the number of fibroblasts and mast cells in the dermis, a decrease in collagen content of the skin is also observed [7]. As a result of this change in collagen content, an increase in laxity and wrinkles can occur.

There are certain chemical changes in the dermal collagen that are age related. Increased collagen glycosylation associated with age maybe is key factor in the formation of cross-link collagen. The dermis also contains minor amounts of glycosaminoglycans, which are closely associated with dermal collagen. Glycosaminoglycans have a high water binding capacity and are essential for normal skin hydration. A significant decrease of glycosaminoglycans, especially hyaluronic acid, might explain the dehydrated, dry, and wrinkled appearance of aging skin.

Collagen is the element that allows skin to undergo changes throughout life. Collagen has been used in many studies as a marker of aging, and today it is considered that collagen deficit is the main reason for skin aging. The skin thickness is directly related to the quantity and quality of collagen. In the 1940s, Albright noted for the first time the existence of marked skin atrophy in postmenopausal women with osteoporosis. Two decades later, McConkey suggested that skin thinning felt by these women was due mainly to a detriment in collagen type I and also that this type of skin was more vulnerable to external aggressions. In the late 1980s, Brincat [2] supports previous findings highlighting the relationship between the decrease in type I collagen content in the skin (declines by 2.1 % per year) and the thickness of the skin (decreases by 1.13 % per year). In the 1990s, using more precise methods, Castelo-Branco et al. [3] corroborated these initial data and its relation with bone mineral density.

25.3 Function Alterations

Marked loss of elasticity that occurs with aging skin is a well-known fact. This is one of the parameters that best correlate with chronological age. Additionally, older people are less prone to skin sensitization and have fewer contact allergies. This fact may be due to a decrease in the number of immunity cells. Besides, older humans sweat less and require a longer period of time to achieve thermal stimulation of the sweat glands. Additionally, there are fewer active glands, with lower secretion. In postmenopausal women, the production of the sebaceous glands is about half that of the previously observed and two times lower than that of men of the same age, but their ability to respond to hormonal stimuli and androgens increases twofold their production.

25.4 Aging, Menopause, and Changes in the Skin and Appendages

The skin undergoes regressive changes with age, although the intensity of these changes varies according to the genetic and environmental factors. In addition, studies with light and electron microscopy have corroborated that there is some hormonal dependence in the composition and preservation of the skin. For example, the impact of thyroid disorders on the skin and appendages is well known. And it has also shown some evolutionary changes related to aging skin with steroid hormones, especially in women as a result of the cessation of ovarian function.

25.5 Estrogen and Skin

Postmenopausal estrogenic deficiency has an intense influence on the skin [8], and, in fact, Black et al. in 1975 showed that skin fibroblasts express estrogen and androgen receptors. Skin, therefore, constitutes a larger female reproductive organ, on which presumably estrogen must have an overt action [9]. Fat and subcutaneous tissues present a significant aromatase activity, which can convert intracellularly estrone and weak androgens to estradiol. The predominant estrogenic receptor in the skin is the beta [10] (reaching high prevalence in the hair follicle) and limited receptor alpha in dermal papilla cells. In sebaceous glands, alpha- and beta-receptors are expressed in similar proportion.

Regarding the action of estrogens on the skin, various in vitro studies have shown that physiological concentrations stimulate the proliferation of keratinocytes and dermal fibroblasts and reduce the activity of matrix metalloproteinase

Table 25.1 Aspects of the skin and appendages influenced by estrogen directly or indirectly

Thickness and degree of hydration of the epidermis	Dunn et al. (1997) [13]
Composition and production of sphingolipids	Lucki and Sewer (2010) [53]
Content of glycosaminoglycans	Stevenson and Thornton (2007) [54]
Number and type of collagen in the skin	Brincat et al. (1983) [51]
Wrinkles	Castelo-Branco et al. (1998) [48]
Laxity	Castelo-Branco et al. (1998) [48]
Activity of sebaceous glands	Bensaleh et al. (2006) [50]
Synchronicity and hair follicle activity	Dao Jr. et al. (2007) [52]
Training and nail quality?	Haenggi et al. (1995) [16]
Scarring of wounds?	Gilliver et al. (2010) [49]

[11]. This activity is involved to some extent in some of the changes that occur in aging. All of the above justifies the hypothesis that includes the skin between the organs that could undergo rapid deterioration. In this sense, Shuster and Black [12] and Castelo-Branco et al. [3, 5] described the curve of skin collagen content, which resembles the curve of evolution of bone mineral density in women suggesting an acceleration in the loss during climacteric. Some studies have shown that such acceleration does not occur if a woman uses HRT5, and this suggests the possibility of maintaining better skin condition prolonging the life span of estrogenic exposure.

The effects of estrogen deprivation in the skin might include some impact on the apparition of wrinkles, dryness, skin atrophy, and consequences such as increased laxity and/or fragility among others (Table 25.1).

Several studies have reported increases in epidermal thickness with only 3 months of use of HRT in postmenopausal women. And one large study, approximately 4,000 women, found that skin dryness was more frequent among women not using HRT13. Later studies with more sophisticated techniques have confirmed that there indeed is a lesser degree of skin hydration in women without estrogen and that there is a significant improvement with HRT. Some authors have suggested that changes in the composition and proportion of sphingolipids that occur after estrogen deficiency could be part of the mechanism for this reduced hydration. Moreover, this reduced skin hydration as well as aesthetic issues could be related to an impairment of the barrier function of the skin.

Moreover, in the dermis, it has been reported that estrogen deprivation accelerates the reduction of glycosaminoglycan content, which also contributes to dehydration and seems to participate in the onset and progression of wrinkles.

25.5.1 Effects on Nails

The nail is composed of a "dead" corneum product, nail plate, and four specialized epithelia: proximal nail fold, matrix, nail bed, and hyponychium.

Nail system is affected during aging: The size of keratinocytes in the nail plate increases, the skin in the nail bed thickens, and elasticity and the number of blood vessels decrease. There are also changes in the chemical composition (Ca and Fe) [14]. Senile nails may appear pale, matte, and opaque, varying in color from white, yellow, black, or gray. Therefore, nail growth decreases by 0.5 % per year from age 25 to 100 years (average growth is 0.1 mm per day in hands and 0.03 mm per day in feet) [15]. One study found that blood flow was reduced up to 30 % in the nail bed in postmenopausal women compared with those who were premenopausal or HRT users [16]. Another study reports that with aging there is a decrease of calcium content in the nails, while magnesium increases [17]. On the other hand, during pregnancy, the nails become brittle and fragile, with cases of onycholysis and leukonychia due to the influence of the hormonal and immune burden [18].

25.5.2 Effects on Pilosebaceous Follicles

Pilosebaceous follicles are formed by the association of sebaceous glands and hair follicles. Isolated sebaceous glands are rare, being located in the oral mucosa, eyelids, nipples, and the female labia. Hair follicles have an intrinsic rhythm alternating regeneration cycles with hair fall cycles. These cycles are called "anagen" (growth), "telogen" (idle), and "catagen" (involution), and its rate can be influenced by hormonal or nutritional factors.

During pregnancy, the proportion of follicles in anagen increase significantly by the effect of higher estrogen concentrations, where as in the postpartum, with the drop in estrogen and changes in growth factors, greater follicle synchronization in fall cycle is observed, being the hair loss clinically detectable. A possible protective effect of estrogen is also indirectly suggested by studies that reported thinner hair and a further decline by the use of tamoxifen [19] and more recently with the use of aromatase inhibitors.

Typically, the secretion of sebaceous glands increases in pregnant women by the action of estrogen and growth factors [18]. Besides, in hyperandrogenic states, hormones have also significant impact on these glands, especially related to the amount and composition of phospholipids. Estrogens increase production of the sebaceous glands, and androgens increase this production in excess causing undesirable states (acne, hirsutism, etc.).

25.5.3 Effects on Eccrine Sweat Glands and Apocrine Glands

The eccrine sweat is a physiological mechanism for regulating body temperature. Eccrine secretion contains water, electrolytes, metals, organic compounds, and macromolecules. Without sweating hyperthermia, exhaustion, heat stroke, and death might occur.

These glands are numerous in soles of the feet, hands, armpits, and forehead and less on the back. It is known that the control and regulation of these glands are by the sympathetic nervous system, which releases acetylcholine. However, there are data showing a modulating effect by sex hormones. Estrogens have the ability to increase potassium conductance in eccrine sweat gland cells by opening K/Ca channels [20]. In addition, estradiol 17-beta may control the intracellular calcium concentration [21], controlling the release of intracellular calcium stores. Several studies have found that during pregnancy there is an overactivity of the eccrine glands in different locations of the body except the hands [18].

The apocrine glands are located mainly in the armpits and perineum. Its activity begins shortly before puberty, and thus its development is believed to be associated with hormonal changes that occur during this period. There is controversy over whether or not the activity in these glands decreases during pregnancy.

25.6 Physiology of Aging

The changes that occur in the skin as a consequence of time define aging skin (Table 25.2).

The biological clock affects both the skin and internal organs in an identical way. However, there are numerous cosmetic techniques to improve the aging aspect, even only in the external component [22].

There are several theories to explain aging; some of them are based on genetic factors limiting the ability of cell proliferation. Other theories are based on the influence of external environmental agents such as exposure to wind, ultraviolet radiation, sun, heat or pollution, toxic habits

Table 25.2 Skin functions that are altered with aging

Decrease of cell turnover	Donofrio (2000) [30]
Decreased barrier function	Breverman and Fonferko (1982) [37]
Decreased elimination of degradation chemical products	Yaar et al. (2003) [23]
Decreased sensory perception	Farage et al. (2009) [22]
Decreased mechanical protection	Breverman and Fonferko (1982) [37]
Delayed wound healing	Frippiat et al. (2001) [34]
Decreased sweat production, tallow, and vitamin D	Farage et al. (2009) [22]
Alteration of DNA repair	Allsopp et al. (1992) [24]
Alteration in the immune response	Arlt and Hewison (2004) [29]
Decreased hormone levels	Phillips et al. (2001) [28]
Alteration in the function of thermoregulation	Holowatz et al. (2010) [55]

(smoking or drinking), sleep disorders, deficient nutrition, and muscle movements [23].

The programmatic theory is based on telomere shortening [24]. Telomeres are the terminal portions of the chromosomes that protect the genic data. During cell mitosis, DNA polymerase is unable to replicate all the terminal base pairs of each chromosome, which defines a progressive shortening with each cell division cycle. Telomerase reverse transcriptase has the ability to replicate these chromosomal ends. The number of telomerases shortens up to 30 % when a person ages, and this leads to DNA instability and interruption of cell cycle or apoptosis.

The reduced ability of cell division is called cell senescence; some authors believe that during the evolution of multicellular organisms, this phenomenon acts as a cancer-preventive mechanism. The aged cells present very short telomeres with irreversible disruption of growth, resistance to apoptosis, and altered cell differentiation. Genes in senescence, involved in the G1 phase and aging cells, lose the ability to induce the genes necessary for advancing the G1 phase of the cell cycle, including c-Fos and certain transcription factors [25]. Other senescence-associated genes that are overexpressed encode various protein products, such as fibronectin and proteases (collagenase and stromelysin) that are involved in the regulation of matrix in the skin structure. This fact and the decreased level of tissue inhibitors of metalloproteinase induce the weakness of skin matrix [26].

During aging, there are decreased secretion and production of several hormones. The best known are estrogen, testosterone, dehydroepiandrosterone (DHEA), and its sulfate (DHEAS) [27, 28]. Other hormones like melatonin, insulin, cortisol, thyroxin, and growth hormone production also decrease with age [29]. Additionally, many cytokines alter its functionality with the decrease of receptor number and increasing senescence of different cells such as fibroblasts. All these changes induce gradually aberrant cellular response to environmental factors that ends in cell death [30].

On the other hand, the stochastic theory is based on the assumption that oxygen consumption is related to aging [31]. Oxygen, although necessary for life, may cause harmful effects such as peroxidation of fatty acid in cell membranes, changes in bases of single-stranded DNA, chromatin change, breaks of DNA, cross-links between DNA proteins, modifications of the carboxyl, and loss of sulfhydryl groups leading to enzyme inactivation and increased proteolysis. Since the efficiency of the antioxidant defense systems is not absolute, in the course of life, cells accumulate molecular oxidative injury that sometimes leads to apoptotic cell death. The immune system plays two special functions: defense against external aggression and internal immune surveillance. With aging, functional B and T lymphocytes alter their activity, and Langerhans cells decrease in number and with associate impaired immune response. These changes contribute to the increased incidence of infections and malignancies in the elderly [32].

25.7 Aging Pathophysiology

The skin aging process involves two pathophysiologic routes: intrinsic aging caused by the decrease in the metabolic functions of the cells due to the time elapsed since birth and the extrinsic aging that is caused by factors out of the subject, i.e., chronic exposure to ultraviolet radiation and pollution (Table 25.3). The most widely accepted theory is that aging is a combination of both during the course of a lifetime.

25.8 Intrinsic Factors

Intrinsic aging affects all skin layers and all structures included in the skin as glands, vessels, nerves, and its different cells. To these changes, alterations caused by hormonal decline are summed. The sum of both will trigger not only aging but also precancerous and tumor cells. In Table 25.4 are summarized the different changes observed with aging in the skin structure.

25.8.1 Epidermis

A flattening of the dermo-epidermal junction with effacement of the dermal papillae and ridge

Table 25.3 Classification of Glogau photoaging

Type 1: age 20–30 years
  Slight changes in photoaging
  Few changes in pigmentation
  No actinic keratoses
  No wrinkles or are minimal
Type 2: age 30–40 years
  Moderate photoaging
  Incipient senile lentigines
  Actinic keratoses palpable but not visible
  Following parallel wrinkles mouth corner
Type 3: age 50–60 years
  Photoaging important
  Dyschromias evident
  Keratosis visible
  Stable wrinkles on the forehead and perioral areas periorbicular
Type 4: age 60 years or more
  Severe photoaging
  Grayish-yellow skin
  Keratosis becoming carcinomas
  Normal skin thickened fibrous
  Total wrinkles around the facial region

Table 25.4 Changes in skin structure with aging

Dermis	Epidermis	Appendages
Hair flat dermal	Atrophy	Depigmented hair
Variable thickness	Fewer fibroblasts	Hair loss
Cells of variable size and shape	Fewer mast	Conversion of terminal hair to fuzz
Occasional nuclear atypia	Fewer vessels	Abnormal nails
Fewer melanocytes	Decreased capillary loops	Fewer glands
Fewer Langerhans cells	Abnormal nerve endings	

interpapillae is observed [33]. In addition, a reduction close to the 50 % in the number of interdigitations is detected from the third to the ninth decade. Consequently, there is a smaller contact area between epidermis and dermis causing increased susceptibility to superficial abrasions and blisters after minimal trauma. In addition, aging is associated with a greater variability in thickness of the epidermis and with an increased size of the corneocytes [34]. The shape of the skin surface is lost with age, and the absorption of hydrophilic substances such as hydrocortisone or benzoic acid is impaired; however, the absorption of hydrophobic substances such as testosterone or estradiol remains unaltered. With aging, the recovery of the barrier function of the stratum corneum is also impaired due to a decrease in the amount of lipids in the lamellar bodies neoformed.

In old age, the skin tends to be dry and crumbly, especially in the lower limbs, which shows a significant decrease in keratin filaments and microfibrils causing an increase of peeling as occurs in ichthyosis vulgaris.

Another function of the epidermis is the production of vitamin D. In the elderly, there is a decrease of production, which added to lower dairy intake, insufficient sun exposure, and sunscreen use causes a decrease in the epidermal level of 7-dehydrocholesterol [22].

25.8.2 Dermis

In the elderly, the decrease in dermal thickness is close to 20 %; although extreme thinning in sun protected areas occurs only after the eighth decade. At these ages, the skin is relatively acellular and avascular. Elastic fibers are lost and wrinkles appear. The number of mast cells is reduced by 50 % with a decreased production of histamine and inflammatory response following exposure to UV radiation. There is thickening of the vascular wall in the microvasculature with reduced perivascular membrane cells that contributes to the brittleness of the vessels.

The loss of vessels, especially the capillary loops in the papillary dermis, causes pallor, decreased temperature, and reduction of cutaneous flow up to 60 %. The reduction of vessels around the hair follicle and glands (eccrine, apocrine, sebaceous) contributes to the progressive atrophy and fibrosis of all these structures. The lower vascular activity also predisposes to poorer control of thermoregulation, which added to the reduction of body fat that promotes heat stroke or hypothermia.

The decrease in number and diameter of elastic fibers begins at 30, and in the elderly people these fibers are often fragmented and associated with small gaps and cysts in the dermo-epidermal junction.

In general, the dermis with aging becomes progressively stiffer, lacks its elasticity, and gradually loses its ability to experience changes in response to stress [35–37].

25.8.3 Changes in Hair

In the fifth decade, half of the population presents 50 % of gray hair, and 100 % have some gray due to the loss of melanocytes in the hair follicle. Further more advanced age is accompanied by a reduction in the amount of hair follicles, partly due to atrophy and fibrosis, and an increase in the proportion of hair follicles (telogen). Baldness is caused by the androgen-dependent conversion of thick and dark terminal hairs in fuzzy, thin, short, and depigmented hairs similar to those present on the forearm [38]. The receding bitemporal hairline begins during adolescence in most women and virtually all men. The hair loss rate and the magnitude of this process vary largely and depend on hereditary factors that at present are unknown. Among women, baldness is a phenomenon less frequent and severe than in men because estrogen prolongs the growth phase (anagen) of the hair cycle. In postmenopausal women, hair loss may be due to a decrease in estrogen levels as well as to a diminished estrogen/androgen ratio. Over 50 % of women at age of 50 have some degree of diffuse alopecia, and over 60 up to 50 % of women have some degree of facial hirsutism.

25.8.4 Cutaneous Nerves and Glands

In the elderly, the amount of eccrine glands decreases around 15 % in most regions of the body. The reduction of spontaneous sweating in response to dry heat is even higher (>70 % compared to young individuals). This fact seems to be related to a decrease in excretion of each single gland. This phenomenon predisposes to heat stroke in older people.

A decrease in size and function of the apocrine glands is also observed in the elderly; the size and number of sebaceous glands do not change with age. The reduction of sebum production by 23 % per decade after 20th in both men and women is due to the simultaneous reduction of gonadal and adrenal androgen production with aging. The clinical burden of this reduction in sebum is unknown and seems to be unrelated to xerosis or seborrheic dermatitis.

The density of Pacini and Meissner corpuscles gradually decreases to about one-third of the initial value between the second and ninth decade and present variations in structure and size [23]. Merkel discs and free nerve endings presented minor changes associated with aging. The decline in the sense perception linked to these changes includes touch, vibratory and corneal sensitivity, the ability to discriminate between two points, and spatial acuteness. The threshold for cutaneous pain perception increases in 20 % in the elderly. All these changes promote the development of traumatic and irritating injuries in older skin.

25.9 Extrinsic Factors

25.9.1 Sun Exposure

One of the most typical lesions of sun-damaged skin is the elastoses (see Figs. 25.4 and 25.6). This process is characterized by the presence of tangled masses of degraded elastic fibers that ends in an amorphous mass. Moreover, in damaged areas by sun, an increase in ground substance and a decrease in the collagen content are observed. An increase in metalloproteinase activity and in the cytokine release may explain these changes. Unlike older skin protected from the sun where hypocellularity is common, in sun-damaged skin the presence of inflammatory cells, including mast cells, histiocytes, and other mononuclear cells, is frequent. In addition, the number of fibroblasts in photodamaged skin is greater than in older skin protected by the sun.

Sun-damaged skin is associated with acanthosis, skin atrophy with the loss of cell polarity and the presence of atypical cells, and reduced number and function of Langerhans cells.

Extrinsic aging develops due to several factors: ionizing radiation, severe physical and psychological stress, alcohol, malnutrition, obesity, and pollution and UV exposure. Of them, UV radiation is the largest contributor to aging.

25.9.2 Tobacco

Another environmental factor that significantly contributes to premature skin aging is the tobacco consumption. The smoker's face and body skin are typical with increased facial wrinkles and ashen-gray look of the skin. Both smoking and UV radiation cause thickening and fragmentation of elastic fibers producing a yellow and thickened skin (elastoses). But while sun elastosis affects mainly the papillary dermis, in the smoker it affects both the papillary and the reticular dermis. Smoke increases the activity of neutrophil elastase, induces dermal chronic ischemia, decreases the levels of vitamin A, increases redox reactions, and reduces the ability to counteract free oxygen radicals and therefore to reverse the DNA lesions [39, 40]. Likewise, smoking induces the activation of MMPs (metalloproteinases) and reduces the hydration of the stratum corneum and accelerates the hydroxylation of estradiol which determines a reduction in the level of estrogen which would increase skin atrophy.

25.9.3 Free Radicals

Free radicals are one of the key factors for understanding the human aging. Within the organism, they are generated intra- or extracellularly [41]. Among the extracellular causes is included the effect of the oxygen on the UV radiation, x-rays, ultrasound, ionizing radiation, photosensitive molecules, tobacco, chemical toxins, and the oxidase system in the macrophage membrane. On the other hand, intracellular free radicals are produced by photochemical reaction from enzymes (i.e., xanthine oxidase) and complexes containing metals such as iron and copper. The human body has mechanisms to neutralize these substances, but under certain conditions an imbalance between production and neutralization may occur [42]. In these circumstances, free radicals acting on physiological pathways induce alterations in telomeres that set the internal clock of human metabolism for chronological aging. Free radicals alter and cause a loss of functional activity in all skin and body structures. They act on carbohydrates, lipids, and proteins; in cellular structures (DNA and lysosomal membrane); and directly on the skin cells: keratinocytes, melanocytes, and fibroblasts.

25.10 Skin Diseases and Aging

Usually, skin diseases are classified according to clinical characteristics (erythema, blistering, coloring, etc.) or in terms of etiology (infectious, genetic, immunological, etc.). However, skin diseases can also be considered according to the period of life in which it most frequently occurs (i.e., pemphigoid increases its incidence gradually since 50). Additionally, some diseases having not a specific age of debut (i.e., psoriasis, Fig. 25.1) may present distinctive characteristics that require specific management in the elderly, and others like neurofibromatosis type I that are

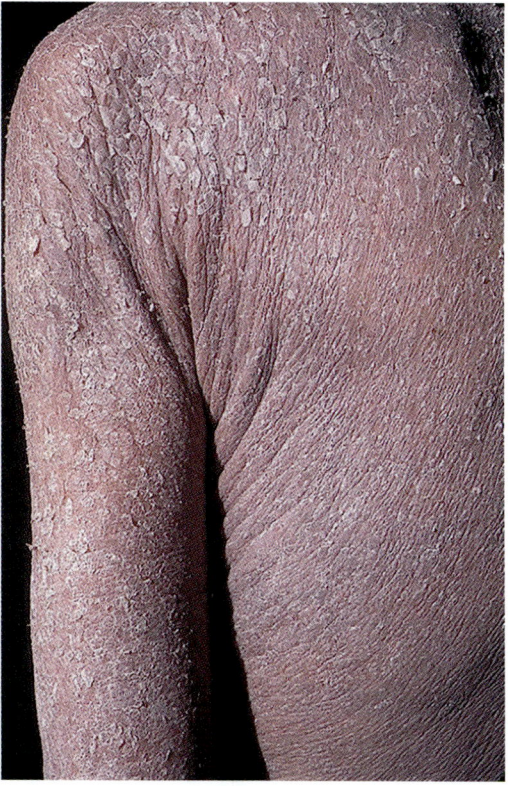

Fig. 25.1 Psoriatic erythroderma

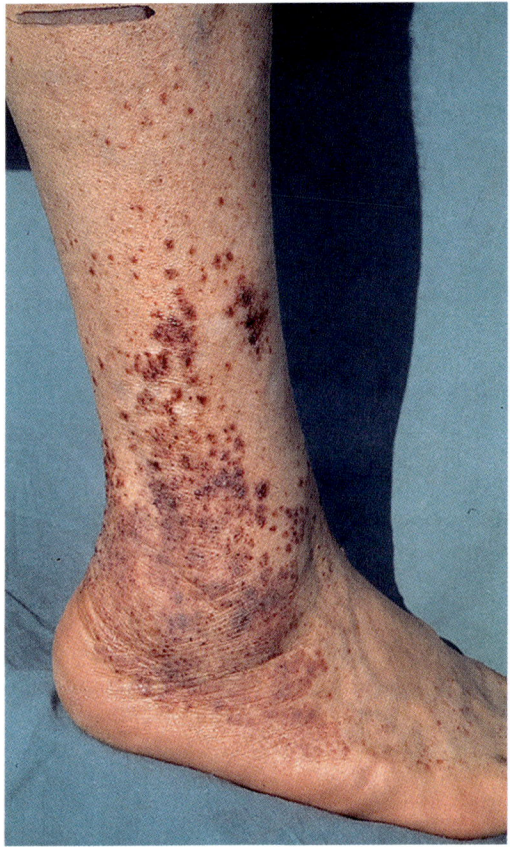

Fig. 25.2 Skin ulcer and vasculitis

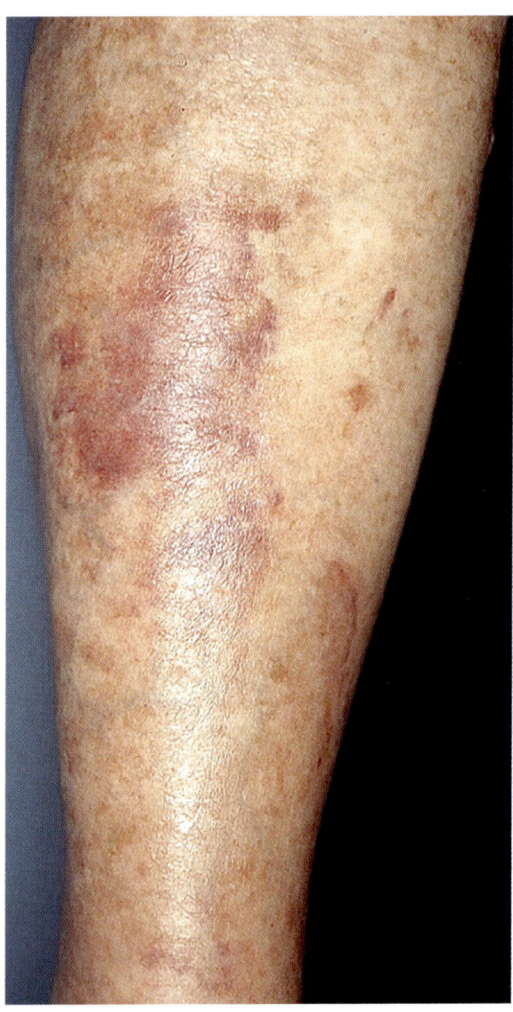

Fig. 25.3 Multiform erythema

present throughout life magnify its manifestations or present new ones.

The reduced ability to respond to inflammation in the aging skin facilitates conditions such as postherpetic neuralgia. Drug intake increases with age, and many adverse events are manifested in the skin; therefore, health-care providers should pay attention to those skin disorders that appear in the elderly in relation to systemic diseases or its treatments, i.e., skin ulcers resulting from vascular insufficiency (Fig. 25.2) or drug reactions such as erythema multiforme (Fig. 25.3). However, the typical skin diseases in aged humans are skin tumors, both benign and malignant due to the immune senescence and the burden of the effects of external agents such as sun, tobacco, or pollution. Multiple actinic keratosis is one of the most representative conditions (Fig. 25.4).

In summary, the years elapsed since birth modify the signs, symptoms, and type of skin diseases. In people over 65 years old, consultations to dermatologist increase by 60 % [43] being the main concerns itching, asteatosis, eczema, pemphigoid, herpes zoster, seborrheic and actinic keratosis, basal and squamous cell carcinoma (Figs. 25.4 and 25.5), and lentigo maligna [44]. Other authors include rosacea and elastoses (Fig. 25.6) to this list [45]. The physiological changes in skin structure and function, with impaired skin barrier, allow the progress of chronic infections (i.e., fungal), irritant dermatitis (i.e., eczema), and pressure ulcers. On the other hand, environmental influences (UV radia-

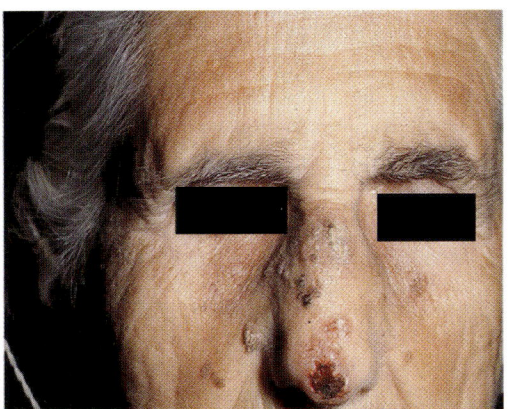

Fig. 25.4 Multiple actinic keratoses and basocellular carcinoma on the nose. The subject also presents with senile elastoses

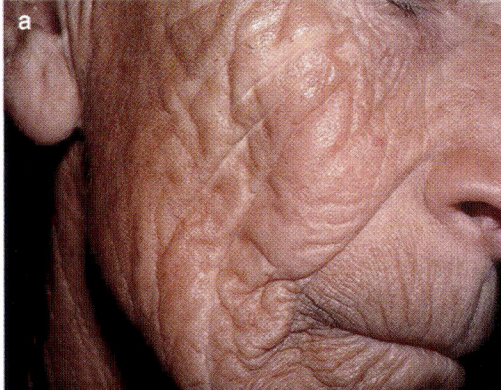

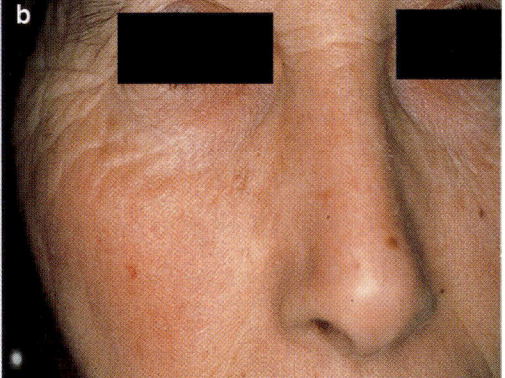

Fig. 25.6 Senile skin with sun elastoses

tion, tobacco, etc.) accumulate its burden over the time promoting cellular alterations that can lead to the appearance of tumors.

25.11 Psychological Impact

Skin diseases of aging affect individuals at the final stages of life when some of them have lost many psychological stimuli yet. On the other hand, to be healthy is strongly related to quality of life. The coincidence of disease and aging has a very high psychic and psychological impact. The implementation of health-related quality-of-life scales in clinical practice might improve this condition [46] since the detection of the psychological impact degree is the first step to individualize the approach to each patient [47].

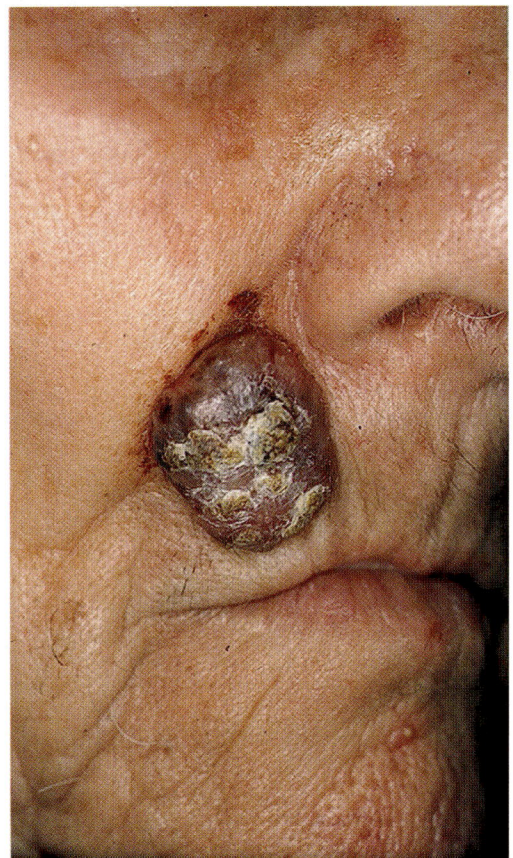

Fig. 25.5 Basocellular carcinoma

References

1. Lovell CR, Smolensky KA, Duance VC, Light ND, Young S, Dyson M. Type I and III collagen content and fibre distribution in normal human skin during ageing. Br J Dermatol. 1987;117:419–28.
2. Brincat M, Kabalan S, Studd JW, Moniz CF, de Trafford J, Montgomery J. Study of the decrease of skin collagen content, skin thickness, and bone mass in the postmenopausal women. Obstet Gynecol. 1987;70:840–5.
3. Castelo-Branco C, Pons F, Gratacos E, Fortuny A, Vanrell JA, González-Merlo J. Relationship between skin collagen and bone changes during aging. Maturitas. 1994;18:199–206.
4. Kohn RR, Schnider SL. Collagen changes in aging skin. New York: Raven Press; 1989. p. 121–42.
5. Castelo-Branco C, Duran M, Gonzales-Merlo J. Skin collagen changes related to age and hormone replacement therapy. Maturitas. 1992;15:113–9.
6. Shuster S, Black MM. The influence of age and sex on skin thickness, skin collagen and density. Br J Dermatol. 1975;93:639–43.
7. Hall DA. The ageing of connective tissue. London: Academic; 1976.
8. Brincat M, Moniz CJ, Studd JW, Darby A, Darby A, Magos A, Emburey G, et al. Long-term effects of the menopause and sex hormones on skin thickness. Br J Obstet Gynaecol. 1985;92(3):256–9.
9. Hall G, Phillps TJ. Estrogen and skin: the effects of estrogen, menopause, and hormone replacement therapy on the skin. J Am Acad Dermatol. 2005;53(4): 55–568; quiz 569–72.
10. Thornton MJ, Taylor AH, Mulligan K, Al-Azzawi F, Lyon CC, O'Driscoll J, et al. The distribution of estrogen receptor beta is distinct to the androgen receptor alpha and the androgen receptor in human skin and the pilosebaceous unit. J Invest Dermatol Symp Proc. 2003;8(1):100–3.
11. Moalli PA, Klingensmith WL, Meyn LA, Zyczynski HM. Regulation of matrix metalloproteinase expression by estrogen in fibroblasts that are derived from the pelvic floor. Am J Obstet Gynecol. 2002;187(1):72–9.
12. Shuster S, Black MM, McVitie E. The influence of age and sex on skin thickness, skin collagen and density. Br J Dermatol. 1975;93(6):639–43.
13. Dunn LB, Damesyn M, Moore AA, Reuben DB, Greendale GA. Does estrogen prevent skin aging? Results from the First National Health and Nutrition Examination Survey (NHANES I). Arch Dermatol. 1997;133(3):339–42.
14. Singh G, Haneef NS, Uday A. Nails changes and disorders among the elderly. Indian J Dermatol Venerol Leprol. 2005;71:386–92.
15. Cohen PR, Scher RK. Nail changes in the elderly. J Geriatric Dermatol. 1993;1:45–53.
16. Haenggi W, Linder HR, Birkhaeuser MH, Scheider H. Microscopic findings of the nail-fold capillaries-dependence on menopausal status and hormone replacement therapy. Maturitas. 1995;22(1):37–46.
17. Ohgitani S, Fujita T, Fujii Y, Hayashi C, Nishio H. Nail calcium content in relation to age and bone mineral density. Clin Calcium. 2008;18(7):959–66.
18. Muallem MM, Rubeiz NG. Physiological and biological skin changes in pregnancy. Clin Dermatol. 2006;24:80–3.
19. Gateley CA, Bundred NJ. Alopecia and breast disease. BMJ. 1997;314(7079):481.
20. Muchekehu RW, Harvey BJ. Estradiol rapidly induces the translocation and activation of the intermediate conductance calcium activated potassium channel in human eccrine sweat gland cells. Steroids. 2009;74(2):212–7. Epub 2008 Nov 5.
21. Muchekehu RW, Harvey BJ. A 17 beta-estradiol rapidly mobilizes intracellular calcium from ryanodine-receptor-gated stores via a PKC – PKA. Cell Calcium. 2008;44(3):276–88. Epub 2008 Jan 22.
22. Farage MA, Miller KW, Berardesca E, Maibach HI. Clinical implications of aging skin: cutaneous disorders in the elderly. Am J Clin Dermatol. 2009;10:73–86.
23. Yaar M, Gilchrest BA, Freedberg IM, Eisen AZ, Wolf K, Austen KF. Dermatology in general medicine, vol. 2. New York: McGraw-Hill; 2003. p. 1386–98.
24. Allsopp RC, Vaziri H, Patterson C, Goldstein S, Younglai EV, Futcher AB, et al. Telomere length predicts replicative capacity of human fibroblasts. Proc Natl Acad Sci U S A. 1992;89:10114–8.
25. Fischer GJ, Talwar HS, Lin J, Lin P, Mcphillips F, Wang Z, et al. Retinoic acid inhibits induction of c-jun protein by ultraviolet radiation that occurs subsequent to activation of mitogen-activated protein kinase pathways in human skin in vivo. J Clin Investig. 1998;101:1432–40.
26. Lahman C, Bergemann IM, Harrison G, Young A. Matrix metalloproteinase and skin aging in smokers. Lancet. 2001;357:935–6.
27. Bolognia JL, Braverman IM, Rousseau ME, Sarrel PM. Skin changes in menopause. Maturitas. 1989;11: 295–304.
28. Phillips TJ, Demircay Z, Sahu M. Hormonal effects on skin aging. Clin Geriatr Med. 2001;17:661–72.
29. Arlt W, Hewison M. Hormones and immune function: implications of aging. Aging Cell. 2004;3:209–16.
30. Donofrio LM. Fat distribution: a morphologic study of the aging face. Dermatol Surg. 2000;26:1107–12.
31. Wenk J, Brenneisen P, Meewes C, Wlaschek M, Peters T, Blaudschun R, et al. UV-induced oxidative stress and photoaging. Curr Probl Dermatol. 2001;29: 83–94.
32. Dewbery C, Norman RA. Skin cancer in elderly patients. Dermatol Clin. 2004;22:93–6.
33. Lavker RM, Zheng PS, Dong G. Aged skin: a study by light, transmission electron, and scanning electron microscopy. J Invest Dermatol. 1987;88:44s–51.
34. Frippiat C, Chen QM, Zdanov S, Magalhaes JP, Magalhaes JP, Remacle J, Toussaint O. Subcytotoxic H_2O_2 stress triggers a release of transforming growth factor-beta. J Biol Chem. 2001;276:2531–7.
35. Swift ME, Burns AL, Gray KL, Di Pietro LA. Age-related alterations in inflammatory response to dermal injury. J Invest Dermatol. 2001;117:1027–35.

36. Yasui T, Takahashi Y, Fukushima S, Ogura Y, Yamashita T, Kuwahara T, et al. Observation of dermal collagen fibres in wrinkled skin using polarization-resolved second harmonic-generation microscopy. T Opt Express. 2009;17:912–23.
37. Breverman IM, Fonferko E. Studies in cutaneous aging I. The elastic fibre network. J Invest Dermatol. 1982;78:434–43.
38. Tobin DJ, Paus R. Graying: geronobiology of the hair follicle pigmentary unit. Exp Gerontol. 2001;36:29–54.
39. Berneburg M, Plettenberg H, Krutmann J. Photoaging of human skin. Photodermatol Photoimmunol Photomed. 2000;16:239–44.
40. Smith JB, Fenske NA. Cutaneous manifestations and consequence of smoking. J Am Acad Dermatol. 1996;34:717–32.
41. O'Hare PM, Fleisher Jr AB, D'Agostino Jr RB, Feldman SR, Hinds MA, Rassette SA, et al. Tobacco smoking contributes little to facial wrinkling. J Eur Acad Dermatol Venereol. 1999;12:133–9.
42. Gniadecka M, Wulf HC, Mortensen NN, Poulsen T. A quantitative assessment of the role of stratum corneum viable epidermis and pigmentation. Acta Derm Venereol. 1996;76:429–32.
43. Kurban RS, Kurban AK. Common skin disorders of aging: diagnosis and treatment. Geriatrics. 1993;48(4):30–1, 5–6, 9–42.
44. Shelley WB, Shelley ED. The ten major problems of aging skin. Geriatrics. 1982;37(9):107–13.
45. Beacham BE. Common dermatoses in the elderly. Am Fam Physician. 1993;47(6):1445–50.
46. Guerra Tapia A, Gonzales Guerra E. Quality of life related to health. In: Guerra Tapia A, editor. Quality of life in dermatology. Madrid: Editorial SANED. 2007; 1:1–3.
47. Guerra Tapia A, Gonzales Guerra E. Quality of life in dermatology. Measurement systems. In: Guerra Tapia A, editor. Psychiatric dermatology: skin of the mind. Editorial Glosa SL. ISBN: 978-84-7429-398-2. Barcelona: 2009; 13–34.
48. Castelo-Branco C, Figueras F, Martinez de Osaba MJ, Vanrell JA. Facial wrinkling in post-menopausal women. Effects of smoking status and hormone replacement therapy. Maturitas. 1998;29(1):75–86.
49. Gilliver SC, Emmerson E, Campbell L, Chambon P, Hardman MJ, Ashcroft GS. 17beta-estradiol inhibits wound healing in male mice via estrogen receptor-alpha. Am J Pathol. 2010;176(6):2707–21.
50. Bensaleh H, Belgnaoui FZ, Douira L, Berbiche L, Senouci K, Hassam B. Skin and menopause. Ann Endocrinol (Paris). 2006;67(6):575–80.
51. Brincat M, Moniz F, Studd JWW, Darby A, Darby AJ, Magos A, Cooper D. Sex hormones and skin collagen content in postmenopausal women. Br Med J. 1983; 287:1337–8.
52. Dao Jr H, Kazin RA. Gender differences in skin: a review of the literature. Gend Med. 2007;4(4):308–28.
53. Lucki NC, Sewer MB. The interplay between bioactive sphingolipids and steroid hormones. Steroids. 2010;75(6):390–9.
54. Stevenson S, Thornton J. Effect of estrogens on skin aging and the potential role of SERMs. Clin Interv Aging. 2007;2(3):283–97.
55. Holowatz LA, Thompson-Torgerson C, Kenney WL. Aging and the control of human skin blood flow. Front Biosci. 2010;15:718–39.

Autoimmune Skin Diseases: Role of Sex Hormones, Vitamin D, and Menopause

26

DeLisa Fairweather

Contents

26.1	Introduction	359
26.2	Sex Differences in the Immune Response	360
26.3	Effect of Menopause on Inflammation	361
26.4	Immune Cells in the Skin	362
26.5	Vitamin D and Skin Inflammation	364
26.6	Vitamin D Deficiency and Rheumatic Autoimmune Disease	365
26.7	Vitamin D Deficiency and Menopause	366
26.8	Skin Manifestations in Rheumatic Autoimmune Diseases	366
26.8.1	Systemic Lupus Erythematosus	366
26.8.2	Rheumatoid Arthritis	367
26.8.3	Sjögren's Syndrome	367
26.8.4	Dermatomyositis	367
26.8.5	Scleroderma	368
26.9	Rheumatic Autoimmune Diseases That Occur Before Menopause	368
26.9.1	Menopause and SLE	368
26.9.2	Menopause and Scleroderma	369
26.10	Rheumatic Autoimmune Diseases That Occur After Menopause	369
26.10.1	Menopause and Rheumatoid Arthritis	369
26.10.2	Menopause and Sjögren's Syndrome	370
26.11	Summary and Future Directions	371
References		373

D. Fairweather, PhD
Department of Environmental Health Sciences,
Johns Hopkins Bloomberg School of Public Health,
615 N. Wolfe Street, Baltimore, MD 21205, USA
e-mail: dfairwea@jhsph.edu

26.1 Introduction

Autoimmune diseases that affect the skin occur predominantly in women and are classified as rheumatic diseases. Autoimmune diseases are the third most common category of disease in the United States after cardiovascular disease and cancer and estimated to affect around 5–8 % of the population [1]. Approximately 80 % of individuals with autoimmune diseases are women [1, 2]. Autoimmune diseases are chronic inflammatory conditions where memory-specific T and B cells and antibodies are directed against self-antigens. Autoimmunity occurs frequently in undiseased individuals, but pathology or overt autoimmune disease only develops when multiple autoantibodies are directed against a target tissue [2, 3]. For this reason, a component of the diagnostic criteria for most autoimmune diseases is based on the presence of particular autoantibodies in the sera. Pathogenic immune complexes (ICs) form when autoantibodies bind self-antigen and activate the complement cascade. Deposition of ICs often damages host tissues by causing direct cytotoxicity to host cells and recruiting inflammation to the damaged site [4, 5].

Historically, rheumatoid factor (RF) has been considered as an autoantibody needed for the formation of ICs [6]. RFs are autoantibodies directed against the Fc portion of IgM or IgG antibodies. The addition of RF to ICs increases their potential for deposition. Roles for RF include enhancing normal immune responses, particularly against infections; promoting complement fixation, antigen presentation, and the avidity of IgG; and improving clearance of ICs by macrophages [7–9]. These roles help clear infections but can also drive autoimmune disease. Several autoimmune diseases have been termed rheumatic diseases because RF autoantibodies are frequently elevated in patients' sera. Rheumatic diseases include systemic lupus erythematosus (SLE), rheumatoid arthritis (RA), (dermato) myositis (DM), Sjögren's syndrome (SS), and scleroderma (Sc) (also called systemic sclerosis). RF occurs in 70–90 % of RA, 60–80 % of SS, 30 % of SLE, 20 % of myositis, and 20 % of systemic sclerosis patients [8, 9]. RF levels have been found to predict the severity of disease in RA and Sjögren's patients suggesting that RF may contribute to the pathogenesis of disease indicating an important role for IC deposition in this process [8, 10]. Rheumatic autoimmune diseases occur more frequently in women; SLE has an incidence of 9:1, Sjögren's syndrome 9:1, systemic sclerosis 4:1, RA 2–3:1, and myositis 2:1 in women versus men [2, 11]. Interestingly, rheumatic diseases have prominent autoimmune skin and/or mucosal manifestations. This chapter will describe our current understanding of the role of sex hormones, vitamin D, and menopause on the development of autoimmune diseases that affect the skin.

26.2 Sex Differences in the Immune Response

An unresolved question is why most autoimmune diseases occur more frequently in women than men. Hashimoto's thyroiditis has an incidence as high as 20:1, Graves' disease 7:1, and autoimmune hepatitis 6:1 in women versus men, for example [2, 11–14]. It is well known that immune responses to antigens differ between men and women. For example, women respond to infection, vaccination, and trauma with increased antibody production [15–18]. Although increased antibody levels protect women from infections, they also increase the risk of developing autoimmune diseases. All researchers agree that estrogen activates B cells resulting in increased levels of antibodies and autoantibodies, while androgens decrease B-cell maturation, reduce B-cell synthesis of antibody, and suppress autoantibody production in humans [19–21]. Microarray and other molecular tools have revealed in recent years how the immune response under normal and pathological conditions is extensively regulated by sex hormones. Sex steroid hormone receptors such as estrogen receptor (ER)-α, ER-β, and androgen receptor are expressed on the cell surface and intracellularly in immune cells. Likewise, cytokine receptors like interleukin (IL)-1 receptor (IL-1R) are found on classic hormone-producing tissues, indicating bidirectional regulation of the immune response [22].

However, studies of sex hormone affects on immune function have been contradictory. In cell culture studies and animal models, estrogen has been shown to induce differentiation of dendritic cells (DCs), stimulate T-cell proliferation, and drive T cells to a T helper (Th) 1 and/or Th17-type adaptive immune response by activating the transcription factor NFκB [5, 19, 23–25]. In other studies, estrogen was found to increase Th2 responses, regulatory T cells (Treg), IL-4-driven alternatively activated M2 macrophages, and the regulatory cytokines IL-4, IL-10, and transforming growth factor (TGF)β [2, 19, 20, 26–33]. These findings are contradictory because Th2 responses transcriptionally downregulate Th1 responses and vice versa. Why in some situations has estrogen been found to increase Th1 responses while in others it increases Th2 responses? One possible explanation lies in the finding that estrogen can inhibit innate Toll-like receptor (TLR) responses thereby reducing interferon (IFN)γ production from macrophages but at the same time increase release of IFN-γ from T cells thereby driving an adaptive Th1 response [2, 6, 21, 28, 30]. Dose may also affect the outcome of estrogen with low doses of estrogen driving Th1 responses and high doses driving Th2 responses [2].

Far less research has been conducted on the effect of androgens on immune cell function, but in general androgens have been found to drive Th1 responses [34–37]. One complication in understanding the role of sex hormones like testosterone on immune cells is that most studies do not interpret data in the context of sex. For example, the sex of cells used in culture experiments is seldom reported [38]. Additionally, effects measured by testosterone may be due to testosterone or estrogen because of aromatase conversion. In support of testosterone increasing Th1 responses and estrogen increasing Th2 responses, we found in a retrospective cohort study of 15,357 adults that more men than women were hospitalized for autoimmune diseases associated with Th1-type pathology, while more women than men had autoimmune diseases associated with a Th2-type response [39]. In particular, Th2-associated rheumatic autoimmune diseases occurred more frequently in women than men (adjusted hazards ratio 2.5, 95 % confidence intervals 1.6–3.9) [39].

Collectively, the data support the idea that estrogen elevates autoantibodies and Th2 responses and promotes fibrosis by stimulating profibrotic IL-4, TGFβ, and fibroblast growth factor, all of which contribute to the increased incidence of autoimmune diseases in women [19, 40, 41].

26.3 Effect of Menopause on Inflammation

Menopause is defined as the final menstrual period without another menstrual period for 12 months [42–44]. The mean age when menopause occurs in Western cultures is between 49 and 52 years [42, 43]. Decreases in estrogen (i.e., estradiol) occur only in the last 6 months before menopause and thereafter [44]. In contrast, testosterone gradually decreases with age in both sexes. There appears to be no period of symptomatic change or "andropause" in men that would be analogous to menopause in women, but instead a steady decline in testosterone levels [45, 46]. After menopause, the primary endogenous source of estrogen is estrone, which is synthesized in adipocytes via aromatase [47]. As in men, testosterone levels decline gradually with age in women [48]. Because autoimmune diseases that affect the skin occur predominantly in women, we will focus on the effect of menopause (rather than andropause) on immune cell function.

Understanding changes in immune function following menopause are complicated by changes that also occur because of aging [49, 50]. Age-related changes in immune function include an impaired ability to respond to new antigens, unsustained memory responses, chronic low-grade inflammation, and an increasing propensity for autoimmune responses [51]. Antibodies and autoantibodies continually increase with age. Additionally, low doses of estrogen are likely to be all that is required to promote B-cell proliferation and autoantibody production past menopause in women (Fig. 26.1). This idea is supported by the finding that hormone replacement therapy (HRT) (lifting estrogen levels to a relatively higher dose) decreases antibody levels in menopausal women [52]. Menopause is also associated with decreases in $CD4^+$ and $CD8^+$ T cells and natural killer (NK) cell activity [47, 53, 54]. Importantly, menopause has been associated with an increase in the cytokines IL-1, IL-6 (IL-1β increases IL-6 levels), and tumor necrosis factor (TNF). These proinflammatory cytokines are associated with driving autoimmune disease in numerous human and animal studies [2]. Importantly, these cytokines are derived mainly from innate immune cells like macrophages and mast cells (MCs). That lower estrogen levels during menopause decrease these cytokines is consistent with the known ability of higher doses of estrogen to downregulate NFκB, Th1 responses, IL-1, and IL-6 via ER-α in various human and murine cell types [55–59]. Thus, during menopause the protective role of estrogen in decreasing innate immune cell activation is lost allowing increased proinflammatory cytokine levels while at the same time autoantibody levels (and ICs) continue to rise (see Fig. 26.1). This type of environment would provide the perfect conditions to promote the development of autoimmune disease. In contrast, in most men androgen levels that promote innate immune cell activation and proinflammatory cytokines are declining past age 50 without the increase in autoantibodies found in women because of estrogen (see Fig. 26.1).

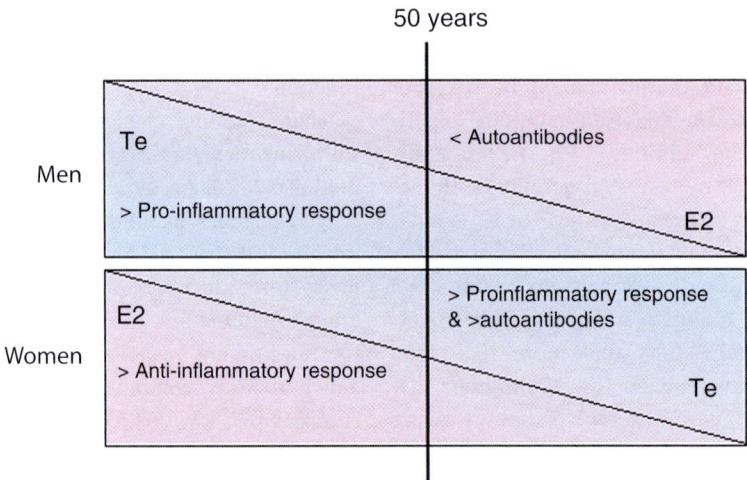

Fig. 26.1 Possible explanation for increased rheumatic autoimmune diseases in women. *Blue* and *pink* represent testosterone (*Te*) and estrogen (*E2*), respectively. As men and women age the estrogen to testosterone ratio alters, with a relatively abrupt decline in estrogen with menopause in women and a gradual decline in testosterone in men. Higher doses of estrogen in premenopausal women promote autoantibody production and fibrosis that lead to SLE and scleroderma. However, lower doses of estrogen after menopause allow continued accumulation of autoantibodies but reduce the protective, anti-inflammatory effects of estrogen, resulting in a proinflammatory immune response that contributes to disease induction in RA, SS, and dermatomyositis. Testosterone in men, regardless of age, reduces autoantibody levels compared to women that protect them from IC-mediated autoimmune diseases

26.4 Immune Cells in the Skin

The skin is the first line of defense against pathogens, toxins, and chemical agents and an important site of immune protection and regulation. The skin was first recognized as an important lymphoid tissue in the 1980s when its link to the lymph system was described as skin-associated lymphoid tissue (SALT) and later as the "skin immune system" [60–62]. Skin has two main layers: the epidermis and the dermis. The epidermis has a number of cells types with immune function including keratinocytes, epidermal DCs called Langerhans cells, γδ T cells known as dendritic epidermal T cells (DETCs), and memory αβ CD8⁺ T cells [62–65]. The epidermis is also where Merkel cells, which communicate with the nervous system, and melanocytes, which provide protection from UV radiation, are found. In contrast, the dermis consists mainly of elastin, collagen fibers, and fibroblasts within an extracellular matrix. Cells with immune function in the epidermis include macrophages, MCs, various DC subtypes, innate lymphoid cells (ILCs), γδ T cells, and αβ T cells [64, 66]. The epidermis is also the site of blood vessels and capillary beds as well as the draining lymphatics.

Keratinocytes not only serve as a protective outer layer of the skin but behave like innate immune cells expressing innate TLRs and Nod-like receptors (NLRs) [62, 64, 67]. They recruit immune cells to the skin by release of chemokines and cytokines like TNF, IL-1α/β, IL-6, IL-18, and IL-33. Interestingly, most of these cytokines are associated with activation of the inflammasome [64, 68]. The inflammasome is an innate immune mechanism of defense within host cells that leads to the production of pro-IL-1β and pro-IL-18 via TLR4 signaling that is activated by caspase-1 resulting in release of active IL-1β and IL-18 from the cell [69]. IL-33 and its receptor ST2 are part of the TLR4/IL-1R signaling family. IL-33 can act synergistically with IL-4 or on its own to induce Th2 responses, while IL-18 (originally named IFN-γ-inducing factor) strongly increases Th1 responses [2, 28, 70]. IL-33 is not only a cytokine but is termed a damage-associated molecular pattern (DAMP) also called an "alarmin" and is released when skin is damaged due to infection, toxins, chemicals, or physical trauma [71]. IL-33 is able to activate skin MCs and type 2 ILCs (Th2-like) via the IL-33R ST2 and to recruit eosinophils to the skin [72]. MCs and ILCs are able to drive immune responses in any direction (i.e., Th1, Th2, Th17) that provides the best protective immune response [64, 66, 73].

Innate lymphoid cells have been identified at many tissues sites, but only recently in the skin [64, 73–76]. ILCs include NK cells, $\gamma\delta$ T cells, as well as a newly defined subtype of ILCs termed ILC1, ILC2, and ILC3, reminiscent of the Th1, Th2, and Th17 classification. ILC1s express the Th1-associated transcription factor Tbet and release IFNγ. This cell population is considered to protect against viral infections where IFNs are needed for viral clearance, and these cells are driven by the classic Th1 cytokine IL-12 or the inflammasome-derived cytokine IL-18. ILC2 include cell types named "nuocytes" and "natural helper cells" and express the Th2-associated transcription factor GATA-3 and produce the Th2 cytokines IL-5, IL-9, and IL-13. ILC2 are promoted by IL-25 and the inflammasome-associated cytokine IL-33 (IL-33 has the closest structural homology to IL-18 and is part of the TLR4/IL-1R signaling family) [72]. ILC2 responses are needed to protect against helminth infections and perform tissue repair but can also promote asthma and tissue scaring/fibrosis. Lastly, ILC3 express the Th17-associated transcription factor RORγt and produce IL-17A, IL-22, and some IFNγ and respond to IL-23 and the inflammasome-derived cytokine IL-1β. This response is important in protecting against bacterial infections and promotes tissue repair but can also lead to fibrosis. Importantly, IL-33 not only increases classic ILC2 and Th2 responses but has also been found to increase Th1 and Th17 responses [72]. This is likely due to ST2 expression on MCs, which are able to promote Th1, Th2, or Th17 responses [66, 72, 77]. MCs are also important in regulating inflammation by responding to vitamin D3 (VitD) (they express the vitamin D receptor) to produce IL-10, a cytokine that downregulates all types of inflammatory responses. They also release TGFβ which can increase Treg populations and drive macrophages to a regulatory myeloid-derived suppressor cell (MDSC) or alternatively activated M2 phenotype [66, 78].

MCs are typically located at sites where the host first encounters pathogens, toxins, and allergens like the skin, respiratory tract, and mucosa (mouth, nose, and bowel) [66, 79]. MCs are able to protect the skin and mucosa from infections of each class of pathogen including viruses, parasites, and bacteria (Th1, Th2, and Th17, respectively) and are specialized to neutralize toxins through the release of detoxifying enzymes [78, 80–84]. MC release of enzymes and profibrotic cytokines like IL-4, TNF, IL-1β, and TGFβ promotes healthy remodeling but can also lead to fibrosis in the skin and other tissue sites [79, 80, 85–87]. MCs are classified as MC_{TC}, MC_T, and MC_C subtypes based on the release of certain proteases. MC_{TC} release tryptase, chymase, carboxypeptidase, and cathepsin G-like proteinase. MC_T cells release only tryptase, while MC_C cells release only chymase and carboxypeptidase but not tryptase [66, 88]. Whereas MC_T cells predominate in the lung and bowel mucosa, MC_{TC} are the main MC type within the skin [66, 88]. Aside from inactivating toxins and promoting remodeling, tryptase and chymase play a role in recruiting inflammation to the skin – in particular, neutrophils, eosinophils, monocyte/macrophages, and T cells. Importantly, chymase is able to cleave pro-IL-1β and pro-IL-18 to their active cytokines without the help of caspase-1 [89, 90]. MCs are resident in the skin but proliferate in response to infection, trauma, and with chronic inflammatory conditions like psoriasis and basal cell carcinoma [66]. MCs also act as antigen presenting cells (APC), along with resident macrophages and DCs; express MHC class I and II, CD80, and CD86; and respond to complement [78, 80]. Skin MCs express a number of receptors that bind antibody including FcϵRI that binds IgE (classic allergy response) and FcγRI and FcγRIIa that bind IgG antibodies and autoantibodies and form ICs [91]. MCs are the key immune cells in the skin that are capable of responding to autoantibodies, which suggests that they may be important in mediating skin-specific autoimmune diseases.

Thus, the most important functions of MCs in promoting autoimmune skin disease include (1) recruiting inflammation to the skin; (2) responding to antibodies, autoantibodies, and ICs; (3) serving as principal cells within the skin involved in TLR4/IL-1R/ST2 signaling and inflammasome activation; and (4) an ability to promote remodeling and fibrosis.

26.5 Vitamin D and Skin Inflammation

Vitamin D is a fat-soluble prohormone that regulates serum calcium levels and bone homeostasis but also functions as a regulator of immune responses and, equally important for this discussion, as a sex steroid. Although most studies examine its role as a regulator of calcium and immune responses, few studies report their findings by sex or interpret their data based on vitamin D as a sex steroid. Most studies also do not emphasize whether women in their studies were pre- or postmenopausal.

Vitamin D is synthesized by keratinocytes in the skin after exposure to the sun (UVB) or from dietary sources and is hydroxylated in the liver by 25-hydroxylase (Cyp2R1) and carried in the bloodstream by vitamin D-binding protein (DBP) to the kidney where it is converted by 25-OH-D-1α-hydroxylase (Cyp27B1) to the active form of vitamin D (i.e., 1α, 25-dihydroxyvitamin D_3), which binds the vitamin D receptor (VDR) [92–94]. VDR is a member of the steroid nuclear receptor superfamily and expressed on the surface of and/or intracellularly in a wide variety of cells including keratinocytes, fibroblasts, and most immune cells [95]. Many tissues not only express the VDR but also express the key enzyme to convert $25(OH)_2D$, the form of vitamin D in the serum, to its active form [96]. This is the form of vitamin D that is used to determine deficiency clinically. Macrophages possess all of the components necessary to import/synthesize cholesterol and convert it to active vitamin D including Cyp2R1 and Cyp27B1, as well as expressing the VDR [97, 98]. Liganded VDR forms a complex with the retinoid X receptor, and this complex has been estimated to regulate around 3 % of the human genome via activation of vitamin D response elements (VDREs) [99]. Many genes that regulate immune function have a VDRE in their promoter, like TNF, for example [97].

Vitamin D via the VDR has important effects on immune cells. In general, vitamin D has been shown in culture studies and animal models to increase Th2 immune responses, IL-10, and Treg and alternatively activate M2 macrophages and TGFβ [97, 100–103]. Additionally, vitamin D is known to mediate protection against infections where it acts on keratinocytes, MCs, macrophages, and DCs to activate innate immune responses. In response to infection, vitamin D upregulates TLR2, TLR4, CD14 (part of TLR4 signaling complex), the inflammasome, IL-1β, TNF, and IFNγ, for example [67, 68, 104–108]. VDRE activation increases many antimicrobial mediators like β-defensin, cathelicidin, and reactive oxygen species. However, the innate responses induced by VDR signaling described here drive Th1 and M1 macrophage responses. This appears contradictory to the ability of vitamin D to upregulate Th2 and regulatory immune responses. Confusion on this topic exists, at least in part, because most studies of vitamin D do not consider their findings in the context of sex. Usually there is no identification of the sex of the cells or animals used to conduct experiments and no interpretation of data taking sex into consideration. Because vitamin D is a sex steroid, sex differences in its effect on immune cells should exist similar to the sex differences observed for estrogens and androgens. A Th2, anti-inflammatory response may be frequently reported for vitamin D because autoimmune diseases that affect mainly women are studied that use female mice. Although few studies examine the issue of sex differences in vitamin D, one study reported that vitamin D administration was only protective in female mice in an animal model of multiple sclerosis, an autoimmune disease that occurs more frequently in women than men [2, 109]. To improve our understanding of the role of vitamin D/VDR on inflammation and autoimmune disease, it is vital that researchers design experiments, analyze data, and report results according to sex. It must also be kept in mind that although many diseases are inhibited by Th2 responses, others like allergy, asthma, and rheumatic autoimmune diseases are promoted by Th2 responses [110, 111].

26.6 Vitamin D Deficiency and Rheumatic Autoimmune Disease

Deficiency in the active form of vitamin D (i.e., $1\alpha,25$-dihydroxyvitamin D_3) is highly prevalent in the United States and worldwide, with roughly 25 % of the population in the United States reported to have inadequate vitamin D levels (<30 ng/mL) while 8 % are at risk for deficiency (Institute of Medicine criterion is <10 ng/mL, but many studies define deficiency as <20 ng/mL) (Table 26.1) [92, 112, 113]. Many but not all epidemiological studies have found an association between low levels of vitamin D and all-cause mortality [114]. Epidemiological studies also provide evidence of a significant association between vitamin D deficiency and an increased risk of autoimmune diseases [115, 116]. However, whether low vitamin D levels cause disease or occur as a result of the disease process is not clear.

Serum vitamin D levels have been found to be deficient or insufficient in patients with SLE [117, 118]. However, SLE patients are recommended to avoid sunlight and use sunscreen, and most SLE occurs in dark-skinned women – factors that can lead to vitamin D deficiency [119, 120]. Additionally, kidney dysfunction is a primary component of SLE [121], a key organ that metabolizes vitamin D to its active form. Administration of active vitamin D to MRL/lpr mice that spontaneously develop a lupus-like disease was found to decrease circulating autoantibodies, proteinuria, and SLE-like skin lesions and improved survival [122, 123], suggesting a relationship between vitamin D levels and the pathogenesis of disease. However, a review of 17 clinical studies found that although vitamin D deficiency is common in SLE, associations between low vitamin D levels and worse disease severity were lacking [118].

Vitamin D deficiency or insufficiency has also been found in RA patients, but in contrast to SLE, lower vitamin D levels are associated with higher disease activity [124, 125]. Additionally, RA patients treated with vitamin D displayed clinical improvement [126], but not all studies agree [118, 127]. Similar to lupus, animal models of RA found that vitamin D administration inhibited disease progression and severity [128, 129]. Psoriasis and psoriatic arthritis are associated with hyperproliferation of keratinocytes, fibrosis, and inflammation involving the skin and joints. Vitamin D supplementation has been used to treat these conditions [118, 130, 131]. Interestingly, a VDR polymorphism has been found that prevents success of vitamin D therapy and is associated with a higher incidence of psoriasis in afflicted individuals [132]. Overall, these data suggest that vitamin D reduces RA and psoriatic arthritis.

What is believed to be an early stage leading to connective tissue disease (CTD) has been termed undifferentiated CTD (UCTD). About 30–40 % of these patients progress to a CTD such as SLE, mixed CTD (MCTD), systemic sclerosis, Sjögren's syndrome, RA, polymyositis/dermatomyositis, and/or systemic vasculitis [127]. One large cohort study examined seasonal variation in vitamin D levels in UCTD patients and found that vitamin D levels fluctuated with seasons but were always lower in UCTD patients than controls, suggesting that vitamin D insufficiency could contribute to the pathogenesis of CTDs [127, 133]. Interestingly, vitamin D insufficiency correlated positively with the probability of developing dermatological symptoms in these patients.

Scleroderma is a chronic autoimmune disease characterized by diffuse skin fibrosis and vasculopathy. Symptoms of scleroderma may occur as part of MCTD. Low circulating vitamin D levels are frequently observed in scleroderma

Table 26.1 Institute of Medicine definition of vitamin D deficiency

Serum 25-hydroxyvitamin D (ng/mL)	Vitamin D status
<12	At risk of deficiency
12–19	At risk of inadequacy
20–50	Sufficient
>50	Possibly harmful

Information obtained from Ross et al. [113]

patients. A number of studies report vitamin D insufficiency in 63–86 % of Sc patients and deficiency in 35–95 % of patients [134–136]. Additionally, patients with vitamin D deficiency have worse disease than those that were vitamin D insufficient, suggesting a role for vitamin D in disease pathogenesis. Dermatologists use the topical form of vitamin D to treat Sc, implicating its importance in reducing disease. TGFβ is a profibrotic cytokine that is believed to be responsible for increasing fibrosis in Sc patients. Vitamin D administered to murine cells has been found to inhibit TGF production [127, 137]. Again, sex of the cells, animals, or patients was not addressed in these studies.

Sjögren's syndrome is characterized by inflammation, dysfunction, and destruction of the exocrine glands, especially the salivary and lacrimal glands, resulting in dry mouth and eyes. However, the lungs, liver, skeletal muscle, and kidneys are often involved [121]. SS can be termed primary SS if it occurs as the only autoimmune disease, but frequently SS is part of an autoimmune disease spectrum and termed secondary SS. Autoimmune diseases that often overlap with SS include SLE, RA, and scleroderma. Several studies found that vitamin D levels are deficient or insufficient in primary SS patients and low levels correlate with disease type and severity [138, 139]. Low vitamin D was found to remain low over a 2-year period of time. Additionally, low vitamin D levels correlated with higher levels of RF in SS patients, suggesting that vitamin D could protect against SS by reducing rheumatoid factor levels (recall that RF helps drive IC formation). Currently there are no data on vitamin D supplementation in SS patients [127]. It is important to point out that low vitamin D in SS patients may be due in part to liver and kidney damage caused by the disease potentially affecting the body's ability to synthesize active vitamin D [121].

26.7 Vitamin D Deficiency and Menopause

Epidemiological data indicate that more than 60 % of postmenopausal women have vitamin D insufficiency and 16 % are vitamin D deficient [127, 140]. With aging dermal and epidermal skin thickness reduces [120]. Consequently, cutaneous vitamin D synthesis decreases with age and following menopause because of smaller stores of the precursor 7-dehydrocholesterol in the skin [141–146]. The elderly may be at additional risk of vitamin D deficiency because of decreased mobility and thereby less sun exposure and potentially due to kidney or liver disease [147].

Thus, it remains unclear whether vitamin D deficiency occurs as a consequence of autoinflammatory damage to the skin and kidney or whether it is caused by low exposure to sunlight (city dwellers and/or geographic location) and the use of sunscreen. What is clear is that vitamin D strongly regulates immune function and particularly immune cells within the skin like MCs, macrophages, and keratinocytes. Even if vitamin D deficiency is caused by autoimmune disease, it could promote disease severity and progression because of its powerful local and systemic effects on inflammation.

26.8 Skin Manifestations in Rheumatic Autoimmune Diseases

26.8.1 Systemic Lupus Erythematosus

The skin represents one of the major organs affected during SLE [148, 149]. Dermatological features of the disease include malar rash and discoid lesions, which form part of the diagnostic criteria for SLE. Twenty percent of all SLE patients present initially with skin manifestations and 50–70 % will eventually develop skin symptoms [150]. Skin manifestations in lupus erythematosus (LE) have been subcategorized as discoid LE (DLE), acute cutaneous LE (ACLE), subacute cutaneous LE (SCLE), and chronic cutaneous LE (CCLE). SCLE occurs most frequently in Caucasian premenopausal women with a mean age at onset of 43 years [149, 151] and so represents an autoimmune disease that usually occurs prior to menopause. SLE also peaks in women around 40 years old, with cutaneous manifestations more common in Caucasian women than men [152]. Most patients with SCLE have only mild systemic disease suggesting a slightly different pathogenesis of disease for SLE versus SCLE.

One of the diagnostic criteria for SLE is photosensitivity, which occurs in up to 70 % of SLE and SCLE patients [153]. UV light is thought to be the main cause of photosensitivity in SLE and SCLE and has been associated with elevated complement, TNF, and IL-1β as well as increased autoantibodies including Ro/SSA [149, 154]. UV is known to activate the inflammasome [155]. For this reason SLE patients are advised to avoid sun exposure. UV activates resident skin cells like keratinocytes, MCs, and fibroblasts and leads to a dominant Th2-type immune response within the skin [148]. Inflammatory cells in the skin of SCLE patients are mainly macrophages, CD4+, and CD8+ T cells but Langerhans cells are absent.

26.8.2 Rheumatoid Arthritis

Compared to other rheumatic autoimmune diseases, RA displays fewer skin lesions as part of its pathology. Dermatological manifestations in RA usually occur in more aggressive and/or chronic forms of RA. There are three main types of pathological patterns: extravascular palisading inflammation, neutrophil-rich and granulomatous vasculitis, and interstitial or subcuticular neutrophilia [156]. All three forms can occur together. Palisading granulomas include rheumatoid nodules that occur in as many as 25 % of patients. Ninety percent of the patients with rheumatoid nodules test positive for RF. Nodules are associated with a clinically poorer outcome. More rarely, severe cases of RA may be associated with neutrophilic dermatitis characterized as symmetrical erythematous papules or plaques on the extensor surfaces of the arms and hands [156]. RA patients often develop cutaneous side effects to drug treatment with the IL-1 blocker anakinra or the TNF inhibitor infliximab. This occurs in 40 % of RA patients and is associated with skin rash, urticaria, vasculitis, and injection site inflammatory reactions [156, 157].

26.8.3 Sjögren's Syndrome

SS is characterized by dry eyes (keratoconjunctivitis sicca) and dry mouth due to inflammation of the lacrimal and salivary glands. Cutaneous manifestations in SS patients include dry skin (xerosis), macular, papular and vesicular rashes, purpura due to vasculitis, thrombotic lesions, and possibly urticaria or allergic skin eruptions [158]. Around 50 % of SS patients complain of dry skin [159]. It remains unclear whether the dysfunction is due to infiltration of the eccrine or sebaceous glands or a primary problem of the glands with secondary inflammation [160]. The immune response includes autoantibody and complement (i.e., IC deposition), increased perivascular DCs, macrophages, and T cells [159]. Hypergammaglobulinemic purpura can occur on the legs, especially after prolonged standing or long airplane rides. The skin lesions are often associated with RF, complement, and ruptured blood vessels suggestive of IC-mediated damage [161]. In a study of a large cohort of patients with hyperglobulinemic purpura without prior diagnosis of SS, around 50 % developed SS later [158, 162].

26.8.4 Dermatomyositis

DM is an autoimmune disease that affects both the skin and muscles as well as having some systemic features. Skin lesions often precede myopathy and may persist well after the muscle disease has been controlled with medication. In a subset of patients, skin manifestations are transient and other patients may have predominantly skin manifestations with little myopathy or vice versa [163]. In general, the course of skin lesions in DM patients does not parallel muscle disease. Cutaneous manifestations in DM are characterized by a heliotropic rash, which is rarely observed in SLE or scleroderma, and Gottron's papules. Gottron's papules are slightly elevated papules or plaques found over bony prominences like phalangeal joints, elbows, knees, and/or feet. It is also characteristic to observe a photosensitive malar rash that is difficult to differentiate from the rash found in

SLE patients. It is also common in DM to develop a psoriasiform dermatitis involving the scalp.

26.8.5 Scleroderma

Scleroderma is characterized by inflammation and fibrosis of the skin but can also involve other organs like the kidney, lung, and heart [121]. The disease is characterized as localized scleroderma (LSc) or systemic scleroderma (SSc) depending on the extent of internal organ involvement [164, 165]. Sclerosis means "thickening" and refers to thickening and hardening of the skin due to fibrosis. The exact relationship between LSc and SSc, or why only the skin appears to be involved in some cases, remains unclear. In the sclerotic stage, there is little inflammation in the skin. In the early inflammatory phase, lymphocytes and MCs are present, but few DCs or Treg [166–170]. The histology of the skin in LSc and SSc appears the same. The immune response has been characterized as predominantly Th2 with elevated levels of IL-2, IL-4, IL-1β, IL-6, and TGFβ [171]. TNF and IL-13, a Th2 cytokine, are elevated in roughly 25 % of SSc patients [172]. The role for autoantibodies in the pathogenesis of disease is unknown, but approximately 95 % of scleroderma patients are positive for antinuclear antibodies (ANA) [173].

26.9 Rheumatic Autoimmune Diseases That Occur Before Menopause

Of rheumatic autoimmune diseases, only two typically peak in appearance before menopause, SLE, and scleroderma. SLE typically presents in females during childbearing years (20s and 30s) [2, 174, 175]. One study found that only 16 % of SLE patients presented after age 50, and in another study the female to male ratio was 13:1 before age 50 but only 3:1 after 50 [176, 177]. Scleroderma disease onset peaks in women from age 30 to 40 years while estrogen levels remain high [164, 178].

26.9.1 Menopause and SLE

SLE has a clear relationship between high estrogen levels and worse disease [2, 6]. Pregnancy increases disease in patients, and in most mouse models of SLE females have worse disease outcomes, administration of estrogen exacerbates disease, and androgen administration ameliorates disease [174]. Polymorphisms in the ER gene have been associated with SLE and estrogen has been found to increase autoantibodies and IC deposition in animal models of lupus [179]. An analysis of 26 articles, comparing men to women with SLE summarized several sex differences. They found that the kidney and skin manifestations were more frequently involved in SLE in males [180]. Men also had decreased Ro/SSA and La/SSB autoantibody levels compared to women, but other autoantibodies like dsDNA and Sm antibodies were higher in men [180]. Additionally, male SLE patients have been found to have higher estrogen to androgen ratios and lower levels of testosterone in their sera [2].

SLE is considered to primarily be driven by Th1-type immune responses increased by TLR activation. Peripheral blood mononuclear cells (PBMCs) from patients display greater serum Th1 and IL-18 levels that correlate with disease activity [181]. However, it is important to realize that IL-18 derives from inflammasome activation, which is not part of a classic IL-12/STAT4-induced Th1 response, and so IL-18 may be responsible for an increased Th1 response [182]. The pathology in SLE is primarily IC-mediated, which is most closely associated with MC and inflammasome activation and Th2 immune responses. Evidence that SLE could be driven by Th2 responses comes from the finding that PBMCs from SLE patients express more TIM-1 (requires a Th2 response) and less TIM-3 (requires a Th1 response) [183].

A number of studies suggest that SLE occurs less frequently following menopause [175]. One line of evidence is the shift in female to male predominance from 13 to 3:1 after 50 years of age [176, 177]. Another comes from a large study of 714 late-onset SLE patients (after 50 years of age) compared to 4,700 younger patients [184].

They found a lower female to male ratio after 50 and a lower incidence of malar rash, photosensitivity, purpura/cutaneous vasculitis, alopecia, and Raynaud's syndrome. A number of small studies examined symptoms in SLE patients for 2–3 years prior to natural menopause and 2–3 years after menopause, and the studies were largely in agreement that there was a decrease in flares, disease activity, proteinuria, autoantibodies, vasculitis, and rash after menopause [185–187]. Patients presenting after menopause had greater RF autoantibodies [184]. Information on HRT remains controversial with some studies finding no effect of HRT on SLE, while others found it to be a risk factor for increased disease [188–190]. However, it must be noted that tissue damage due to SLE is greater after menopause [191, 192], perhaps because of long-term damage over time and gradually increasing ICs (see Fig. 26.1).

26.9.2 Menopause and Scleroderma

Scleroderma is regarded as the prototypic fibrotic disease [193]. Although a relatively uncommon disease, it has the highest case-specific mortality of any of the autoimmune rheumatic diseases because of vascular and fibrotic complications. Patients with systemic sclerosis have a fourfold increase in mortality compared to the general population, with approximately a third of deaths due to cardiovascular diseases including atherosclerosis [194, 195]. A number of cytokines are believed to drive extracellular matrix remodeling and fibrosis during scleroderma including TNF, IL-1β, IL-4, IL-13, IL-33, and TGFβ [196, 197]. Studies of human scleroderma and animal models have revealed elevated expression of profibrotic cytokines like TGFβ and elevated numbers of MCs, eosinophils, and basophils (blood MCs) – cells and cytokines associated with Th2 responses [170, 172, 198]. A recent study found that scleroderma patients had elevated expression of TLR4 on fibroblasts that when cultured were more sensitive to TGFβ and produced greater amounts of collagen [198]. Approximately 95 % of scleroderma patients are positive for ANA [173], and ICs are known to contribute to systemic vasculitis symptoms in these patients [199–201]. A common outcome of IC deposition in tissues is remodeling and fibrosis [2, 6].

Scleroderma occurs more frequently in women than men with ranges of 3:1–14:1 reported [164, 178, 202, 203]. Estrogen has well-defined roles in increasing Th2 responses and antibody and autoantibody levels and in driving profibrotic responses associated with TNF, IL-4, and TGFβ production suggesting that estrogen could contribute to pathology in scleroderma [2, 6]. In support of this idea is data indicating that scleroderma disease onset peaks in women from age 30 to 40 years, when estrogen levels are high [164, 178]. However, data are scarce on the effect of menopause on scleroderma. Studies aimed at examining the role of osteoporosis in scleroderma patients have reported that earlier menopause in women with scleroderma may be a risk factor for developing osteoporosis [204].

26.10 Rheumatic Autoimmune Diseases That Occur After Menopause

The remaining three rheumatic autoimmune diseases, RA, dermatomyositis, and Sjögren's syndrome, peak after menopause suggesting a protective role for estrogen. Little information is available regarding sex differences or effects of menopause on dermatomyositis, so the following discussion will focus on RA and SS.

26.10.1 Menopause and Rheumatoid Arthritis

The most common age of onset of disease in RA is around 60 years of age (about 10 years after menopause) [205]. The female to male ratio in RA is about 1:1 prior to 50 years of age but goes up to 3:2 after 50 [206, 207]. A key diagnostic feature and biomarker of early disease are anticyclic citrullinated autoantibodies. Like SLE, pathology in RA joints is driven by IC-mediated damage resulting in inflammation consisting of

T cells, macrophages, and MCs [6]. TNF, IL-1β, and IL-6 are elevated during disease and suggest activation of the inflammasome. TNF and IL-1β are also profibrotic and lead to joint remodeling and damage. Although estrogen is likely to increase autoantibodies and ICs in women with RA, animal models of arthritis have shown that estrogen protects against disease by decreasing proinflammatory cytokines [208]. Clinical studies of RA patients found that IFNγ levels were higher than IL-4 in inflamed joints [209]. This could be due to an increased Th1-type immune response or to inflammasome activity via IL-18. Interestingly, two studies found that RA patients had higher circulating levels of IL-4 characteristic of a Th2-type immune response [210, 211]. Inflammasome activation of MCs and alternatively activated macrophages is characteristic of a mixed Th1/Th2 environment which is likely to occur at the transition to menopause in women when the ratio of estrogen to testosterone decreases (see Fig. 26.1) [78, 182].

Evidence in support of a protective role for high estrogen levels in RA is the finding that up to two-thirds of young RA patients that become pregnant undergo partial or total remission of disease [212], and disease onset is less likely during pregnancy [213]. Additionally, women report that RA symptoms are lower during the postovulatory phase of the menstrual cycle and during pregnancy, when estrogen levels are high (progesterone is likely to also be important in mediating these effects but is not discussed in this chapter; see [214]) [212, 215]. It has been shown that RA patients with an onset after 50 years of age have a worse functional outcome, more frequent acute onset of disease, more involvement of large proximal joints like the shoulders, and greater systemic manifestations including increased osteoporosis and cardiovascular disease [6, 206, 207]. Additionally, the incidence of RA continues to rise with age [216, 217]. HRT has been found to protect against the development of RA in some studies but not in others [218–221]. It is important to realize that oral administration of a hormone is not likely to provide the same immune stimulus as naturally and locally produced hormone, which could explain, at least in part, why HRT is not always found to reduce the risk for developing RA. Overall, the data suggest that estrogen levels observed during peak childbearing years protect against RA. Most of the pathology of RA is driven by ICs and autoantibody levels increase with age. So perhaps it just "takes time" to develop RA. However, the role of estrogen and menopause in RA is not as clear as it is for SLE or scleroderma.

26.10.2 Menopause and Sjögren's Syndrome

SS is characterized by chronic inflammation of the exocrine salivary and lacrimal (tear) glands resulting in dry mouth and eyes [222]. Although SS primarily involves the salivary and lacrimal glands, many other organs are affected including skin, joints, kidneys, lungs, and muscle. SS can occur as a primary condition or in association with other autoimmune diseases – primarily the rheumatic diseases SLE, RA, scleroderma, and dermatomyositis. Autoantibodies in SS include ANA, particularly against ribonuclear proteins (e.g., anti-Ro/SSA) and RF. The double name Ro and SSA or La and SSB derives from the description of these autoantibodies by two different research groups – one to define SLE patients ("Ro" and "La") and the other in association with SS (SSA and SSB). Ro and La follow the early convention of naming new autoantigens from the surname letters of the donor of the serum [223]. Plasma cells within the salivary glands of SS patients have been found to produce Ro/SSA and La/SSB autoantibodies [224]. The inflammatory infiltrate in SS includes T and B cells, DCs, and macrophages as well as IC deposition, apoptosis, and remodeling [223].

Similar to SLE, Sjögren's syndrome is more common in women than men with a ratio of 9:1 [225]. RFs are detected in around 60 % of SS patients, but their frequency has been reported to be higher in men in some studies [226]. ANA autoantibodies, which are not specific to SS, are significantly higher in women with Sjögren's in many studies [227–230]. SSA autoantibodies, which are disease specific, are also reported to be elevated in women with SS compared to men [228, 231, 232]. Similar to RA, SS peaks shortly after menopause around age 55 suggesting a protective role for estrogen [233]. Female mice have been found to have greater lacrimal and salivary gland inflammation than males in an animal model of Sjögren's [234]. In another mouse model of SS, females were found to have greater salivary gland inflammation, a more predominant Th2 and Th17 response, and more B cells than males [235]. More recently ovariectomy of adult female mice (modeling menopause) in a SS model significantly increased inflammation in the lacrimal (tear) gland that preceded apoptosis [236]. Estrogen replacement of ovariectomized mice in these studies reversed this effect reducing T- and B-cell infiltration, suggesting that estrogen reduces tear gland inflammation during SS. Thus, reduced levels of estrogen with menopause could decrease the protective effect of estrogen including its proliferative effects on glandular cells leading to increased apoptosis [237, 238]. In support of this idea, low salivary estrogen levels have been found to correlate with a feeling of dry mouth in healthy menopausal women [239].

Another theory to explain the sex difference suggests that lower estrogen levels in females after menopause reduce salivary gland-specific TGFβ production allowing increased inflammation (TGFβ is associated with increased Treg). Microarray conducted on normal salivary glands from men and women without SS found that women had lower expression of TGFβ [240]. Female mice where TGFβ receptor I was inactivated in the salivary gland developed inflammation and an increased Th1-type immune response [241], suggesting that this mechanism could influence inflammation. In contrast, testosterone has been found to increase TGFβ expression in the lacrimal gland and to suppress inflammation in a mouse model of SS [242].

Not only is estrogen lower following menopause, but also the adrenal prohormone dehydroepiandrosterone (DHEA), which is only about half the level in SS patients that it is in healthy age- and sex-matched controls [243]. DHEA is important for the repair and renewal of acinar cells of the labial salivary glands and impaired levels of DHEA can lead to apoptosis of the cells [238]. DHEA has been used as a therapy in SS patients, where administration reduced symptoms of dry mouth [244]. This could lead to upregulation of TLR and activation of the inflammasome leading to inflammation. The inflammasome does appear to be activated during SS in humans and animal models [245, 246]. Genetic polymorphisms in IL-1β or IL-1 receptor antagonist (an inhibitor of IL-1R signaling) are known to affect SS [247, 248]. Additionally, IL-18, a component of the inflammasome, was found to be present in macrophages within inflammatory foci of the salivary gland of SS patients, and circulating IL-18 levels were elevated in SS patients compared to controls [249]. Interestingly, serum IL-18 levels were strongly correlated with SSA/Ro and SSB/La autoantibodies. Although SS has traditionally been considered a Th1-driven immune response, this could be due to IL-18 rather than the classical Th1 pathway. Th2 responses clearly increase autoantibody levels and the inflammasome is associated with Th2 responses, MCs, and M2 macrophages [2, 4, 28]. Additional support for the idea that SS could be a Th2-driven disease comes from the finding that SS patients had significantly higher levels of circulating IL-13, a definitive Th2 cytokine, compared to controls [250].

26.11 Summary and Future Directions

Autoimmune diseases that affect the skin occur predominantly in women with rheumatic autoimmune diseases such as SLE, RA, Sjögren's syndrome, scleroderma, and dermatomyositis. Common immune mechanisms drive pathology in all rheumatic diseases and include MC and macrophage activation of the inflammasome, vitamin D deficiency, elevated autoantibodies and IC deposition, and elevated levels of proinflammatory and profibrotic cytokines like TNF and IL-1β. Evidence to date suggests that cutaneous manifestations in SLE and scleroderma are lower following menopause, suggesting that high levels of estrogen that are present during peak childbearing years contribute to disease pathogenesis. The primary pathology in SLE and scleroderma is ICs and fibrosis, respectively. Estrogen is well known to increase the autoantibodies and profibrotic cytokines needed to promote these diseases.

In contrast, Sjögren's syndrome, RA, and dermatomyositis peak after menopause. Understanding how the menopausal transition affects inflammation in this case is complicated by changes in the immune response that occur with aging. However, low levels of estrogen are able to promote B-cell proliferation and antibody production, and autoantibody levels in women continue to increase with age. Additionally, lower estrogen levels reduce the protective effects of estrogen that were present prior to menopause and allow increased activation of innate immune cells resulting in elevated proinflammatory and profibrotic cytokines. The skin is particularly susceptible to the effects of fluctuating estrogen and vitamin D levels because skin immune cells and keratinocytes are directly influenced by these sex steroids. It is not clear yet whether vitamin D deficiency causes rheumatic autoimmune diseases or occurs as a result of autoimmune damage to the skin and kidneys reducing production of the active form of the hormone. Regardless of when it occurs, low vitamin D levels are likely to affect the pathogenesis of disease because of the potent regulatory effects vitamin D has on immune and skin cells.

Although some aspects of the immune response important in driving autoinflammation in the skin are known, there are many gaps that still need to be addressed (Table 26.2). Published studies need to be reanalyzed according to sex and age and new studies designed that examine whether sex differences exist. All clinical, animal, and culture studies must report the sex used for the study. Vitamin D needs to be understood as a sex steroid that is expected to have different effects on inflammation according to sex, just as estrogens and androgens induce different affects. Additionally, the skin is an organ that is centrally involved in regulating vitamin D levels in the body and should be considered when attempting to understand the effects of vitamin D deficiency or insufficiency on chronic inflammatory diseases. We need a better understanding of the role of MCs in autoimmune skin diseases, since they are the primary immune cells responding to ICs within the skin. We also need studies that examine the role of IL-33/ST2, the inflammasome, and ILCs in the skin during rheumatic autoimmune diseases. And finally, we need to define the relationship of ER, AR, and VDR signaling on immune cells and how differing ratios of estrogen to testosterone, as occurs following menopause and with aging, and differing vitamin D levels affect skin inflammation. This knowledge would improve our ability to treat these diseases with vitamin D supplementation and HRT.

Table 26.2 Areas that need research

Clinical, animal model, and cell culture studies need to report the sex used in experiments and analyze data according to sex
We need to determine the relationship between VDR, ER, and AR signaling and its effect on immune and other cells like keratinocytes in the skin
As the primary cells that respond to autoantibodies and ICs, we need a better understanding of MC function in the skin in rheumatic autoimmune diseases
Determine the role of the inflammasome in the autoimmune skin disease
We need a better understanding of the role of newly identified immune cells and cytokines in the skin (e.g., ILCs, IL-33, ST2) on the pathogenesis of autoimmune skin disease
Clinical studies need to report and analyze data according to age or menopause status (i.e., before and after 50 years of age), especially in women
We need more data on sex differences in skin manifestations for rheumatic autoimmune diseases
Studies need to be conducted to ascertain the role of kidney and skin damage and inflammation on vitamin D deficiency
Do vitamin D deficiency definitions proposed by the Institute of Medicine, which are based on bone health, correlate to pathology in autoimmune diseases?

Funding This work was supported by a National Institutes of Health (NIH) award from the National Heart, Lung, and Blood Institute (HL111938) and an American Heart Association Grant-in-Aid (12GRNT12050000).

References

1. Jacobson DL, Gange SJ, Rose NR, Graham NMH. Epidemiology and estimated population burden of selected autoimmune disease in the United States. Clin Immunol Immunopathol. 1997;84:223–43.
2. Fairweather D, Frisancho-Kiss S, Rose NR. Sex differences in autoimmune disease from a pathologic perspective. Am J Pathol. 2008;173:600–9.
3. Notkins AL. Pathogenic mechanisms in autoimmune disease. Autoimmun Rev. 2004;3(Suppl):S7–9.
4. Fairweather D, Frisancho-Kiss S, Njoku DB, Nyland JF, Kaya Z, Yusung SA, Davis SE, Frisancho JA, Barrett MA, Rose NR. Complement receptor 1 and 2 deficiency increases coxsackievirus B3-induced myocarditis and heart failure by increasing macrophages, IL-1β and immune complex deposition in the heart. J Immunol. 2006;176:3516–24.
5. Wahren-Herlenius M, Dorner T. Immunopathogenic mechanisms of systemic autoimmune disease. Lancet. 2013;382:819–31.
6. Fairweather D, Petri MA, Coronado MJ, Cooper Jr LT. Autoimmune heart disease: role of sex hormones and autoantibodies in disease pathogenesis. Expert Rev Clin Immunol. 2012;8:269–84.
7. Carson DA, Chen PP, Fox RI, Kipps TJ, Jirik F, Goldfien RD, Silverman G, Radoux V, Fong S. Rheumatoid factor and immune networks. Ann Rev Immunol. 1987;5:109–26.
8. Newkirk MM. Rheumatoid factors: host resistance or autoimmunity? Clin Immunol. 2002;104:1–13.
9. Dorner T, Egerer K, Feist E, Burmester GR. Rheumatoid factor revisited. Curr Opin Rheumatol. 2004;16:246–53.
10. Firestein GS. Evolving concepts of rheumatoid arthritis. Nature. 2003;423:356–61.
11. Zandman-Goddard G, Peeva E, Shoenfeld Y. Gender and autoimmunity. Autoimmun Rev. 2007;6:366–72.
12. Beeson PB. Age and sex associations of 40 autoimmune diseases. Am J Med. 1994;96:457–62.
13. Whitacre CC. Sex differences in autoimmune disease. Nat Immunol. 2001;2:777–80.
14. Gleicher N, Barad DH. Gender as a risk factor for autoimmune diseases. J Autoimmun. 2007;28:1–6.
15. Styrt B, Sugarman B. Estrogens and infection. Rev Infect Dis. 1991;13:1139–50.
16. Flanagan KL, Klein SL, Skakkebaek NE, Marriott I, Marchant A, Selin L, Fish EN, Prentice AM, Whittle H, Benn CS, Aaby P. Sex differences in the vaccine-specific and non-targeted effects of vaccines. Vaccine. 2011;16:2349–54.
17. Lang TJ. Estrogen as an immunomodulator. Clin Immunol. 2004;113:224–30.
18. Cook IF. Sexual dimorphism of humoral immunity with vaccines. Vaccine. 2008;26:3551–5.
19. Straub RH. The complex role of estrogens in inflammation. Endocr Rev. 2007;28:521–74.
20. Rubtsov A, Rubtsova K, Kappler JW, Marrack P. Genetic and hormonal factors in female-biased autoimmunity. Autoimm Rev. 2010;9:494–8.
21. Lahita RG. Sex hormones and immune function. In: Legato MJ, editor. Principles of gender-specific medicine. 2nd ed. MA: Elsevier; 2010. p. 615–26.
22. Wilder RL. Neuroendocrine-immune system interactions and autoimmunity. Annu Rev Immunol. 1995;13:307–38.
23. Carreras E, Turner S, Frank MB, Knowlton N, Osban J, Centola M, Park CG, Simmons A, Alberola-lla J, Kovats S. Estrogen receptor signaling promotes dendritic cell differentiation by increasing expression of the transcription factor IRF4. Blood. 2010;115:238–46.
24. Khan D, Dai R, Karpuzoglu E, Ahmed SA. Estrogen increases, whereas IL-27 and IFN-gamma decrease, splenocyte IL-17 production in WT mice. Eur J Immunol. 2010;40:2549–56.
25. Wang Y, Cela E, Gagnon S, Sweezey NB. Estrogen aggravates inflammation in *Pseudomonas aeruginosa* pneumonia in cystic fibrosis mice. Respir Res. 2010;30:166.
26. Polanczyk MJ, Carson BD, Subramanian S, Afentoulis M, Vandenbark AA, Ziegler SF, Offner H. Cutting edge: estrogen drives expansion of the CD4 + CD25+ regulatory T-cell compartment. J Immunol. 2004;173:2227–30.
27. Polanczyk MJ, Hopke C, Huan J, Vandenbark AA, Ziegler SF, Offner H. Enhanced FoxP3 expression and Treg cell function in pregnant and estrogen-treated mice. J Neuroimmunol. 2005;170:85–92.
28. Frisancho-Kiss S, Davis SE, Nyland JF, Frisancho JA, Cihakova D, Rose NR, Fairweather D. Cutting edge: cross-regulation by TLR4 and T cell Ig mucin-3 determines sex differences in inflammatory heart disease. J Immunol. 2007;178:6710–4.
29. Xia X, Zhang S, Yu Y, Zhao N, Liu R, Liu K, Chen X. Effects of estrogen replacement therapy on estrogen receptor expression and immunoregulatory cytokine secretion in surgically induced menopausal women. J Reprod Immunol. 2009;81:89–96.
30. Pulendran B, Tang H, Manicassamy S. Programming dendritic cells to induce Th2 and tolerogenic responses. Nat Immunol. 2010;11:647–55.
31. Dinesh RK, Hahn BH, Singh RP. PD-1, gender and autoimmunity. Autoimm Rev. 2010;9:583–7.
32. Sellner J, Kraus J, Awad A, Milo R, Hemmer B, Stuve O. The increasing incidence and prevalence of female multiple sclerosis- a critical analysis of potential environmental factors. Autoimmun Rev. 2011;10:495–502.
33. Papenfuss TL, Powell ND, McClain MA, Bedarf A, Singh A, Gienapp IE, Shawler T, Whitacre CC. Estriol generates tolerogenic dendritic cells in vivo that protect against autoimmunity. J Immunol. 2011;186:3346–55.
34. Giron-Gonzalez JA, Moral FJ, Elvira J, Garcia-Gil D, Guerrero F, Gavilan I, Escobar L. Consistent production of a higher Th1:Th2 cytokine ratio by stimulated T cells in men compared with women. Eur J Endocrinol. 2000;143:31–6.
35. Giltay EJ, Fonk JC, von Blomberg BM, Drexhage HA, Schalkwijk C, Gooren LJ. In vivo effects of sex steroids in lymphocyte responsiveness and

immunoglobulin levels in humans. J Clin Endocrinol Metab. 2000;85:1648–57.
36. Loria RM. Immune up-regulation and tumor apoptosis by androstene steroids. Steroids. 2002;67:953–66.
37. Desai KV, Michalowska AM, Kondaiah P, Ward JM, Shih JH, Green JE. Gene expression profiling identifies a unique androgen-mediated inflammatory/immune signature and a PTEN (phosphatase and tensin homolog deleted on chromosome 10)-mediated apoptotic response specific to the rat ventral prostate. Mol Endocriniol. 2004;18:2895–907.
38. Miller VM. Why are sex and gender important to basic physiology, translational and individualized medicine? Am J Physiol Heart Circ Physiol. 2014;306:H781–8.
39. Dube SR, Fairweather D, Pearson WS, Felitti VJ, Anda RF, Croft JB. Cumulative childhood stress and autoimmune diseases in adults. Psychomatic Med. 2009;71:243–50.
40. Gharaee-Kermani M, Hatano K, Nozaki Y, Phan SH. Gender-based differences in bleomycin-induced pulmonary fibrosis. Am J Pathol. 2005;166:1593–606.
41. Pennell LM, Galligan CL, Fish EN. Sex affects immunity. J Autoimmun. 2012;38:J282–91.
42. Kato I, Toniolo P, Akhmedkhanov A, Koenig KL, Shore R, Zeleniuch-Jacquotte A. Prospective study of factors influencing the onset of natural menopause. J Clin Epidemiol. 1998;51:1271–6.
43. Jacobsen BK, Heuch I, Kvale G. Age at natural menopause and all-cause mortality: a 37-year follow-up of 19,731 Norwegian women. Am J Epidemiol. 2003;157:923–9.
44. Harlow SD, Gass M, Hall JE, Lobo R, Maki P, Rebar RW, Sherman S, de Sluss PM, Villiers TJ. Executive summary of the stages of reproductive aging workshop + 10: addressing the unfinished agenda of staging reproductive aging. J Clin Endocrinol Metab. 2012;97:1159–68.
45. Vermeulen A. Declining androgens with age: an overview. In: Vermeulien A, Oddens BJ, editors. Androgens and the aging male. New York: Parthenon Publishing; 1996. p. 3–14.
46. Pines A. Male menopause: is it a real clinical syndrome? Climacteric. 2011;14:15–7.
47. Bove R. Autoimmune diseases and reproductive aging. Clin Immunol. 2013;149:251–64.
48. Davison SL, Bell R, Donath S, Montalto JG, Davis SR. Androgen levels in adult females: changes with age, menopause, and oophorectomy. J Clin Endocrinol Metab. 2005;90:3847–53.
49. Weiskopf D, Weinberger B, Grubeck-Loebenstein B. The aging of the immune system. Transpl Int. 2009;22:1041–50.
50. Gameiro CM, Romao F, Castelo-Branco C. Menopause and aging: changes in the immune system- a review. Maturitas. 2010;67:316–20.
51. Goronzy JJ, Weyand CM. Understanding immunosenescence to improve responses to vaccines. Nat Immunol. 2013;14:428–36.
52. Blum M, Zacharovich D, Pery J, Kitai E. Lowering effect of estrogen replacement treatment on immunoglobulins in menopausal women. Rev Fr Gynecol Obstet. 1990;85:207–9.
53. White HD, Crassi KM, Givan AL, Stern JE, Gonzalez JL, Memoli VA, Green WR, Wira CR. CD3+ CD8+ CTL activity within the human female reproductive tract: influence of stage of the menstrual cycle and menopause. J Immunol. 1997;158:3017–27.
54. Shakhar K, Shakhar G, Rosenne E, Ben-Eliyahu S. Timing within the menstrual cycle, sex and the use of oral contraceptives determine adrenergic suppression of NK cell activity. Br J Cancer. 2000;83:1630–6.
55. Evans MJ, Eckert A, Lai K, Adelman SJ, Harnish DC. Reciprocal antagonism between estrogen receptor and NF-κB activity in vivo. Circ Res. 2001;89:823–30.
56. Demyanets S, Pfaffenberger S, Kaun C, Rega G, Speidl WA, Kastl SP, Weiss TW, Hohensinner PJ, Dietrich W, Tschuggel W, Bochkov VN, Awad EM, Maurer G, Huber K, Wojta J. The estrogen metabolite 17β-dihydroequilenin counteracts interleukin-1α induced expression of inflammatory mediators in human endothelial cells in vitro via NF-κB pathway. Thromb Haemost. 2006;95:107–16.
57. Feldman I, Feldman GM, Mobarak C, Dunkelberg JC, Leslie KK. Identification of proteins within the nuclear factor-kappa B transcriptional complex including estrogen receptor-alpha. Am J Obstet Gynecol. 2007;196:394.e1–11.
58. Paimela T, Ryhanen T, Mannermaa E, Ojala J, Kalesnykas G, Salminen A, Kaarniranta K. The effect of 17beta-estradiol on IL-6 secretion and NF-kappaB DNA-binding activity in human retinal pigment epithelial cells. Immunol Lett. 2007;110:139–44.
59. Liu H-B, Loo KK, Palaszynski I, Ashouri J, Lubahn DB, Voskuhl RR. Estrogen receptor α mediates estrogen's immune protection in autoimmune disease. J Immunol. 2003;171:6936–40.
60. Streilein JW. Skin-associated lymphoid tissues (SALT): origins and functions. J Invest Dermatol. 1983;80:12S–6.
61. Bos JD, Kapsenberg ML. The skin immune system (SIS): its cellular constituents and their interactions. Immunol Today. 1986;7:235–40.
62. Nestle FO, Di Meglio P, Qin J-Z, Nickoloff BJ. Skin immune sentinels in health and disease. Nat Rev Immunol. 2009;9:679–91.
63. Grice EA, Segre JA. The skin microbiome. Nat Rev Microbiol. 2011;9:244–53.
64. Heath WR, Carbone FR. The skin-resident and migratory immune system in steady state and memory: innate lymphocytes, dendritic cells and T cells. Nat Immunol. 2013;14:978–85.
65. Klechevsky E. Human dendritic cells- stars in the skin. Eur J Immunol. 2013;43:3147–55.
66. Harvima IT, Nilsson G. Mast cells as regulators of skin inflammation and immunity. Acta Derm Venereol. 2011;91:644–50.

67. Schauber J, Dorschner RA, Coda AB, Buchau AS, Liu PT, Kiken D, Helfrich YR, Kang S, Elalieh HZ, Steinmeyer A, Zugel U, Bikle DD, Modlin RL, Gallo RL. Injury enhances TLR2 function and antimicrobial peptide expression through a vitamin D-dependent mechanism. J Clin Invest. 2007;117:803–11.
68. Feldmeyer L, Keller M, Niklaus G, Hohl D, Werner S, Beer H-D. The inflammasome mediates UVB-induced activation and secretion of interleukin-1β by keratinocytes. Curr Biol. 2007;17:1140–5.
69. Wen H, Miao EA, Ting JP-Y. Mechanisms of NOD-like receptor-associated inflammasome activation. Immunity. 2013;39:432–41.
70. Liew FY. IL-33: a Janus cytokine. Ann Rheum Dis. 2012;71(Supp II):i101–4.
71. Yu S-L, Wong C-K, Tam L-S. The alarmin functions of high-mobility group box-1 and IL-33 in the pathogenesis of systemic lupus erythematosus. Expert Rev Clin Immunol. 2013;9:739–49.
72. Imai Y, Yasuda K, Sakaguchi Y, Haneda T, Mizutani H, Yoshimoto T, Nakanishi K, Yamanishi K. Skin-specific expression of IL-33 activates group 2 innate lymphoid cells and elicits atopic dermatitis-like inflammation in mice. Proc Natl Acad Sci U S A. 2013;110:13921–6.
73. Philip NH, Artis D. New friendships and old feuds: relationships between innate lymphoid cells and microbial communities. Immunol Cell Biol. 2013;91:225–31.
74. Pantelyushin S, Haak S, Ingold B, Kulig P, Heppner FL, Navarini AA, Vecher B. Rorγt+ innate lymphocytes and γδ T cells initiate psoriasiform plaque formation in mice. J Clin Invest. 2012;122:2252–6.
75. Cai Y, Shen X, Ding C, Qi C, Li K, Li X, Jala VR, Zhang HG, Wang T, Zheng J, Yan J. Pivotal role of dermal IL-17-producing γδ T cells in skin inflammation. Immunity. 2011;35:596–610.
76. Kim BS, Siracusa MC, Saenz SA, Noti M, Monticelli LA, Sonnenberg GF, Hepworth MR, van Voorhees AS, Comeau MR, Artis D. TSLP elicits IL-33-independent innate lymphoid cell responses to promote skin inflammation. Sci Transl Med. 2013;5:170ra116.
77. Martin SFF. Allergic contact dermatitis: xenoinflammation of the skin. Curr Opin Immunol. 2012;24:720–9.
78. Fairweather D, Frisancho-Kiss S. Mast cells and inflammatory heart disease: potential drug targets. Cardiovasc Hematol Disord Drug Targets. 2008;8:80–90.
79. Kennelly R, Conneely JB, Bouchier-Hayes D, Winter DC. Mast cells in tissue healing: from skin to the gastrointestinal tract. Curr Pharm Des. 2011;17:3772–5.
80. Frisancho-Kiss S, Nyland JF, Davis SE, Barrett MA, Gatewood SJL, Njoku DB, Cihakova D, Silbergeld EK, Rose NR, Fairweather D. Cutting edge: T cell Ig mucin-3 reduces inflammatory heart disease by increasing CTLA-4 during innate immunity. J Immunol. 2006;176:6411–5.
81. Maurer M, Lopez Kostka S, Sievenhaar F, Moelle K, Metz M, Knop J, von Stebut E. Skin mast cells control T cell-dependent host defense in *Leishmania major* infections. FASEB J. 2006;20:2460–7.
82. Siebenhaar F, Syska W, Weller K, Magerl M, Zuberbier T, Metz M, Maurer M. Control of *Pseudomonas aeruginosa* skin infections in mice is mast cell-dependent. Am J Pathol. 2007;170:1910–6.
83. Metz M, Margeri M, Kuhl NF, Valeva A, Bhakdi S, Maurer M. Mast cells determine the magnitude of bacterial toxin-induced skin inflammation. Exp Dermatol. 2008;18:160–6.
84. Metz M, Piliponsky AM, Chen C-C, Lammel V, Abrink M, Pejler G, Tsai M, Galli SJ. Mast cells can enhance resistance to snake and honeybee venoms. Science. 2006;313:526–30.
85. Fairweather D, Frisancho-Kiss S, Yusung SA, Barrett MA, Davis SE, Gatewood SJL, Njoku DB, Rose NR. IFN-γ protects against chronic viral myocarditis by reducing mast cell degranulation, fibrosis, and the profibrotic cytokines TGF-β1, IL-1β, and IL-4 in the heart. Am J Pathol. 2004;165:1883–94.
86. Huttunen M, Aalto M-L, Harvima RJ, Horsmanheimo M, Harvina IT. Alterations in mast cells showing tryptase and chymase activity in epithelializating and chronic wounds. Exp Dermatol. 2000;9:258–65.
87. Weller K, Foitzik K, Paus R, Syska W, Maurer M. Mast cells are required for normal healing of skin wounds in mice. FASEB J. 2006;20:2366–8.
88. Irani A-MA, Bradford TR, Kepley CL, Schechter NM, Schwartz LB. Detection of MC_T and MC_{TC} types of human mast cells by immunohistochemistry using new monoclonal anti-tryptase and anti-chymase antibodies. J Histochem Cytochem. 1989;37:1509–15.
89. Mizutani H, Schechter NM, Lazarus G, Clack RA, Kupper TS. Rapid and specific conversion of precursor interleukin 1β (IL-1β) to an active IL-1 species by human mast cell chymase. J Exp Med. 1991;174:821–5.
90. Omoto Y, Tokime K, Yamanaka K, Habe K, Morioka T, Kurokawa I, Tsutsui H, Yamanishi K, Nakanishi K, Mizutani H. Human mast cell chymase cleaves pro-IL-18 and generates a novel and biologically active IL-18 fragment. J Immunol. 2006;177:8315–9.
91. Pullen NA, Falangea YT, Morales JK, Ryan JJ. The Fyn-STAT5 pathway: a new frontier in IgE- and IgG-mediated mast cell signaling. Front Immunol. 2012;3:117.
92. Lavie CJ, Lee JH, Milani RV. Vitamin D and cardiovascular disease: will it live up to the hype? J Am Coll Cardiol. 2011;58:1547–56.
93. Plum LA, DeLuca HF. Vitamin D, disease and therapeutic opportunities. Nat Rev Drug Disc. 2010;9:941–55.
94. Zittermann A, Gummert JF. Sun, vitamin D, and cardiovascular disease. J Photochem Photobiol. 2010;101:124–9.
95. Norman AW. Minireview: vitamin D receptor: new assignments for an already busy receptor. Endocrinology. 2006;147:5542–8.
96. Mason RS, Reichrath J. Sunlight vitamin D and skin cancer. Anti-Cancer Agents Med Chem. 2013;13:83–97.

97. Bikle DD. Vitamin D regulation of immune function. In: Litwack G, editor. Vitamins and hormones: vitamins and the immune system, vol. 86. Amsterdam: Elsevier; 2011. p. 1–21.
98. Onyimba JA, Coronado MJ, Garton AE, Kim JB, Bucek A, Bedja D, Gabrielson KL, Guilarte TR, Fairweather D. The innate immune response to coxsackievirus B3 predicts progression to cardiovascular disease and heart failure in male mice. Biol Sex Differ. 2011;2:2.
99. Lisse TS, Hewison M, Adams JS. Hormone response element binding proteins: novel regulators of vitamin D and estrogen signaling. Steroids. 2011;76:331–9.
100. Litwack G, editor. Vitamins and hormones: vitamins and the immune system, vol. 86. Amsterdam: Elsevier; 2011.
101. Topiliski I, Flaishon L, Naveh Y, Harmelin A, Levo Y, Shacher I. The anti-inflammatory effects of 1,25-dihydroxyvitamin D3 on Th2 cells in vivo are due in part to the control of integrin-mediated T lymphocyte homing. Eur J Immunol. 2004;34:1068–76.
102. Gregori S, Casorati M, Amuchastegui S, Smiroldo S, Davalli AM, Adorini L. Regulatory T cells induced by 1 alpha,25-dihydroxyviatin D3 and mycophenolate mofetil treatment mediate transplantation tolerance. J Immunol. 2001;167:1945–53.
103. Daniel C, Sartory NA, Zahn N, Radeke HH, Stein JM. Immune modulatory treatment of trinitrobenzene sulfonic acid colitis with calcitriol is associated with a change of a T helper (Th) 1/Th17 to a Th2 and regulatory T cell profile. J Pharmacol Exp Ther. 2008;324:23–33.
104. Rook GA, Steele J, Fraher L, Barker S, Karmiali R, O'Riordan J, Stanford J. Vitamin D3, gamma interferon, and control of proliferation of *Mycobacterium tuberculosis* by human monoctyes. Immunology. 1986;57:159–63.
105. Wang TT, Nestel FP, Bourdeau V, Nagai Y, Wang Q, Liao J, Tavera-Mendoza L, Lin R, Hanrahan JW, Mader S, White JH. Cutting edge: 1,25-dihydroxyvitamin D3 is a direct inducer of antimicrobial peptide gene expression. J Immunol. 2004;173:2909–12.
106. Baroni E, Biffi M, Benigni F, Monno A, Carlucci D, Carmeliet G, Bouillon R, D'Abrosio D. VDR-dependent regulation of mast cell maturation mediated by 1,25-dihydroxyvitamin D3. J Leukoc Biol. 2007;81:250–62.
107. Liu PT, Stenger S, Li H, Wenzel L, Tan BH, Krutzik SR, Ochoa MT, Shauber J, Wu K, Meinken C, Kamen DL, Wagner M, Bals R, Steinmeyer A, Zugel U, Gallo RL, Eisenberg D, Hweison M, Hollis BW, Adams JS, Bloom BR, Modlin RL. Toll-like receptor triggering of a vitamin D-mediated human antimicrobial response. Science. 2006; 311:1770–3.
108. Liu PT, Stenger S, Tan DH, Modlin RL. Cutting edge: vitamin D-mediated human antimicrobial activity against *Mycobacterium tuberculosis* is dependent on the induction of cathelicidin. J Immunol. 2007;179:2060–3.
109. Spach KM, Hayes CE. Vitamin D3 confers protection from autoimmune encephalomyelitis only in female mice. J Immunol. 2005;175:4119–26.
110. Brehm JM, Schuemann B, Fuhlbrigge AL, Hollis BW, Strunk RC, Zeiger RS, Weiss ST, Litonjua AA. Serum vitamin D levels and severe asthma exacerbations in the Childhood Asthma Management Program study. J Allergy Clin Immunol. 2010; 126:52–8.
111. Wittke A, Weaver V, Mahon BD, August A, Cantorna MT. Vitamin D receptor-deficient mice fail to develop experimental allergic asthma. J Immunol. 2004;173:3432–6.
112. Looker AC, Johnson CL, Lacher DA, Pfeiffer CM, Schleicher RL, Sempos CT. Vitamin D status: United States, 2001–2006. NCHS Data Brief. 2011; 59:1–8.
113. Ross AC, Taylor CL, Yaktine AL, Del Valle HB, editors. Dietary reference intakes: calcium and vitamin D. Washington, DC: The National Academies Press; 2011.
114. Melamed ML, Michos ED, Post W, Astor B. 25-hydroxyvitamin D levels and the risk of mortality in the general population. Arch Intern Med. 2008; 168:1629–37.
115. Cutolo M. Vitamin D and autoimmune rheumatic diseases. Rheumatology (Oxford). 2009;48:210–2.
116. Ascherio A, Munger KL, Simon KC. Vitamin D and multiple sclerosis. Lancet Neurol. 2010;9:599–612.
117. Muller K, Kriegbaum NJ, Baslund B, Sorensen OH, Thymann M, Bentzen K. Vitamin D3 metabolism in patients with rheumatic diseases: low serum levels of 12-hydroxyvitamin D3 in patients with systemic lupus erythematosus. J Clin Rheumatol. 1995;14:397–400.
118. Cutolo M, Plebani M, Shoenfeld Y, Adorini L, Tincani A. Vitamin D endocrine system and the immune response in rheumatic diseases. In: Latwick G, editor. Vitamins and hormones: vitamins and the immune system. Amsterdam: Elsevier; 2011. p. 327–51.
119. Clemens TL, Adams JS, Henderson SL, Holick MF. Increased skin pigment reduces the capacity of skin to synthesize vitamin D3. Lancet. 1982;1:74–6.
120. Tang JY, Fu T, Lau C, Oh DH, Bikle DD, Asgari MM. Vitamin D in cutaneous carcinogenesis. J Am Acad Dermatol. 2012;67:803.e1–12.
121. Kronbichler A, Mayer G. Renal involvement in autoimmune connective tissue diseases. BMC Med. 2013;11:95.
122. Lemire JM, Ince A, Takashima M. 1,25-Dihydroxyvitamin D3 attenuates the expression of experimental murine lupus of MRL/l mice. Autoimmunity. 1992;12:143–8.
123. Schoenfeld N, Amital H, Shoenfeld Y. The effect of melanism and vitamin D synthesis on the incidence of autoimmune disease. Nat Clin Pract Rheumatol. 2009;5:99–105.
124. Oelzner P, Muller A, Deschner F, Huller M, Abendroth K, Hein G, Stein G. Relationship between disease activity and serum levels of vitamin D

125. Cutolo M, Otsa K, Laas K, Yprus M, Lehtme R, Secchi ME, Sulli A, Paolino S, Seriolo B. Circannual vitamin D serum levels and disease activity in rheumatoid arthritis: Northern versus Southern Europe. Clin Exp Rheumatol. 2006;24:702–4.

126. Andjelkovic Z, Vojinovic J, Pejnovic N, Popovic M, Dujic A, Mitrovic D, Pavlica L, Stefanovic D. Disease modifying and immunomodulatory effects of high dose 1 alpha (OH) D3 in rheumatoid arthritis patients. Clin Exp Rheumatol. 1999;17:453–6.

127. Zold E, Barta Z, Bodolay E. Vitamin D deficiency and connective tissue disease. In: Latwick G, editor. Vitamins and hormones: vitamins and the immune system. Amsterdam: Elsevier; 2011. p. 261–86.

128. Cantorna MT, Hayes CE, DeLuca HF. 1,25-Dihydrooxycholecalciferol inhibits the progression of arthritis in murine models of human arthritis. J Nutr. 1998;128:68–72.

129. Larsson P, Mattsson L, Klareskog L, Johnsson C. A vitamin D analogue (MC 1288) has immunomodulatory properties and suppresses collagen-induced arthritis (CIA) without causing hyper calcaemia. Clin Exp Immunol. 1998;114:277–83.

130. Huckins D, Felson DT, Holick M. Treatment of psoriatic arthritis with oral 1,25-dihydroxyvitamin D3: a pilot study. Arthritis Rheum. 1990;33:1723–7.

131. Gaal J, Lakos G, Szodoray P, Kiss J, Horvath I, Horkay E, Nagy G, Szegedi A. Immunological and clinical effects of alphacalcidol in patients with psoriatic arthropathy: results of an open, follow-up pilot study. Acta Derm Venereol. 2009;89:140–4.

132. Dayangac-Erden D, Karaduman A, Erdem-Yurter H. Polymorphisms of vitamin D receptor gene in Turkish familial psoriasis patients. Arch Dermatol Res. 2007;99:487–91.

133. Zold E, Szodoray P, Gaal J, Kappelmayer J, Csathy L, Gymesi E, Zeher M, Szegedi G, Bodolay E. Vitamin D deficiency in undifferentiated connective tissue disease. Arthritis Res Ther. 2008;10:R123.

134. Calzolari G, Data V, Carignola R, Angeli A. Hypovitaminosis D in systemic sclerosis. J Rheumatol. 2009;36:2844.

135. Vacca A, Cormier C, Piras M, Mathieu A, Kahan A, Allanore Y. Vitamin D deficiency and insufficiency in 2 independent cohorts of patients with systemic sclerosis. J Rheumatol. 2009;36:1924–9.

136. Caramaschi P, Dalla GA, Ruzzenente O, Volpe A, Rvagnani V, Tinazzi I, Barausse G, Bambara LM, Biasi D. Very low levels of vitamin D in systemic sclerosis patients. Clin Rheumatol. 2010;29:1419–25.

137. Artaza JN, Norris KC. Vitamin D reduces the expression of collagen and key profibrotic factors by inducing an antifibrotic phenotype in mesenchymal multipotent cells. J Endocrinol. 2009;200:207–21.

138. Muller K, Oxholm P, Sorensen OH, Thymann M, Hoier-Madsen M, Bendtzen K. Abnormal vitamin D3 metabolism in patients with primary Sjögren's syndrome. Ann Rheum Dis. 1990;49:682–4.

139. Bang B, Asmussen K, Sorensen OH, Oxholm P. Reduced 25-hydroxyvitamin D levels in primary Sjögren's syndrome. Correlations to disease manifestations. Scand J Rheumatol. 1999;28:180–3.

140. Aguado P, del Campo MT, Garces MV, Gonzalez-Casaus ML, Bernad M, Gijon-Banos J, Martin Mola E, Torrijos A, Martinez ME. Low vitamin D levels in outpatient postmenopausal women from a rheumatology clinic in Madrid, Spain: their relationship with bone mineral density. Osteoporos Int. 2000;11:739–44.

141. Lagunova Z, Porojnicu AC, Lindberg F, Hexeberg S, Moan J. The dependency of vitamin D status on body mass index, gender, age and season. Anticancer Res. 2009;29:3710–20.

142. Need AG, Morris HA, Horowitz M, Nordin C. Effects of skin thickness, age, body fat, and sunlight on serum 25-hydroxyvitamin D. Am J Clin Nutr. 1993;58:882–5.

143. Nordin BE, Polley KJ. A cross-sectional, longitudinal, and intervention study on 557 normal postmenopausal women. Calcif Tissue Int. 1987;41 Suppl 1:S1–59.

144. Webb AR, Pilbean C, Hanafin N, Holick MF. An evaluation of the relative contributions of 25-hydroxyvitamin D in an elderly nursing home ooulation in Boston. Am J Clin Nutr. 1990;51:1075–81.

145. Gonzalez G, Alvarado JN, Rojas A, Navarrete C, Velasquez CG, Arteaga E. High prevalence of vitamin D deficiency in Chilean healthy postmenopausal women with normal sun exposure: additional evidence for a worldwide concern. Menopause. 2007;14:455–61.

146. Vieth R, Ladak Y, Walfish PG. Age-related changes in the 25-hydroxyvitamin D versus parathyroid hormone relationship suggest a different reason why older adults require more vitamin D. J Clin Endocrinol Metab. 2003;88:185–91.

147. Hocher B, Reichetzeder C. Vitamin D and cardiovascular risk in postmenopausal women: how to translate preclinical evidence into benefit for patients. Kidney Int. 2013;84:9–11.

148. Sticherling M. Lupus erythematosus: chronic cutaneous lupus erythematosus. In: Hertl M, editor. Autoimmune diseases of the skin. 3rd ed. Vienna: Springer-Verlag; 2011. p. 193–213.

149. Pellowski DM, Kihslinger JE, Sontheimer RD. Lupus erythematosus: subacute cutaneous and systemic lupus erythematosus. In: Hertl M, editor. Autoimmune diseases of the skin. 3rd ed. Vienna: Springer-Verlag; 2011. p. 216–41.

150. Costner MI, Sontheimer RD, Provost TT. Lupus erythematosus. In: Sontheimer RD, Provost TT, editors. Cutaneous manifestations of rheumatic diseases. Philadelphia: Williams and Wilkins; 2003. p. 15–64.

151. Southheimer RD, Thomas JR, Gilliam JN. Subacute cutaneous lupus erythematosus: a cutaneous marker for a distinct lupus erythematosus subset. Arch Dermatol. 1979;115:1409–15.

152. Tan TC, Fang H, Magder LS, Petri MA. Differences between male and female systemic lupus erythematosus in a multiethnic population. J Rheumatol. 2012;39:759–69.
153. Kind P, Lehmann P, Plewig G. Phototesting in lupus erythematosus. J Invest Dermatol. 1993;100:53S–7.
154. Mond CB, Perterson MG, Rothfield NF. Correlation of anti-Ro antibody with photosensitivity rash in systemic lupus erythematosus patients. Arthritis Rheum. 1989;32:202–4.
155. Nasti TH, Timares L. Inflammasome activation of IL-1 family mediators in response to cutaneous photodamage. Photchem Photobiol. 2012;88:1111–25.
156. Frances C, Kluger N. Skin manifestations of rheumatic diseases. In: Sontheimer RD, Provost TT, editors. Cutaneous manifestations of rheumatic diseases. Philadelphia: Williams and Wilkins; 2011. p. 405–33.
157. Lee HH, Song IH, Friedrich M, Gauliard A, Detert J, Rowert J, AUdring H, Kary S, Burmester GR, Sterry W, Worm M. Cutaneous side-effects in patients with rheumatic disease during application of tumour necrosis factor-alpha antagonists. Br J Dermatol. 2007;156:486–91.
158. Fox RI, Fox CM. Sjögren's syndrome. In: Sontheimer RD, Provost TT, editors. Cutaneous manifestations of rheumatic diseases. Philadelphia: Williams and Wilkins; 2011. p. 283–324.
159. Alexander EL, Provost TT. Cutaneous manifestations of primary Sjögren's syndrome: a reflection of vasculitis and association with anti-Ro (SSA) antibodies. J Invest Dermatol. 1983;80:386–91.
160. Tappinos NI, Plihronis M, Tziofas AG, Moutsopoulos HM. Sjogern's syndrome. Autoimmune epithelitis. Adv Exp Med Biol. 1999;455:127–34.
161. Fox RI, Chen PP, Carson DA, Fong S. Expression of a cross reactive idiotype on rheumatoid factor in patients with Sjögren's syndrome. J Immunol. 1986;136:477–83.
162. Kyle R, Gleich G, Baynd E, Vaughan JH. Benign hyperglobulinemic purpura of Waldenstrom. Medicine (Baltimore). 1971;50:113–23.
163. Vleugels RA, Callen JP. Dermatomyositis. In: Hertl M, editor. Autoimmune diseases of the skin. 3rd ed. Vienna: Springer-Verlag; 2011. p. 243–66.
164. Kellet CV, Orteu H, Dutz JP. Scleroderma: localized scleroderma. In: Sontheimer RD, Provost TT, editors. Cutaneous manifestations of rheumatic diseases. Philadelphia: Williams and Wilkins; 2011. p. 137–72.
165. Hunzelmann N, Krieg T. Scleroderma: progressive systemic scleroderma. In: Sontheimer RD, Provost TT, editors. Cutaneous manifestations of rheumatic diseases. Philadelphia: Williams and Wilkins; 2011. p. 173–91.
166. Milano A, Pendergrass SA, Sargent JL, George LK, McCalmont TH, Connolly MK, Whitfield ML. Molecular subsets in the gene expression signatures of scleroderma skin. PLoS One. 2008;3:e2696.
167. Whittaker SJ, Smith NP, Jones RR. Solitary morphoea profunda. Br J Dermatol. 1989;120:431–40.
168. Antiga E, Quaglino P, Bellandi S, Volpi W, Del Bianco E, Comessatti A, Osella-Abate S, De Simone C, Marzano A, Bernengo MG, Fabbri P, Caproni M. Regulatory T cells in the skin lesions and blood of patients with systemic sclerosis and morphoea. Br J Dermatol. 2010;162:1056–63.
169. Aiba S, Tabata N, Ohtani H, Tagami H. Cd34+ spindle-shaped cells selectively disappear from the skin lesion of scleroderma. Arch Dermatol. 1994;130: 593–7.
170. Kubo M, Ihn H, Yamane K, Tamaki K. Up-regulated expression of transforming growth factor beta receptors in dermal fibroblasts in skin sections from patients with localized scleroderma. Arthritis Rheum. 2001;44:731–4.
171. Ihn H, Sato S, Fujimoto M, Kikuchi K, Takehara K. Demonstration of interleukin-2, interleukin-4 and interleukin-6 in sera from patients with localized scleroderma. Arch Dermatol Res. 1995;287:193–7.
172. Hasegawa M, Sato S, Nagaoka T, Fujimoto M, Takehara K. Serum levels of tumor necrosis factor and interleukin-13 are elevated in patients with localized scleroderma. Dermatology. 2003;207:141–7.
173. Shanmugam VK, Swistowski DR, Saddic N, Wang H, Steen VD. Comparison of indirect immunofluorescence and multiplex antinuclear antibody screening in systemic sclerosis. Clin Rheumatol. 2011;30: 1363–8.
174. Schwartzman-Morris J, Putterman C. Gender differences in the pathogenesis and outcome of lupus and lupus nephritis. Clin Dev Immunol. 2012;2012: 604892.
175. Sammaritano LR. Menopause in patients with autoimmune diseases. Autoimmun Rev. 2012;11: A430–6.
176. Font J, Pallares L, Cervera R, Lopez-Soto A, Navarro M, Bosch X, Ingelmo M. Systemic lupus onset in the elderly: clinical and immunological characteristics. Ann Rheum Dis. 1991;50:702–5.
177. Ho CTK, Mok CC, Lau CS, Wong RWS. Late onset systemic lupus erythematosus in southern Chinese. Ann Rheum Dis. 1998;57:437–40.
178. Peterson LS, Nelson AM, Su WP, Mason T, O'Fallon WM, Gabriel SE. The epidemiology of morphea (localized scleroderma in Olmstead County 1960–1993. J Rheumatol. 1997;24:73–80.
179. Wang J, Nuite M, McAlindon TE. Association of estrogen and aromatase gene polymorphisms with systemic lupus erythematosus. Lupus. 2010;19: 734–40.
180. Lu L-J, Wallace DJ, Ishimori ML, Scofield RH, Weisman MH. Male systemic lupus erythematosus: a review of sex disparities in this disease. Lupus. 2010;19:119–29.
181. Akahoshi M, Nakashima H, Tanaka Y, Kohsaka t, Nagano S, Ohgami E, Arinobu Y, Yamaoka K, Niiro H, Shinozaki M, Hirakata H, Horiuchi T, Otsuka T,

181. Niho Y. Th1/Th2 balance of peripheral T helper cells in systemic lupus erythematosus. Arthritis Rheum. 1999;42:1644–8.
182. Palma G, Barbieri A, Bimonte S, Palla M, Zappavigna S, Caraglia M, Ascierto PA, Ciliberto G, Arra C. Interleukin 18: friend or foe in cancer. Biochem Biophys Acta. 2013;1836:296–303.
183. Wang Y, Meng J, Wang X, Liu S, Shu Q, Gao L, Ju Y, Zhang L, Sun W, Ma C. Expression of human TIM-1 and TIM-3 on lymphocytes from systemic lupus erythematosus patients. Scand J Immunol. 2007;67:63–70.
184. Boddaert J, Huang DLT, Amoura Z, Wechler B, Godeau P, Piette JC. Late onset systemic lupus erythematosus: a personal series of 47 patients and pooled analysis of 714 cases in the literature. Medicine. 2004;83:348–59.
185. Mok CC, Lau CS, Ho CT, Wong RW. Do flares of systemic lupus erythematosus decline after menopause? Scand J Rheumatol. 1999;28:357–62.
186. Sanchez-Guerrero J, Villegas A, Mendoza-Feuntes A, Romero-Diaz J, Moreno-Coutino G, Cravioto MC. Disease activity during the premenopausal and post menopausal periods in women with SLE. Am J Med. 2001;111:464–8.
187. Namjou B, Scofield RH, Kelly JA, Goodman EL, Aberle T, Bruner GR, Harley JB. The effects of previous hysterectomy on lupus. Lupus. 2009;18:1000–5.
188. Cooper GS, Dooley MA, Treadwell EL, St Claire W, Gilkeson GS. Hormonal and reproductive risk factors for development of SLE: results of a population based case-control study. Arthritis Rheum. 2002;46:1830–9.
189. Costenbader KH, Feskanich D, Stampfer MJ, Kalson EW. Reproductive and menopausal factors and risk of SLE in women. Arthritis Rheum. 2007;56:1251–62.
190. Buyon JP, Petri M, Kim MY, Kalunian KC, Grossman J, Hahn BH, Merrill JT, Sammaritano L, Lockshin M, Alarcon GS, Manzi S, Belmont HM, Askanase AD, Sigler L, Dooley MA, von Feldt J, McCune WJ, Friedman A, Wachs J, Cronin M, Hearth-Holmes M, Tan M, Licciardi F. The effect of combined estrogen and progesterone hormone replacement therapy on disease activity in systemic lupus erythematosus. Ann Intern Med. 2005;142:953–62.
191. Urowitz MB, Ibanez D, Jerome D, Gladman DD. The effect of menopause on disease activity in systemic lupus erythematosus. J Rheumatol. 2006;33:2193–8.
192. Fernandez M, Calvo-Alen J, Alarcon G, Roseman JM, Bastian HM, Fessler BJ, McGwin Jr G, Vila LM, Sanchez ML, Reveille JD. Systemic lupus erythematosus in a multiethnic US cohort (LUMINA): XXI. Disease activity, damage accrual, and vascular events in pre-and postmenopausal women. Arthritis Rheum. 2005;52:1655–64.
193. Sticherling M. Systemic sclerosis- dermatological aspects. Part 1: pathogenesis, epidemiology, clinical findings. J Dtsch Dermatol Ges. 2012;10:705–18.
194. Toms TE, Panoulas VF, Kitas GD. Dyslipidaemia in rheumatological autoimmune diseases. Open Cardiov Med J. 2011;5:64–75.
195. Au K, Singh MK, Bodukam V, Bae S, Maranian P, Ogawa R, Spiegel B, McMahon M, Hahn B, Khanna D. Atherosclerosis in systemic sclerosis: a systemic review and meta-analysis. Arthritis Rheum. 2011;63:2078–90.
196. Viswanath V, Phiske MM, Gopalani VV. Systemic sclerosis: current concepts in pathogenesis and therapeutic aspects of dermatological manifestations. Indian J Dermatol. 2013;58:255–68.
197. Greenblatt MB, Aliprantis AO. The immune pathogenesis of scleroderma: context is everything. Curr Rheumatol Rep. 2013;15:297.
198. Battacharyya S, Kelly K, Melichian DS, Tamaki Z, Fang F, Su Y, Feng G, Pop RM, Budinger GRS, Mutlu GM, Lafyatis R, Tadstake T, Feghali-Bostwick C, Varga J. Toll-like receptor 4 signaling augments transforming growth factor-β responses: a novel mechanism for maintaining and amplifying fibrosis in scleroderma. Am J Pathol. 2013;182:192–205.
199. Giuggioli D, Manfredi A, Colaci M, Manzini CU, Antonelli A, Ferri C. Systemic sclerosis and cryoglbulinemia: our experience with overlapping syndrome of scleroderma and sever cryoglobulinemic vasculitis and review of the literature. Autoimmun Rev. 2013;12:1058–63.
200. Reddi DM, Cardona DM, Burchette JL, Puri PK. Scleroderma and IgG4-related disease. Am J Dermatopathol. 2013;35:458–62.
201. Quemeneur T, Mouthon L, Cacoub P, Meyer O, Michon-Pasturel U, Vanhille P, Hatron P-Y, Guillevin L, Hachull E. Systemic vasculitis during the course of systemic sclerosis: report of 12 cases and review of the literature. Medicine. 2013;92:1–9.
202. Nguyen C, Berenzne A, Baubet T, Mestre-Stanislas C, Rannou F, Papelard A, Merell-Dubois S, Revel M, Guillevin L, Poiraudeau S, Mouthon L, Groupe Francais de recherché sur la Sclerodermie. Association of gender with clinical expression, quality of life, disability, and depression and anxiety in patients with systemic sclerosis. PLoS One. 2011;6:e17551.
203. Lawrence RC, Helmick CG, Arnett FC, Deyo RA, Felson DT, Giannini EH, Heyse SP, Hirsch R, Hochberg MC, Hunder GG, Liang MH, Pillemer SR, Steen VD, Wolfe F. Estimates of the prevalence of arthritis and selected musculoskeletal disorders in the United States. Arthritis Rheum. 1998;41:778.
204. Loucks J, Pope JE. Osteoporosis in scleroderma. Semin Arhtits Rheum. 2004;34:678–82.
205. Pikwer M, Nilsson J-A, Bergstrom U, Jacobsson LTH, Turesson C. Early menopause and severity of rheumatoid arthritis in women older than 45 years. Arthritis Res Ther. 2012;14:R190.

206. Deal CL, Meenan RF, Goldenberg DL, Anderson JT, Sack B, Pastan RS, et al. The clinical features of elderly-onset rheumatic arthritis: a comparison with younger onset disease of similar duration. Arthritis Rheum. 1985;28:987–94.
207. Turkcapar N, Demir O, Atli T, Kopuk M, Turgay M, Kinikli G, et al. Late onset rheumatoid arthritis: clinical and laboratory comparisons with younger onset patients. Arch Gerontol Geriatr. 2006;42:225–31.
208. Nielsen RH, Christiansen C, Stolina M, Karsdal MA. Oestrogen exhibits type II collagen protective effects and attenuates collagen-induced arthritis in rats. Clin Exp Immunol. 2008;152:21–7.
209. Dolhain RJ, van der Heiden AN, ter Haar NT, Breedveld FC, Miltenburg AM. Shift toward T lymphocytes with a T helper 1 cytokine-secretion profile in the joints of patients with rheumatoid arthritis. Arthritis Rheum. 1996;39:1961–9.
210. Haddad A, Bienvenu J, Moissec P. Increased production of a Th2 cytokine profile by activated whole blood cells from rheumatoid arthritis patients. J Clin Immunol. 1998;18:399–403.
211. Van Roon JA, Verhoef CM, van Roy JL, Gmelig-Meyling FH, Huber-Bruning O, Lafever FP, Bijlsma JW. Decrease in peripheral type 1 over type 2 T cell cytokine production in patients with rheumatoid arthritis correlates with an increase in severity of disease. Ann Rheum Dis. 1997;56:656–60.
212. Ostenson M, Aune B, Husby G. Effect of pregnancy and hormonal changes on the activity of rheumatoid arthritis. Scand J Rheumatol. 1983;12:69–72.
213. Silman A, Kay A, Brennan P. Timing of pregnancy in relation to the onset of rheumatoid arthritis. Arthritis Rheum. 1992;35:152–5.
214. Hughes GC. Progesterone and autoimmune disease. Autoimmun Rev. 2012;11:A502–14.
215. Latman NS. Relation of menstrual cycle phase to symptoms of rheumatoid arthritis. Am J Med. 1983;74:957–60.
216. Linos A, Worthington JW, O'Fallon WM, Kurland LT. The epidemiology of rheumatoid arthritis in Rochester, Minnesota: a study of incidence, prevalence, and mortality. Am J Epidemiol. 1980;111:87–98.
217. Dugowson CE, Koepsell TD, Voigt LF, Bley L, Nelson JL, Daling JR. Rheumatoid arthritis in women: incidence rate in group health cooperative, Seattle, Washington, 1987–1989. Arthritis Rheum. 1991;34:1502–7.
218. Brennan P, Bankhead C, Silman A, Symmons D. Oral contraceptives and rheumatoid arthritis: results from a primary care-based incident case-control study. Semin Arthritis Rheum. 1997;26:817–23.
219. Hannaford PC, Kay CR, Hirsch S. Oral contraceptives and rheumatoid arthritis: new data from the Royal College of General Practitioners' oral contraception study. Ann Rheum Dis. 1990;49:744–6.
220. Vandenbroucke JP, Valkenburg HA, Boersma JW, Cats A, Festen JJ, Huber-Bruning O, Rasker JJ. Oral contraceptives and rheumatoid arthritis: further evidence for a preventative effect. Lancet. 1982;2:839–42.
221. Costenbader KH, Manson JE. Do female hormones affect the onset or severity of rheumatoid arthritis? Arthritis Rheum. 2008;59:299–301.
222. Wallace DJ. The Sjögren's Book. Oxford: Oxford University Press; 2012.
223. Mackay IR. Pathogenesis of Sjögrens. In: Wallace DJ, editor. The Sjögren's book. Oxford: Oxford University Press; 2012. p. 17–30.
224. Tegner P, Halse AK, Haga HJ, Jonsson R, Wahren-Herlenius M. Detection of anti-Ro/SSA and anti-La/SSB autoantibody-producing cells in salivary glands from patients with Sjögren's syndrome. Arthritis Rheum. 1998;41:2238–48.
225. Fox RI. Sjögren's syndrome. Lancet. 2005;366: 321–31.
226. Diaz-Lopez C, Geli C, Corominas H, Malat N, Diaz-Torner C, Llobet JM, de la Serna AR, Laiz A, Moreno M, Vasquez G. Are there clinical or serological differences between male and female patients with primary Sjögren's syndrome? J Rheumatol. 2004;31:1352–5.
227. Brennan M, Fox P. Sex differences in primary Sjögren's syndrome. J Rheumatol. 1999;26:2373–6.
228. Drosos A, Tsiakou E, Tsifetaki N, Politi EN, Siamopoulou-Mavridou A. Subgroups of primary Sjögren's syndrome. Sjögren's syndrome in male and pediatric Greek patients. Ann Rheum Dis. 1997;56:333–5.
229. Horvath IF, Szodoray P, Zeher M. Primary Sjögren's syndrome in men: clinical and immunological characteristics based on a large cohort of Hungarian patients. Clin Rheumatol. 2008;27:1479–83.
230. Ramos-Casals M, Solans R, Rosas J, Camps MT, Gil A, Del Pino-Montes J, Jimenez-Alonso J, Mico ML, Beltran J, Belenguer R, Pallares L, GEMESS Study Group. Primary Sjögren syndrome in Spain: clinical and immunologic expression in 1010 patients. Medicine (Baltimore). 2008;87:210–9.
231. Molina R, Provost T, Arnett F, Bias WB, Hochberg MC, Wilson RW, Alexander EL. Primary Sjögren's syndrome in men. Clinical, serologic, and immunogenetic features. Am J Med. 1986;80:23–31.
232. Goeb V, Salle V, Duhaut P, Jouen F, Smail A, Ducroix J-P, Tron F, Le Loet X, Vittecoq O. Clinical significance of autoantibodies recognizing Sjögren's syndrome A (SSA), SSB, calpastatin, and alpha-fodrin in primary Sjögren's syndrome. Clin Exp Immunol. 2007;148:281–7.
233. Allan TR, Parke A. Gynecological issues, including pregnancy. In: Wallace DJ, editor. The Sjögren's book. Oxford: Oxford University Press; 2012. p. 113–23.
234. Toda I, Sullivan BD, Rocha EM, da Silveira LA, Wickham LA, Sullivan DA. Impact of gender on exocrine gland inflammation in mouse models of Sjögren's syndrome. Exp Eye Res. 1999;69:355–66.
235. Cihakova D, Talor MV, Barin JG, Baldeviano GC, Fairweather D, Rose NR, Burek CL. Sex differences in a murine model of Sjorgren syndrome. Ann NY Acad Sci. 2009;1173:378–83.

236. Mostafa S, Seamon V, Azzarolo AM. Influence of sex hormones and genetic predisposition in Sjögren's syndrome: a new clue to the immunopathogenesis of dry eye disease. Exp Eye Res. 2012;96:88–97.
237. Toda I, Sullivan BD, Wickham LA, Sullivan DA. Gender- and androgen-related influence on the expression of proto-oncogene and apoptotic factor mRNAs in lacrimal glands of autoimmune and non-autoimmune mice. J Steroid Biochem Mol Biol. 1999;71:49–61.
238. Konttinen YT, Fuellen G, Bing Y, Porola P, Stegaev V, Trokovic N, Falk SSI, Szodoray P, Takakubo Y. Sex steroids in Sjögren's syndrome. J Autoimmun. 2012;39:49–56.
239. Agha-Hosseini F, Mirzaii-Dizgah I, Mansourian A, Khayamzadeh M. Relationship of stimulated saliva 17beta-estradiol and oral dryness feeling in menopause. Maturitas. 2009;62:197–9.
240. Michael D, Soi S, Cabera-Perez J, Weller M, Alexander S, Alevizos I, Illei GG, Chiorini JA. Microarray analysis of sexually dimorphic gene expression in human minor salivary glands. Oral Dis. 2011;17:653–61.
241. Nandula SR, Amarnath S, Molinolo A, Bandyopadhyay BC, Hall B, Goldsmith CM, Zheng C, Larsson J, Sreenath T, Chen W, Ambudkar IS, Karlsson S, Baum BJ, Kulkarni AB. Female mice are more susceptible to developing inflammatory disorders due to impaired transforming growth factor β signaling in salivary glands. Arthritis Rheum. 2007;56:1798–805.
242. Rocha EM, Wickham LA, Huang Z, Toda I, Gao J, da Silveira LA, Sullivan DA. Presence and testosterone influence on the levels of anti- and pro-inflammatory cytokines in lacrimal tissues of a mouse model of Sjögren's syndrome. Adv Exp Med Biol. 1998;438:485–91.
243. Valtysdottir ST, Wide L, Hallgren R. Low serum dehydroepiandrosterone sulfate in women with primary Sjögren's syndrome as an isolated sign of impaired HPA axis function. J Rheumatol. 2001;28:1259–65.
244. Forsblad-d'Elia H, Carlsten H, Labrie F, Konttinen YT, Ohlsson C. Low serum levels of sex steroids are associated with disease characteristics in primary Sjögren's syndrome: supplementation with dehydroepiandrosterone restores the concentrations. J Clin Endocrinol Metab. 2009;94:2044–51.
245. Chen YT, Lazarev S, Bahrami AF, Noble LB, Chen FY, Zhou D, Gallup M, Yadav M, McNamara NA. Interleukin-1 receptor mediates the interplay between CD4+ T cells and ocular resident cells to promote keratinizing squamous metaplasia in Sjögren's syndrome. Lab Invest. 2012;92:556–70.
246. Yamada A, Arakaki R, Kudo Y, Ishimaru N. Targeting IL-1 in Sjögren's syndrome. Exp Opin Ther Targets. 2013;17:393–401.
247. Perrier S, Coussediere C, Dubost JJ, Albuisson E, Sauvezie B. IL-1 receptor antagonist (IL-1RA) gene polymorphism in Sjögren's syndrome and rheumatoid arthritis. Clin Immunol Immunopathol. 1998;87:309–13.
248. Muraki Y, Tsutsumi A, Takahashi R, Suzuki E, Hayashi T, Chino Y, Goto D, Matsumoto I, Murata H, Noguchi E, Sumida T. Polymorphisms of IL-1 beta gene in Japanese patients with Sjögren's syndrome and systemic lupus erythematosus. J Rheumatol. 2004;31:720–5.
249. Bombardieri M, Barone F, Pittoni V, Alessandri C, Conigliaro P, Blades MC, Priori R, McInnes IB, Valesini G, Pitzalis C. Increased circulating levels and salivary gland expression of interleukin-18 in patients with Sjögren's syndrome: relationship with autoantibody production and lymphoid organization of the periductal inflammatory infiltrate. Arthritis Res Ther. 2004;6:R447–56.
250. Spadaro A, Rinaldi T, Riccieri V, Taccari E, Valesini G. Interleukin-13 in autoimmune rheumatic diseases: relationship with the autoantibody profile. Clin Exp Rheumatol. 2002;20:213–6.

Part V

Menopause, Quality of Life, and Healthy Aging

Postmenopausal Vulva and Vagina

27

Miranda A. Farage, Kenneth W. Miller, and Howard I. Maibach

Contents

27.1	**Introduction**	385
27.2	**Vulvar Skin Physiology**	386
27.3	**Vulvovaginal Atrophy**	387
27.4	**Urogenital Infections**	388
27.4.1	Urinary Tract Infections	388
27.4.2	Sexually Transmitted Infections	388
27.4.3	Desquamative Inflammatory Vaginitis (DIV)	388
27.5	**Urinary Incontinence**	389
27.6	**Vulvar Dermatoses**	392
27.7	**Summary**	392
References		393

M.A. Farage, MSc, PhD (✉)
Clinical Innovative Sciences, The Procter and Gamble Company, 6110 Center Hill Avenue, Cincinnati, OH 45224, USA
e-mail: Farage.m@pg.com

K.W. Miller, PhD
Global Product Stewardship, The Procter and Gamble Company, Cincinnati, OH USA
e-mail: Miller.kw.1@pg.com

H.I. Maibach, MD
Department of Dermatology, University of California, School of Medicine, San Francisco, CA, USA
e-mail: MaibachH@derm.ucsf.edu

27.1 Introduction

Menopause occurs when ovarian function ceases and estradiol production decreases to miniscule levels. Although peripheral androgen conversion by the adrenals continues to produce a low level of estrogen after menopause, overall circulating levels decline dramatically from greater than 120 pg/mL to about 18 pg/mL [1]. The perimenopausal transition begins sometime after the age of 45 and lasts about 4 years. A constellation of symptoms emerges as follicular function declines. The most notable is menstrual cycle irregularity, reflecting an increase in the number anovulatory cycles and cycles with a prolonged follicular phase. Other symptoms can include cramps, bloating or breast tenderness, vasomotor symptoms ("hot flashes"), migraine headaches, and vaginal dryness. Menopause has transpired when a woman has not menstruated for a year [2]. Median age of menopause in a multiethnic sample of American women was 51.4 years [3].

Vulvovaginal and urethral epithelia have high levels of estrogen receptors that mediate hormonal action on the tissue. Consequently, the dramatic drop in circulating estrogen that accompanies menopause profoundly affects urogenital tissue structure and function. This chapter discusses postmenopausal vulvovaginal changes, with an emphasis on alterations in vulvar skin physiology, tissue atrophy, urinary changes, and susceptibility to infection. Vulvar dermatoses that are more common in older women are also discussed.

27.2 Vulvar Skin Physiology

Skin hydration, coefficient of friction, and permeability of vulvar skin differ from that of exposed skin (reviewed in [4, 5]). Although menopause affects these parameters on exposed skin, age-related effects on vulvar skin appear negligible (Table 27.1). In brief, keratinized skin of the labia majora is more hydrated than forearm skin as measured by trans-epidermal water loss [6], and its coefficient of friction is higher [7]. Following menopause, small differences in these parameters have been measured on exposed skin, but changes in the water barrier function and friction coefficient of vulvar skin are insignificant [7].

Skin penetration of hydrocortisone and testosterone also has been compared on the forearm and on the vulva. (For perspective, penetration of testosterone but not hydrocortisone is mediated by androgen receptors.) In young women, vulvar skin is more permeable to hydrocortisone than forearm skin; however, following menopause, skin penetration of this steroid drops on the forearm but not on the vulva. By contrast, comparable testosterone penetration rates were measured at both sites in younger women, and menopause had no impact on testosterone penetration at either site [8].

Studies with the model irritant, sodium lauryl sulfate, revealed differences in susceptibility to skin irritation between exposed skin and vulvar

Table 27.1 Comparative skin physiology and menopausal status

Site	Menopausal status[a]	Observation	Significance[b]	Reference
Water barrier function (TEWL, $g/m^2 \cdot h$)				
Forearm	Premenopausal	3.7±0.4	$p<0.05$	Elsner and Maibach [6]
	Postmenopausal	2.6±0.3		
Vulva	Premenopausal	14.8±1.5	n.s.	
	Postmenopausal	13.5±1.8		
Friction coefficient, μ				
Forearm	Premenopausal	0.49±0.02	$p<0.05$	Elsner et al. [7]
	Postmenopausal	0.45±0.01		
Vulva	Premenopausal	0.60±0.04	n.s.	
	Postmenopausal	0.60±0.06		
Hydrocortisone penetration (% dose absorbed)				
Forearm	Premenopausal	2.8±2.4	n.s.	Oriba et al. [8]
	Postmenopausal	1.5±1.1		
Vulva	Premenopausal	8.1±4.1	$p<0.01$	Schagen van Leeuwen et al. [9]
	Postmenopausal	4.4±2.8		
Testosterone penetration (% dose absorbed)				
Forearm	Premenopausal	20.2±8.1	n.s.	Oriba et al. [8]
	Postmenopausal	14.7±4.2		
Vulva	Premenopausal	26.7±8.0	n.s.	
	Postmenopausal	24.6±5.5		
Visual erythema scores (scored on day 2 after 24-h postexposure to 1 % sodium lauryl sulfate)				
Forearm	Premenopausal	9	$p=0.03$	Elsner et al. [10]
	Postmenopausal	5		
Vulva	Premenopausal	0	n.s.	
	Postmenopausal	0		

Adapted with kind permission from Miranda Farage and Howard Maibach [11]
[a]Group sizes (water barrier function and friction parameters): premenopausal, 34 subjects, postmenopausal, 10 subjects. Group sizes (hydrocortisone and testosterone penetration): 9 subjects in each age group visual erythema score to sodium lauryl sulfate. Sodium lauryl sulfate application: 10 subjects per age group
[b]n.s. not significant

skin. Forearm skin was far more susceptible to the model irritant, aqueous sodium lauryl sulfate (1 % w/v): this agent caused intense erythema on the forearms of premenopausal women but no visually discernible response on the vulva in either pre- or postmenopausal women [10].

27.3 Vulvovaginal Atrophy

Vulvovaginal atrophy often develops as hormonal stimulation declines through the menopausal transition (reviewed in [11, 12]). Reportedly, 10–50 % of postmenopausal women exhibit clinical signs and symptoms (Table 27.2) [14–16].

Table 27.2 Signs and symptoms of urogenital atrophy

	Signs	Symptoms
Vulvar changes	Sparse pubic hair	Itching, burning, soreness
	Shrunken labia	
	Inelastic labial skin	
	Introital narrowing or stenosis	
	Peri-introital lacerations	
	Phimotic clitoral hood	
	Fibrosed glans clitoris	
	Irritation of the posterior fourchette	
Vaginal changes	Smooth, pale, friable vaginal mucosa	Vaginal dryness
	Limited vaginal secretions	Coital discomfort or dyspareunia
	Vaginal pH >4.5	Malodorous discharge (in cases of infection)
	Higher proportion of immature basal cells on Pap smear	Burning leukorrhea (desquamative inflammatory vaginitis)
Urinary changes	Eversion of urethral mucosa	Urinary frequency
	Ecchymoses	Dysuria
		Nocturia
		Urinary tract infection

Adapted with permission from Farage et al. [13]

Pubic hair becomes sparse, the labia majora lose subcutaneous fat, and the labia minora and vestibule atrophy [17, 18]. In addition, the introitus narrows, the clitoral hood may become phimotic, and the exposed glans clitoris may fibrose. At the cytological level, estrogen-induced parakeratosis of vulvar stratum corneum, which is highest in the third decade of life, is rarely observed by the eighth decade [19].

Vaginal changes also ensue. The vaginal vault becomes shorter and narrower, losing its typical folds (rugae). Blood flow decreases and vaginal lubrication declines. As the epithelium thins, it becomes susceptible to friction-induced bleeding. Moreover, the loss of a glycogen-rich environment both disfavors colonization by lactic acid-producing microbes [20] and reduces hydrogen ion production by vaginal epithelial cells [21, 22]. Consequently, vaginal pH rises above 4.5, which heightens susceptibility to vaginal infection. A Papanicolaou smear of the upper third of the vagina reveals a higher proportion of parabasal cells and lower levels of superficial squamous cells [23–25].

Genital symptoms include decreased vaginal secretions, vaginal irritation, vulvar pruritus, dyspareunia, and postcoital bleeding [12]. Urinary symptoms include urethral discomfort, increased frequency, and dysuria [12]. If the vulvovaginal microbiota becomes disturbed, malodorous vaginal discharge, vulvovaginal inflammation, or recurrent urinary tract infection may accompany atrophic changes. In the patient free of infection, a vaginal pH of greater than 5 is a sign of hypoestrogenism [20, 23].

Only about 25 % of women who experience symptoms mention them to their health-care provider, as many consider their discomfort to be an inevitable consequence of aging. However, urinary pain, vulvovaginal irritation, or dyspareunia secondary to vaginal atrophy may prompt a woman to seek treatment. Low-dose, intravaginal estrogen therapy ameliorates vulvovaginal atrophy without significant systemic side effects and is the conservative and recommended choice when hormone supplementation is considered solely for the relief of this condition [26, 27]. Randomized trials of an ultralow-dose, 10-μg estradiol tablet demonstrated efficacy in normalizing vaginal pH and vaginal cytology and in reducing the most bothersome symptoms of atrophy [28, 29]. This dose exhibited low overall systemic absorption and was associated with no significant evidence of endometrial hyperplasia [28]. The North American Menopause Society concludes that opposing progestogen is generally not indicated at the low estrogen doses administered locally for vaginal atrophy [26, 27].

Intravaginal administration of dehydroepiandrosterone (DHEA), an androgenic sex steroid precursor, has been proposed as an alternative approach to treating postmenopausal vaginal atrophy and associated sexual dysfunction [30, 31]. Locally applied DHEA is converted by vaginal cells to estrogens and androgens without affecting serum concentrations of estradiol or testosterone, thereby avoiding effects on other organs [32]. In randomized trials, treatment improved clinical signs of atrophy (pH, cytology, vaginal secretions, and epithelial thickness) and measures of sexual health [30, 31]. However, in contrast to intravaginal estradiol therapy, which requires application of a tablet two to three times a week, DHEA requires daily dosing of a cream preparation, a regimen that women may find more onerous [33]. The North American Menopause Society (NAMS) Web site (menopause.org) is a good source of information on treatment options for health conditions associated with menopause.

27.4 Urogenital Infections

27.4.1 Urinary Tract Infections

Escherichia coli is the primary organism involved in urinary tract infections (UTIs), and the vagina is a reservoir for urethral colonization [34–36]. As circulating estrogen declines, cell densities of lactic acid-producing microbes fall, and the incidence of vaginal colonization with *E. coli* rises [37]. This elevates the risk of UTIs. Insulin-dependent diabetes and a prior history of recurrent UTIs are associated with higher risk of UTIs after menopause [38]. Although the number of studies is limited [39, 40], a meta-analysis found evidence that intravaginal estradiol therapy may reduce the risk of urinary tract infection [41]. However, the therapy does not have regulatory approval in the USA for this indication.

27.4.2 Sexually Transmitted Infections

Many people remain sexually active in old age and can be at risk of acquiring sexually transmitted infection. Transmission of genital herpes simplex remains pertinent, and both women with an intact cervix and women who have undergone a hysterectomy can acquire trichomonadal, gonorrheal, or chlamydial infection. With advent of modern treatment, HIV/AIDS is now a chronic illness in the developed world; infected people can now live into their 70s or longer and may transmit the disease. The use of condoms should be encouraged. Sexually transmitted infection among older adults is a sensitive subject that may be facilitated in the clinical setting with a non-threatening conversation and by using patient education pamphlets.

27.4.3 Desquamative Inflammatory Vaginitis (DIV)

Women over age 40 can suffer from desquamative inflammatory vaginitis, a rare inflammatory vaginal infection that occurs primarily in white women [42, 43]. It produces a copious, purulent discharge, and the vulva and vaginal vault appear glazed due to epithelial sloughing. Vaginal pH is greater than 4.5, but the "whiff test" is negative (no fishy odor when a drop of vaginal secretion is added to 10 % aqueous potassium hydroxide). Microscopy reveals an outpouring of inflammatory white cells (a hallmark sign), a paucity of lactobacilli, large numbers of other bacteria, and a preponderance of immature, squamous vaginal epithelial cells. Typical treatment is a 2-week course of clindamycin. Prognosis is good if there is a favorable initial response, but in some cases, long-term maintenance therapy is required.

27.5 Urinary Incontinence

Urinary incontinence is underreported condition. It may emerge prior to menopause, but incidence increases with age. Reported prevalence rates vary depending on the condition (stress, urge, or mixed incontinence) and demographic variables (age, race, parity, body mass index, etc.) [44]. Reported rates range from 10 to 40 % among subgroups of community-dwelling individuals [45, 46] and from 43 to 77 % among nursing home residents [47].

Stress and urge incontinence have different symptoms and underlying pathology (Table 27.3). Stress incontinence involves the uncontrolled loss of urine induced by sudden pressure on the abdominal organs (such as a cough, a sneeze, heavy lifting, exercise, or coital penetration). It stems from a weakened sphincter at the junction of the bladder and urethra. Stress incontinence may be first experienced by younger women aged 30–50 when the bladder sphincter is weakened by childbirth. However, its incidence peaks during the perimenopausal period (between the ages 45 and 49) [46], possibly because aging manifests the underlying weakness. Another important factor is obesity, which places additional stress on the bladder. Obese women (BMI ≥30) have twice the risk of developing stress incontinence independent of age and parity. Epidemiological data indicate that each 5-unit increase in BMI is associated with 20–70 % increase in urinary incontinence risk [48].

Urogenital prolapse, the downward descent of the internal urogenital organs toward the vagina due to weakened support, can coexist with stress incontinence. Relaxation of the musculature of the vaginal vault and weakening of the pelvic muscles due to childbirth contributes to urogenital prolapse.

Mild stress incontinence is manageable with pelvic muscle training (Kegel exercises), by limiting fluid intake, by more frequent voiding, and with the use of feminine pads. Pelvic floor muscle exercises are more effective in younger than older women [49]. Devices for stress incontinence include pessaries and urethral orifice plugs, but most women are disinclined to use them.

Table 27.3 Types of urinary incontinence in adult women[a]

	Stress	Urge
Patient population	Women aged 30–50, especially those who have given birth. Incidence rises with age	Older, usually postmenopausal women (>age 50)
Symptoms	Uncontrolled urine loss when sudden pressure is applied to the bladder (e.g., sneezing, coughing, lifting heavy objects, intercourse)	Increased frequency and urgency Inability to suppress urine loss
Causes	Weakness of the sphincter muscle at the junction of the bladder neck and the urethra	Overactive bladder muscle (i.e., stronger, more frequent bladder contractions at lower urine volumes); weakened outlet
Risk factors	Childbirth; obesity; genital prolapse; Caucasian race	Childbirth may contribute to the problem in younger women by weakening the outlet; the risk after age 50 is independent of childbearing history and may reflect age-related changes
Mechanism	Nerve or sphincter muscle damage or damage to the connective tissue supporting the bladder neck	Impaired nerve-brain reflexes regulating bladder wall contractions; shortening and thinning of the urethra after menopause; slower and less efficient voiding (retention). Childbirth may weaken the outlet, making the impact of bladder contractions more apparent
Treatment	Pelvic floor muscle training (Kegel exercises)	Behavioral modifications
	Surgery (least conservative)	Antimuscarinic drugs

Adapted from Farage et al. [13]
[a]Mixed stress-urge occurs in 30 % of cases

Duloxetine, a serotonin and noradrenaline reuptake inhibitor used to treat mood disorder, reduces the frequency of stress incontinence in randomized controlled trials in younger and postmenopausal women [9, 50, 51]. It is approved for this indication in Europe but not in the USA. In overweight or obese women, weight loss is a first-line intervention for stress urinary incontinence. For severe cases of stress incontinence, surgery is the least conservative remaining option for therapy; however, a paucity of data exists on the effectiveness of surgery in the older postmenopausal patient.

Urge incontinence involves the strong urge to urinate and inability to voluntarily control urine loss. Urge incontinence is unpredictable and more distressing when involving large urine losses. An abnormality in the sensory reflex mechanism causes heightened contractions (spasms) in the bladder wall, exerting pressure on the bladder neck and creating a feeling of urgency at lower urine volumes than is typical. Childbirth may contribute to sphincter weakness, so that the impact of bladder contractions is more apparent.

Several therapeutic approaches exist for this condition. Efficacious antimuscarinic drugs (e.g., oxybutynin, Tolterodine) block cholinergic muscarinic receptors associated with uncontrolled bladder contractions [52]. Common side effects are dry mouth and constipation. Anticholinergic drugs are contraindicated in patients with documented untreated narrow-angle glaucoma. Behavioral interventions include moderating fluid intake (although low intakes may increase contractions at lower urine volumes); bladder retraining through scheduled voids and conscious urge suppression; limiting caffeine, alcohol, and diuretics; and adding dietary fiber or probiotics to avoid constipation. Kegel exercises may alleviate the contribution of a weakened sphincter but will not affect bladder contractions.

Interstitial cystitis is a poorly understood condition with symptoms that may contribute to urinary frequency and urge incontinence (reviewed in [53, 54]). One prevailing theory is that compromise of the protective mucus layer of bladder mucosa (possibly from prior injury, subclinical infection, or autoimmune destruction) is a precipitating event. Potassium ions, present at high concentration in urine, cross this "leaky" epithelium, triggering chronic inflammation, injury, and neuronal damage to the bladder interstitium. Interstitial cystitis manifests as symptoms of urgency, frequency, burning pain associated with bladder filling, and dysuria. Patients with interstitial cystitis but not those with healthy bladders are sensitive to instilled potassium (potassium sensitivity test), which elicits reduced bladder capacity and pain. In the early stages of the condition, the patient may not recognize the increased voiding as dysfunctional; however, pain and greater frequency develop as the disease progresses. Most patients with this condition also experience dyspareunia. Interstitial cystitis often coexists with vulvodynia [55–57] and that both conditions may have a neurogenic component [58]. Because interstitial cystitis is associated with bladder pain, dysuria, high voiding frequency, low void volumes, and nocturia, it shares the symptomatic characteristics of overactive bladder syndrome or urge incontinence.

For the active, community-dwelling older woman with urinary incontinence [59], feminine protection is the self-treatment option of choice. She will search for other options only when symptoms become too difficult to manage or when she fears her symptoms signal pathology. Consequently, it is up to the clinician to broach the subject sensitively as part of the medical history: simple algorithms (such as the Three Incontinence Questions [3IQ] questionnaire [60]) can be offered to assist the patient in defining the nature and cause of her symptoms (stress, urge, or mixed incontinence).

For the older woman unable to maintain adequate perineal hygiene independently, incontinence dermatitis can become a significant problem. Several factors contribute to its development [59] (see Chap. 17 in this book) (Fig. 27.1). First, chronic exposure to urinary moisture makes the skin more susceptible to friction damage; in the older adult, excess skin hydration is dissipated more slowly than in younger people [61]. Bacterial action on the urine generates urinary ammonia, which elevates the local pH; this alters skin barrier function and

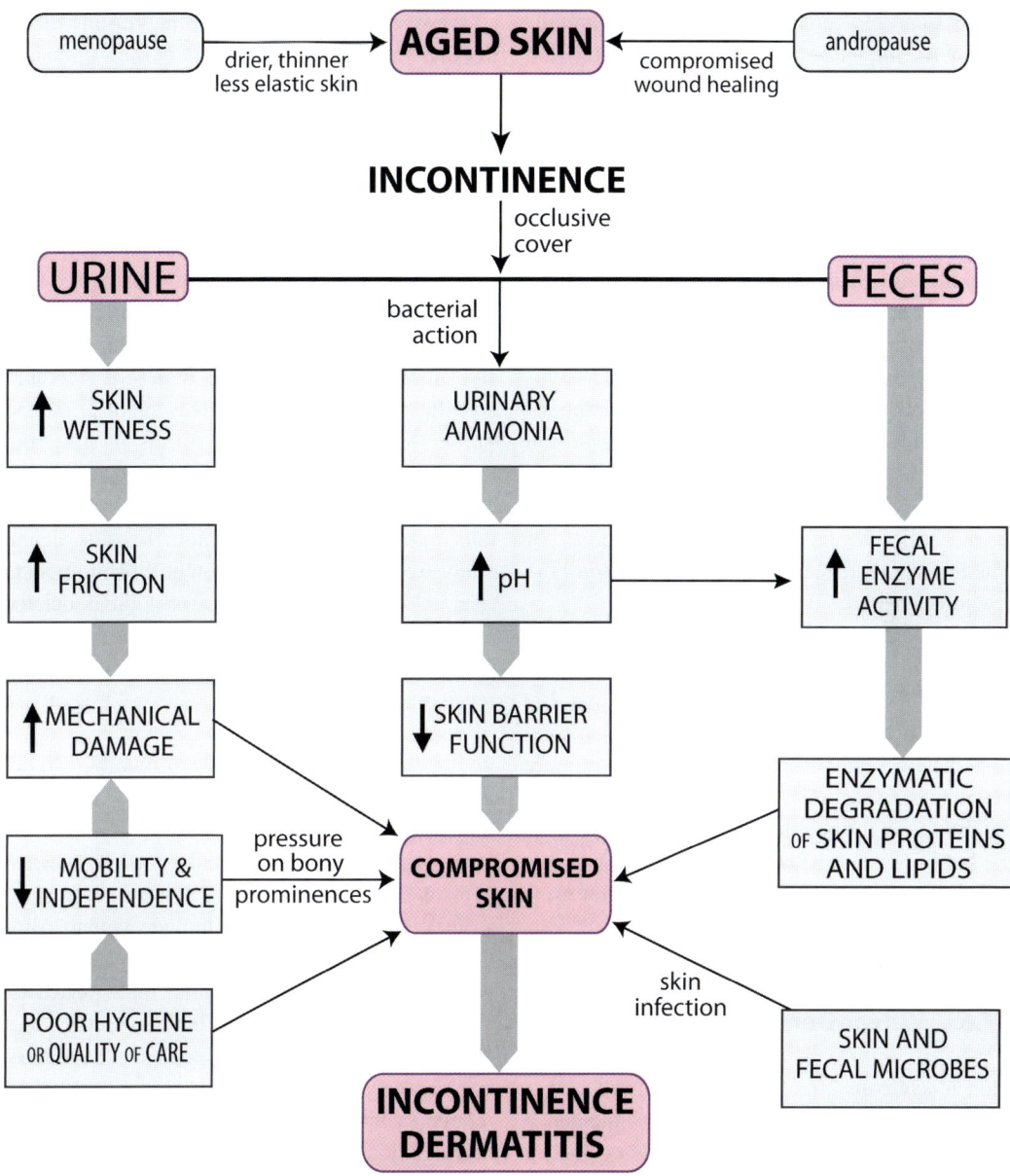

Fig. 27.1 Risk factors for incontinence dermatitis in the older person

activates fecal enzymes, which further compromise skin integrity and increase skin susceptibility to microbial infection [62–65]. Atrophied genital tissue is especially susceptible to pH changes and to enzymatic action. Moreover, in the incapacitated patient, reduced mobility creates higher shear forces on the tissue, a trigger for the development of decubitus ulcers (pressure sores). Lastly, those with impaired cognition may be unable to alert caregivers to incontinent episodes. These factors underscore the need for vigilant hygiene and physical assistance for the older adult with incontinence.

In community-dwelling individuals receiving home care, helpful interventions include prompted or timed toileting, use of incontinence garments, use of antimuscarinic drugs where appropriate [66, 67], and assistance with perineal care. In nursing homes, urine containment with incontinence products is a first-line intervention. Catheterization is sometimes used but carries the risk of infection. Behavioral interventions such as prompted voiding and timed voiding are used to a limited degree, and antimuscarinics are only an adjunct treatment [68]. Prompted voiding involves caregivers checking and querying patients, giving toileting prompts, and reinforcing initiative on the part of the patient. In randomized trials, prompted voiding over the course of 3 months was associated with small improvements in daytime incontinence in nursing homes where the population had substantial cognitive and mobility limitations [69]. Timed voiding is bringing the patient to the toilet at fixed intervals regardless of whether she requests it or has voided during the previous interval.

In the USA, an estimated 16 billion dollars annually is spent on urinary incontinence management [70]; in nursing homes, an hour per day is spent on dealing with incontinence at a total cost per incontinent patient of approximately $10,000 per year [37]. By 2030, it is estimated that one in eight people worldwide will be over the age of 65, and the economic impact of incontinence management will become even more significant [71].

27.6 Vulvar Dermatoses

Lichen sclerosus affects the skin and the vulvovaginal mucosa (reviewed in [72]). Incidence peaks bimodally, rising in adolescents and in peri- or postmenopausal women. Symptoms are intense vulvar itch, soreness, pain, and dyspareunia, but there is no abnormal vaginal discharge. White polygonal plaques with a wrinkled appearance appear bilaterally on the vulva; the labia, vestibule, and introitus as well as the perineum can be affected. Advanced disease is typified by a "keyhole" or "figure-eight" configuration of sclerotic tissue surrounding the introitus and anus. Potent topical corticosteroids or macrolides are used to manage symptoms and retard disease progression.

Erosive lichen planus is a rare, chronic disorder that affects only the mucosa of the vagina and vulvar vestibule; vulvar skin is unaffected [72]. Peak incidence is between the ages of 30 and 70. Signs and symptoms include intense vulvar itch and pain, dyspareunia, excessive discharge, and postcoital bleeding. Discharge is due to erosive shedding, and the vaginal epithelium may bleed upon speculum insertion. These signs and symptoms mimic those of desquamative inflammatory vaginitis, but the distinguishing features of erosive lichen planus are the absence of infection and the presence of white, lacy plaques on the vulvar vestibule and inner aspects of the labia minora. White plaques on the oral mucosa (buccal mucosa, gingiva, palate, or tongue) are a common extragenital manifestation. Erosive lichen planus requires the use of potent topical steroids (e.g., clobetasol propionate) or topical macrolides (tacrolimus). Oral corticosteroids (e.g., prednisone) are a second-line treatment for more recalcitrant cases.

27.7 Summary

Vulvovaginal atrophy secondary to hypoestrogenism affects 10–50 % of postmenopausal women. Genital symptoms include vulvar irritation and pruritus, decreased vaginal secretions, vaginal burning, dyspareunia, and postcoital bleeding; urinary symptoms include urethral discomfort, frequency, and dysuria. Low-dose, intravaginal estrogen therapy is an option to relieve symptoms of vulvovaginal atrophy and improve quality of life. Although the risk factors and precipitating events vary, postmenopausal women are also more likely to experience stress or urge incontinence. Stress incontinence, linked to childbirth or obesity, is uncontrolled urine loss provoked by abdominal pressure on a weakened bladder sphincter. Urge incontinence is the inability to suppress voiding and is likely due to age-related changes in the nervous system that cause abnormal bladder spasms; however, interstitial cystitis, thought to result from a disrupted bladder mucosal barrier, mimics some of the symptoms of urge incontinence. Women are unlikely to seek treatment until their symptoms become highly disruptive: health-care providers can assist by sensitively broaching the subject and by providing literature that describes these conditions and available treatment options. Vigilant perineal hygiene in the older person who is unable to care for herself is critical to avoiding incontinence dermatitis. Lastly, certain rare infections and vulvar dermatoses are more prevalent in postmenopausal women. Desquamative inflammatory vaginitis is a persistent inflammatory vaginal infection that erodes the vaginal mucosa and requires aggressive antibiotic treatment. Lichen sclerosus is a vulvar dermatosis of the skin as well as the mucosa. White, wrinkled polygonal plaques manifest bilaterally and may become sclerotic. Erosive lichen planus affects only the mucosa and causes discharge with shedding of the vaginal epithelium. Although its signs and symptoms mimic those of desquamative inflammatory vaginitis, its distinguishing features are the absence of infection and the presence of white, lacy plaques on the vulvar vestibule and inner aspects of the labia minora. Potent topical corticosteroids are used in treatment of both these dermatoses.

References

1. Pandit L, Ouslander JG. Postmenopausal vaginal atrophy and atrophic vaginitis. Am J Med Sci. 1997;314(4):228–31.
2. Burger HG. The menopausal transition. Baillieres Clin Obstet Gynaecol. 1996;10(3):347–59.
3. Gold EB, Bromberger J, Crawford S, Samuels S, Greendale GA, Harlow SD, Skurnick J. Factors associated with age at natural menopause in a multiethnic sample of midlife women. Am J Epidemiol. 2001;153(9):865–74.
4. Oriba HA, Elsner P, Maibach HI. Vulvar physiology. Semin Dermatol. 1989;8(1):2–6.
5. Farage MA, Maibach HI. Morphology and physiological changes of genital skin and mucosa. Curr Probl Dermatol. 2011;40:9–19. doi:10.1159/000321042.
6. Elsner P, Maibach HI. The effect of prolonged drying on transepidermal water loss, capacitance and pH of human vulvar and forearm skin. Acta Derm Venereol. 1990;70(2):105–9.
7. Elsner P, Wilhelm D, Maibach HI. Frictional properties of human forearm and vulvar skin: influence of age and correlation with transepidermal water loss and capacitance. Dermatologica. 1990;181(2):88–91.
8. Oriba HA, Bucks DA, Maibach HI. Percutaneous absorption of hydrocortisone and testosterone on the vulva and forearm: effect of the menopause and site. Br J Dermatol. 1996;134(2):229–33.
9. Schagen van Leeuwen JH, Lange RR, Jonasson AF, Chen WJ, Viktrup L. Efficacy and safety of duloxetine in elderly women with stress urinary incontinence or stress-predominant mixed urinary incontinence. Maturitas. 2008;60(2):138–47. doi:10.1016/j.maturitas.2008.04.012.
10. Elsner P, Wilhelm D, Maibach HI. Effect of low-concentration sodium lauryl sulfate on human vulvar and forearm skin. Age-related differences. J Reprod Med. 1991;36(1):77–81.
11. Farage MA, Maibach H. Lifetime changes in the vulva and vagina. Arch Gynecol Obstet. 2006;273(4):195–202. doi:10.1007/s00404-005-0079-x.
12. Bachmann GA, Nevadunsky NS. Diagnosis and treatment of atrophic vaginitis. Am Fam Physician. 2000;61(10):3090–6.
13. Farage MA, Miller KW, Ledger WL. Confronting the challenges of postmenopausal urogenital health. Aging Health. 2010;6(5):611–26.
14. Greendale GA, Judd HL. The menopause: health implications and clinical management. J Am Geriatr Soc. 1993;41(4):426–36.
15. Stenberg A, Heimer G, Ulmsten U, Cnattingius S. Prevalence of genitourinary and other climacteric symptoms in 61-year-old women. Maturitas. 1996;24(1–2):31–6.
16. van Geelen JM, van de Weijer PH, Arnolds HT. Urogenital symptoms and resulting discomfort in non-institutionalized Dutch women aged 50–75 years. Int Urogynecol J Pelvic Floor Dysfunct. 2000;11(1):9–14.
17. Erickson KL, Montagna W. New observations on the anatomical features of the female genitalia. J Am Med Womens Assoc. 1972;27(11):573–81.
18. Jones IS. A histological assessment of normal vulval skin. Clin Exp Dermatol. 1983;8(5):513–21.
19. Nauth HF, Boger A. New aspects of vulvar cytology. Acta Cytol. 1982;26(1):1–6.
20. Caillouette JC, Sharp Jr CF, Zimmerman GJ, Roy S. Vaginal pH as a marker for bacterial pathogens and menopausal status. Am J Obstet Gynecol. 1997;176(6):1270–5; discussion 1275–7.
21. Gorodeski GI. Effects of estrogen on proton secretion via the apical membrane in vaginal-ectocervical epithelial cells of postmenopausal women. Menopause. 2005;12(6):679–84.
22. Gorodeski GI, Hopfer U, Liu CC, Margles E. Estrogen acidifies vaginal pH by up-regulation of proton secretion via the apical membrane of vaginal-ectocervical epithelial cells. Endocrinology. 2005;146(2):816–24.
23. Brizzolara S, Killeen J, Severino R. Vaginal pH and parabasal cells in postmenopausal women. Obstet Gynecol. 1999;94(5 Pt 1):700–3.

24. Hess R, Austin RM, Dillon S, Chang CC, Ness RB. Vaginal maturation index self-sample collection in mid-life women: acceptability and correlation with physician-collected samples. Menopause. 2010;15 (4 Pt 1):726–9.
25. McEndree B. Clinical application of the vaginal maturation index. Nurse Pract. 1999;24(9):48, 51–2, 55–6.
26. North American Menopause Society. Estrogen and progestogen use in postmenopausal women: 2010 position statement of The North American Menopause Society. Menopause. 2010;17(2):242–55.
27. Sturdee DW, Panay N. Recommendations for the management of postmenopausal vaginal atrophy. Climacteric J Int Menopause Soc. 2010;13(6):509–22. doi:10.3109/13697137.2010.522875.
28. Panay N, Maamari R. Treatment of postmenopausal vaginal atrophy with 10-mug estradiol vaginal tablets. Menopause Int. 2012;18(1):15–9. doi:10.1258/mi.2012.011120.
29. Simon J, Nachtigall L, Gut R, Lang E, Archer DF, Utian W. Effective treatment of vaginal atrophy with an ultra-low-dose estradiol vaginal tablet. Obstet Gynecol. 2008;112(5):1053–60.
30. Labrie F, Archer D, Bouchard C, Fortier M, Cusan L, Gomez JL, Girard G, Baron M, Ayotte N, Moreau M, Dube R, Cote I, Labrie C, Lavoie L, Berger L, Gilbert L, Martel C, Balser J. Intravaginal dehydroepiandrosterone (prasterone), a physiological and highly efficient treatment of vaginal atrophy. Menopause. 2009;16(5):907–22.
31. Labrie F, Archer D, Bouchard C, Fortier M, Cusan L, Gomez JL, Girard G, Baron M, Ayotte N, Moreau M, Dube R, Cote I, Labrie C, Lavoie L, Berger L, Gilbert L, Martel C, Balser J. Effect of intravaginal dehydroepiandrosterone (prasterone) on libido and sexual dysfunction in postmenopausal women. Menopause. 2009;16(5):923–31.
32. Labrie F, Cusan L, Gomez JL, Cote I, Berube R, Belanger P, Martel C, Labrie C. Effect of intravaginal DHEA on serum DHEA and eleven of its metabolites in postmenopausal women. J Steroid Biochem Mol Biol. 2008;111(3–5):178–94.
33. Panjari M, Davis SR. Vaginal DHEA to treat menopause related atrophy: a review of the evidence. Maturitas. 2011;70(1):22–5. doi:10.1016/j.maturitas.2011.06.005.
34. Navas-Nacher EL, Dardick F, Venegas MF, Anderson BE, Schaeffer AJ, Duncan JL. Relatedness of Escherichia coli colonizing women longitudinally. Mol Urol. 2001;5(1):31–6. doi:10.1089/10915360 1750124285.
35. Norinder BS, Luthje P, Yadav M, Kadas L, Fang H, Nord CE, Brauner A. Cellulose and PapG are important for Escherichia coli causing recurrent urinary tract infection in women. Infection. 2011;39(6):571–4. doi:10.1007/s15010-011-0199-0.
36. Farage MA, Miller KW, Sobel JD. The vaginal microbiota in menopause. In: Farage MA, Miller KW, Maibach H, editors. Textbook of aging skin. Berlin: Springer; 2010. p. 883–93.
37. Borrie MJ, Davidson HA. Incontinence in institutions: costs and contributing factors. CMAJ. 1992;147(3):322–8.
38. Jackson SL, Boyko EJ, Scholes D, Abraham L, Gupta K, Fihn SD. Predictors of urinary tract infection after menopause: a prospective study. Am J Med. 2004;117(12):903–11.
39. Eriksen B. A randomized, open, parallel-group study on the preventive effect of an estradiol-releasing vaginal ring (Estring) on recurrent urinary tract infections in postmenopausal women. Am J Obstet Gynecol. 1999;180(5):1072–9.
40. Raz R, Stamm WE. A controlled trial of intravaginal estriol in postmenopausal women with recurrent urinary tract infections. N Engl J Med. 1993;329(11):753–6.
41. Cardozo L, Lose G, McClish D, Versi E, de Koning Gans H. A systematic review of estrogens for recurrent urinary tract infections: third report of the hormones and urogenital therapy (HUT) committee. Int Urogynecol J Pelvic Floor Dysfunct. 2001;12(1):15–20.
42. Sobel JD, Reichman O, Misra D, Yoo W. Prognosis and treatment of desquamative inflammatory vaginitis. Obstet Gynecol. 2011;117(4):850–5. doi:10.1097/AOG.0b013e3182117c9e.
43. Sobel JD. Desquamative inflammatory vaginitis: a new subgroup of purulent vaginitis responsive to topical 2% clindamycin therapy. Am J Obstet Gynecol. 1994;171(5):1215–20.
44. Mallett VT. Female urinary incontinence: what the epidemiologic data tell us. Int J Fertil Womens Med. 2005;50(1):12–7.
45. Anger JT, Saigal CS, Litwin MS. The prevalence of urinary incontinence among community dwelling adult women: results from the National Health and Nutrition Examination Survey. J Urol. 2006;175(2):601–4.
46. Hannestad YS, Rortveit G, Sandvik H, Hunskaar S. A community-based epidemiological survey of female urinary incontinence: the Norwegian EPINCONT study. Epidemiology of Incontinence in the County of Nord-Trondelag. J Clin Epidemiol. 2000;53(11):1150–7.
47. Offermans MP, Du Moulin MF, Hamers JP, Dassen T, Halfens RJ. Prevalence of urinary incontinence and associated risk factors in nursing home residents: a systematic review. Neurourol Urodyn. 2009;28(4):288–94.
48. Subak LL, Richter HE, Hunskaar S. Obesity and urinary incontinence: epidemiology and clinical research update. J Urol. 2009;182(6 Suppl):S2–7.
49. Choi H, Palmer MH, Park J. Meta-analysis of pelvic floor muscle training: randomized controlled trials in incontinent women. Nurs Res. 2007;56(4):226–34. doi:10.1097/01.NNR.0000280610.93373.e1.
50. Cardozo L, Lange R, Voss S, Beardsworth A, Manning M, Viktrup L, Zhao YD. Short- and long-term efficacy and safety of duloxetine in women with predominant stress urinary incontinence. Curr Med Res Opin. 2010;26(2):253–61. doi:10.1185/03007990903438295.

51. Li J, Yang L, Pu C, Tang Y, Yun H, Han P. The role of duloxetine in stress urinary incontinence: a systematic review and meta-analysis. Int Urol Nephrol. 2013;45(3):679–86. doi:10.1007/s11255-013-0410-6.
52. Malone-Lee JG, Walsh JB, Maugourd MF. Tolterodine: a safe and effective treatment for older patients with overactive bladder. J Am Geriatr Soc. 2001;49(6):700–5.
53. Dasgupta J, Tincello DG. Interstitial cystitis/bladder pain syndrome: an update. Maturitas. 2009;64(4):212–7. doi:10.1016/j.maturitas.2009.09.016.
54. Butrick CW, Howard FM, Sand PK. Diagnosis and treatment of interstitial cystitis/painful bladder syndrome: a review. J Womens Health (Larchmt). 2010;19(6):1185–93. doi:10.1089/jwh.2009.1702.
55. Kahn BS, Tatro C, Parsons CL, Willems JJ. Prevalence of interstitial cystitis in vulvodynia patients detected by bladder potassium sensitivity. J Sex Med. 2010;7(2 Pt 2):996–1002. doi:10.1111/j.1743-6109.2009.01550.x.
56. Parsons CL, Bullen M, Kahn BS, Stanford EJ, Willems JJ. Gynecologic presentation of interstitial cystitis as detected by intravesical potassium sensitivity. Obstet Gynecol. 2001;98(1):127–32.
57. Peters K, Girdler B, Carrico D, Ibrahim I, Diokno A. Painful bladder syndrome/interstitial cystitis and vulvodynia: a clinical correlation. Int Urogynecol J Pelvic Floor Dysfunct. 2008;19(5):665–9. doi:10.1007/s00192-007-0501-y.
58. Bullones Rodriguez MA, Afari N, Buchwald DS. Evidence for overlap between urological and nonurological unexplained clinical conditions. J Urol. 2013;189(1 Suppl):S66–74. doi:10.1016/j.juro.2012.11.019.
59. Farage MA, Miller KW, Berardesca E, Maibach HI. Incontinence in the aged: contact dermatitis and other cutaneous consequences. Contact Dermatitis. 2007;57(4):211–7. doi:10.1111/j.1600-0536.2007.01199.x.
60. Brown JS, Bradley CS, Subak LL, Richter HE, Kraus SR, Brubaker L, Lin F, Vittinghoff E, Grady D. The sensitivity and specificity of a simple test to distinguish between urge and stress urinary incontinence. Ann Intern Med. 2006;144(10):715–23.
61. Roskos KV, Guy RH. Assessment of skin barrier function using transepidermal water loss: effect of age. Pharm Res. 1989;6(11):949–53.
62. Berg RW. Etiology and pathophysiology of diaper dermatitis. Adv Dermatol. 1988;3:75–98.
63. Berg RW, Buckingham KW, Stewart RL. Etiologic factors in diaper dermatitis: the role of urine. Pediatr Dermatol. 1986;3(2):102–6.
64. Buckingham KW, Berg RW. Etiologic factors in diaper dermatitis: the role of feces. Pediatr Dermatol. 1986;3(2):107–12.
65. Andersen PH, Bucher AP, Saeed I, Lee PC, Davis JA, Maibach HI. Faecal enzymes: in vivo human skin irritation. Contact Dermatitis. 1994;30(3):152–8.
66. Burgio KL, Goode PS, Richter HE, Markland AD, Johnson 2nd TM, Redden DT. Combined behavioral and individualized drug therapy versus individualized drug therapy alone for urge urinary incontinence in women. J Urol. 2010;184(2):598–603. doi:10.1016/j.juro.2010.03.141.
67. Burgio KL, Locher JL, Goode PS, Hardin JM, McDowell BJ, Dombrowski M, Candib D. Behavioral vs drug treatment for urge urinary incontinence in older women: a randomized controlled trial. JAMA. 1998;280(23):1995–2000.
68. Fink HA, Taylor BC, Tacklind JW, Rutks IR, Wilt TJ. Treatment interventions in nursing home residents with urinary incontinence: a systematic review of randomized trials. Mayo Clin Proc. 2008;83(12):1332–43.
69. Hu TW, Igou JF, Kaltreider DL, Yu LC, Rohner TJ, Dennis PJ, Craighead WE, Hadley EC, Ory MG. A clinical trial of a behavioral therapy to reduce urinary incontinence in nursing homes. Outcome and implications. JAMA. 1989;261(18):2656–62.
70. Wilson L, Brown JS, Shin GP, Luc KO, Subak LL. Annual direct cost of urinary incontinence. Obstet Gynecol. 2001;98(3):398–406.
71. Farage MA, Miller KW, Berardesca E, Maibach HI. Psychosocial and societal burden of incontinence in the aged population: a review. Arch Gynecol Obstet. 2008;277(4):285–90. doi:10.1007/s00404-007-0505-3.
72. Farage MA, Miller KW, Ledger WJ. Determining the cause of vulvovaginal symptoms. Obstet Gynecol Surv. 2008;63(7):445–64.

Physical Activity and Quality of Life During Menopausal Transition and Postmenopause

28

Kirsi Mansikkamäki and Riitta M. Luoto

Contents

28.1 Menopausal Symptoms and Quality of Life 397

28.2 Measurement of Quality of Life 398

28.3 Physical Activity, Menopausal Symptoms, and Quality of Life 399

28.4 Physical Activity and Quality of Life During Menopause: Evidence from Experimental Studies 400

28.5 Physical Activity and Change in Quality of Life: Evidence from Cohort Studies 401

28.6 Future Studies 402

References 403

K. Mansikkamäki, MS (✉)
UKK Institute for Health Promotion,
Tampere University of Applied Sciences,
Kaupinpuistonkatu 1, Tampere 33500, Finland
e-mail: kirsi.mansikkamaki@uta.fi

R.M. Luoto, MD, PhD
UKK Institute for Health Promotion,
Tampere, Finland
e-mail: riitta.luoto@uta.fi

28.1 Menopausal Symptoms and Quality of Life

Women experience menopause between 40 and 58 years of age, the median age being 51 years [1]. Due to the long duration of menopausal transition, the impact of menopause for women's subjective health may be large [2]. Menopause may be associated with many symptoms and poor perceived health, which subsequently has an effect to quality of life [3, 4]. Menopause is also associated with a number of physical, psychological, and social changes [5].

Typical symptoms during menopausal transition are hot flushes, night sweats, vaginal dryness, and sleep disturbance [3, 4]. In addition, menopausal women commonly report a variety of other symptoms, including sexual dysfunction, depression, anxiety, memory loss, fatigue, headache, joint pains, and weight gain, but they may relate to aging as well as menopause itself. Evidence from population-based cohort and cross-sectional studies support associations between menopausal status and vasomotor symptoms, vaginal dryness, and sleep disturbance. However, associations between menopause and mood symptoms, cognitive disturbances and somatic complaints are inconclusive [2].

Over one-third of the premenopausal, half of the perimenopausal, and 54 % of both postmenopausal and hysterectomized Finnish women reported bothersome symptoms [6]. The difference between pre- and perimenopausal women was largest and statistically most significant in the case of back pain and hot flushes. Physically active women reported fewer somatic symptoms than did women with a sedentary lifestyle [6].

Some studies have found that menopause is associated with poor quality of life [7], but not all [5]. Menopausal transition is not to be avoided, but it seems that if women do not have severe subjective menopausal symptoms, menopausal transition does not affect her quality of life. However, if menopause-related symptoms are severe, menopausal transition is related to poorer quality of life. Avis et al. [8] found in a longitudinal study (SWAN) that menopausal transition showed little impact on health-related quality of life (HRQL) when adjusted for symptoms, medical conditions, and stress. In Avis et al.'s study, even controlling for wide range of variables, late peri- and postmenopausal women were more likely to report reduced functioning on the role-physical domain of HRQL than premenopausal women.

Mishra et al. [9] also found significant declines in the physical health domains on the SF-36 quality of life scale among women who remained perimenopausal over 2 years, compared to women who remained premenopausal. It is possible that these findings are due to health problems that may co-occur with menopause and/or aging. In Avis et al.'s study [8], findings support the role of symptoms in relation to HRQL. They found that vaginal dryness, urine leakage, poor sleep, and depression were highly related to all SF-36 domains and same kind of findings have Kumari et al. [5] by women who experienced vasomotor symptoms or depression showed significant declines on the SF-36. In Avis et al's study, they conclude that changes in HRQL over the menopausal transition are largely explained by symptoms related to menopause and/or aging such as vasomotor symptoms, vaginal dryness, urine leakage, problems with sleeping, health conditionings such as arthritis, and depressed mood and stress [8]. All these findings highlight the importance of controlling for important covariates in assessing the impact of the menopausal transition on HRQL.

28.2 Measurement of Quality of Life

In this chapter, we discuss a conception of "quality of life" meaning women's own perception of her well-being. Health-related quality of life (HRQL) definition comes from PRO Harmonization Group and is stated as "HRQL represents the patients' evaluation of the impact of a health condition and its treatment on daily life" [10]. In Short Form (SF-36) scale, there are 36 items assessing eight dimensions of quality of life. Each scale is scored from 0 to 100, in which 100 being the most favorable score. Other quality of life questionnaires that are included to this review are Women's Health Questionnaire (WHQ) and MENQOL, which are menopause-specific quality of life questionnaires and focused on psychological as well as physical items (Table 28.1). In our previous longitudinal study [11], we used global quality of life scale,

Table 28.1 Quality of life measurement scales

Dimensions	A 36-item Short Form Health Survey SF-36 [28]	Menopausal quality of life, MENQOL [26]	Women's Health Questionnaire, WHQ [28]
1	Physical functioning	Vasomotor function	Depressed mood
2	Role function physical	Psychosocial function	Somatic symptoms
3	Mental health	Physical function	Memory/concentration
4	Role function emotional	Sexual function	Vasomotor symptoms
5	Social functioning	–	Anxiety/fears
6	Bodily pain	–	Sexual behavior
7	Vitality	–	Sleep problems
8	General health	–	Menstrual symptoms
9	–	–	Attractiveness

Ladder of Life scale, which was modified by Andrews and Withey in 1976. Respondents were asked to evaluate their quality of life during the previous month. The scale was from 0 to 10 with 0 meaning worst possible quality of life and 10 meaning best possible quality of life. This quality of life scale is self-anchoring because ratings are made relative to each person's conception of her best or worst quality of life.

28.3 Physical Activity, Menopausal Symptoms, and Quality of Life

Physical activity has been shown to enhance quality of life among midlife women [12, 13], and some studies suggest that physical activity is associated with a decrease of hot flushes [14, 15]. How might physical activity affect to occurrence of hot flushes? During menopause, estrogen concentrations decrease, and consequently the level of neurotransmitter β-endorphin, which is known to affect thermoregulation, decreases. It is also known that physical activity increases hypothalamic β-endorphin production and thereby may affect and stabilize thermoregulation [16] and diminish hot flushes. On the other hand, physical activity raises acutely core body temperature and thus could theoretically increase the occurrence of vasomotor symptoms [17]. The other explanations include association between physical activity, mood, and weight. Maintaining or increasing physical activity level during menopausal transition period and postmenopause has been suggested to reduce a variety of psychological symptoms, including anxiety, stress, and depression [18].

Physical activity and weight is an interesting issue when vasomotor symptoms are considered. One possible mechanism in how physical activity could affect frequency of hot flushes is controlling body weight [14, 17]. Obesity was long time thought to be a protective factor against vasomotor symptoms, because androgens are aromatized into estrogens in body fat. Women with more adipose tissue would be expected to have a lower risk of vasomotor symptoms because of higher levels of estrogen [17]. However, several studies have found that obesity may be a risk factor rather than a protective characteristic during the menopause. Evidence indicates that higher body mass index and body fat in particular are associated with greater vasomotor symptom reporting and primarily hot flushes [19]. Davis et al. [20] suggests that obesity is an independent risk factor for experiencing severe menopausal symptoms. These findings are consistent with a thermoregulatory model of vasomotor symptoms in which body fat acts as an insulator, rendering vasomotor symptoms, a putative heat dissipation event, more likely.

Weight gain during menopause is not related to menopause itself but rather to aging [20]. The hormonal changes across the menopausal transition substantially contribute to increased central abdominal fat and abdominal obesity. Reduction in weight and abdominal circumference has been associated at least partly with reduction in vasomotor symptoms among overweight and obese women [21]. Although there are multiple observational studies which have documented that women with a higher BMI report more frequent or severe hot flushes during menopause, the mechanisms underlying this association are still poorly understood. Recently proposed explanations for the observed association between BMI and hot flushes include alterations in leptin and other cytokines expressed by adipocytes that affect thermoregulatory function [22]. Finally, women who are overweight or obese may differ in psychological or social factors that affect their subjective experience of and willingness to report symptoms such as hot flushes [21].

Symptoms that are related to menopause (hot flushes, night sweats, vaginal dryness) may have a negative impact on women's health-related quality of life [23]. If the symptoms are a result of the loss of estrogen, replacing estrogen using hormonal therapy, symptoms could disappear and improve quality of life. Hess et al. [24] found in their study that poor HRQL does not increase likelihood of initiating hormonal therapy, nor is hormonal therapy use associated with HRQL improvements. Women who initiated hormonal therapy and reported frequent menopausal symptoms reported an improvement in vitality compared with those who initiated hormonal therapy and did not report a frequent symptom. In Hess et al.'s study [24], it showed that hormonal therapy does not affect the overall feeling of "wellness" but only the symptoms which bothered their life. Similar conclusions were made in a review by Utian and Woods [25]; health-related as well as menopause-related quality of life benefits are contingent of symptoms status. Severely symptomatic women experience a significant improvement in their health-related and menopause-related quality of life, but in clinical trials women without severe symptoms at baseline do not experience an increase in quality of life [25].

28.4 Physical Activity and Quality of Life During Menopause: Evidence from Experimental Studies

Efficacy of yoga, exercise, and usual activity for the improvement of menopause-related QoL in women with vasomotor symptoms was studied in a randomized controlled trial by Reed et al. [26]. The report is part of a trial in which the main aim was to study efficacy of omega-3 treatment for vasomotor symptoms [27]. The instruction of the yoga intervention was provided during weekly 90-min classes, and daily home practice was instructed for 20 min on days when class was not attended. Women in the exercise intervention group were expected to perform resistance exercise training sessions three times per week with targeted training heart rate 50–60 % of the heart rate reserve for the first month and 60–70 % for the next 2 months. The exercise took 40–60 min per session, and the aim was to achieve the energy expenditure goal of 16 kcal/kg. The usual activity group was instructed to continue their usual physical activity and not to begin any new physical exercise. Women in all three groups received either placebo that contained olive oil or an active omega-3 capsule. The Menopausal Quality of Life Questionnaire (MENQOL) was used to evaluate menopause-related QoL in 29 items. Scoring generates a total score and four domain scores (vasomotor, physical, psychosocial, sexual functioning) (see Table 28.1).

The yoga intervention was found to have significantly greater improvement in MENQOL scores at 12 weeks when compared with the usual activity group, additionally no group differences were observed between exercise and usual activity or omega-3 and placebo [26]. According to the results, for yoga compared to usual activity, baseline to 12-week improvements were seen for MENQOL total, vasomotor symptom domain, and sexuality domain scores. However, for women who underwent exercise and omega-3 therapy compared with control subjects, improvements in baseline to 12-week total MENQOL scores were not observed. Exercise showed benefit in the MENQOL physical domain score at 12 weeks. As conclusion, yoga appears to improve menopausal quality of life among healthy sedentary women in spite of modest effect.

A Finnish trial studied quality of life effects of moderate-intensity aerobic training [28]. Women aged 43–63 years, with weekly severe hot flashes, no current use of hormone replacement therapy, and sedentary (physical exercise <2 times/week), were recruited into a randomized controlled trial. Outcomes were hot flushes and health-related quality of life (HRQL). Intervention included moderate-intensity aerobic training for 6 months, four times per week walking for 50 min at 60 % of VO_2max. Control group continued their usual activities. Hot flashes were reported by mobile phone twice a day. Health-related quality of life was estimated by the Short Form-36 Health survey and Women's Health Questionnaire. Results of the study showed that decrease in the nighttime hot flashes was larger among the intervention group than among the control group, but not during daytime. At the end of intervention, women reported significantly fewer nighttime hot flashes (43 %) than the control women (54 %). Significant differences between the groups in SF-36 score changes were found in physical functioning, general health, vitality, and in WHQ depression.

Imayama et al. studied individual and combined effects of dietary weight loss and/or exercise interventions on HRQOL and psychosocial factors (depression, anxiety, stress, social support) in a randomized trial setting [29]. Overweight or obese postmenopausal women were randomly assigned to 12 months of dietary weight loss, moderate-to-vigorous aerobic exercise, combined diet and exercise, or control groups. According to their results, the combined diet + exercise group improved four aspects of HRQOL (physical functioning, role-physical, vitality, and mental health) and stress, whereas the diet group increased vitality score, but HRQOL did not change differently in the exercise group compared with controls. In Imayama et al.'s study, a combined diet and exercise intervention had larger positive effects on HRQOL than that from exercise or diet alone [29].

The importance of weight loss was also found in an experimental study by Guimaraes and Baptista [30]. In their study, at least moderate-intensity PA for 60 min/day had favorable influence on the prevention of menopausal symptoms and on QOL, particularly in the psychological and social domains. The influence of habitual PA was partially associated with a decrease in the symptoms of menopause and/or with weight loss.

To summarize, results from experimental studies show beneficial effects of physical activity on quality of life, independent of dose, type, or other details of physical activity.

28.5 Physical Activity and Change in Quality of Life: Evidence from Cohort Studies

A total of 1,165 Finnish women aged 45–64 years from a national representative population-based study were followed up for 8 years [11]. Ordinal logistic regression analysis was used to measure the effect of menopausal status on global quality of life. Other variables included in the analyses were age, education, change of physical activity as assessed with metabolic equivalents, change of weight, and hormone therapy use. According to the results, peri- or postmenopausal women increased their physical activity (28 %) during the 8-year follow-up period slightly more often than premenopausal (18 %) women. Menopausal status was not significantly correlated with change of QoL. QoL of the most highly educated women was more likely to improve than among the less educated. Women whose physical activity increased or remained stable had higher probability for improved QoL than women whose physical activity decreased. Women whose weight remained stable during follow-up also improved their QoL compared to women who gained weight. Women who had never used hormone therapy had 1.3 greater odds for improved QoL. As conclusion, the study showed that improvement of global QoL is correlated with stable or increased physical activity, stable weight, and high education, but not with change in menopausal status.

Change in global quality of life is more associated with change in physical activity than change in menopausal status [11]. However, women whose physical activity or weight remained the same, physical activity increased or women who were the most highly educated, had improved QoL over time.

Mishra et al. [9] in their longitudinal study with 2 years of follow-up found that certain domains of QoL decline with aging and physical aspects of general health and well-being measured by SF-36 scale declined during the menopausal transition. Women who were perimenopausal for at least a year reported greater decline in their physical health and psychosomatic domains than did premenopausal women [9]. In Smith-DiJulio et al.'s longitudinal study [31], it was found that negative life events predicted decreased well-being in menopausal transition, but factors associated with the menopausal transition did not. They also found that women's sense of mastery and satisfaction with her life and ability to use available social support predicted increased well-being. These findings suggest also that for most women, the menopausal transition is not a predictor of well-being when considered in a broader life context.

Physical activity has been reported to decrease with age [32], but in Luoto et al.'s study [28], it seems that women in menopausal transition changed their behavior into another direction. Increased motivation for lifestyle modification during menopausal transition could explain this increasing physical activity.

Elavsky et al. [12] found in a longitudinal study of middle-aged women that physical activity improves physical self-worth and positive affect and that the improvements in affect lead to improvements in QoL. In Moilanen et al.'s study [11], those women who decreased their physical activity had deterioration in QoL than did women whose physical activity remained stable. Women who increased their physical activity improved their QoL. In the study by Elavsky et al. [12], increase in physical activity mediated positive affect and therefore had a positive effect on QoL. Some other studies claim that physical activity alleviates menopausal symptoms (hot flushes) and so improves QoL [15, 33].

In an Australian longitudinal study, women were followed annually for 13 years of time to study duration of menopausal symptoms. In Col et al.'s study, the duration of menopausal symptoms was found to be longer than expected, over 5 years. The only factor which was associated with duration of hot flushes was regular exercise, which was associated with shorter symptom duration [2].

It is hypothesized that endorphin concentration in the hypothalamus decreases and estrogen production declines, facilitating the release of norepinephrine and serotonin. Exercise may have ameliorating effects on vasomotor symptoms by increasing the presence of hypothalamic and peripheral ß-endorphin production. Through these mechanisms, exercise may help to stabilize the thermoregulatory center and diminish the risk of hot flushes [34]. The relationship between physical activity and QoL during the menopause is complex and may involve a number of alternative mechanisms, physiological or psychological or both.

Women who gained weight were more likely to report deterioration in QoL. This is consistent with other studies [28, 35]. The 8-year follow-up study by Dennerstein et al. [33] found that increase of body mass index was associated with decline in self-rated health. Whether this is because of their knowledge of the relationship between body fatness and chronic disease or whether it reflects a problem with body image is unknown. In the study by Sammel et al. [35], the major predictors of weight gain among menopausal women were quality of life and other psychological factors including depressed mood and anxiety. One might speculate some causality between these factors; did weight gain lead to decline in QoL or did poorer QoL lead to weight gain?

The Study of Women's Health Across the Nation (SWAN) [36], which is a multiethnic cohort study, found that women who had gained weight during the study period reported more vasomotor symptoms (hot flushes) than women whose weight remained stable. Thurston and Joffe [37] summarized association between obesity and vasomotor symptoms from SWAN studies and found that obesity is a key factor of occurrence of vasomotor symptoms. One possible explanation mechanism could be thermoregulatory model of vasomotor symptoms, in which adipose tissue acts as an insulator, preventing the heat dissipating action of vasomotor symptoms, thereby increasing their occurrence or severity. Abdominal adiposity and particularly subcutaneous adiposity were associated with increased likelihood of hot flushes [37]. Lean women have more hot flushes at the time of menopause [38], and they have been shown to use hormone replacement therapy more frequently [39], although opposite results also exist [40]. Stadberg et al. [41] found that a higher BMI was correlated with a higher climacteric symptom score. They thought that possible reason maybe that overweight women sweat more often because of their extra weight load and obesity is also associated with less exercise and poorer general health. Overweight could also be viewed as a lifestyle factor with less concern about health and lower self-esteem [42].

28.6 Future Studies

A positive association between physical activity and perception of QoL during menopause is found in a number of studies with experimental or nonexperimental design. Future studies could address the recent possibilities of more precise exposure evaluation with objective physical activity measurement instead of self-reported physical activity. Due to the current understanding of physical activity's ability to prevent breast cancer [43], even women using hormone therapy for menopausal symptoms might benefit from an increase in physical activity.

References

1. Zapantis G, Santoro N. The menopausal transition: characteristics and management. Best Pract Res Clin Endocrinol Metab. 2003;17:33–52.
2. Col NF, Guthrie JR, Politi M, Dennerstein L. Duration of vasomotor symptoms in middle-aged women: a longitudinal study. Menopause. 2009;16:453–7.
3. Utian W. Psychosocial and socioeconomic burden of vasomotor symptoms in menopause: a comprehensive review. Health Qual Life Outcomes. 2005;3:47.
4. McVeigh C. Perimenopause: more than hot flushes and night sweats for some Australian women. J Obstet Gynecol Neonatal Nurs. 2005;34:21–7.
5. Kumari M, Stafford M, Marmot M. The menopausal transition was associated in a prospective study with decreased health functioning in women who report menopausal symptoms. J Clin Epidemiol. 2005;58: 719–27.
6. Moilanen J, Aalto AM, Hemminki E, Aro AR, Raitanen J, Luoto R. Prevalence of menopause symptoms and their association with lifestyle among Finnish middle-aged women. Maturitas. 2010;67(4):368–74.
7. Blumel JE, Castelo-Branco C, Binfa L, Gramegna G, Tacla X, Aracena B, Cumsille MA, Sanjuan A. Quality of life after the menopause : a population study. Maturitas. 2000;34:17–23.
8. Avis NE, Colvin A, Bromberger JT, Hess R, Matthews KA, Ory M, Schocken M. Change in health-related quality of life over menopausal transition in multiethnic cohort of middle-aged women: Study of Women's Health Across the Nation (SWAN). Menopause. 2009;16:860–9.
9. Mishra GD, Brown WJ, Dobson AJ. Physical and mental health: changes during menopause transition. Qual Life Res. 2003;12:405–12.
10. Zöllner YF, Acquadro C, Schaefer M. Literature review of instrument to assess health-related quality of life during and after menopause. Qual Life Res. 2005;14:309–27.
11. Moilanen JM, Aalto A-M, Raitanen J, Hemminki E, Aro AR, Luoto R. Physical activity and change in quality of life during menopause – an 8 year follow-up study. Health Qual Life Outcomes. 2012;10:8. http://www.hqlo.com/content/10/1/8.
12. Elavsky S. Physical activity, menopause and quality of life: the role of affect and self-worth across time. Menopause. 2009;16:265–71.
13. Courneya KS, Tamburrini AL, Woolcott CG, McNeely ML, Karvinen K, Campbell KL, McTiernan A, Friedenreich CM. The Alberta physical activity and breast cancer prevention trial: quality of life outcomes. Prev Med. 2011;52:26–32.
14. Gold EB, Sternfeld B, Kelsey JL, Brown C, Mouton C, Reame N, Salamone L, Stellato R. Relation of demographic and lifestyle factors to symptoms in a? multi-racial/ethnic population of women 40–55 years of age. Am J Epidemiol. 2000;152:463–73.
15. Ivarsson T, Spetz A-C, Hammar M. Physical exercise and vasomotor symptoms in postmenopausal women. Maturitas. 1998;29:139–46.
16. Hammar M, Berg G, Lindgren R. Does physical exercise influence the frequency of postmenopausal hot flushes? Acta Obst Gyn Scand. 1990;69:409–12.
17. Thurston RC, Hadine J. Vasomotor symptoms and menopause: findings from Study of Women's Health Across the Nation. Obstet Gynecol Clin North Am. 2011;38:489–501.
18. Nelson DB, Sammel MD, Freeman EW, Lin H, Gracia CR, Schmitz KH. Effect of physical activity on menopausal symptoms among urban women. Med Sci Sports Exerc. 2008;40:50–8.
19. Thurston RC, Sowers MF, Sternfeld B, Gold EB, Bromberger J, Chang Y, Joffe H, Crandall CJ, Waetjen LE, Matthews KA. Gains in body fat and vasomotor symptom reporting over menopausal transition. Am J Med. 2009;170:766–74.
20. Davis SR, Castelo-Branco C, Chedraui P, Lumsden MA, Nappi RE, Shab D, Villaseca P. Understanding weight gain at menopause. Climacteric. 2012;15:419–29.
21. Huang AJ, Subak LL, Wing R, West DS, Hernandez AL, Macer J, Grady D. An intensive behavioral weight loss intervention and hot flushes in women. Arch Intern Med. 2010;170:1161–7.
22. Alexander C, Cochran CJ, Gallicchio L, Miller SR, Flaws JA, Zacur H. Serum leptin levels, hormone levels, and hot flashes in midlife women. Fertil Steril. 2009. doi:10.1016/j.fertnstert/2009.04.001. published online May 22, 2009.
23. Hlatky MA, Boothroyd D, Vittinghoff E, Sharp P, Whooley MA. Quality of life and depressive symptoms in postmenopausal women after receiving hormone therapy: results from the Heart and Estrogen/Progestin Replacement Study (HERS) trial. JAMA. 2002;287:591–7.
24. Hess R, Colvin A, Avis NE, Bromberger JT, Schocken M, Johnston JM, Matthews KA. The impact of hormone therapy on health-related quality of life: longitudinal results from the Study of Women's Health Across the Nation. Menopause. 2008;15(3):422–8. doi:10.1097/gme.0b013e31814faf2b. PubMed PMID: 18467950.
25. Utian WH, Woods NF. Impact of hormone therapy on quality of life after menopause. Menopause. 2013;20: 1098–105.
26. Reed SD, Guthrie KA, Newton KM, Anderson GL, Booth-LaForce C, Caan B, et al. Menopausal quality of life: RCT of yoga, exercise, and omega-3 supplements. Am J Obstet Gynecol. 2014;210:244.e1–11. Epub 2014 Jan 3.
27. Cohen LS, Joffe H, Guthrie KA, Ensrud KE, Freeman M, Carpenter JS, et al. Efficacy of omega-3 for vasomotor symptoms treatment: a randomized controlled

trial. Menopause. 2014;21(4):347–54. PubMed PMID: 23982113.
28. Luoto R, Moilanen J, Heinonen R, Mikkola T, Raitanen J, Tomas E, Ojala K, Mansikkamäki K, Nygård CH. Effect of aerobic training on hot flushes and quality of lif-- randomized controlled trial. Ann Med. 2012;44(6):616–26. doi:10.3109/07853890.2011.583674.
29. Imayama I, Alfano CM, Kong A, Foster-Schubert KE, Bain CE, Xiao L, et al. Dietary weight loss and exercise interventions effects on quality of life in overweight/obese postmenopausal women: a randomized controlled trial. Int J Behav Nutr Phys Act. 2011;8:118.
30. Guimaraes ACA, Baptista F. Influence of habitual physical activity on the symptoms of climacterium/menopause and the quality of life of middle-aged women. Int J Women's Health. 2011;3:319–28.
31. Smith-DiJulio K, Woods Fugate N, Mitchell ES. Wellbeing during the menopausal transition and early postmenopause: a longitudinal analysis. Menopause. 2008;15:1095–102.
32. Pedersen P, Kjœller M, Ekholm O, Grœnbaek M, Curtis T. Readiness to change level of physical activity in leisure time among physically inactive Danish adults. Scand J Public Health. 2009;37:785–92.
33. Dennerstein L, Lehert P, Guthrie JR, Burger HG. Modeling women's health during the menopausal transition: a longitudinal analysis. Menopause. 2007;14:53–62.
34. Reid RL, Hoff JD, Yen SS, Lee CH. Effects of exogenous beta h-endorphin on pituitary hormone secretion and its disappearance rate in normal human subjects. J Clin Endocrinol Metab. 1981;52:1179–83.
35. Sammel MD, Grisso JA, Freeman EW, Hollander L, Liu L, Liu S, et al. Weight gain among women in the late reproductive years. Fam Pract. 2003;20:401–11.
36. Thurston RC, Sowers MF, Chang Y, Sternfeld B, Gold EB, Johnston JM, et al. Adiposity and reporting of vasomotor symptoms among midlife women. The study of women's health across the nation. Am J Epidemiol. 2008;167:78–85.
37. Thurston RC, Joffe H. Vasomotor symptoms and menopause: findings from the Study of Women's Health across the Nation. Obstet Gynecol Clin North Am. 2011;38(3):489–501. doi:10.1016/j.ogc.2011.05.006. Review.
38. Erlik Y, Meldrum DR, Judd HL. Estrogen levels in postmenopausal women with hot flushes. Obstet Gynecol. 1982;59:403–7.
39. Jalava-Broman J, Mäkinen J, Ojanlatva A, Jokinen K, Sillanmäki L, Rautava P. Treatment of climacteric symptoms in Finland prior to the controversial reports on hormone therapy. Acta Obstet Gynecol. 2008;87:682–6.
40. Den Tonkelaar I, Seidell J, van Noord P. Obesity and fat distribution in relation to hot flushes in Dutch women from the DOM-project. Maturitas. 1996;23:301–5.
41. Stadberg E, Mattson L, Milsom I. Factors associated with climacteric symptoms and the use of hormone replacement therapy. Acta Obstet Gynecol Scand. 2000;79:286–92.
42. Kirchengast S. Relations between antropometric characteristic and degree of severity of climacteric syndrome in Australian women. Maturitas. 1993;17:167–80.
43. Thomson CA, McCullough ML, Wertheim BC, Chlebowski RT, Martinez ME, Stefanick ML, et al. Nutrition and physical activity cancer prevention guidelines, cancer risk, and mortality in the women's health initiative. Cancer Prev Res (Phila). 2014;7(1):42–53. doi:10.1158/1940-6207.CAPR-13-0258.

Quality of Life

29

Maria Celeste O. Wender
and Patrícia Pereira de Oliveira

Contents

29.1	Cervantes Scale	408
29.2	Women's Health Questionnaire (WHQ)	410
29.3	The Utian Menopause Quality Of Life Score (UQOL)	411
29.4	Menopause-Specific Quality Of Life Questionnaire (MENQOL)	411
29.5	The Menopausal Quality Of Life Scale (MQOL)	412
29.6	The Menopause Rating Scale (MRS)	412
29.7	Qualifemme	413
29.8	Summary	413
References		413

M.C.O. Wender, MD, PhD (✉)
Department of Obstetrics and Gynecology,
Menopause Clinic of Hospital de Clinicas de Porto
Alegre, Federal University of Rio Grande do Sul
Rua 14 de julho 746/4, Porto Alegre,
Rio Grande do Sul 91340430, Brazil
e-mail: mceleste@ufrgs.br

P.P. de Oliveira
Department of Medicine, University Unochapecó,
Chapecó, Santa Catarina, Brazil
e-mail: patriciapoliveira@hotmail.com

Although the concept of quality of life (QOL) has been defined in several different ways by different authors and studies, these definitions generally agree as to the importance of self-esteem and personal well-being to QOL and often involve concepts such as functional capacity, socioeconomic status, emotional state, social interaction, intellectual activity, self-care, family support, health status, cultural, ethical and religious values, lifestyle habits, satisfaction with one's job and with life in general, and the environment in which one lives [1]. The World Health Organization (WHO) Quality of Life Group [2] has adopted a multidimensional definition of the concept and has suggested that QOL consists of an "individual's perception of their position in life in the context of the culture and value system in which they live and in relation to their goals, expectations, standards and concerns."

A number of assessment instruments have been developed to transform subjective QOL information into objective and measurable parameters which could be used to evaluate individuals and populations. To facilitate the standardization and implementation of these instruments, efforts must be made to ensure that they are easy to administer and have valid psychometric properties for assessing QOL in different populations [3, 4]. The fact that these instruments are generally developed for use in a single culture and tend to be heavily language-based may lead to significant communication and cultural biases [5]. Therefore, whenever such instruments must be used in a different language from the one in which they were initially developed, not only must they be translated, but their cultural and psychometric properties must also be reevaluated [3, 4, 6].

QOL questionnaires and scales may be either specific or generic [6–8]. Specific instruments allow for a more in-depth understanding of the relationship between menopausal symptoms and QOL, while generic instruments investigate the physical and mental factors that influence QOL during the climacteric and are not restricted to particular aspects of this stage of life. Recent studies suggest that instruments of both types should be used in combination to increase the accuracy of the assessment and that qualitative assessment methods should be added to QOL assessment batteries so as to provide a more multidimensional, liberal, and subjective picture of QOL [9].

Generic instruments usually perform a global assessment of important facets of QOL and evaluate physical, social, psychological, and spiritual domains. Some of the most widely used generic QOL questionnaires are the World Health Organization Quality of Life (WHOQOL) assessment instrument, the Medical Outcomes Study 36-item Short Form Health Survey (SF-36) [10], the Nottingham Health Profile (NHP), and the Quality of Well-being (QWB) scale. The best known of these instruments is probably the WHOQOL-100. This 100-item instrument was originally developed by the WHO [2, 9], and, due to the length of application, has recently been adapted into a shorter version, known as the WHOQOL-bref. The latter instrument contains 26 items, of which two are general questions about QOL. The remaining items represent each of the 24 domains assessed by the WHOQOL-100. The instrument assesses four major domains: physical, psychological, social relationships, and environment. The domains are assessed by a series of questions referring to the previous 2 weeks, which investigate the following concepts: perception of QOL; satisfaction with health status; the impact of pain on daily activities; need for medical and health-care services; ability to enjoy life; concentration abilities; feelings of safety; characteristics of the environment; self-esteem; financial status; leisure activities; ability to move freely; satisfaction with sleep patterns, work, personal, and sexual relationships, and the use of means of transportation. The abbreviated version of the questionnaire was developed using data from a study involving 20 health centers in 18 countries [2].

Specific instruments, on the other hand, were designed to assess particular aspects of QOL, such as health-related quality of life, and to be more sensitive in detecting change following interventions. Such instruments may aim to assess specific areas of life (functional capacity, sexual functions, social relations, etc.), populations (youth, elderly, climacteric women, etc.), diseases (diabetes, breast cancer, etc.), or other life changes (such as pain following a therapeutic intervention).

The assessment of the menopausal transition and of postmenopausal women has been the subject of a number of debates and discussions in the literature. The menopausal transition marks a period of physiological changes which take place as women approach reproductive senescence. Evidence supports the clinical importance of the transition for many women as a period of significant changes in health status and of the appearance of symptoms (i.e., vasomotor symptoms, sleep disturbances, depression) which may influence women's quality of life [11–13]. Perimenopausal women may exhibit great symptom variability, and their experience of this stage in life may be subjected to various cultural influences. The WHO defines menopause as the cessation of menstruation for at least 12 consecutive months, which generally occurs at approximately 50 years of age [14]. Among the many factors associated with QOL and aging, previous physical and emotional health, social insertion, and experience with major life events are some of the most relevant.

Some of these factors are assessed by instruments that investigate the impact of climacteric symptoms on QOL, such as the health-related quality of life in the Spanish women through and beyond menopause (The Cervantes Scale), Women's Health Questionnaire (WHQ), Utian

Table 29.1 Comparison between measures of quality of life during the climacteric and menopause

Instrument	Author	Domains	Score
Cervantes Scale (CS)	Palacios et al. [17]	Four Menopause and health Sexuality Relationship with partner Psychological	Responses are scored on a scale of 0–5. Since the CS is a negative scale, its "positive items" (numbers 4, 8, 13, 15, 20, 22, 26, and 30) should be reverse scored before statistical analysis. Its total score can range from zero to 155 points.
WHQ	Hunter et al. [21]	Nine Mood Somatic symptoms Vasomotor symptoms Anxiety and fears Sexual behavior Sleep problems Menstrual symptoms Memory and concentration Attractiveness	Four-point scale Yes, definitely Yes, sometimes No, not much No, not at all
UQOL	Utian et al. (1970–2000) [23]	Four Occupational quality of life Health-related quality of life Emotional quality of life Sexual quality of life	Fully phrased statements (symptoms and feelings)
MENQOL	Primary Care Research Group of the University of Toronto, Canada (1992) Hilditch et al. [24]	Four Vasomotor Psychosocial Physical Sexual	Seven-point scale ranging from "not at all bothered" to "extremely bothered"
MQOL	Jacobs et al. [25]	Four Physical Vasomotor Psychosocial Sexual	Six-point scale ranging from "I am never like this" to "I am always like this" For the general quality of life item, participants are asked to rate their own quality of life on a scale from 1 to 100
MRS	Schneider and Sodergren (1996) [26]	Three Psychological Somato-vegetative Urogenital	Five-point scale ranging from asymptomatic to severe
Qualifemme	Le Floch et al. [30]	Four Climacteric Psychosocial Somatic Urogenital	10 mm visual analogue scale

Quality of Life (UQOL), the Menopause-Specific Quality of Life Questionnaire (MENQOL), the Menopause Quality of Life Scale (MQOL), Menopause Rating Scale (MRS), and the Qualifemme (Table 29.1).

A recent meta-analysis [15] sought to identify the most appropriate and psychometrically sound instruments for assessing QOL in women in the postmenopause. The analysis included studies of the following scales: WHQ, MRS,

MENQOL, MQOL, the MENCAV scale, UQOL, and MENQOL-Intervention. The MENQOL-Intervention questionnaire is a modified version of the MENQOL which takes into account the influence of treatment side effects on QOL and patient outcome [16]. Of the seven measures discussed in the meta-analysis, the WHQ appeared to be the most psychometrically robust. However, the results of the study also showed that most of the specific instruments for assessing QOL during menopause need to be further evaluated and that their psychometric properties must be investigated in more diversified samples and cross-cultural studies. Another interesting publication has reviewed the validated instruments available to measure QOL, discussed the results of clinical trials of HT which have used validated instruments to assess QOL, and investigated the effect of HT on QOL [6].

29.1 Cervantes Scale

The Cervantes Scale (CS) was developed and validated between 2001 and 2002 for use in Spanish pre- and perimenopausal women. It is a self-administered instrument that assesses QOL and the factors that may influence it during those periods [17]. Initially, the instrument was composed of 94 questions distributed into eight domains; however, its final version only included 31 questions, divided into the following four domains: menopause and health (15 items), sexuality (4 items), relationship with partner (3 items), and psychological (9 items) [17, 18].

The "menopause and health" domain assesses changes in QOL due to signs and symptoms that are common in women between the ages of 45 and 64 years and is the most susceptible to improvement through treatment interventions. It comprises the following three subdomains: vasomotor symptoms (three items), health (five items), and aging (seven items). The "sexuality" domain assesses sexual satisfaction and interest, as well as changes in the frequency of sexual relationships. The "relationship with partner" domain assesses marital satisfaction and the patient's role in her relationship. The "psychological" domain assesses changes in QOL due to anxiety and depression. Responses are scored on a scale of 0–5. Since the CS is a negative scale, its "positive items" (numbers 4, 8, 13, 15, 20, 22, 26, and 30) should be reverse scored before statistical analysis. The total score may range from 0 to 155, where higher scores are indicative of worse quality of life [17].

In Brazil, Lima and colleagues [19] conducted a cross-sectional study in which the scale was translated to Brazilian Portuguese and adapted both culturally and psychometrically for use in the local population. The study involved 180 women aged between 45 and 64 years, recruited from outpatient clinics in university hospitals (68.3 %) or from private clinics (31.7 %) in a city in southern Brazil. Participants had a mean age of 52.3 ± 5 years and most were Caucasian individuals (90.0 %) with primary level education (52.2 %) who earned up to four minimum wages per month (47.3 %). Women who were illiterate, had significant visual impairment and severe and/or untreated illnesses, or used antidepressants were excluded from the study. The translation and cultural adaptation of the scale were performed according to Wild et al. [3]. Sociodemographic, clinical, and behavioral data were collected from all participants, and individuals were administered the following questionnaires: the Brazilian Portuguese version of the CS, the WHQ, and the WHOQOL-bref. The latter two instruments were used as comparative standards for the newly adapted scale, as they had already been validated for use in the Brazilian population. The psychometric assessment of the Brazilian version of the CS was conducted using Cronbach's alpha to investigate internal consistency, the intraclass correlation coefficient to assess reproducibility, and correlations between the CS and other QOL assessment instruments to verify construct, convergent, criterion, and concurrent validity. Discriminant validity was assessed based on the use of t-tests and ANOVA to analyze population characteristics. Sixty-six women (36.6 %) were also readministered the scale after a 2-week interval. Most women were not being treated for any chronic illnesses (53.3 %), but among those

Table 29.2 Correlations between domains and subdomains of the Cervantes Scale

Cervantes Scale domains	A r / p	B r / p	C r / p	D r / p	E r / p	F r / p	G r / p	Total
Menopause and health (A)	1							
Vasomotor symptoms (B)	0.74 <0.001	1						
Health (C)	0.86 <0.001	0.54 <0.001	1					
Aging (D)	0.88 <0.001	0.46 <0.001	0.62 <0.001	1				
Psychological (E)	0.72 <0.001	0.38 <0.001	0.73 <0.001	0.64 <0.001	1			
Sexuality (F)	0.23 0.002	0.06 0.427	0.08 0.278	0.35 <0.001	0.34 <0.001	1		
Relationship with partner (G)	0.09 0.214	−0.03 0.652	0.07 0.384	0.15 0,040	0.24 0.001	0.60 <0.001	1	
Total score	0.88 <0.001	0.56 <0.001	0.77 <0.001	0.83 <0.001	0.88 <0.001	0.56 <0.001	0.43 <0.001	1

Reprinted from Lima et al. [18]
r correlation coefficient

who were undergoing such treatment, the most commonly reported illness was hypertension (66.6 % of women receiving chronic treatment). Only 15 % of participants were smokers, and 28.3 % reported to drinking alcoholic beverages. A significant portion of participants was sedentary (49.4 %). A total of 33.9 % of the women interviewed menstruated without the need for any treatment, while 25.6 % of participants were receiving hormone treatment (a total of 47.7 % of postmenopausal participants were in the latter group). Natural menopause was reported by 26.1 % of women. Their mean menopausal age was 48.1 ± 4.1 years. Surgical menopause (hysterectomy) was reported by 22.2 % of women, while 12.8 % were uncertain of when menopause occurred, and 38.9 % were still menstruating regularly. Of the 85 % of women who reported to having climacteric symptoms, 51 % reported hot flashes. The Cronbach's alpha for the total scale score was 0.83, and the internal consistency of each of the four domains was as following: menopause and health (0.81), psychological (0.84), sexuality (0.79), and relationship with partner (0.73). The intraclass correlation coefficient for the test-retest reliability of the CS was $r=0.94$; 95% CI: 0.89 – 0.96 ($p<0.001$). Most of the correlations between total CS scores and scores on its domains and subdomains were statistically significant. However, no correlations were found between the sexuality domain and the vasomotor symptoms and health subdomains, the relationship with partner and menopause and health domains, and the vasomotor symptoms and health subdomains. The strongest correlations were identified between total CS score and the menopause and health and psychological domains (Table 29.2). The Pearson's correlation coefficient between total CS scores and scores on the WHQ and WHOQOL-bref was $r=0.79$ and $r=-0.71$, respectively, significant at $p<0.001$ (Table 29.3). These results show the construct, convergent, criterion, concurrent, and discriminant validity of the Brazilian version of the CS. No part of the instrument had to be modified for cultural appropriateness. In conclusion, this study produced a version of the CS that was very similar to the original instrument and was easily understood by all participants.

However, given the sociocultural diversity of the Brazilian population and the complexity of the transcultural questionnaire adaptation process, the questionnaire should be further tested in different regions in the country.

Table 29.3 Correlations between domains and subdomains of the Cervantes Scale, the Women's Health Questionnaire, and the WHOQOL-BREF

Cervantes Scale domains	Women's Health Questionnaire	WHOQOL-BREF
Menopause and health	0.71	−0.58
Vasomotor symptoms	0.46	−0.30
Health	0.60	−0.48
Aging	0.67	−0.59
Psychological	0.68	−0.63
Sexuality	0.47	−0.48
Relationship with partner	0.29	−0.35
Total Cervantes Scale score	0.79	−0.71

Reprinted from Lima et al. [18]
The values represent the correlation coefficient
$p < 0.001$ for all correlations

The CS has adequate psychometric properties (internal consistency, reproducibility, and validity) for assessing QOL and health during the climacteric. It is also sensitive in detecting the effect of a number of non-climacteric related factors on QOL. Lastly, the scale has proved adequate for assessing QOL in women with varying sociodemographic, clinical and behavioral characteristics.

In an attempt to develop a shorter version of the CS, Pérez-López and colleagues [20] selected 10 of the 31 items that comprised the original scale based on their clinical relation to menopausal symptoms and administered the new version of the instrument to 1,739 middle-aged women. Scale reliability was assessed using internal consistency (Cronbach's alpha values) and the intraclass correlation coefficient (ICC). The new instrument (CS-10) had a mean (±SD) ICC of 0.45 ± 0.06 and a Cronbach's alpha of 0.778, indicating satisfactory internal consistency. The median [interquartile range] total CS-10 score for the entire sample was 10.0 [12–0], and median scores for pre-, peri-, and post-menopausal women were as follows: 8.0 [2], 9.0 [9–0], and 14.0 [14–0], respectively. Median CS-10 scores increased significantly according to menopausal status, marital status, and ethnicity.

A multiple linear regression analysis determined that lower QOL was related to older age, greater parity, longer time since menopause, greater body mass index, ethnicity (American women of African descent), and smoking.

These preliminary findings suggest that the CS-10 may make significant contributions to daily clinical practice and contribute to a more precise diagnosis of menopausal symptoms.

29.2 Women's Health Questionnaire (WHQ)

The *Women's Health Questionnaire* (WHQ) was developed in 1986 in England by Myra Hunter to assess physical and emotional symptoms, as well as changes in the health status of climacteric women (45–64 years of age). The instrument was developed through the study of 682 patients of an ovarian cancer screening clinic in a London hospital [21].

The WHQ avoids an overemphasis on postmenopausal symptoms and aims to assess global changes in women's lives. It is used in a number of countries worldwide and has been translated into languages such as French, Swedish, Afrikaans, Bulgarian, Danish, Dutch, Belgian Dutch, Australian English, Canadian English, German, Italian, and Spanish [21, 22]. The instrument was also the first measure of QOL to be included in the International Health-related Quality of Life Outcomes database (IQOD). The IQOD was created to develop reference values, establish item banking, and to allow for the psychometric validation of linguistically validated QOL instruments using pooled data form international studies. The database contains baseline QOL, sociodemographic, and clinical data from international clinical or epidemiological studies (see http://www.iqod.org).

The WHQ consists of 36 signs and symptoms which the respondent is asked to rate on a 5-point Likert severity scale ranging from 0 to 4. Scores can be summed to provide both factor and total scores. Higher scores are indicative of more suffering and functional impairment. The WHQ assesses the following themes:

somatic symptoms, depressed mood, memory and concentration, anxiety and fears, sexual behavior, vasomotor symptoms, sleep problems, menstrual symptoms, and attractiveness [8].

29.3 The Utian Menopause Quality Of Life Score (UQOL)

The UQOL scale assesses the impact of menopausal symptoms based on the respondent's self-evaluation of her personal well-being. The current version of the UQOL was adapted from the original Utian questionnaire, which was developed in the United States in 1970 to assess well-being in participants of a study comparing estrogen therapy to placebo [23]. To validate the instrument according to modern psychometric principles, the original UQOL was systematically reviewed and revised by a panel of expert judges, comprising two psychologists who specialized in behavioral medicine, one psychiatrist, and one reproductive endocrinologist [23].

The instrument that resulted from this process was evaluated in a preliminary study of 327 peri- and postmenopausal women aged between 46 and 65 years, recruited from 11 communities in Eastern and Central-Western United States. The women were administered a measure of QOL which was found to have four factors, each of which corresponded to one domain of QOL. The final version of the tool developed in the study contained 23 items and was validated in a geographically and socioeconomically diverse population using the well-recognized SF-36 scale [10] The UQOL assesses the following four areas: occupational QOL, health QOL, emotional QOL, and sexual QOL. Items are rated on a five-point Likert scale, and scores on the items corresponding to each domain are summed to provide factor scores. Negatively worded items must be reverse scored before data analysis. The Cronbach's alpha for the total scale has been reported at 0.830, which shows adequate reliability.

Although the UQOL has satisfactory psychometric properties, it cannot be considered a measure of menopause-related QOL, as its items are more consistent with the assessment of general QOL. Therefore, the authors of the UQOL recommend that their scale be used in combination with other instruments that provide a more specific assessment of climacteric symptoms. In conclusion, although the UQOL consists of an adequate measure of QOL, it should not be the only instrument used in studies that aim to investigate the impact of menopausal symptoms on QOL, regardless of whether participants are receiving hormone therapy (HT).

29.4 Menopause-Specific Quality Of Life Questionnaire (MENQOL)

The MENQOL is a self-administered instrument which was developed specifically to assess QOL during menopause [24]. It was developed in the 1990s by a group of Canadian researchers, and since then, its psychometric properties have been extensively examined. The MENQOL was developed through a study of 88 women aged between 47 and 62 years, all of whom had an intact uterus and had not received HT in the previous 6 months. These women were administered an instrument containing a list of 106 menopause symptoms to be rated according to their severity. Symptoms were identified based on the scientific literature and on the clinical experience of the authors, who consisted of eight doctors and two QOL specialists. Participants were asked whether they had experienced each one of the symptoms listed and required to rate each symptom on a 7-point Likert severity scale. The questionnaire originally investigated the following five domains: physical, vasomotor, psychosocial, sexual, and working life. However, the latter domain was later dropped from the scale, after a validation study showed that its contribution to score variability was negligible. The resulting instrument contained 29 items divided into four domains (physical, vasomotor, psychosocial, and sexual), as well as one question about general QOL. Items were scored on a scale of one ("not at all bothered") to eight ("extremely bothered"). The total score for each domain was calculated based on the mean ratings of all items corresponding to that factor [24].

Like the WHQ, the MENQOL does not provide a global score, and the relative contribution of each subscale to total QOL is unknown.

29.5 The Menopausal Quality Of Life Scale (MQOL)

The Menopausal Quality of Life Scale (MQOL) was developed in the Plymouth University (United Kingdom) Psychology Department by Pamela Jacobs and colleagues [25]. The questionnaire was developed to achieve the following major objectives: (1) to analyze the impact of menopause on health-related QOL (HRQOL); (2) to assess the impact of work, age, and medical history on HRQOL during menopause; (3) to investigate differences in HRQOL based on self-rated menopausal status; and (4) to examine the effects of HT on QOL during perimenopause.

The study was originally conducted on 32 women recruited through advertisements around the university campus and in local newspapers. A second wave of participants consisting of 29 women who participated in focus groups was later recruited for the study. The final sample was composed of 61 women with a mean age of 48 years, of whom 43 % were receiving HT, 13 % had a prior history of HT, and 44 % had never used HT. These studies produced a 63-item questionnaire which assessed the following seven domains: energy, sleep, appetite, cognition, feelings, social interaction, and symptom impact. Each item was scored on a six-point Likert scale, and to decrease response bias, 34 items were negatively worded while 29 were positively worded. A total of 99 individuals responded to the questionnaire. Participants had a mean age of 50 years, and 30 % of them were found to be HT users, while 8 % had a prior history of HT. After psychometric analysis, 15 items were excluded from the questionnaire, so that the final version of the MQOL contained a total of 48 items. A new study [26] was then conducted using the 48-item MQOL in addition to a measure of general HRQOL (a global measure of GQOL (H-scale) in which participants were asked to rate their overall QOL on a 100-point scale [26]. The global H scale has named end points ("perfect quality of life" and "might as well be dead"), separated by seven additional quantifiers. The presence of such quantifiers has been found to be associated with greater reliability and of an assessment of responder preference when compared with simple endpoint labeling. These instruments were administered to 1,188 women with a mean age of 51, of whom 22.5 % were receiving HT. A principal component analysis of the complete data set and of participant subsamples found that a general "severity" factor accounted for 35 % of the variability in MQOL scores. Further analyses led the authors to conclude that the MQOL should provide a global score rather than separate subscores for each of the seven domains. The Cronbach's alpha coefficients for each factor ranged from 0.91 to 0.69, showing adequate internal consistency. Correlations between domain scores were also satisfactory, with the energy and social interaction scores having a correlation of 0.68, the energy and symptom impact domains correlating at 0.68, the symptom impact and social interaction factors having a correlation of 0.67, and the cognition and feelings scores correlating at 0.65. In light of these results, the authors concluded that all factors should have equal weight in the composite QOL score and determined that they should all be summed to provide a global measure of QOL [24].

29.6 The Menopause Rating Scale (MRS)

The MRS was developed to address the lack of standardized measures to assess the severity of aging symptoms and their impact on QOL. The MRS was developed in the early 1990s based on data obtained from a representative sample of 500 German women aged between 45 and 60 years [27]. Although it was initially designed to be completed by the doctor in charge of treatment, methodological criticisms led the instrument to be adapted to a self-administered format [28]. The scale was internationally well accepted, and after being translated from the original

German to English, the MRS was adapted for use in Brazilian Portuguese, English, French, Indonesian, Italian, Mexican, Argentinian, Spanish, Swedish, and Turkish [29].

The instrument consists of 11 questions that probe the following three symptom domains: somato-vegetative, urogenital, and psychological. Items are assessed on a scale of 0 to 3, where higher scores denote greater perceived symptom severity (a score of 0 indicates no complaints, while 4 suggests very severe symptoms). The participant answers each item according to their personal experience of each symptom, and the scores for all items within each subscale are added up to provide factor scores. The total scale score is obtained by summing up the subscale scores. The urogenital factor was found to explain 59 % of the variance in total MRS scores [29].

29.7 Qualifemme

The Qualifemme was developed in France with the aim of assessing the influence of menopausal on QOL. The instrument was initially composed of 32 items drawn from previously translated and validated measures of HRQOL. The items were linguistically validated into French [30] and analyzed by a group of menopause specialists with the aim of adding clinical experience to the instrument. Items were rated on a visual analogue scale. The Qualifemme scores of 351 women aged between 41 and 68 years were analyzed to reveal five factors: general (9 items), pyschological (12 items), vasomotor (2 items), urogenital (6 items), and a final factor corresponding to pain and hair and skin problems (3 items). The scale had satisfactory internal consistency, and a factor with a Cronbach's alpha of 0.87 was found to explain 46 % of the variance in Qualifemme scores. A second study of 58 women aged between 51 and 73 years was performed to determine the scale's reliability. Test-retest analyses were conducted on a sample of 62 individuals, and the Pearson correlation between scores at the two time points was found to range from 0.84 to 0.98. Strong correlations were also found between raw and standardized scores on the Qualifemme ($r=0.99$ $p<0.001$). As a result of statistical analyses, the scale was reduced from 32 to 15 items, while maintaining its psychometric properties [30].

29.8 Summary

The past decades have seen a significant increase in the importance given to QOL in both community and health-care settings. Increases in QOL have been associated with decreased morbidity and mortality rates and, therefore, have been a major aim of a number of health-care policies and programs. Although much has been done in the way of defining and operationalizing the concept of QOL, an optimal assessment tool for this variable has yet to be found.

A number of assessment instruments have been developed to assess QOL in specific patient groups so as to obtain more relevant data on which to base health-care policies targeting improvements in population health. Assessments of QOL may be especially relevant for climacteric/menopausal women due to the influence of their symptoms on general well-being. Although there is no universally accepted tool to assess QOL in these individuals, since several factors may limit the cross-cultural applicability of the existing assessment methods, the present results suggest that, when assessing specific populations, it is important to use validated scales.

References

1. Verlade-Jurado E, Avila-Figueroa C. Methods for quality of life assessment. Salud Publica Mex. 2002;44(4):349–61.
2. WHOQOL GROUP. The development of the World Health Organization quality of life assessment instrument (the WHOQOL). In: Orley J, Kuyken W, editors. Quality of life assessment: international perspectives. Heidelberg: Springer Verlag; 1994. p. 41–60.
3. Wild D, Grove A, Martin M, Eremenco S, McElroy S, Verjee-Lorenz A, et al. Principles of good practice for the translation and cultural adaptation process for Patient-Reported Outcomes (PRO) measures: report of the ISPOR task force for translation and cultural adaptation. Value Health. 2005;8(2):94–104.

4. Guillemin F, Bombardier C, Beaton D. Cross-cultural adaptation of health-related quality of life measures: literature review and proposed guidelines. J Clin Epidemiol. 1993;46(12):1417–32.
5. Ferraz MB, Oliveira LM, Araujo PM, Atra E, Tugwell P. Crosscultural reliability of the physical ability dimension of the health assessment questionnaire. J Rheumatol. 1990;17(6):813–7.
6. Utian WH, Woods NF. Impact of hormone therapy on quality of life after menopause. Menopause. 2013;20(10):1098–105.
7. Silva Filho CR, Baracat EC, Conterno Lde O, Haidar MA, Ferraz MB. Climacteric symptoms and quality of life: validity of women's health questionnaire. Rev Saude Publica. 2005;39(3):333–9.
8. Hunter M. The women's health questionnaire : a measure of mid-aged women's perceptions of their emotional and physical health. Psychol Health. 1992;7(7):45–54.
9. Fleck MPA, Leal OF, Louzada S, Xavier M, Chachamovich E, Vieira G, et al. Development of the Portuguese version of the OMS evaluation instrument of quality of life. Rev Bras Psiquiatr. 1999;21(1):19–28.
10. Ware Jr JE, Sherbourne CD. The MOS 36-item short-form health survey (SF-36). I. Conceptual framework and item selection. Med Care. 1992;30(6):473–83.
11. Harlow SD, Gass M, Hall JE, Lobo R, Maki P, Rebar RW, et al. Executive summary of the Stages of Reproductive Aging Workshop + 10: addressing the unfinished agenda of staging reproductive aging. J Clin Endocrinol Metab. 2012;97(4):1159–68.
12. Bromberger JT, Schott LL, Kravitz HM, Sowers M, Avis NE, Gold EB, et al. Longitudinal change in reproductive hormones and depressive symptoms across the menopausal transition: results from the Study of Women's Health Across the Nation (SWAN). Arch Gen Psychiatry. 2010;67(6):598–607.
13. Woods NF, Mitchell ES. Sleep symptoms during the menopausal transition and early postmenopause: observations from the Seattle Midlife Women's Health Study. Sleep. 2010;33(4):539–49.
14. Fritz MA, Speroff L. Clinical gynecologic endocrinology and infertility. 8th ed. Philadelphia: Lippincott Williams & Wilkins; 2010.
15. Shin H, Shin HS. Measurement of quality of life in menopausal women: a systematic review. West J Nurs Res. 2012;34(4):475–503.
16. Lewis JE, Hilditch JR, Wong CJ. Further psychometric property development of the menopause-specific quality of life questionnaire and development of a modified version, MENQOL-intervention questionnaire. Maturitas. 2005;50(3):209–21.
17. Palacios S, Ferrer-Barriendos J, Parrilla JJ, Castelo-Branco C, Manubens M. Design of a new specific quality of life scale for menopause in Spanish language, the Cervantes Scale. Climateric. 2002;5(supplement 1):159.
18. Lima JE, Palacios S, Wender MC. Quality of life in menopausal women: a Brazilian Portuguese version of the Cervantes Scale. Sci World J. 2012;2012:620519.
19. Lima JEM. Tradução, adaptação cultural e validação da versão em português brasileiro da Escala Cervantes de Qualidade de Vida Relacionada com a Saúde da Mulher durante a Perimenopausa e na Pós-menopausa. Brazil: Universidade Federal do Rio Grande do Sul; 2009. Master's thesis.
20. Perez-Lopez FR, Fernandez-Alonso AM, Perez-Roncero G, Chedraui P, Monterrosa-Castro A, Llaneza P. Assessment of menopause-related symptoms in mid-aged women with the 10-item Cervantes Scale. Maturitas. 2013;76(2):151–4.
21. Hunter M, Battersby R, Whitehead M. Relationships between psychological symptoms, somatic complaints and menopausal status. Maturitas. 1986;8(3):217–28.
22. Hunter MS. The Women's Health Questionnaire (WHQ): Frequently Asked Questions (FAQ). Health Qual Life Outcomes. 2003;1;41.
23. Wulf H. Utian and Nancy Fugate Woods. Impact of hormone therapy on quality of life after menopause. Menopause. 2013;20(10):1098–1105.
24. Hilditch JR, Lewis J, Peter A, van Maris B, Ross A, Franssen E, et al. A menopause-specific quality of life questionnaire: development and psychometric properties. Maturitas. 1996;24(3):161–75.
25. Jacobs PA, Hyland ME, Ley A. Self-rated menopausal status and quality of life in women aged 40–63 years. Br J Health Psychol. 2000;5(4):395–411.
26. Hyland ME, Sodergren SC. Development of a new type of global quality of life scale, and comparison of performance and preference for 12 global scales. Qual Life Res. 1996;5(5):469–80.
27. Hauser GA, Huber IC, Keller PJ, Lauritzen C, Schneider HPG. Evaluation der klinischen Beschwerden (Menopause rating scale). Zentralbl Gynakol. 1994;116:16–23.
28. Schneider HP, Heinemann LA, Rosemeier HP, Potthoff P, Behre HM. The Menopause Rating Scale (MRS): reliability of scores of menopausal complaints. Climacteric. 2000;3(1):59–64.
29. Heinemann LA, Potthoff P, Schneider HP. International versions of the Menopause Rating Scale (MRS). Health Qual Life Outcomes. 2003;1:28.
30. Le Floch JP, Colau JC, Zartarian M. Validation d'une méthode d'évaluation de la qualité de vie en ménopause. Ref Gynecol Obstet. 1994;2(2):179–88.

Vasomotor Symptoms

Maria Celeste O. Wender
and Patrícia Pereira de Oliveira

Contents

30.1 The Physiopathology of VMS 416
30.2 Epidemiology 418
30.3 Hormone and Nonhormonal Therapy 421
30.3.1 Hormone Therapy 421
30.3.2 Nonhormonal Therapy 425

References 428

M.C.O. Wender, MD, PhD (✉)
Department of Obstetrics and Gynecology,
Menopause Clinic of Hospital de Clinicas de Porto Alegre, Federal University of Rio Grande do Sul
Rua 14 de julho 746/4, Porto Alegre,
Rio Grande do Sul 91340430, Brazil
e-mail: mceleste@ufrgs.br

P.P. de Oliveira, PhD
Department of Medicine, University Unochapecó,
Chapecó, Santa Catarina, Brazil
e-mail: patriciapoliveira@hotmail.com

The menopausal transition can be categorized into several stages and is accompanied by significant psychological, organic, and metabolic changes. Menopausal symptoms refer to the symptoms experienced during the menopausal transition and after menopause. The current nomenclature for female reproductive senescence is confusing; however, in 2001 a revision of the terminology was proposed by the Stages of Reproductive Aging Workshop (STRAW) group [1, 2]. Menopause is defined as amenorrhea for 12 months following the final menstrual period and can be classified into natural or surgical menopause. Natural menopause is defined as the permanent cessation of menstruation resulting from the loss of ovarian follicular activity without other obvious pathological or physiological causes. Surgical menopause is defined as the cessation of menstruation resulting from the removal of the uterus, with or without bilateral oophorectomy. The menopausal transition comprehends the period between the first variations in menstrual cycle length and the final menstrual period.

The first menopausal symptoms to appear, and the most detrimental to women's well-being, are usually vasomotor in nature. The most commonly reported menopausal vasomotor symptoms (VMS) are hot flashes or flushes. These are experienced by approximately 50–80 % of women during the menopausal transition [3–5] and constitute one of the main reasons for seeking medical attention [6]. Hot flashes are among the most commonly reported VMS and consist of

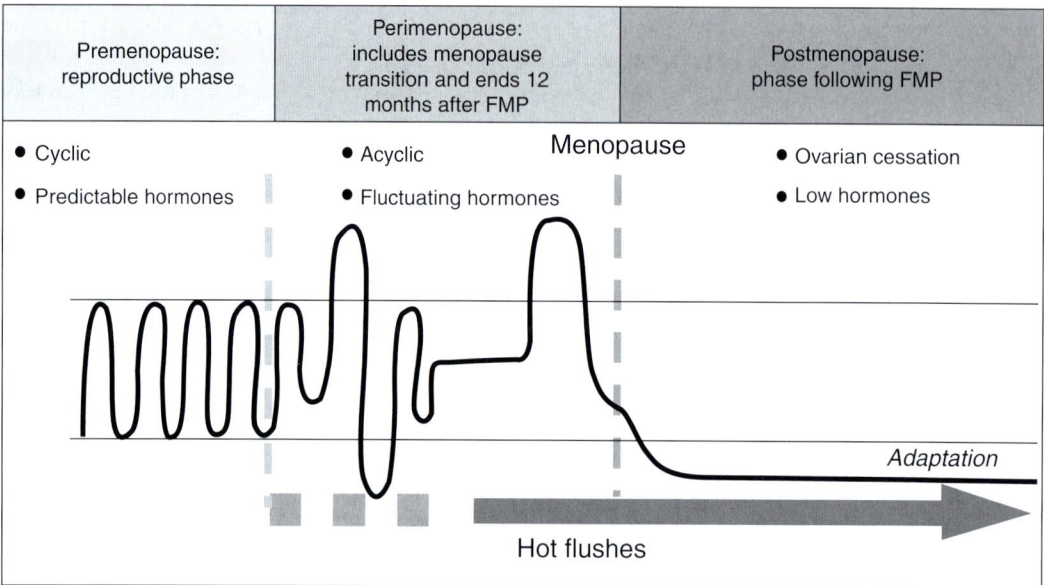

Fig. 30.1 Relationship between estrogen and a woman's reproductive phases and the occurrence of hot flushes. The reproductive phase is characterized by cyclic and predictable estrogen levels. During perimenopause, hormones fluctuate and become acyclic. During this period, many women experience VMS; although severe, the frequency is transient. During the postmenopausal period, women can experience severe and persistent VMS due to the declining levels of ovarian hormones. For most women, VMS eventually diminish over time. *FMP* final menstrual period (Reprinted with permission from Deecher and Dorries [5], With kind permission from Springer Science + Business Media)

recurrent sensations of intense heat on the skin around the head, neck, anterior thorax, and back. These may be accompanied by sweating, palpitations, nausea, dizziness, chills, pressure, or pain in the head and chest; changes in breathing patterns or heart rate; and sleep alterations [5, 7, 8]. These episodes generally last from 1 to 5 min but may continue for as long as 15 min in some cases [9]. Another frequent vasomotor symptom is commonly known as "night sweats." Hot flashes and intense sensations of heat are common causes of insomnia in climacteric women [10]. VMS tend to decrease in intensity over the first 5 years after the menopausal transition and appear to peak in late perimenopause and early postmenopause, that is, in the years around the end of the menstrual cycle [4–6] (Fig. 30.1). In a small percentage of cases, these symptoms may occur prior to premenopausal menstrual changes or even decades after the menopausal transition [4]. On average, moderate or severe hot flashes continue for nearly 5 years after menopause [1, 2, 4, 11]. However, more than one-third of women experience moderate to severe hot flashes for 10 years or more after menopause [11]. These symptoms may be worse or more persistent in women with early or surgical menopause [5, 6].

30.1 The Physiopathology of VMS

The physiopathological mechanisms that underlie VMS are not entirely known. Although altered estrogen levels due to decreased ovarian function are known to contribute significantly to the development of VMS, they are not the sole cause of these phenomena [5, 6, 12, 13]. Studies have found that the combination of high FSH and low E2 concentrations may be associated with a higher probability of VMS, especially in perimenopausal women with non-ovulating cycles; however, not all women who exhibit these alterations report VMS [2, 13, 14].

Body temperature is maintained through a dynamic equilibrium between internal and external factors. Symptomatic postmenopausal women have been found to display a narrowing of the thermoneutral zone or the range of temperatures in which the body can be maintained without triggering thermoregulatory homeostatic mechanisms such as sweating or shivering [13].

The thermoregulatory system monitors and maintains body temperature through the interaction of three main elements: the brain, the internal abdominal cavity, and the peripheral vascular system. When body temperature drops below the optimum level for normal physiological functioning, peripheral vasoconstriction and shivering may occur so as to conserve heat and increase body temperature. Conversely, when body temperature rises above the optimum level, peripheral vasodilation and sweating may take place, so as to facilitate heat loss through the skin [5]. These phenomena are controlled by a hypothalamic nucleus (anterior hypothalamus/preoptic area) which is responsible for maintaining body temperature within the thermoneutral zone, an optimal temperature range whose limits vary slightly over the circadian cycle [7, 12–14]. The hypothalamic thermoregulatory center is also sensitive to variations in monoamine neurotransmitters, such as serotonin and noradrenaline; to changes in gonadal steroids, such as progesterone and the luteinizing hormone; and to some medications and medical conditions [4, 5, 15, 16].

Information about changes in body temperature reaches the brain through heat- and cold-sensitive fibers in the central nervous system, in deep tissues, and in the skin. The temperature sensors involved in the activation of thermoregulatory responses are located deep within the body (in the gastrointestinal tract and other internal organs, in intra-abdominal veins, and in the spinal medulla) as well as in peripheral organs (skin) [5]. The preoptic area sends fibers to effector structures in the brain stem and the medulla through the medial forebrain bundle. These projections control heat loss effectors in the lateral hypothalamus, the periaqueductal gray, and the reticular formation, which are responsible for peripheral vasodilation and sweating. Body temperature is essentially maintained by changes in cutaneous and subcutaneous blood flow and sweating. If body temperature rises above the normal level, peripheral vasodilation is triggered, leading to an increase in blood flow (sympathetic nervous system). When temperature drops below the thermoregulatory limit, there is a reduction in blood flow to peripheral tissues, so as to maintain body heat [13, 14, 17].

The exact physiopathological mechanisms behind VMS have not been completely elucidated. Of the three most prominent hypotheses for the origin of VMS, the one proposed by Tataryn et al. [18] appears to be the most accepted. According to this theory, stimulation by beta-2-adrenergic receptors may lead to increased sympathetic activity during the menopausal transition, which could lead to a reduction in the thermoneutral zone. VMS could therefore consist of large responses to small variations in body temperature [13]. Significant decreases in cardiac vagal control have been found to occur during hot flashes, which may help elucidate the physiology of hot flashes [19]. These responses could involve intense sensations of heat, skin flushing, and increased blood flow leading to changes in heart rate and blood pressure, all of which are commonly associated with hot flashes. Conversely, reductions in body temperature may induce an exaggerated vasodilation, leading to chills and sweating [5].

Another hypothesis suggests that a decrease in the responsiveness of peripheral vascular systems (skin) to temperature variations could interfere with the speed and efficiency of vessel responses, leading to exaggerated reactions to stimuli and, consequently, VMS. Perimenopausal fluctuations and a postmenopausal decrease in estradiol levels could contribute to this disequilibrium, reducing blood vessel elasticity and leading to inadequate responses to variations in body temperature [5].

A third hypothesis associates the occurrence of VMS with neurochemical alterations secondary to gonadal hormone variations. These hypotheses have served as the basis for the development of medications that aim to control VMS by normalizing norepinephrine and/or 5-HT levels [5].

30.2 Epidemiology

VMS appear to vary according to race and ethnicity, with African-American women being more likely to report such symptoms and Chinese and Japanese women being less likely to do so [4, 6]. In the Ovarian Aging Study cohort, both obese and nonobese African-American women as well as obese white women were found to be significantly more prone to hot flashes than nonobese white women (interaction, $p=0.01$) [11]. The reasons for these differences are not entirely clear, although E2 levels, body mass index (BMI), hormone use, and socioeconomic status are thought to be risk factors for VMS. The possible role of a soy-rich diet, such as that seen in Asian cultures, is still a controversial topic [4]. Gene variants in estrogen α-receptors and in enzymes involved in the synthesis of and conversion between more and less potent estrogens have been associated with varying probabilities of VMS in different ethnic and racial groups due to their impact on steroid hormone activity. A number of studies have investigated the contribution of polymorphisms in estrogen receptors and in nucleotides involved in the synthesis and metabolism of different estrogens (E2, estrogen, estriol) to the development of VMS. Although the results of these studies are not definitive, they appear to suggest that associations between genetics and VMS may be observed both at a central (brain) and peripheral level (autonomic nervous system, vascular system, or other structures involved in VMS) [4].

The SWAN Genetics Study [20] identified important associations between genetic sex steroid hormone pathway variants and measures of health status. The study describes selected genetic characteristics of health-related attributes during the menopausal transition in African-American, Caucasian, Chinese, and Japanese women. The sample consisted of menstruating women aged 42–52 years, living in the community, who were not using exogenous hormones. The genotypes and haplotypes of six genes (27 single nucleotide polymorphisms [SNPs]) in the sex steroid hormone pathway were found to be associated with circulating hormone concentrations, menstrual cycle profiles, and health-related outcomes, including lipid levels, diabetes mellitus, depressive symptoms, measures of cognition, bone mineral density (BMD), and vasomotor symptoms. Allele frequencies and distances differed significantly between the four ethnic groups evaluated, which resulted in variable patterns of association between genetic variables and the health-related measures evaluated. Several SNPs were associated with health outcomes, and some associations were significantly more prominent in specific ethnicities. For instance, ESR1 rs3798577 was related to circulating estradiol concentrations, indicators of ovarian aging, high-density lipoprotein (HDL) cholesterol, apolipoprotein A-1, insulin sensitivity, and lumbar spine BMD. CYP1A1 rs2606345 was found to be associated with estrogen metabolite concentrations, vasomotor symptoms, and depressive symptoms. In Chinese women, statistically significant associations were found between ESR2 rs1256030 and HDL cholesterol, lumbar spine BMD, hip BMD, and metabolic syndrome [20].

Obesity has also been considered a risk factor for VMS [4, 6]. Although obesity used to be considered protective against VMS due to the aromatization of androgens to estrogens in adipose tissue, recent studies have found that obesity may actually be a risk factor for these symptoms during perimenopause and early menopause. This association is consistent with a thermoregulatory model of VMS, even though the mechanisms underlying this interaction remain unclear. The adipose tissue may act as an insulator and prevent the dissipation of the heat caused by VMS, increasing their frequency and severity and possibly having an impact on other neuroendocrine processes. Every 1-SD increase in total and subcutaneous abdominal adiposity was associated with a proportional increase in the odds of hot flashes in age- and site-adjusted models (odds ratio [OR]=1.28; 95 % CI: 1.06–1.55 and OR=1.30; 95 % CI: 1.07–1.58, respectively). Visceral adiposity was not associated with susceptibility to hot flashes [21]. This phenomenon may be more applicable to women in the beginning of the menopausal transition [4]. Body fat gains were associated with a higher frequency of hot flashes during the menopausal transition. However, the association between changes in body fat distribution and night sweats was not statistically significant [22]. Bioimpedance studies have found that, regardless of BMI, a higher percentage of fat mass was associated with a greater likelihood of VMS, even after controlling for other confounders. Lean mass was not found to be related to VMS. Studies using abdominal tomography have also shown that high abdominal adiposity, especially if subcutaneous, is associated with more complaints about hot flashes in women who report higher gains in body fat from 1 year to the next [2].

Lifestyle may also be related to the occurrence of VMS. Among the lifestyle factors studied in relation to these symptoms, smoking deserves special attention [4, 6, 23]. In fact, SWAN results show that both active smoking and passive exposure to smoke are associated with a greater likelihood of VMS. It has been hypothesized that the association between smoking and VMS may be attributable to the antiestrogenic effects of cigarette smoking. On the other hand, the study also found that variations in endogenous E2 levels did not account for the association between smoking and VMS [23].

Other lifestyle factors, such as diet and physical activity, have shown weaker associations with VMS. Dietary factors, such as total kilocalories, fats, fibers, caffeine, alcohol, vitamins, or isoflavones (genistein), consumed have shown no relationship with VMS in the SWAN study [24, 25]. The same has been found for physical activity [26]. However, it is possible that the latter may have a dual and opposing influence on VMS (positive effect on mood and body weight and negative effect on core body temperature, which could increase the occurrence of symptoms) [25].

Mood and negative emotions, especially anxiety, also appear to influence the intensity of VMS [4, 6, 11]. Although this interaction has not been extensively studied, it is thought that the influence of physiological and psychological factors may be both combined and bidirectional [4]. Studies suggest that VMS may precede, follow, or occur simultaneously with depression, which suggests a number of possible causal relationships. Other factors, including social variables such as childhood abuse or neglect, low socioeconomic status, low education, and income, may also have a negative influence on the intensity of VMS. To examine whether women were more likely to experience a major depressive episode during perimenopause or postmenopause compared to the premenopausal period, 221 premenopausal women were analyzed. The results showed that women were two to four times more likely to experience a major depressive episode when they were in perimenopausal (OR=2.27) or postmenopausal (OR=3.57), even after controlling for several factors associated with depression, such as history of major depression at baseline, annual psychotropic medication use, high BMI, upsetting life events, and frequent VMS [27]. On the other hand, a second study assessed a randomly identified, population-based cohort of midlife women, who were followed for 6 years to estimate the association between anxiety and menopausal hot flashes in the early transition to menopause. At the end of the study, 32 % of the women were in the early transition stage, and 20 % were in the late menopausal transition or postmenopausal. A total of 37 % of the premenopausal women, 48 % of those in the early transition, 63 % of women in the late transition, and 79 % of the postmenopausal women reported to experiencing hot flashes. Anxiety scores were significantly associated with the occurrence, severity, and frequency of hot flashes (each outcome at $P<0.001$). The study also revealed that women with moderate and high anxiety were three and five times more likely, respectively, to report hot flashes than women in the normal anxiety range [28].

A multicenter study conducted on 896 Chilean, Ecuadorian, Panamanian, and Spanish women in the peri- and postmenopausal period aimed to assess the association between climate (altitude, temperature, humidity, and annual temperature range) and the occurrence of hot flashes and/or night sweats. A total of 58.5 % (524/896) of the sample reported regular symptoms, and higher symptom prevalence was found in women living in places with higher temperatures and lower altitudes [29].

Overall, studies show that, although quality of life may not be influenced by menopause itself, it may be significantly lower in women who report VMS [4]. This relationship may be due to the impact of such symptoms on life and general health, as VMS may influence sleep quality, mood, and cognition and interact with other medical conditions. There appears to be a strong association between VMS and the quality and continuity of sleep (difficulty falling or remaining asleep or trouble waking up) [4]. For instance, the sleep disturbances caused by VMS may be an important risk factor for depression. Conversely, the serotonergic and noradrenergic symptoms commonly associated with depression may also influence the development of VMS [4]. In the SWAN study, difficulty sleeping was reported by 37.7 % of 12,603 women (78.5 % of those participating in this cross-sectional survey), 40–55 years old. These prevalence rates increased between pre- and late perimenopause. Late perimenopausal and surgically menopausal women were the most likely to report difficulty sleeping. The study suggested that women who begin the menopausal transition at an earlier age may experience more frequent and/or severe sleep symptoms [30]. Additionally, an experimental model of leuprolide-induced hot flashes has demonstrated a causal relationship between hot flashes and poor sleep quality [31].

Cognitive performance may also be impaired during the perimenopausal period, and there have been reports of temporary reductions in learning ability which subsequently resolve in the postmenopausal period [4, 32, 33]. In the Rochester Investigation of Cognition Across Menopause [33], 117 middle-aged women were recruited and categorized into the following stages: late reproductive ($n=34$), early menopausal transition ($n=28$), late menopausal transition ($n=41$), or early postmenopause ($n=14$). Women in the first year postmenopause performed significantly worse than women in the late reproductive and late menopausal transition stages on measures of verbal learning, verbal memory, and motor function. They also performed significantly worse than women in the late menopausal transition stage on attention/working memory tasks. In a separate study, a cohort of 1,903 midlife US women were followed longitudinally for 6 years and asked whether the symptoms reported during the menopausal transition negatively affected cognitive performance. The study also investigated whether these symptoms were responsible for the negative effect of perimenopause on cognitive processing speed. After adjustment for demographic variables, the results showed that women with concurrent depressive symptoms scored 1 point lower on the Symbol Digit Modalities Test (SDMT) ($p<0.05$) than those without such symptomatology. On the East Boston Memory Test, the rate of learning in women with anxiety symptoms was 0.09 lower at each assessment ($p=0.03$) and was found to be equivalent to 53 % of the mean learning rate for the cohort as a whole. The SDMT learning rate was 1.00 point smaller in late perimenopause than during premenopause ($p=0.04$); statistical adjustment for symptoms did not attenuate this negative effect. Depressive and anxiety symptoms had a small negative effect on processing speed. The authors concluded that depression, anxiety, sleep disturbance, and VMS did not account for the decrement in SDMT learning observed during late perimenopause [32]. Although these changes are not directly related to VMS, these findings suggest that physiological changes associated with these phenomena may have an impact on cognitive function [4].

The Women's Health Initiative (WHI) and the Heart and Estrogen/Progestin Replacement Study (HERS) have also investigated the relationship between VMS and other medical conditions. These studies found that the presence of moderate and severe VMS may be associated with cardiovascular disease (CVD). Results also showed that CVD was more frequent among symptomatic women undergoing hormone therapy (HT) [34–36]. The SWAN Heart Study assessed 588 women and found that those with hot flashes displayed medial carotid thickening (a marker of atherosclerosis), a symptom which had been previously reported mostly in overweight and obese women. Women reporting hot flashes, and in the case of IMT more frequent hot flashes, had poorer endothelial function, greater aortic calcification, and greater IMT when compared to individuals without hot flashes, even after controlling for demographic confounds, other known cardiovascular risk factors, as well as E2 levels. These findings support the association between VMS and CVD [37, 38].

Women with VMS also appear to have lower mineral bone density (MBD) than asymptomatic women, with reductions in spine and hip density being more common in the postmenopausal period and lower femoral neck density being more frequent in premenopausal women [4].

30.3 Hormone and Nonhormonal Therapy

Many treatments may help control VMS. However, it is important to weigh the risks and benefits of each treatment on a case-by-case basis and to discuss treatment preferences with the patient in order to select the most adequate option. Estrogen has been used as a hormone supplement, and many studies indicate that it is superior to placebo in alleviating VMS, reducing the frequency of hot flashes by 77 % or by approximately 2.5–3 hot flashes daily. However, recent studies have reported adverse effects of estrogen, raising important concerns about its use [39]. There has been an increasing amount of literature on nonhormonal agents for the treatment of hot flashes. Conventional nonhormonal treatments (CNHT) and complementary and alternative medicines (CAM) have both been studied for their ability to relieve VMS. CNHT are neuroactive agents considered to be safe in cases in which estrogens are contraindicated, such as psychotropic medications like selective serotonin reuptake inhibitors, serotonin-norepinephrine reuptake inhibitors, and gabapentin. CAM are defined as a group of healthcare systems, practices and products which are not normally considered to be conventional medicine: herbal products, acupuncture, vitamins, exercise, yoga, and many others. Another promising nonpharmacological therapy which is currently under investigation involves stellate ganglion blocking [40].

30.3.1 Hormone Therapy

Hormone therapy (HT) appears to have greater efficacy than nonhormonal therapy in the control of VMS [39, 41]. Its effect has been confirmed in women of all ages, and it has been found to reduce symptoms in up to 80 % of those treated [6]. Although its prescription should still be evaluated on an individual basis, its benefits appear to outweigh its risks in symptomatic women younger than 60 years or those who are less than 10 years postmenopause [42]. To assess the cardiovascular risks of HT, 1,006 women aged between 45 and 48 years who were in the perimenopausal or early menopausal stages were randomly assigned to HT or placebo (combined HT for women with an intact uterus and estrogen alone for women who had undergone hysterectomies). Patients were then followed for 16 years. After 10 years of treatment, it was found that women who began HT in early menopause appear to have a lower risk of cardiovascular events (HR 0.48, 95 % CI 0.26–0.87, $p=0.015$) and lower mortality rates (0.57, 0.30–1.08), $p=0.084$), without a concomitant increase in the risk of any type of cancer (0.92, 0.58–1.45, $p=0.71$), including breast cancer (0.58, 0.27–1.27, $p=0.17$), deep vein thrombosis (2.01, 0.18–22.16), or strokes (0.77, 0.35–1.70), than those who did not receive such a treatment [23].

To minimize adverse events, the lowest effective dose should be used for the shortest amount of time and only when there are no contraindications (see list). The choice to undergo HT is an individualized one, and the impact of treatment on health and quality of life should always be considered. The duration of treatment must always be discussed with the patient, and she should also be informed of her personal risk, which is calculated based on factors such as age and years since menopause, and of the increased risk of venous thromboembolism, stroke, ischemic disease, and breast cancer associated with HT [42].

Although there is no consensus regarding the ideal duration of treatment, the North American Menopause Society (NAMS) suggests a maximum treatment duration of 5 years, although the chance of symptom recurrence remains stable at approximately 50 %, regardless of patient age and treatment duration [43].

According to the last HT Position Statement of NAMS [43], HT should be primarily recommended for the treatment of VMS and never as the main intervention in the management of CVD or osteoporosis or the prevention of dementia, even though HT has proved to be effective and adequate for the prevention of osteoporosis-related fractures in at-risk women aged 60 years or less and to lead to a lower cardiovascular risk and reduced mortality rates when initiated less than 10 years postmenopause [42–45]. According to the global consensus statement on menopausal hormone therapy, women with premature ovarian insufficiency should be prescribed systemic HT until they reach the mean natural menopausal age [42, 43].

Absolute contraindications for HT [46, 47]:
- History of breast cancer
- Coronary disease
- History of stroke or thromboembolism
- Active liver disease
- Being at risk for any one of these complications

Estrogen therapy is the gold standard for managing VMS [39, 41]. Studies suggest that HT is more effective than other treatments in reducing hot flushes. Oral 17-β-estradiol and progestogen decrease the number of episodes by as much as −16.8/day (−23.4 to −10.2 mean difference in number of hot flushes per day), while the use of soy isoflavones has only been found to decrease the number of daily hot flushes by a mean of −1.22 (−2.02 to −0.42) [48]. In non-hysterectomized women, it should be prescribed in combination with a progestogen due to the risk of hyperplasia or endometrial cancer [14, 17–19, 22]. As well as relieving VMS, HT may also have positive effects on urinary and sexual function, bone health, mood disturbances, and quality of life [18, 19, 22], as well as on muscle and joint pain and sleep disturbances [19]. However, HT should not be used as primary therapy for these conditions.

The use of low-dose topical estrogen may improve sexual satisfaction by increasing vaginal lubrication, blood flow, and sensitivity, although it has not been associated with a longer period of sexual activity. Topical estrogen has been found to alleviate the symptoms caused by a hyperactive bladder and to have a positive effect on repeated urinary infection [49]. Ultralow-dose estradiol-releasing vaginal rings and oral oxybutynin appeared to be similarly effective in decreasing the number of daily voids in postmenopausal women with overactive bladder [49]. However, it should not be used as the main treatment for sexual dysfunction, decreased libido, or urinary tract dysfunctions [43].

The risk of breast cancer in HT users aged 50 years or older has been the object of constant discussion. This risk appears to be especially associated with the combined use of estrogen and progestogen and may be influenced by treatment duration. Overall, the risk of breast cancer in these patients appears to be low and to decrease when treatment is discontinued. However, there are no data supporting its use in patients with a history of breast cancer [42, 43]. Although the WHI study did not primarily focus on the effect of HT on VMS, it was able to provide important information on this subject. The study assessed the impact of isolated (equine estrogen 0.625 mg/day) and combined (associated with medroxyprogesterone acetate 2.5 mg/day) estrogen therapy on the reduction of cardiovascular events (CVE) in postmenopausal women aged between 50 and 79 years. Although the study found a decrease in the risk of fractures and colon cancer, a 5.2-year follow-up showed an increased risk of breast cancer, coronary artery disease or CAD, stroke, and venous thromboembolism (VTE), which required one of the arms of the study to be interrupted in 2002. Although estrogen and progestogen therapy (EPT) did not significantly increase the risk of breast cancer until the fourth year of use, individuals receiving this treatment had an overall higher rate of abnormal mammography results [34].

In the original WHI study, the total rate of CAD was $39 \times 33/10{,}000$ people/year in the EPT and placebo groups, respectively (HR 1.24; CI 1.00–1.54). Estrogen therapy (ET) was not associated with increased rates of CAD (HR 0.91; CI 0.75–1.12) and appeared to have a protective influence in younger women (50–59 years) and those with less than 10 years of menopause [34]. A 31 % increase in the risk of stroke was observed in the EPT group, and a 39 % increase was found in the ET group regardless of age and other risk factors, although no excess risk was seen in the younger patient group [14]. The rate of VTE was higher in the EPT than in the placebo group (34×16/10,000 people/year, with HR 2.06; CI 1.60–2.70) [34]. It is important to note that each case should be carefully analyzed before HT is prescribed, since some methodological issues (such as the high mean age of women involved in studies, long duration of menopause, overweight/obesity, and smoking rates) may limit the generalization of the findings reported to the general population. A recent placebo-controlled randomized clinical trial (RCT) conducted on 1,006 women between the ages of 45 and 59 years investigated the occurrence of cardiovascular events in recently menopausal women (less than 2 years) undergoing HT (2 mg 17β estradiol + 1 mg norethisterone acetate, administered in triphasic regimen, or 2 mg 17β estradiol in hysterectomized women) [44]. After 10 years of treatment, there was a significant reduction in the risk of death, cardiac insufficiency, and acute myocardial infarction but no apparent increase in the risk of cancer, VTE, and stroke, suggesting that early HT may offer more benefits than risks for healthy women.

The data on the association between HT and the risk of ovarian cancer are somewhat conflicting. The use of HT for less than 5 years was associated with an RR of 1.03 for ovarian cancer, while individuals who had been receiving HT for over 10 years had an RR of 1.21. ET was associated with a higher risk of ovarian cancer than EPT [43]. The WHI found that EPT did not lead to a statistically significant increase in the incidence of ovarian cancer after a mean of 5.6 years of use (4.2 cases per 10,000 in the EPT group versus 2.7 cases per 10,000 per year in the placebo group) [50]. As the incidence of ovarian cancer was rare, the risk for the disease was considered small. However, women with other risk factors for ovarian cancer (for instance, a family history of cancer or a BRCA mutation) should be informed of the possible association between increased cancer risk and HT before starting treatment [43, 45].

The effect of HT on the incidence of lung cancer has also been investigated. However, there does not appear to be a consensus as to the relationship between these variables. While a meta-analysis reported an increase in the risk of lung adenocarcinoma in HT patients [51], another suggested that HT may have a protective effect against lung cancer in nonsmokers [52]. In the WHI study, post hoc analyses after an average of 7.1 years of HT found that the incidence of non-small cell lung cancer was not significantly higher in the EPT group (HR, 1.28, CI 95%, 0.94–1.73, $p=0.12$), although the number of lung cancer deaths (HR, 1,87, 95 % CI, 1.22–2.88, $p=0.004$) and of poorly differentiated and metastatic tumors were both higher in the EPT group (HR 1,87, $p=0.004$; CI, 1.22–2.88 95 %). However, it is important to note that all women diagnosed with cancer had a current or past history of smoking or were over 60 years old [27]. These results highlight the need to motivate tobacco users to quit smoking and suggest that current or past smokers who receive EPT should be carefully monitored during treatment [43, 45].

HT (estrogen plus progestin) does not appear to influence the risk of colorectal, esophageal, and endometrial cancer. However, weak evidence (small case-control studies) suggests that HT users may experience a reduction in the risk of stomach cancer and an increase in the risk of spleen cancer [53].

The route of hormone administration should also be carefully selected due to the association between certain forms of administration and specific medical conditions. The oral administration (OA) of estrogen may lead to an increase in sex hormone-binding globulin (SHBG) and thyroid binding globulins (TBG), reducing their bioavailability. Therefore, although OA may have a greater impact than transdermal administration (TDA), women who are being treated for hypothyroidism may need to increase their medication upon beginning orally administered HT [6].

The effects of TDA appear to be more stable, leading to quick and reliable results which are maintained for 3–7 days depending on drug formulation. These factors have great therapeutic importance. Hormones can also be administered through adhesive patches, gels, or sprays [6].

Combined estrogen and progestogens (E+P) should always be used in non-hysterectomized women to avoid the risk of endometrial cancer, but they may be used in isolation for the control of VMS. However, the maintenance of drug treatment may be confounded by adverse events such as weight gain, edema, and mood disturbances [4]. The most frequently used progestogens are medroxyprogesterone acetate (MPA) 1.5–10 mg; cyproterone acetate (CPA) 2–5 mg: nomegestrol acetate 5 mg; dydrogesterone 10 mg; norgestimate, trimegestone, norethisterone acetate 5–10 mg; and norethindrone 0.35–0.7 mg/day (minimal dosage) or 12 days a month (other dosages). Natural progesterone protects the endometrium and has only a small influence on lipid parameters. It is generally given in doses of 100–300 mg/day [43, 54]. The Kronos Early Estrogen Prevention Study (KEEPS), a recently conducted 4-year, randomized, double-blinded, placebo-controlled clinical trial, assessed the effects of low-dose oral or transdermal (skin patch) estrogen and cyclic monthly progesterone on healthy women aged 42 years to within 3 years after menopause [55]. The trial did not include women with evidence of cardiovascular disease, levels of plasma cholesterol or triglycerides which would normally be treated with lipid-lowering drugs, severe obesity, or heavy smoking. In the primary study, 727 participants were randomized into three groups: 0.45 mg a day of an oral conjugated equine estrogen (o-CEE), 50 μg a day of transdermal estradiol (t-E2), or a placebo. Women on active estrogens received 200 mg of micronized progesterone (MP) for 12 days each month. Both HT groups had reduced menopause symptoms, improvements in lubrication, and decreased pain during intercourse. However, the t-E2 group also had improved arousal and libido, while the o-CEE group did not. The carotid ultrasound results showed similar rates of arterial wall thickness progression in all three treatment groups over the 4 years of study [55].

Daily and continuous use of progesterone has been shown to be able to induce endometrial atrophy and, consequently, reduce vaginal bleeding in approximately 70–80 % of women after 6 months of treatment. The new progestogens (nomegestrol, norgestimate, dydrogesterone, and trimegestone) have a low androgenic effect and high selectivity for the progesterone receptor, leading to fewer negative effects on lipid profiles. Patients who have a low tolerance to monthly progestogen therapy should be prescribed continuous estrogen associated with progestogens (at doses equivalent to MPA 10 mg/day) for 15 days every 60 or 90 days. In women with a uterus, 0-CEE with cyclic MP has been found to have the most favorable effect on HDL-C, without an accompanying increase in the risk of endometrial hyperplasia [56]. However, the PEPI trial observed modest yet significant differences in hemostasis changes between different types and regimens of progestogen in postmenopausal women using CEE [57]. Nevertheless, in non-hysterectomized women, CEE with cyclic micronized progesterone (MP) has been found to have the most favorable effects on HDL-C, without leading to an excess risk of endometrial hyperplasia [55].

A recent Cochrane review of the short- and long-term effects of tibolone [58] found that the drug was superior to placebo in decreasing the frequency of VMS (two RCTs, $n=847$, OR 0.42; 95% CI 0.25–0.69); however, the 2.5 mg/day dose of the drug – the only one to significantly outperform the placebo – was also found to increase vaginal bleeding (7 RCTs, $n=7,462$; OR 2.75, 95% CI 1.99–3.80). When compared to 2 equipotent doses of EPT, tibolone was more effective in reducing vaginal bleeding (15 RCTs, $n=6,342$; OR 0.32, 95% CI 0.24–0.42) but had a lower impact on the frequency of VMS (two RCTs, $n=545$, OR 4.16, 95% CI 1.50–11. Two large RCTs comparing tibolone with placebo have also provided important data on the long-term effects of the drug [58]. An RCT of 3,098 women with breast cancer and menopause symptoms found an increase in cancer recurrence approximately 3.1 years into treatment (OR 1.50; 95% CI 1.21–1.85), which caused the trial to be interrupted [54]. The same RCT observed an excess risk of stroke in tibolone-treated patients

(OR 2.18, 95 % CI 1.12–4.21). The low number of events also precluded analyses of the impact of tibolone versus placebo on endometrial cancer rates (seven RCTs, $n=8,152$; OR 1.98; 95 % CI 0.73–5.32). The authors concluded that, even though 2.5 mg/day tibolone was associated with a lower incidence of vaginal bleeding, it proved to be less effective than EPT in decreasing VMS. The drug also appears to have less long-term safety than previously thought, since, according to a recent study, it may lead to an increase in the risk of breast cancer in women with a prior history of the disease and to an increased risk of stroke in women aged over 60 years [58].

In another randomized study, tibolone reduced the risk of fracture and breast cancer and possibly colon cancer, although it led to an increased risk of stroke in older women with osteoporosis [59]. The study involved 4,538 women between the ages of 60 and 85 years and had a bone mineral density T score of -2.5 or less at the hip or spine or a T score of -2.0 or less and radiologic evidence of a vertebral fracture, all of whom underwent a median of 34 months of treatment. The tibolone group received once-daily tibolone (at a dose of 1.25 mg), while the other group received placebo. A decreased risk of vertebral (70 cases versus 126 cases per 1,000 person-years, relative hazard, 0.55; 95 % CI 0.41–0.74; $p<0.001$) and nonvertebral fractures (122 cases versus 166 cases per 1,000 person-years, relative hazard, 0.74; 95 % CI, 0.58–0.93; $p=0.01$) was found in the tibolone group. The latter group also had a decreased risk of invasive breast cancer (relative hazard, 0.32; 95 % CI, 0.13–0.80; $p=0.02$) and colon cancer (relative hazard, 0.31; 95 % CI, 0.10–0.96; $p=0.04$). However, the tibolone group was also revealed to have an increased risk of stroke (relative hazard, 2.19; 95 % CI, 1.14–4.23; $p=0.02$), which led to the study being interrupted.

Many drug combinations can be used to treat VMS, and the choice of treatment should only be made after assessing each individual case. Treatment should always begin with the lowest possible dose, and the conventional dosage should only be employed if symptoms are unresponsive to therapy [6, 60]. If the only symptoms reported are vaginal dryness or discomfort during intercourse, low-dose topical estrogen therapy should be prescribed [42].

There is no evidence of the safety and efficacy of "bioidentical" hormones, and their use should therefore be avoided [6, 42, 45]. Even though the FDA-approved bioidentical hormones may be preferred over standard hormone replacement treatments due to their physiologic benefits and safety profiles, the Endocrine Society has voiced concerns that patients may be receiving potentially misleading or false information about the benefits and risks of "bioidentical hormones" [61].

30.3.2 Nonhormonal Therapy

Although there are no comparative studies of the effectiveness of non-estrogen treatment, options tend to be less effective in controlling VMS [62]. Nonhormonal methods usually reduce symptoms by 50–60 %, which may be considered acceptable by a number of women who do not want to or cannot receive HT [63, 64].

A meta-analysis of nonhormonal treatments for VMS [48] found that the selective serotonin (SSRIs) and norepinephrine (SNRIs) reuptake inhibitors gabapentin and clonidine are somewhat effective in reducing symptoms, although their effect on both the frequency and severity of VMS is lower than that of estrogen therapy [39, 41]. Currently, paroxetine (7.5 mg/day) is the only Food and Drug Administration-approved nonhormonal treatment for moderate to severe VMS [65].

Antidepressants (SSRIs and SNRIs) have shown some success in the control of VMS [40, 48, 61]. SSRIs act by increasing extracellular serotonin concentrations (5-HT), and SNRIs have the double effect of increasing 5-HT and norepinephrine (NE) levels, both of which are involved in hypothalamic thermoregulation [40]. After improvement, treatment should be gradually withdrawn. Clinical trials of paroxetine, venlafaxine, and desvenlafaxine have shown that these drugs may provide adequate symptom control [45, 48, 64, 66].

Special care should be taken when prescribing SSRIs to women who use tamoxifen. By interacting with cytochrome p450 (CYP2D6), these drugs may irreversibly inhibit the metabolism of tamoxifen to endoxifen, interfering with the efficacy of this treatment in patients with breast cancer. Venlafaxine and desvenlafaxine are the least potent inhibitors of this process [40].

Paroxetine doses of 10 mg to 12.5 mg/day appear to provide adequate VMS control (in up to 62 % of cases). Higher doses do not increase its efficacy but may lead to additional side effects (headaches, nausea, insomnia, somnolence) [40, 48]. A Canadian cohort study of breast cancer patients treated with tamoxifen who were also receiving paroxetine showed that death risk in these patients increased proportionately with the duration of treatment and ranged from 25 to 75 % [64]. In this study, of 2,430 women treated, 15.4 % died of breast cancer during mean follow-up 2.38 ± 2.59 years. After some adjustments, absolute increases of 25, 50, and 75 % in the proportion of time on tamoxifen with overlapping use of paroxetine were associated with 24, 54, and 91 % increases in the risk of death from breast cancer, respectively ($p<0.05$). In this way, it was estimated that the use of paroxetine for 41 % of tamoxifen treatment would result in one additional breast cancer death for every 19.7 patients so treated within 5 years of cessation of tamoxifen (95 % CI, 12.5–46.3).

Venlafaxine (75 mg/day) has also proved to be effective in controlling VMS in women with breast cancer [67]. When this drug reaches the liver, it is metabolized by CYP2D6 to desvenlafaxine, which interacts less with cytochrome p450 and, consequently, does not interfere with tamoxifen treatment. Doses of 100 and 150 mg/day have been found to decrease hot flashes by up to 65.4 and 66.6 %, respectively, after 12 weeks of treatment [66]. Desvenlafaxine is a novel serotonin-norepinephrine reuptake inhibitor which is highly selective for serotonin and norepinephrine transporters and has a weak or no affinity for dopamine receptors and transporters. The results of two double-blind, randomized, placebo-controlled trials revealed that, after 12 weeks of treatment, the groups treated with desvenlafaxine at doses of 100, 150, or 200 mg reported a more significant decrease in the number of hot flushes than the placebo group. Its tolerability profile is consistent with that of other serotonin-norepinephrine reuptake inhibitors [66, 68]. Desvenlafaxine 100 mg/day was superior to placebo in reducing the average daily number of hot flushes at weeks 4 ($p=0.013$) and 12 ($p=0.005$) of treatment, achieving a 64 % decrease from baseline at week 12, and the 75 % responder rate was significantly higher for desvenlafaxine 100 mg (50 %) compared with placebo (29 %; $p=0.003$; number needed to treat=4.7) at week 12. The average daily severity of hot flushes was also significantly lower in the desvenlafaxine 100-mg group than in the placebo group at week 12 ($p=0.020$) [68]. There is no evidence for an increased risk of cardiovascular, cerebrovascular, or hepatic events associated with the use of desvenlafaxine 100 mg/day for the treatment of menopausal VMS [69].

Fluoxetine at 20 mg/day and citalopram 10–30 mg/day are effective to a lesser extent than other antidepressants, probably due to their lower affinity for NE receptors [40]. The same phenomenon may explain the lower effectiveness of escitalopram 10–20 mg/day [5]. Sertraline (25–100 mg/day) has not been found to be effective in controlling VMS [70]. However, some studies showed a significant improvement of hot flushes with 50 mg/day sertraline in normal postmenopausal women and in women with tamoxifen treatment for breast cancer [71, 72]. Moreover, when compared with women in a placebo group, those who used sertraline were more likely to report gastrointestinal complaints, dry mouth, dizziness, and sexual function [68, 71, 72].

A multisite, randomized, placebo-controlled clinical trial with enrollment stratified by race (African-American and white) was conducted at four MsFlash network sites [73]. All eligible women were randomized in equal proportions to escitalopram 10 mg/day or to a matching placebo pill. At week 8, the reduction in the frequency of hot flashes was greater in the escitalopram group than in the placebo group (−4.60, SD 4.28, and −3.20, SD 4.76, respectively, $p=0.004$). The results also showed that 55 % of the escitalopram group (versus 36 % of the placebo group) reported >= 50 % decreases in hot flash frequency ($p = 0.009$). Between-group differences in decreases in the severity/frequency and bother of hot flashes were also found to be significant ($p = 0.003$ and $p = 0.013$, respectively) [73].

Randomized clinical trials with neuroendocrine agents showed a modest reduction in VMS and other frequent menopausal symptoms [40]. Studies of gabapentin have found the drug to be effective in treating VMS. Two double-blind, randomized, placebo-controlled trials have shown a significant reduction in the frequency and severity of hot flushes in women treated with 900 mg/day gabapentin [74, 75]. Although it was primarily developed to treat dizziness, the drug has also shown to be effective in treating neuropathic pain, migraines, essential tremor, bipolar disorder, uremic pruritus, and fibromyalgia, as well as VMS in postmenopausal women (off-label indication) [4, 19, 32, 74]. Although its mechanism of action is still unknown, the drug appears to reduce symptoms by up to 72 % [76]. Even though the required dosage (900 mg/day) may have low tolerability and lead to reduced treatment adherence [61], a new slow release formula has been found to reduce hot flashes and improve sleep quality while causing less side effects than the current reference drug. The most commonly reported side effects of gabapentin with this dose are dizziness (18 %), loss of balance (14 %), and somnolence (12 %) [74, 77].

Studies have also suggested that clonidine may be moderately effective in treating VMS (reducing symptoms by up to 38 %) but often at the cost of significant side effects such as hypotension, dry mouth, constipation, and sedation [6, 53, 61]. An 8-week treatment with oral clonidine, 0.1 mg/d, has been found to be effective against tamoxifen-induced hot flashes in postmenopausal women with breast cancer in a randomized, double-blind, placebo-controlled clinical trial (38 % versus 24 %, CI for difference, 3–27 %). Patients receiving clonidine were more likely than those receiving placebo to report difficulty sleeping (41 % compared with 21 %; $p = 0.02$) [78]. The International Menopause Society [42] recommends that patients with mild to moderate VSM who cannot receive HT should be treated with clonidine. If the drug is unavailable or ineffective, venlafaxine and gabapentin should be considered. For breast cancer patients treated with tamoxifen, the Comité de l'évolution des pratiques en oncologie (CEPO) [79] recommends that venlafaxine, citalopram, clonidine, gabapentin, and pregabalin be used for the treatment of hot flashes. However, the use of paroxetine and fluoxetine should be avoided due to their detrimental impact on the efficacy of tamoxifen. In patients with breast cancer who are not being treated with tamoxifen, venlafaxine, paroxetine, citalopram, clonidine, gabapentin, and pregabalin may all be effectively used in treating hot flashes. Fluoxetine, sertraline, phytoestrogens, black cohosh, and St. John's wort should not be used to treat hot flashes, given the lack of evidence for their therapeutic efficacy in breast cancer survivors [79].

Black cohosh and phytoestrogens have been found to be comparable to placebo in treating VMS [19, 33, 41]. *Cimicifuga racemosa* (black cohosh) is not considered a phytoestrogen and is a partial serotonin agonist. However, it only has a modest effect on VMS [41, 80]. A recent study is conducted on 351 women aged between 45 and 55 years with two or more VMS per day – of whom 52 % were in the menopausal transition stage and 48 % were postmenopausal – to test the comparative efficacy of three herbal regimens (black cohosh, 160 mg daily; multibotanical with black cohosh, 200 mg daily, and nine other ingredients; or multibotanical plus dietary soy counseling), hormone therapy (conjugated equine estrogen, 0.625 mg daily, with or without medroxyprogesterone acetate, 2.5 mg daily), and a placebo in relieving VMS [41]. The number and intensity of VMS per day as well as the Wiklund Vasomotor Symptom Subscale scores did not differ between the herbal intervention groups and placebo at 3, 6, or 12 months or for the average overall scores obtained at all follow-up time points ($p > 0.05$ for all comparisons) with one exception: At 12 months, symptom intensity was significantly worse in individuals assigned to the multibotanical plus soy intervention than in the placebo group ($p = 0.016$). The difference in the number of VMS per day reported by individuals in the placebo group and those exposed to any of the herbal treatments, at any time point in the study, was less than one symptom per day. The average follow-up scores of individuals in these groups differed by less than 0.55 symptom per day. The difference between hormone therapy and placebo groups was of −4.06 vasomotor symptoms per day for the average of all follow-up scores (95 % CI, −5.93 to −2.19 symptoms per day; $p<0.001$) [41]. These drugs consist of nonsteroidal molecules similar to estradiol and diethylstilbestrol and should be avoided in breast cancer patients, as they can antagonize the effects of tamoxifen and aromatase inhibitors. These substances have also been found to have estrogen-like effects at a cellular level. Botanical products containing soy isoflavones or red clover may have widely varying levels of bioavailability, as well as a wider action spectrum than estradiol and estrogen depending on β-receptor activation [40]. However, the long-term safety of these treatments is virtually unknown [61].

Some studies suggest that low-intensity exercise, such as yoga, may reduce SVM and improve psychological well-being. To assess the efficacy of yoga in reducing VMS, a systematic review and meta-analysis were performed using articles from the Medline, Scopus, Cochrane Library, and PsycINFO databases [81]. The study only selected RCT that assessed the effect of yoga on the main psychological, somatic, vasomotor, and/or urogenital symptoms of menopause. Standardized mean differences (SMD) were calculated for each outcome. Five RCTs with a total of 582 participants were included in the systematic review, while four RCTs with a total of 545 participants were included in the meta-analysis. The study found moderate evidence of a short-term effect on psychological symptoms (SMD=−0.37 95% CI −0.67 to −0.07, $p=0.02$) but no significant evidence of the effect of yoga on psychological, somatic, vasomotor, or urogenital menopause symptoms. Yoga was also found to have no serious adverse effects [81].

Few RCTs have produced reliable evidence of the effect of aerobic exercise on VMS, although some studies suggest that aerobic exercise may improve well-being and quality of life in women with such symptoms. To assess the effectiveness of exercise in controlling or reducing VMS in peri- and postmenopausal women, a systematic review [82] of studies (including but not limited to RCTs) comparing the efficacy of exercise with that of other treatments or with the absence of treatment was recently published. No significant between-group differences on VMS were found in studies comparing exercise and no treatment/control groups (three studies; SMD=−0.14; 95% CI: −0.54 to −0.26), exercise and HT (three studies; SMD=0.49, 95 %, CI: −0.27 to −1.26), and exercise and yoga (two studies; SMD=−0.09, 95% CI: −0.64 to −0.45), although comparisons were based on small samples.

Stellate ganglion blockade was found to be effective in reducing vasomotor symptoms and sleep quality in a study of 13 women who were breast cancer survivors (age range 38–71 years) and reported severe hot flushes [83, 84]. Lipov et al. [83] found that this treatment led to a stabilization of hot flushes and long-term reduction in these symptoms in a 24-week follow-up study, while Haest et al. [84] found that the effect on sleep quality was maintained, but the impact on hot flushes was reduced, after this treatment.

References

1. Soules MR, Sherman S, Parrott E, Rebar R, Santoro N, Utian W, et al. Executive summary: Stages of Reproductive Aging Workshop (STRAW). Fertil Steril. 2001;76(5):874–8.
2. Soules MR, Sherman S, Parrott E, Rebar R, Santoro N, Utian W, et al. Executive summary: Stages of Reproductive Aging Workshop (STRAW). Climacteric. 2001;4(4):267–72.
3. Joffe H, Groninger H, Soares CN, Nonacs R, Cohen LS. An open trial of mirtazapine in menopausal women with depression unresponsive to estrogen replacement therapy. J Womens Health Gend Based Med. 2001;10(10):999–1004.
4. Thurston RC, Joffe H. Vasomotor symptoms and menopause: findings from the Study of Women's Health across the Nation. Gynecol Clin North Am. 2011;38(3):489–501.
5. Deecher DC, Dorries K. Understanding the pathophysiology of vasomotor symptoms (hot flushes and night sweats) that occur in perimenopause, menopause, and postmenopause life stages. Arch Womens Ment Health. 2007;10(6):247–57.
6. Santoro N. Symptoms of menopause: hot flushes. Clin Obstet Gynecol. 2008;51(3):539–48.

7. Freedman RR. Hot flashes revisited. Menopause. 2000;7(1):3–4.
8. Miller EH. Women and insomnia. Clin Cornerstone. 2004;6(Suppl 1B):S8–18.
9. Voda AM. Climacteric hot flash. Maturitas. 1981;3(1):73–90.
10. Soares CN. Insomnia in women: an overlooked epidemic? Arch Womens Ment Health. 2005;8(4):205–13.
11. Freeman EW, Sammel MD, Sanders RJ. Risk of long-term hot flashes after natural menopause: evidence from the Penn Ovarian Aging Study cohort. Menopause. 2014 [Epub ahead of print]
12. Freedman RR. Hot flashes: behavioral treatments, mechanisms, and relation to sleep. Am J Med. 2005;118(Suppl 12B):124–30.
13. Freedman RR, Krell W. Reduced thermoregulatory null zone in postmenopausal women with hot flashes. Am J Obstet Gynecol. 1999;181(1):66–70.
14. Freedman RR, Norton D, Woodward S, Cornelissen G. Core body temperature and circadian rhythm of hot flashes in menopausal women. J Clin Endocrinol Metab. 1995;80(8):2354–8.
15. Rebar RW, Spitzer IB. The physiology and measurement of hot flushes. Am J Obstet Gynecol. 1987;156(5):1284–8.
16. Berendsen HH. The role of serotonin in hot flushes. Maturitas. 2000;36(3):155–64.
17. Meldrum DR, Erlik Y, Lu JK, Judd HL. Objectively recorded hot flushes in patients with pituitary insufficiency. J Clin Endocrinol Metab. 1981;52(4):684–8.
18. Tataryn IV, Lomax P, Bajorek JG, Chesarek W, Meldrum DR, Judd HL. Postmenopausal hot flushes: a disorder of thermoregulation. Maturitas. 1980;2(2):101–7.
19. Thurston RC, Christie IC, Matthews KA. Hot flashes and cardiac vagal control: a link to cardiovascular risk? Menopause. 2010;17(3):456–61.
20. Sowers MR, Wilson AL, Karvonen-Gutierrez CA, Kardia SR. Sex steroid hormone pathway genes and health-related measures in women of 4 races/ethnicities: the Study of Women's Health Across the Nation (SWAN). Am J Med. 2006;119(9 Suppl 1):S103–10.
21. Thurston RC, Sowers MR, Sutton-Tyrrell K, Everson-Rose SA, Lewis TT, Edmundowicz D, et al. Abdominal adiposity and hot flashes among midlife women. Menopause. 2008;15(3):429–34.
22. Thurston RC, Sowers MR, Sternfeld B, Gold EB, Bromberger J, Chang Y, et al. Gains in body fat and vasomotor symptom reporting over the menopausal transition: the study of women's health across the nation. Am J Epidemiol. 2009;170(6):766–74.
23. Gold EB, Block G, Crawford S, Lachance L, FitzGerald G, Miracle H, et al. Lifestyle and demographic factors in relation to vasomotor symptoms: baseline results from the Study of Women's Health Across the Nation. Am J Epidemiol. 2004;159(12):1189–99.
24. Gold EB, Leung K, Crawford SL, Huang MH, Waetjen LE, Greendale GA. Phytoestrogen and fiber intakes in relation to incident vasomotor symptoms: results from the Study of Women's Health Across the Nation. Menopause. 2013;20(3):305–14.
25. Gold EB, Colvin A, Avis N, Bromberger J, Greendale GA, Powell L, et al. Longitudinal analysis of the association between vasomotor symptoms and race/ethnicity across the menopausal transition: study of women's health across the nation. Am J Public Health. 2006;96(7):1226–35.
26. Gibson C, Matthews K, Thurston R. Daily physical activity and hot flashes in the Study of Women's Health Across the Nation (SWAN) Flashes Study. Fertil Steril. 2014;101(4):1110–6.
27. Bromberger JT, Meyer PM, Kravitz HM, Sommer B, Cordal A, Powell L, et al. Psychologic distress and natural menopause: a multiethnic community study. Am J Public Health. 2001;91(9):1435–42.
28. Freeman EW, Sammel MD, Lin H, Gracia CR, Kapoor S, Ferdousi T. The role of anxiety and hormonal changes in menopausal hot flashes. Menopause. 2005;12(3):258–66.
29. Hunter MS, Gupta P, Chedraui P, Blumel JE, Tserotas K, Aguirre W, et al. The International Menopause Study of Climate, Altitude, Temperature (IMS-CAT) and vasomotor symptoms. Climacteric. 2013;16(1):8–16.
30. Kravitz HM, Ganz PA, Bromberger J, Powell LH, Sutton-Tyrrell K, Meyer PM. Sleep difficulty in women at midlife: a community survey of sleep and the menopausal transition. Menopause. 2003;10(1):19–28.
31. Joffe H, White DP, Crawford SL, McCurnin KE, Economou N, Connors S, et al. Adverse effects of induced hot flashes on objectively recorded and subjectively reported sleep: results of a gonadotropin-releasing hormone agonist experimental protocol. Menopause. 2013;20(9):905–14.
32. Greendale GA, Wight RG, Huang MH, Avis N, Gold EB, Joffe H, et al. Menopause-associated symptoms and cognitive performance: results from the study of women's health across the nation. Am J Epidemiol. 2010;171(11):1214–24.
33. Weber MT, Rubin LH, Maki PM. Cognition in perimenopause: the effect of transition stage. Menopause. 2013;20(5):511–7.
34. Rossouw JE, Anderson GL, Prentice RL, LaCroix AZ, Kooperberg C, Stefanick ML, et al. Risks and benefits of estrogen plus progestin in healthy postmenopausal women: principal results from the Women's Health Initiative randomized controlled trial. JAMA. 2002;288(3):321–33.
35. Hulley S, Grady D, Bush T, Furberg C, Herrington D, Riggs B, et al. Randomized trial of estrogen plus progestin for secondary prevention of coronary heart disease in postmenopausal women. Heart and Estrogen/progestin Replacement Study (HERS) research group. JAMA. 1998;280(7):605–13.
36. Grady D, Herrington D, Bittner V, Blumenthal R, Davidson M, Hlatky M, et al. Cardiovascular disease outcomes during 6.8 years of hormone therapy: Heart and Estrogen/progestin Replacement Study follow-up (HERS II). JAMA. 2002;288(1):49–57.

37. Thurston RC, Sutton-Tyrrell K, Everson-Rose SA, Hess R, Powell LH, Matthews KA. Hot flashes and carotid intima media thickness among midlife women. Menopause. 2011;18(4):352–8.
38. Thurston RC, Sutton-Tyrrell K, Everson-Rose SA, Hess R, Matthews KA. Hot flashes and subclinical cardiovascular disease: findings from the Study of Women's Health Across the Nation Heart Study. Circulation. 2008;118(12):1234–40.
39. Maclennan AH, Broadbent JL, Lester S, Moore V. Oral oestrogen and combined oestrogen/progestogen therapy versus placebo for hot flushes. Cochrane Database Syst Rev. 2004; (4):CD002978.
40. Villaseca P. Non-estrogen conventional and phytochemical treatments for vasomotor symptoms: what needs to be known for practice. Climacteric. 2012; 15(2):115–24.
41. Newton KM, Reed SD, LaCroix AZ, Grothaus LC, Ehrlich K, Guiltinan J. Treatment of vasomotor symptoms of menopause with black cohosh, multibotanicals, soy, hormone therapy, or placebo: a randomized trial. Ann Intern Med. 2006;145(12):869–79.
42. de Villiers TJ, Gass ML, Haines CJ, Hall JE, Lobo RA, Pierroz DD, et al. Global consensus statement on menopausal hormone therapy. Climacteric. 2013;16(2):203–4.
43. North American Menopause Society. The 2012 hormone therapy position statement of: The North American Menopause Society. Menopause. 2012;19(3):257–71.
44. Schierbeck LL, Rejnmark L, Tofteng CL, Stilgren L, Eiken P, Mosekilde L, et al. Effect of hormone replacement therapy on cardiovascular events in recently postmenopausal women: randomised trial. BMJ. 2012;345:e6409.
45. Sturdee DW, Pines A, International Menopause Society Writing G, Archer DF, Baber RJ, Barlow D, et al. Updated IMS recommendations on postmenopausal hormone therapy and preventive strategies for midlife health. Climacteric. 2011;14(3):302–20.
46. Fichera M, Rinaldi N, Tarascio M, Taschetta S, Caldaci LM, Catavorello A, et al. Indications and contraindications of hormone replacement therapy in menopause. Minerva Ginecol. 2013;65(3):331–44.
47. Wender MCO, Freitas F, De Castro JAS, Caran JZ, De Oliveira PP. Climatério. In: Freitas FM CH, Rivoire WA, Passos EP, editors. Rotinas em ginecologia. 6th ed. Porto Alegre: Artmed; 2011. p. 700–22.
48. Nelson HD, Vesco KK, Haney E, Fu R, Nedrow A, Miller J, et al. Nonhormonal therapies for menopausal hot flashes: systematic review and meta-analysis. JAMA. 2006;295(17):2057–71.
49. Nelken RS, Ozel BZ, Leegant AR, Felix JC, Mishell Jr DR. Randomized trial of estradiol vaginal ring versus oral oxybutynin for the treatment of overactive bladder. Menopause. 2011;18(9):962–6.
50. Anderson GL, Judd HL, Kaunitz AM, Barad DH, Beresford SA, Pettinger M, et al. Effects of estrogen plus progestin on gynecologic cancers and associated diagnostic procedures: the Women's Health Initiative randomized trial. JAMA. 2003;290(13):1739–48.
51. Greiser CM, Greiser EM, Doren M. Menopausal hormone therapy and risk of lung cancer-systematic review and meta-analysis. Maturitas. 2010;65(3): 198–204.
52. Oh SW, Myung SK, Park JY, Lym YL, Ju W. Hormone therapy and risk of lung cancer: a meta-analysis. J Womens Health (Larchmt). 2010;19(2):279–88.
53. Umland EM. Treatment strategies for reducing the burden of menopause-associated vasomotor symptoms. J Manag Care Pharm. 2008;14(3 Suppl):14–9.
54. Kenemans P, Bundred NJ, Foidart JM, Kubista E, von Schoultz B, Sismondi P, et al. Safety and efficacy of tibolone in breast-cancer patients with vasomotor symptoms: a double-blind, randomised, non-inferiority trial. Lancet Oncol. 2009;10(2):135–46.
55. Wolff EF, He Y, Black DM, Brinton EA, Budoff MJ, Cedars MI, et al. Self-reported menopausal symptoms, coronary artery calcification, and carotid intima-media thickness in recently menopausal women screened for the Kronos early estrogen prevention study (KEEPS). Fertil Steril. 2013;99(5): 1385–91.
56. The Postmenopausal Estrogen/Progestin Interventions (PEPI) Trial. The Writing Group for the PEPI Trial. Effects of estrogen or estrogen/progestin regimens on heart disease risk factors in postmenopausal women. JAMA. 1995;273(3):199–208.
57. Smith NL, Wiley JR, Legault C, Rice KM, Heckbert SR, Psaty BM, et al. Effect of progestogen and progestogen type on hemostasis measures in postmenopausal women: the Postmenopausal Estrogen/ Progestin Intervention (PEPI) study. Menopause. 2008;15(6):1145–50.
58. Formoso G, Perrone E, Maltoni S, Balduzzi S, D'Amico R, Bassi C, et al. Short and long term effects of tibolone in postmenopausal women. Cochrane Database Syst Rev; 2012;(2):CD008536.
59. Cummings SR, Ettinger B, Delmas PD, Kenemans P, Stathopoulos V, Verweij P, et al. The effects of tibolone in older postmenopausal women. N Engl J Med. 2008;359(7):697–708.
60. Palacios S. Advances in hormone replacement therapy: making the menopause manageable. BMC Womens Health. 2008;8:22.
61. Thacker HL. Assessing risks and benefits of nonhormonal treatments for vasomotor symptoms in perimenopausal and postmenopausal women. J Womens Health (Larchmt). 2011;20(7):1007–16.
62. Stearns V. Clinical update: new treatments for hot flushes. Lancet. 2007;369(9579):2062–4.
63. Stearns V, Slack R, Greep N, Henry-Tilman R, Osborne M, Bunnell C, et al. Paroxetine is an effective treatment for hot flashes: results from a prospective randomized clinical trial. J Clin Oncol. 2005; 23(28):6919–30.
64. Kelly CM, Juurlink DN, Gomes T, Duong-Hua M, Pritchard KI, Austin PC, et al. Selective serotonin reuptake inhibitors and breast cancer mortality in women receiving tamoxifen: a population based cohort study. BMJ. 2010;340:c693.

65. FDA. FDA approves the first non-hormonal treatment for hot flashes associated with menopause 2013 [Oct 7 2013]. Available from: http://www.fda.gov/newsevents/newsroom/pressannouncements/ucm359030.htm
66. Archer DF, Seidman L, Constantine GD, Pickar JH, Olivier S. A double-blind, randomly assigned, placebo-controlled study of desvenlafaxine efficacy and safety for the treatment of vasomotor symptoms associated with menopause. Am J Obstet Gynecol. 2009;200(2):172.e1–10.
67. Loprinzi CL, Kugler JW, Sloan JA, Mailliard JA, LaVasseur BI, Barton DL, et al. Venlafaxine in management of hot flashes in survivors of breast cancer: a randomised controlled trial. Lancet. 2000;356(9247):2059–63.
68. Speroff L, Gass M, Constantine G, Olivier S, Study I. Efficacy and tolerability of desvenlafaxine succinate treatment for menopausal vasomotor symptoms: a randomized controlled trial. Obstet Gynecol. 2008;111(1):77–87.
69. Archer DF, Pinkerton JV, Guico-Pabia CJ, Hwang E, Cheng RF, Study I. Cardiovascular, cerebrovascular, and hepatic safety of desvenlafaxine for 1 year in women with vasomotor symptoms associated with menopause. Menopause. 2013;20(1):47–56.
70. Kerwin JP, Gordon PR, Senf JH. The variable response of women with menopausal hot flashes when treated with sertraline. Menopause. 2007;14(5):841–5.
71. Gordon PR, Kerwin JP, Boesen KG, Senf J. Sertraline to treat hot flashes: a randomized controlled, double-blind, crossover trial in a general population. Menopause. 2006;13(4):568–75.
72. Kimmick GG, Lovato J, McQuellon R, Robinson E, Muss HB. Randomized, double-blind, placebo-controlled, crossover study of sertraline (Zoloft) for the treatment of hot flashes in women with early stage breast cancer taking tamoxifen. Breast J. 2006;12(2):114–22.
73. Freeman EW, Guthrie KA, Caan B, Sternfeld B, Cohen LS, Joffe H, et al. Efficacy of escitalopram for hot flashes in healthy menopausal women: a randomized controlled trial. JAMA. 2011;305(3):267–74.
74. Pandya KJ, Morrow GR, Roscoe JA, Zhao H, Hickok JT, Pajon E, et al. Gabapentin for hot flashes in 420 women with breast cancer: a randomised double-blind placebo-controlled trial. Lancet. 2005;366(9488):818–24.
75. Guttuso Jr T, Kurlan R, McDermott MP, Kieburtz K. Gabapentin's effects on hot flashes in postmenopausal women: a randomized controlled trial. Obstet Gynecol. 2003;101(2):337–45.
76. Yadav M, Volkar J. Potential role of gabapentin and extended-release gabapentin in the management of menopausal hot flashes. Int J Gen Med. 2013;6:657–64.
77. Butt DA, Lock M, Lewis JE, Ross S, Moineddin R. Gabapentin for the treatment of menopausal hot flashes: a randomized controlled trial. Menopause. 2008;15(2):310–8.
78. Pandya KJ, Raubertas RF, Flynn PJ, Hynes HE, Rosenbluth RJ, Kirshner JJ, et al. Oral clonidine in postmenopausal patients with breast cancer experiencing tamoxifen-induced hot flashes: a University of Rochester Cancer Center Community Clinical Oncology Program study. Ann Intern Med. 2000;132(10):788–93.
79. L'Esperance S, Frenette S, Dionne A, Dionne JY. Comite de l'evolution des pratiques en o. Pharmacological and non-hormonal treatment of hot flashes in breast cancer survivors: CEPO review and recommendations. Support Care Cancer. 2013;21(5):1461–74.
80. Geller SE, Shulman LP, van Breemen RB, Banuvar S, Zhou Y, Epstein G, et al. Safety and efficacy of black cohosh and red clover for the management of vasomotor symptoms: a randomized controlled trial. Menopause. 2009;16(6):1156–66.
81. Cramer H, Lauche R, Langhorst J, Dobos G. Effectiveness of yoga for menopausal symptoms: a systematic review and meta-analysis of randomized controlled trials. Evid Based Complement Alternat Med. 2012;2012:863905.
82. Daley AJ, Stokes-Lampard HJ, Macarthur C. Exercise to reduce vasomotor and other menopausal symptoms: a review. Maturitas. 2009;63(3):176–80.
83. Lipov EG, Joshi JR, Xie H, Slavin KV. Updated findings on the effects of stellate-ganglion block on hot flushes and night awakenings. Lancet Oncol. 2008;9(9):819–20.
84. Haest K, Kumar A, Van Calster B, Leunen K, Smeets A, Amant F, et al. Stellate ganglion block for the management of hot flashes and sleep disturbances in breast cancer survivors: an uncontrolled experimental study with 24 weeks of follow-up. Ann Oncol. 2012;23(6):1449–54.

The Menopausal Transition and Women's Health

31

Nancy Fugate Woods and Ellen Sullivan Mitchell

Contents

31.1	Introduction	433
31.2	Early Contributions to Menopausal Transition Research	434
31.3	New Understandings of the Menopausal Transition and Early Postmenopause	435
31.3.1	Staging Reproductive Aging	435
31.4	Endocrine Changes During the Menopausal Transition and Early Postmenopause	438
31.5	Symptoms During the Menopausal Transition and Early Postmenopause	439
31.5.1	Hot Flashes	439
31.5.2	Sleep Symptoms	441
31.5.3	Depressed Mood	442
31.5.4	Cognitive Symptoms	442
31.5.5	Pain Symptoms	443
31.5.6	Sexual Desire	443
31.6	Interference with Daily Living and Symptoms	443
31.6.1	Clusters of Symptoms During the Menopausal Transition	444
31.7	Stress and the Menopausal Transition	445
31.8	Well-Being	445
31.9	The Menopausal Transition and Healthy Aging	446
31.9.1	Metabolic Changes	446
31.9.2	Lipid Patterns	446
31.9.3	Glucose and Insulin	447
31.9.4	Thrombotic Changes	447
31.9.5	Inflammatory Responses	447
31.10	Metabolic Syndrome	448
31.11	Summary	448
References		448

31.1 Introduction

Experiencing menopause is a common experience for the majority of women from Western countries who survive to their mid-50s, yet scientific work about the natural menopausal transition and its consequences for women's health was limited until the 1990s. Stimulated by concern about the aging of the world's population, during the past three decades, researchers have focused increasingly on understanding the natural menopausal transition [1]. Understanding the menopausal transition and related physiologic changes is critical to comprehending healthy aging. Moreover, many women view the menopausal transition as an opportunity to reappraise their health and health-related behavior patterns [2].

N.F. Woods, PhD, BSN, MN (✉)
Biobehavioral Nursing, University of Washington,
NE Pacific St., Seattle, WA 98195, USA
e-mail: nfwoods@uw.edu

E.S. Mitchell, PhD, BSN, MN
Family and Child Nursing, University of Washington,
Seattle, WA, USA
e-mail: nellem@uw.edu

In order to comprehend the menopausal transition and its consequences for health, researchers have engaged women recently in contributing to knowledge about menopause by:

- Focusing research on the general population of women, not only women seeking health care
- Using longitudinal study designs to track processes occurring with women's midlife development
- Reflecting on the menopausal transition from an integrative (e.g., biopsychosociocultural) framework and from a feminist perspective that puts women at the center of investigations
- Valuing the importance of a lifespan perspective by recognizing that women's experiences earlier in the lifespan are influential in midlife and old age [3]
- Considering population-specific experiences of the menopausal transition, including those of diverse ethnic groups, age cohorts who experience different lives, and women around the globe

The purposes of this chapter are to:

1. Review recent history of research on the menopausal transition and early postmenopause
2. Describe approaches to staging the menopausal transition and their application in recent research
3. Summarize current understanding of endocrine changes occurring during the menopausal transition and early postmenopause
4. Characterize symptoms women experience (hot flashes, sleep disruption, mood changes, cognitive changes, pain, sexual desire changes) and their correlates during the menopausal transition and postmenopause
5. Chart the relationship of the menopausal transition to healthy aging

31.2 Early Contributions to Menopausal Transition Research

Early contributions to understanding the menopausal transition included studies such as those conducted by Neugarten and colleagues, who examined the meanings of the menopausal transition for a cohort of midlife women born in the 1940s [4]. This cohort expressed concerns about adopting to the "empty nest" after their children left home. With the advent of the Women's Movement of the 1960s and 1970s in the USA and around the world, investigators began to study women born in the Post-World War II era. In 1981, Massachusetts Women's Health Study investigators began tracking a population of white women in the state of Massachusetts for 10 years. Participants were between 45 and 55 years of age at recruitment, identified through census lists for the state. Investigators charted the course of hot flashes and their relationship to use of health services. They found that depression occurred during this period but was strongly related to life events [5, 6]. In another early effort (1983), Matthews and colleagues studied women from the state of Pennsylvania (The Healthy Women Study) to determine the natural history of the menopausal transition and behavioral and biological changes that occurred during the MT and postmenopause and their effects on cardiovascular disease risk [7]. The Melbourne Midlife Women's Health Project was launched in Australia at about the same time as the Massachusetts Women's Health Study using a similar approach. Investigators recruited women 45–55 years of age and measured symptoms, hormone levels, and their relationship to quality of life, bone mineral density, body composition, cardiovascular disease risk, and memory [8]. In 1989, the Seattle Midlife Women's Health Study investigators initiated recruitment of women 35–55 years of age selected from census tracts in the city of Seattle [9, 10], and in 1994, the investigators for the multisite Study of Women and Health Across the Nation (SWAN) began recruitment of a multiethnic cohort [11]. In Sweden, Collins and her colleagues began studying midlife women in this same era, focusing on stress related to work as well as hormonal changes they experienced [12]. In addition, the 1946 British Birth Cohort Study investigators included measures related to menopause and led a series of analyses of these data [13, 14]. These contemporaneous efforts led to active collaboration among many of the researchers who were anxious to share what they were learning and the methods they were using and provide support for one another.

During the same era, researchers such as Ann Voda worked to understand symptom experiences related to the menopausal transition and expand our knowledge of women's experiences of hot flashes from their own point of view as well as their physiologic correlates [15]. Other investigators began investigating questions about physiologic changes in women's menstrual cycles and hormonal patterns [16–18].

Despite this work, the US National Institutes of Health did not have a research agenda for women's health until the early 1990s [19]. In 1993, the National Institutes of Health cosponsored the first workshop on menopause, proposing a specific research agenda [20]. From the early 1990s, researchers studying the menopausal transition have made remarkable contributions. The Study of Women and Health Across the Nation, launched shortly after the NIH-sponsored conference on menopause, has played a significant role in expanding our understanding of the menopausal transition and early postmenopause and its relationship to healthy aging. Also of note was a transformative view of the menopausal transition as a normal developmental experience, supplanting notions of the menopausal transition and postmenopause as a pathology in search of a cure [21, 22].

31.3 New Understandings of the Menopausal Transition and Early Postmenopause

31.3.1 Staging Reproductive Aging

Efforts to identify stages of reproductive aging have facilitated ability of researchers around the globe to compare data from women within the same stage or across stages of the menopausal transition and clinicians to use staging to help women make decisions, for example, about screening for bone density or managing fertility during the menopausal transition. Although research on staging reproductive aging is in early development, there have been several useful discoveries about approaches that clinicians and women, themselves, can use to determine at what point they are in the transition to menopause. Early efforts to "stage" the menopausal transition relied on questions asking women about their menstrual cycles. For example, Massachusetts Women's Health Study investigators asked women whether they had had a period in the past three months and were cycling regularly, classifying these women as premenopausal, indicating that women had not yet reported irregularity of their cycles. Women who had reported irregularity of their cycles and 3–11 months of amenorrhea were considered in "perimenopause" (now referred to as the menopausal transition). Those who had not menstruated in the past year were classified as "postmenopausal" [23]. Similar questions were used to stage reproductive aging for participants in the Melbourne Midlife Women's Health Project [24].

Mitchell and colleagues used data from menstrual calendars and questionnaires to propose an initial model that specified an early, middle, and late transition stage [25]. In this staging system, changes in flow and small changes in cycle length preceded changes in regularity of cycles and skipping periods.

In 2001, the Staging Reproductive Aging Workshop [26] convened investigators and clinicians from the USA and Australia to develop criteria to use in staging reproductive aging. Stages were anchored to the final menstrual period (FMP) such that stage +1 and stage +2 represented early and late postmenopause, respectively, and stages −1 and −2 represented the late and early menopausal transition (see Fig. 31.1 below for the provisional staging system developed by the STRAW conference group in 2001).

Mitchell and colleagues modified their framework following the Staging Reproductive Aging Workshop (STRAW) (see Soules et al. [26] for details) and in collaboration with the ReSTAGE investigators. Figure 31.2 includes a menstrual calendar from a woman in the late reproductive stage (STRAW -3), showing regularity of her menstrual cycles over a year. Figure 31.3 includes data

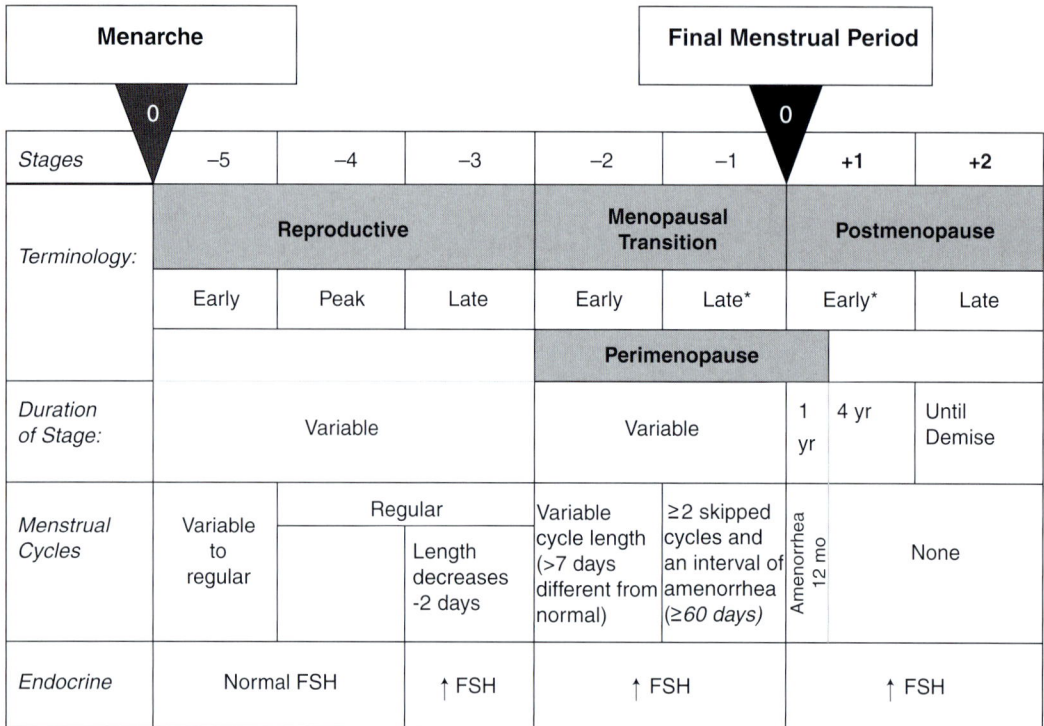

Fig. 31.1 Proposed staging system for the menopausal transition (Reprinted from fertility and sterility, 76/5, Soules et al. [26], Copyright 2001, with permission from Elsevier)

Fig. 31.2 Menstrual calendar, late reproductive stage

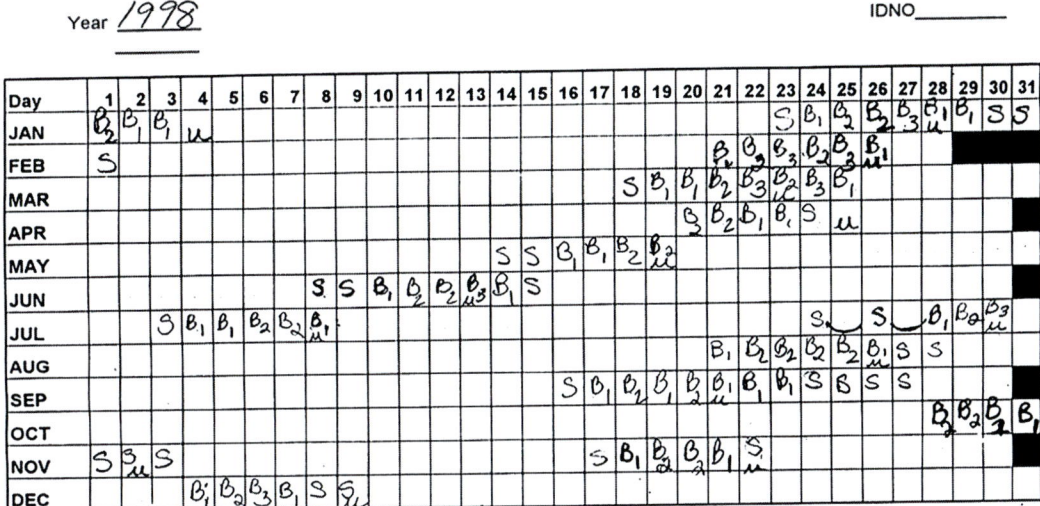

Fig. 31.3 Menstrual calendar, early menopausal transition stage

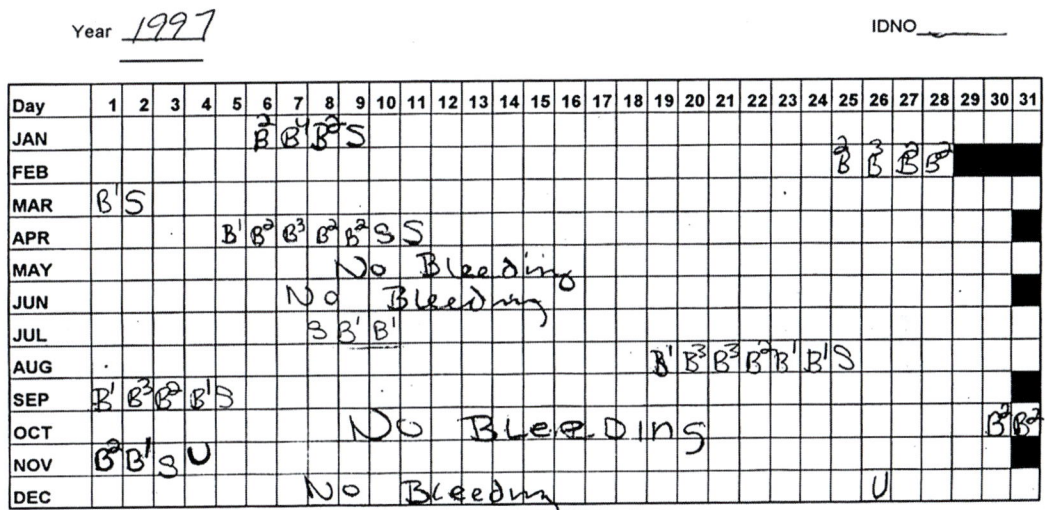

Fig. 31.4 Menstrual calendar, late menopausal transition stage

from a woman who is experiencing irregularity of 7 days or more between consecutive menstrual cycles, indicating that she is now in the early menopausal transition stage. Figure 31.4 illustrates cycles for a woman who has begun skipping periods with at least 60 days of amenorrhea between periods, the criterion for late menopausal transition stage. Later the ReSTAGE project investigators analyzed data from the Melbourne Women's Health Project, the Study of Women and Health Across the Nation (SWAN), the Tremin Trust Data, and the Seattle Midlife Women's

Table 31.1 Age of onset and duration of menopausal transition stages: observations from the Seattle Midlife Women's Health Study (2011)

	Early menopausal transition stage	Late menopausal transition stage	Early postmenopause
Age of onset	N=125	N=131	N=112
M,SD	46.3, 3.6	49.5, 2.8	52.1, 2.9
Median	46.8	49.8	52.4
Duration	N=83	N=82	–
M, SD,	2.9, 1.5	2.5, 1.3	
Median	2.6	2.3	
Range	0.2–6.5	0.4–7.0	

Health Study. They validated that a break in cyclicity manifested by a difference of 7 or more days in cycle length between sequential cycles that reoccurred within the next 10 bleeding segments was a good indicator for the beginning of the early phase of the menopausal transition. Moreover, their work indicated that a period of 60 or more days of amenorrhea that reoccurred within the next 10 bleeding segments for women less than 45 years of age signaled the entry into the late stage of the menopausal transition [27–30].

Women do not experience the final menstrual period at the same age, nor do they experience the stages of reproductive aging at specific ages. Table 31.1 includes the ages of onset and duration of the stages of the menopausal transition based on the Seattle Midlife Women's Health Study. Of interest is that the early stage required an average of 2.9 years and the late stage an average of 2.5 years. When the early and late menopausal transition stages for women in the SMWHS were added together, the average duration of the menopausal transition (early + late) was 5.3 years, (SD=1.8 years with a range from 1.1 to 9.8 years) (Mitchell and Woods, unpublished data). Similar data from other longitudinal cohorts will support the universality or variability in these data across populations.

31.4 Endocrine Changes During the Menopausal Transition and Early Postmenopause

Staging reproductive aging, anchored by changes observed in menstrual cycle regularity, provided a framework within which to examine changes occurring in the ovarian (estrogens, progesterone, testosterone, Mullerian-inhibiting hormone (MIH), and inhibins) and pituitary hormones (FSH and LH). Santoro's early and careful description of endocrine levels across the menstrual cycles of women approaching menopause and those who had experienced their final menstrual period stimulated awareness of the changes in endocrine levels, including the realization that some women experienced episodes of hyper-estrogen levels before their final period [16].

SWAN investigators found there was a period of approximately four years during which the maximal changes occur at the greatest rate in both FSH and estradiol, with the changes in FSH preceding the changes in estradiol. After this 4-year period of maximum changes, both FSH and E2 levels stabilize [31, 32]. Acceleration of the FSH rise occurs 2 years before the FMP with deceleration beginning immediately before the FMP and stabilizing 2 years after the FMP [32], consistent with earlier findings of Sowers and colleagues [33]. Estradiol concentrations did not change substantially until about 2 years before the FMP when it began decreasing with the maximal rate of change occurring at the FMP and then decelerating to achieve stability about 2 years after FMP. Obesity, smoking behavior, and being Chinese or Japanese were associated with variation in estradiol levels, but not with the pattern of estradiol change. In obese women, initial acceleration of FSH occurred slightly later (at 5.45 years before FMP) and was attenuated compared to that observed in nonobese women.

In the daily hormone sub-study of SWAN, Santoro found that cycles become anovulatory prior to the FMP with progesterone levels dropping as women ovulated more irregularly or ceased ovulation [34]. Although the precise cause of menstrual cessation is not yet clear, we know that estradiol levels drop as ovulation decreases in frequency and FSH rises in response to ovarian signals from inhibins and Anti-Müllerian Hormone [32–36]. AMH is produced in growing ovarian follicles, a direct indicator of ovarian reserve, and becomes nondetectable 5 years prior to the final menstrual period. Inhibin B is produced by small antral follicles, indicating growth of the antral follicle cohort. Inhibin B suppresses FSH secretion through negative feedback to the pituitary and declines to undetectable levels 4–5 years prior to the final menstrual period [37]. Work is still underway to determine which, if any, of these indicators is the best marker for predicting menopause.

Androgens, including testosterone and DHEAS, have also been studied in the SWAN population, revealing a rise in DHEAS during the late menopausal transition stage, followed by a decline during the early postmenopause [38, 39], Approximately 85 % of women had an increase in DHEAS between pre/early menopausal transition and late menopausal transition/early postmenopause [39]. DHEAS provides an important source of estrogen for women during the postmenopause as it is converted to estrone. Testosterone levels were relatively stable in the Melbourne Midlife Women's Health cohort and the SWAN cohort [32, 38, 40].

Cortisol has also been shown to rise between the early menopausal transition stage and late menopausal transition stage in one study [41], but such a rise was not seen in the SWAN study [38]. Effects of both estrogens and androgens on women's health after menopause have been explored recently and are discussed later in this chapter.

Lasley et al. [42] investigated the impact of adrenal contributions to sex steroids in the SWAN participants, finding that DHEAS, DHEA, and androstenediol increase at their greatest rate and are at peak variability during the years immediately before menopause when estradiol levels are low. Androstenediol is a prohormone for peripheral conversion to bioactive steroids, acting as a signal transducer in estrogen and androgen receptors. Adiol levels increase fivefold at the same time circulating estradiol levels are decreasing. Lasley proposed that disappearance of inhibin B rising FSH triggers an increase in delta-5 (androstenediol) production, producing a transition in metabolism from estrogenic to androgenic. SWAN participants exhibited high levels of androstenediol, about 100 time the levels of E2. Lasley proposed that the higher levels of Adiol, which has lower estrogenic bioactivity than estradiol, may be needed to compensate for lower estradiol levels during this period. Although the clinical significance of this increase in Adiol is not known at this time, the higher concentration of Adiol in the presence of lower estradiol levels in the years prior to the FMP could contribute to total circulating estrogen ligand pool in women during the MT.

Adrenal androgen dynamics may be key to understanding development of the metabolic syndrome. The relationship of both ovarian and adrenal steroids to health during the menopausal transition and postmenopause is not fully understood, and to date most researchers have studied changes in individual hormones and the ratio of estradiol to testosterone. As discussed later, it is may be the ratio of testosterone to estradiol that is the most important predictor of changes in cardiovascular disease risk. In addition, the promise of more sensitive assays for androgens and a more full understanding of the role of adrenal androgens as precursors of estrogens will enhance our concepts of endocrine changes during the menopausal transition on many health outcomes during the postmenopause.

31.5 Symptoms During the Menopausal Transition and Early Postmenopause

31.5.1 Hot Flashes

Women experience a variety of symptoms during the menopausal transition, including hot flashes and night sweats, often referred to as vasomotor symptoms. A hot flash is a sensation of intense heat, often accompanied by sweating and flushing. Hot flashes occur in an effort to dissipate heat characterized by vascular dilation. Voda [19] characterized the menopausal hot flash from women's own experiences, exploring the question "who is the woman who has hot flashes and what are the characteristics of the hot flashes?" Using data from daily self-reports, she sought to describe the frequency, duration, trigger, origin, spread, intensity, and method of coping with hot flashes. She found that no single pattern characterized women's experiences. Although the majority of hot flashes began on the upper body, for example, the chest or face, some women noted their hot flashes started in other parts of their body. Hot flashes tended to spread to other areas on the upper body but for some women spread to the legs and arms or back. On average, a hot flash lasted about 3 min. Women distinguished between mild, moderate, and severe hot flashes. Their coping strategies related to the duration and severity of their hot flashes. Internal strategies included ingesting a cold beverage. External strategies involved fanning oneself, showering, or opening a window. Some hot flash triggers included sleeping, work activities, recreation and relaxation, and housework. Voda's study emphasized the variability in women's hot flash experiences and how they managed them. In collaboration with Kay and others, Voda extended this work to characterize the experiences of both Mexican American and Anglo women [43]. They found that although Anglo women experienced hot flashes negatively, Mexican American women found positive components of meaning, for example, they viewed menopause as a natural part of life, indicating they could no longer have children, and meaning they could be confident they would not become pregnant again [43].

Hot flashes that women reported in laboratory studies were associated with a rise in skin temperature and skin conductance levels, elevated heart rate and respiratory rate, and reduced blood pH. Laboratory studies also revealed autonomic nervous system activation, such as occurs with a stress response, in mediating vasodilation and elaboration of norepinephrine following the hot flash [44–46]. Potent vasodilators such as calcitonin gene-related peptide are released during hot flashes, but not during exercise or sweating [47]. Although the etiology of hot flashes and the mechanisms stimulating vasodilation remain unclear, most investigators suggest that estrogen withdrawal or changing estrogen levels is involved.

The effects of changing estrogen levels on blood vessel structure and function are beginning to be characterized by SWAN investigators focusing on the relationship of the menopausal transition and associated physiological changes to heart disease risk. Thurston et al. [48] found that women who had hot flashes experience lower heart rate variability during the flash, indicating that the parasympathetic nervous system, which helps influence return to normal heart rate after a stressful experience, may function differently in women with hot flashes than in women who do not have hot flashes. Woods and colleagues found that women experiencing a cluster of symptoms with severe hot flashes had higher norepinephrine levels than those experiencing low severity symptoms [49]. Thurston also found that women who have hot flashes have less expansion of their arteries when blood flow is increased than do women without hot flashes [47]. Hot flashes also have been linked to calcification of the aorta seen in heart disease [48, 50] and increased carotid intima-medial thickness among midlife women [51]. There is also an association with adiposity and hot flashes that suggests that women with greater adiposity experience more severe hot flashes [52–55]. In contrast, when hot flash monitors are used to measure sternal skin conductance, higher BMI and waist circumference were associated with fewer hot flashes, but only among older women in the study [52]. In addition, there is evidence that women who experienced hot flashes have higher levels of tPA and factor VII than those without hot flashes [56]. Taken together, this work is beginning to suggest the role of hot flashes as a marker for subclinical heart disease.

Hot flashes are associated with both increased FSH and lower estrogen levels and also are associated with increased bone turnover during the menopausal transition. During the early and late stages of the menopausal transition, women with the most frequent hot flashes tended to have higher N-telopeptide levels, a marker of bone loss [57]. Moreover, low estrogen levels as well as higher FSH levels have been associated with higher levels of interleukins, for example, IL1B, linking both gonadotropins and estrogen to immune response [58] as well as to hot flashes.

As Voda found, hot flashes may be barely noticeable or severe, resulting in a high degree of variability of the experience among women [19, 59]. For some, hot flashes are associated with impaired quality of life, disturbed sleep, irritability, and depressed mood, among other symptoms [60]. Thurston found that women who were most bothered by hot flashes were those with more negative affect, greater symptom sensitivity, sleep problems, poorer health, duration of hot flashes, younger age, and African American race. Bother associated with night sweats was associated with sleep problems and night sweats duration [60]. For many women, hot flashes are sufficiently bothersome to lead them to seek health care during the menopausal transition [61, 62]. Although the majority of women in most population-based studies experience hot flashes [63], it is unclear how long they persist. Barnabei and colleagues [64] found that between 23 and 37 % of participants in the Women's Health Initiative Study who were in their 60s and 11–20 % of women in their 70s reported hot flashes. Some participants in the Melbourne study reported hot flashes for as long as 10 years after the FMP, although the average duration was 5 years [65].

In the Seattle Midlife Women's Health Study, hot flash severity increased as women entered the late menopausal transition stage or early postmenopause. Those who used hormone therapy, had a longer duration of the early menopausal transition stage, were older at the time of their final menstrual period, and had higher levels of FSH had more severe hot flashes. Anxiety was also associated with hot flash severity. Older age at entry into the early menopausal transition stage and higher urinary estrogen (estrone) levels were associated with decreased hot flash severity.

Psychosocial/mood (stress, depressed mood) and lifestyle variables (BMI, activity level, sleep, alcohol use) were not associated with hot flash severity in this study [59]. In contrast, in daily diary studies, women reported negative affect on the same day and the day after they reported hot flashes, suggesting that negative cognitive appraisal of hot flashes and perhaps other associated symptoms are linked to subsequent experiences of negative affect [66]. Other investigations have revealed that body mass index (BMI) [67], anxiety [68, 69], and other lifestyle behaviors have been associated with hot flash severity. As one example, women who smoked reported more severe hot flashes [67].

31.5.2 Sleep Symptoms

In addition to hot flashes, women commonly experience sleep symptoms during the menopausal transition and early postmenopause. Shaver was the first to study sleep during the perimenopause using polysomnographic methods in a sleep laboratory, discovering the relationship between sleep problems and ongoing stressful life events and anxiety [70–73]. In the Seattle Midlife Women's Health Study, women who experienced more severe difficulty going to sleep had several other symptoms such as anxiety, reported more stress, had a history of sexual abuse, rated their own health more poorly, and had greater caffeine intake and less alcohol use than women who did not have this problem. Neither estrogen nor FSH was related to difficulty getting to sleep. On the other hand, women who had more severe awakening during the night were older, were more likely to be in the late MT stage and early postmenopause, had higher FSH and lower estrogen (estrone) levels, and reported more severe hot flashes, depressed mood, anxiety, joint pain, backache, perceived stress, poorer overall health, less alcohol use, and a history of sexual abuse. Women who had more severe problems with awakening early (and not getting back to sleep) were older, reported more severe hot flashes, depressed mood, anxiety, joint pain, backache, and perceived stress, rated their health more poorly, and had higher epinephrine and lower urinary estrogen levels [74]. These findings are consistent with those of other contemporary studies [75–77]. Moreover, in the Seattle Midlife Women's Health Study, sleep symptoms were related to other symptoms, including hot flashes, depressed mood, anxiety, and pain [74, 78]. Recent findings from a study of relationships between menopausal transition-related symptoms and EEG sleep measures indicate that hot flashes were associated with longer sleep time. Women with higher anxiety symptoms had longer sleep latency and lower sleep efficiency only if they also had hot flashes. Hot flashes and mood symptoms were unrelated to either delta sleep ratio or REM latency [79]. In this same study, elevated beta EEG power in the NREM and REM sleep in women during late perimenopause (late MT) and early postmenopause exceeded levels in pre (late reproductive stage) and early perimenopause (early MT). Elevated beta EEG power indicates increased arousal and disturbed sleep quality during the late perimenopause (late MT) and early postmenopause [80]. Sleep symptoms during the MT may be amenable to symptom management strategies that take into account women's experiences of arousal and their ability to regulate it as well as efforts to promote women's general health rather than focusing only on the MT.

31.5.3 Depressed Mood

Depressed mood is also a commonly experienced symptom during the menopausal transition and early postmenopause. In the Seattle Midlife Women's Health Study, age was associated with slightly lower depressed mood (CES-D) scores. Being in the late MT stage was significantly related to experiencing depressed mood, although there was no effect of being in the early MT stage or the early postmenopause. Hot flash severity, life stress, family history of depression, history of postpartum blues, sexual abuse history, BMI, and use of antidepressants were also individually related to depressed mood. Neither FSH nor estrogen was related to depressed mood [81–83]. Several investigator groups have now identified the menopausal transition as a period of vulnerability to depressed mood [84–87]. There is a suggestion that variability of hormonal levels (estrogen, FSH) is related to depressed mood, although there is no evidence that estrogen levels themselves are related [87–89]. Of interest is that testosterone rise has been associated with depressed mood in a subset of the SWAN study participants [85] and DHEAS associated with depressed mood symptoms but not major depression in the Penn Ovarian Aging Study participants [90]. A recent assessment of SWAN participants who responded to a Structured Clinical Interview for DSM-IV Axis Disorders (SCID) revealed that compared to women who were premenopausal, those who were in the perimenopause or early postmenopause were 2–4 times more likely to experience a major depressive episode, even when prior depression history, upsetting life events, psychotropic medication use, hot flashes, and serum levels or changes in reproductive hormone levels were taken into account. Although women in the late menopausal transition stage are vulnerable to depressed mood, factors that account for depressed mood earlier in the lifespan continue to have an important influence and should be considered in studies of etiology and therapeutics. Of interest is that depressive symptoms during midlife are related to progression of coronary artery calcification, a risk factor for cardiovascular disease [91].

31.5.4 Cognitive Symptoms

Women complain of forgetfulness and difficulty concentrating commonly during this period of life. Seattle Midlife Women's Health Study participants who experienced more severe difficulty concentrating were slightly older, reported more anxiety, depressed mood, nighttime awakening, perceived stress, poorer perceived health, and were employed. The best predictors of forgetfulness included slightly older age, hot flashes, anxiety, depressed mood, awakening during the night, perceived stress, poorer perceived health, and history of sexual abuse.

Menopausal transition-related factors were not significantly associated with difficulty concentrating or forgetfulness. Considering women's ages and the context in which they experience the menopausal transition may be helpful in understanding women's experiences of cognitive symptoms [92]. Studies of functional changes in memory during the menopausal transition indicate that aside from a period of slightly reduced learning, there are no significant changes in memory function during this period of the lifespan. The minor slowing of learning during the late menopausal transition stage disappears during the early postmenopause [93–95].

31.5.5 Pain Symptoms

Although women experience pain symptoms throughout the lifespan, there is some evidence that pain symptoms are influenced by estrogen [96]. In the Seattle Midlife Women's Health Study, women experienced a slight increase in back pain with age and a significant increase in back pain during the early and late MT stages and early postmenopause, but estrogen, FSH, and testosterone levels were unrelated to back pain [78]. Perceived stress and lower overnight urinary cortisol levels were associated with more severe back pain; history of sexual abuse and catecholamines did not have a significant effect. Those most troubled by symptoms of hot flashes, depressed mood, anxiety, nighttime awakening, and difficulty concentrating reported significantly greater back pain. Of the health-related factors, having worse perceived health, exercising more, using analgesics, and having a higher BMI were associated with more back pain, but alcohol use and smoking did not have significant effects. Having more formal education was associated with less back pain, but parenting, having a partner, and employment were unrelated. Age was associated with increased severity of joint pain, but menopausal transition-related factors, such as stage or hormone levels, were unrelated. Symptoms of hot flashes, nighttime awakening, depressed mood, and difficulty concentrating were each significantly associated with joint pain, as was poorer perceived health, more exercise, higher BMI, and greater analgesic use. History of sexual abuse was the only stress-related factor significantly related to joint pain severity. Based on these findings which are consistent with those of others [97–100], clinicians working with women traversing the menopausal transition should be aware that managing back and joint pain symptoms among midlife women requires consideration of their changing biology as well as their ongoing life challenges and health-related behaviors. Moreover, the relationship between pain and sleep symptoms should be considered, including sleep hygiene interventions [78].

31.5.6 Sexual Desire

There is a great deal of interest in the effects of the menopausal transition on sexual desire. In the Seattle Midlife Women's Health Study, women experienced a significant decrease in sexual desire during the late MT stage and early PM [100]. Those with higher urinary estrone (E1G) and testosterone (T) reported significantly higher levels of sexual desire, whereas those with higher FSH levels reported significantly lower sexual desire. Women using hormone therapy also reported higher sexual desire. Those reporting higher perceived stress reported lower sexual desire, but history of sexual abuse did not have a significant effect. Those most troubled by symptoms of hot flashes, fatigue, depressed mood, anxiety, difficulty getting to sleep, early morning awakening, and awakening during the night also reported significantly lower sexual desire, but there was no effect of vaginal dryness. Women with better perceived health reported higher sexual desire, and those reporting more exercise and more alcohol intake also reported greater sexual desire. Having a partner was associated with lower sexual desire. Women's sexual desire during the menopausal transition and early postmenopause is related to both her biology as well as the social situation in which she finds herself [101–103].

31.6 Interference with Daily Living and Symptoms

In addition to rating symptoms as severe or bothersome, many women indicate their symptoms interfere with many aspects of their daily lives, for

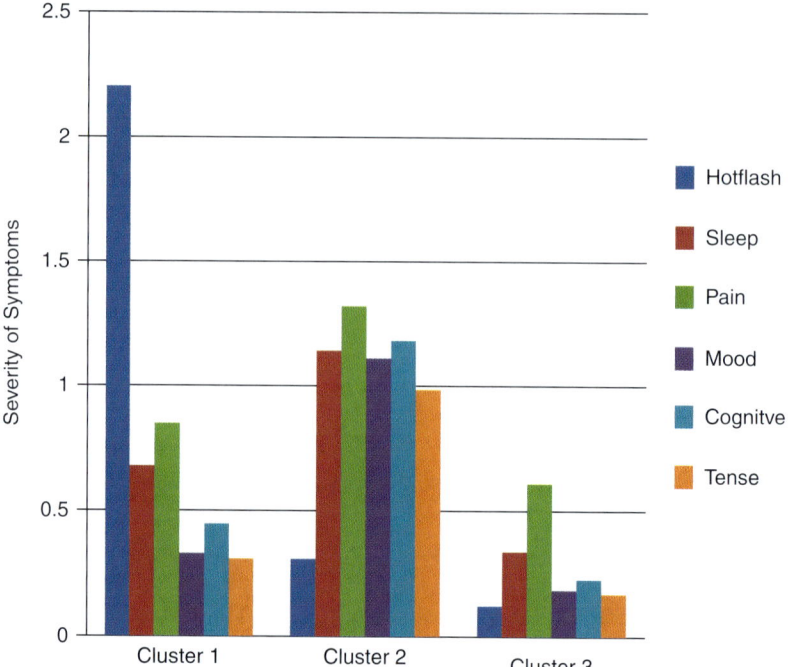

Fig. 31.5 Severity of Symptoms by Symptom Clusters Identified in the Seattle Midlife Women's Health Study

example, work and relationships with family and friends [104]. In an effort to determine which sets of symptoms were most challenging for women, participants in the Seattle Midlife Women's Health Study rated the degree to which how they felt each day interfered with their ability to work and their relationships. Hot flashes, depressed mood, anxiety, sleep problems, cognitive symptoms, and pain symptoms each contributed to interference, but the most influential factors interfering with work were stress levels and difficulty concentrating. The most influential factors interfering with relationships were stress, depressed mood, and problems concentrating [105].

31.6.1 Clusters of Symptoms During the Menopausal Transition

As studies of the menopausal transition and symptoms have progressed, it is increasingly evident that women experience multiple symptoms with some experiencing multiple severe symptoms. Moreover, researchers studying symptom have identified the importance of studying co-occurring symptoms or symptom clusters as a basis for identifying mechanisms that may be common to several symptoms or explain relationships among symptoms. As an example, Joffe and colleagues have found that induced hot flashes objectively recorded influence sleep efficiency, creating fragmentation. Subjective hot flashes are associated with perceived poor sleep quality [106]. In addition, investigators studying symptom clusters are concerned about identifying therapeutics that will maximize effects of an intervention on all or most symptoms and minimize the likelihood that a therapy will have positive effects on one symptom but exacerbate others [107]. Cray and colleagues identified three clusters of symptoms women experienced during the menopausal transition and early postmenopause [108]. Among these were clusters of (1) low severity symptoms of all types (hot flashes, mood, sleep disruption, cognitive, pain, and tension symptoms; (2) moderately severe hot flashes along with moderate levels of other symptoms; and (3) low severity hot flashes with moderate levels of all other symptoms (Fig. 31.5). The high hot flash cluster versus the low symptom severity cluster was associated with being in the late menopausal transition stage as well as with higher levels of FSH, lower levels of estrogen, higher norepinephrine, and lower epinephrine levels. The moderate severity symptom cluster versus the low severity cluster was associated only with having lower epinephrine levels [109].

In contrast to a symptom cluster, a syndrome is a pattern of symptoms that is presumably disease-specific and results from a common underlying mechanism. Avis and colleague demonstrated a lack of evidence for a "menopausal syndrome" despite some evidence linking some of the symptoms in clusters to endocrine dynamics during the menopausal transition [110].

Given the global nature of health care, it is important to focus on women's experiences of menopause in many parts of the world. To date much of this body of work has been conducted in economically developed countries, often incorporating measures common to Western cultures. A detailed review of the symptoms women experience around the globe is beyond the scope of this chapter. Nonetheless, Leidy Sievert [111] has led development of research culminating in identification of ways in which diverse populations of women experience menopause. Her work includes a biocultural model in which environment, culture, and biology intersect to influence the expression of hot flashes. Leidy Sievert elaborates that environment prompts consideration of the climate and altitude in which women live their lives and that culture warrants consideration of practices related to marriage, religion, attitudes, medicalization, hysterectomy practices, smoking, reproductive patterns, and diet. Finally, because different populations of the world have different genetic characteristics, they also may have differing hormone levels and sweating patterns. Thus, the variation across populations and the variation within populations of women are complex and together influence women's individual experiences. Indeed, Leidy Sievert points out that cross-country comparative studies illustrate the differences between cultures, while cross-cultural study of menopause can facilitate understanding of women's place in society and the influence of social context on symptom experience [112]. In a comparison of symptom experiences across countries, women from different countries report some similar symptoms but may cluster their symptoms differently. For example, expression of somatic with emotional complaints varies across populations, possibly reflecting comfort with expression of emotional symptoms [113]. Both Avis [110] and Locke [114] have provided compelling data about the diversity of the menopause experience and associated symptoms.

31.7 Stress and the Menopausal Transition

Given the nature of symptoms that women experience during the menopausal transition, one might ask whether the menopausal transition, itself, is stressful. We found that there was little change in perceived stress during the early and late menopausal transition stages. Instead, as women aged, those who were employed and had a history of sexual abuse and depressed mood experienced greater stress. Those who experienced an improvement in the burdens associated with their roles, more social support and more adequate incomes reported less stress. Those who appraised aging changes in their bodies as negative and perceived their health as poorer had higher stress levels [115]. These findings are consistent with findings of other studies of women that implicate exposure to stress to symptom experience during this part of the lifespan. Clinicians working with women traversing the menopausal transition should remain vigilant to the social circumstances of women's lives, as well as focusing on the social and endocrine features of this transition. Of interest is that when we asked women who had participated in the Seattle Midlife Women's Health Study for 15 years what was the most challenging aspect of their lives during that period, only one said that it was the menopausal transition (Woods and Mitchell, unpublished).

31.8 Well-Being

Despite the symptoms women experience and their experiences of stress during this period of the lifespan, women report high levels of well-being. Although entry to the early transition stage had no effect on well-being, being in the late MT stage predicted a decrease in well-being, but this decrease in well-being did not persist into the early postmenopause. Well-being also was lower in women taking hormones, replicating findings from the Women's Health Initiative. The significant variability in women's well-being was more affected by life events other than the menopausal transition and by the personal resources available to meet transition demands [116].

31.9 The Menopausal Transition and Healthy Aging

31.9.1 Metabolic Changes

There is a growing understanding of the relationship of the menopausal transition to healthy aging. Among this body of work are studies linking dimensions of the menopausal transition to health outcomes through metabolic changes affecting bone, muscle, and fat. During the menopausal transition and early postmenopause, women experience changes in body composition affecting both lean body mass (bone density, muscle mass) and fat deposition (subcutaneous and intra-abdominal). Bone loss accelerates in the late menopausal transition and continues in the early PM in both the spine and hip areas. For some women, the decrease in bone mass may lead to osteoporosis. Women also lose skeletal muscle mass [117], the consequences of which may be linked to outcomes during the postmenopausal period, such as development of sarcopenia. Loss of muscle may lead to losses observed in physical functioning in postmenopausal women in hand grip, ability to move from sitting to standing position, velocity, and perceived physical functioning. Moreover, greater losses have been observed in women with hysterectomy compared to those experiencing a natural menopause [117]. The role of muscle in glucose metabolism as well as in physical functioning has not yet been considered fully in longitudinal studies of the menopausal transition.

Table 31.2 Indicators of metabolic syndrome

Abdominal obesity (waist >35 in.)
Atherogenic dyslipidemia with triglycerides >150 mg/dl, HDL <50 mg/dl, elevated LDL, and small dense LDL
Hypertension B/P >130/85 mmHg
Fasting blood glucose >110 mg/dl
Insulin resistance and glucose intolerance
Prothrombotic state
Proinflammatory state

Women accumulate an average increase in fat mass of approximately 3.4 KG over a 6-year period [117]. Changes in hypothalamic-pituitary-ovarian hormones are related to changing fat metabolism. Increases in FSH were associated with changes in levels of substances which regulate appetite, fat deposition, and inflammation: increases of FSH were positively associated with leptin and adiponectin and negatively associated with ghrelin [118]. As changes occur in both intra-abdominal and subcutaneous fat mass, women experience changes in lipid patterns, glucose levels and insulin resistance, and thrombotic and inflammatory responses.

As seen in Table 31.2, a condition labeled metabolic syndrome includes several risk factors for cardiovascular disease. Many of these risk factors become more prevalent as women complete the menopausal transition. Changes in lipid patterns, glucose and insulin, and thrombotic and inflammatory processes that comprise the metabolic syndrome become more prevalent as women reach the late menopausal transition stage and postmenopause.

31.9.2 Lipid Patterns

The SWAN study cohort experienced changing levels of lipids during the late stage of the menopausal transition and early postmenopause, consistent with cross-sectional findings from an earlier study [119]. Total cholesterol, low-density lipoprotein cholesterol, triglycerides, and lipoprotein(a) levels peaked during the late MT and early PM. HDL cholesterol also peaked during this period [120]. Greater increases in ghrelin levels over the MT were associated with increases in low-density lipoprotein cholesterol [121]. The hormonal changes during the menopausal transition and early postmenopause have been implicated in changes in fat deposition and lipid metabolism. In SWAN participants, FSH was associated with increased total cholesterol and LDL cholesterol. Estradiol was associated with increased triglycerides, lower LDL, higher HDL, and testosterone with greater BMI, higher triglyceride levels. Sex hormone-binding globulin (SHBG) was associated with lower waist circumference, BMI, total cholesterol, LDL, and HDL levels. Free androgen index (FAI, a measure of bioavailable androgen) was associated with greater waist circumference, BMI, total cholesterol, triglycerides [122].

31.9.3 Glucose and Insulin

In another longitudinal study, increases in leptin over the menopausal transition were associated with glucose, insulin, and insulin resistance and also with greater diastolic blood pressure. Larger decreases in adiponectin over the menopausal transition were associated with greater increases in insulin and insulin resistance as well as increases in systolic blood pressure and greater decreases in HDL-C [123]. FSH has been associated with increased insulin resistance and lower insulin levels and testosterone with higher glucose levels. SHBG is associated with lower insulin, glucose, homeostatic measurement of insulin resistance measures (HOMA-IR), and free androgen with greater insulin, glucose, and HOMA-IR levels [122].

31.9.4 Thrombotic Changes

Studies of hemostatic factors and hormone levels during the menopausal transition revealed that both testosterone and estrogen play important roles. Androgens (testosterone and free androgen index (FAI) were positively associated with plasminogen activator inhibitor type I (PAI-1) and tissue plasminogen activator (t(PA)). FAI was positively associated with C-reactive protein (hs-CRP). Lower SHBG levels which were associated with greater levels of bioavailable testosterone were also associated with higher levels of PAI-1, hs-CRP, and factor VIIc [124]. Androgens were strongly associated with fibrinolytic and inflammation markers, even when considering age, body size, smoking, and race-ethnicity in the SWAN cohort [124].

Estrogen was significantly related to some hemostatic factors in the SWAN cohort: lower estradiol was associated with higher PAI-1 and t(PA), but not with fibrinogen, factor VII, c or hs-CRP. Elevated FSH was related to higher levels of PAI-1, factor VII levels and to lower fibrinogen, and hs-CRP. Transitions to postmenopause were not associated with different levels of hemostatic factors. Endogenous estrogens may be associated with lower CVD risk via fibrinolytic but not coagulation or inflammatory mechanisms [123].

31.9.5 Inflammatory Responses

Changes in intra-abdominal fat metabolism during this period of life have been associated with inflammatory markers and adipokines. Increase in intra-abdominal fat from premenopause to postmenopause was correlated positively with the change in serum alpha amylase (SAA), C-reactive protein (CRP), tissue plasminogen activator (tPA), and leptin and negatively correlated with the change in adiponectin [125]. These are each involved in regulation of fat metabolism, inflammation, and appetite. During the menopausal transition, women also experience changing levels of inflammatory markers, including IL-6. To date there are no longitudinal data available from the SWAN cohort. Nonetheless, a recent report indicates that there are between-group differences among women who have not yet begun the menopausal transition, women in the transition, and women in early and late postmenopause. IL-4 was higher in late postmenopausal women, and IL-2 was higher in the early postmenopause as was granulocyte-macrophage colony-stimulating factor (GM-CSF). Age was negatively related to IL-6, but the menopausal transition and postmenopause were unrelated. Estradiol was negatively related to

IL-6 levels and weakly negatively related to IL-2, IL-8, and GM-CSF [126]. Results from longitudinal studies are needed to clarify the relationship between the menopausal transition and these immune indicators.

31.10 Metabolic Syndrome

There is mounting evidence that the endocrine changes during the menopausal transition have important effects on risk factors for heart disease, in particular, the metabolic syndrome. As discussed earlier, higher free androgen and lower SHBG levels play an important role in CV risk factors for women during the menopausal transition. Recent evidence suggests that an increasing ratio of testosterone to estrogen is implicated in development of metabolic syndrome. Women with low sex hormone-binding globulin, free androgen index, and high total T at baseline experienced increased risk of metabolic syndrome over 5 years of follow-up. Both baseline total T:E2 ratio and its rate of change were associated with the increased incident metabolic syndrome [127].

31.11 Summary

Recently completed research on the menopausal transition and early postmenopause has contributed to understanding of the stages of the reproductive aging, endocrine changes accompanying these stages, symptoms and their correlates, and the relationship of the menopausal transition and accompanying physiologic changes to healthy aging. Future work remains to enhance health promotion for midlife women as well as their efforts to manage their symptoms.

References

1. He W, Sengupta M, Velkoff, VA, Debarros KA. U.S. Census Bureau, current population reports. P23-209, 65+ in the United States: 2005. Washington DC: US Government Printing Office; 2005.
2. Kaufert P, Boggs P, Ettinger B, Woods NF, Utian WH. Women and menopause: beliefs, attitudes, and behaviors. The North American menopause Society 1997 Menopause Survey. Menopause. 1998;5(4):197–202.
3. Mishra GD, Cooper R, Kuh D. A life course approach to reproductive health: theory and methods. Maturitas. 2010;65:92–7.
4. Neugarten B. The awareness of middle age. In: Neugarten B, editor. Middle age and aging. Chicago: University of Chicago Press; 1968. p. 93–8.
5. McKinlay S, McKinlay J. Selected studies of the menopause. J Biosoc Sci. 1973;5:533–55.
6. McKinlay SM, Brambilla DJ, Posner JG. The normal menopause transition. Maturitas. 1992;14(2):103–15.
7. Matthews K, Wing R, Kuller L, Meilahn EN, Kelsey SF, Costello EJ, et al. Influences of natural menopause on psychological characteristics and symptoms of middle-aged healthy women. J Consult Clin Psychol. 1990;58:345–51.
8. Guthrie JR, Dennerstein L, Taffe JR, Lehert P, Burger HG. Hot flushes during the menopause transition: a longitudinal study in Australian-born women. Menopause. 2005;12:460–7.
9. Woods NF, Mitchell ES. Women's images of midlife: observations from the Seattle Midlife Women's Health Study. Health Care Women Int. 1997;18:439–53.
10. Woods NF, Mitchell ES. Anticipating menopause: observations from the Seattle Midlife Women's Health Study. Menopause. 1999;6:167–73.
11. Sowers M, Crawford S, Sternfeld B, Morganstein D, Gold E, Greendale G, et al. 2000. In: Lobo R, Kelsey J, Marcus R, editors. Menopause: biology and pathobiology. San Diego: Academic; 2000. p. 175–88.
12. Collins A, Landgren BM. Reproductive health, use of estrogen and experience of symptoms in perimenopausal women: a population-based study. Maturitas. 1994;20:101–11.
13. Mishra GD, Cooper R, Tom SE, Kuh D. Early life circumstances and their impact on menarche and menopause. Womens Health. 2009;5(2):175–90.
14. Kuh D, Hardy R. Women's health in midlife: findings from a British birth cohort study. J Br Menopause Soc. 2003;9(2):55–60.
15. Voda AM. Climacteric hot flash. Maturitas. 1981;3:73–90.
16. Santoro N, Brown JR, Adel T, Skurnick J. Characterizaton of reproductive hormonal dynamics in the perimenopause. J Clin Endocrinol Metab. 1996;81:1495–501.
17. Santoro N. The menopause transition: an update. Hum Reprod Update. 2002;8:155–60.
18. Reame NE, Kelche RP, Beitins IZ, Yu MY, Zawacki CM, Padmanabhan V. Age effects of follicle-stimulating hormone and pulsatile luteinizing hormone secretion across the menstrual cycle of premenopausal women. J Clin Endocrinol Metab. 1996;81(4):1512–8.
19. U. S. Public Health Services. Opportunities for Research on Women's Health. Bethesda: National Institutes of Health; 1992.
20. National Institute on Aging. Workshop on Menopause: Current Knowledge and Recommendations for Research. National Institutes of Health, Bethesda, MD. 1993.

21. MacPherson KI. Menopause as disease: the social construction of a metaphor. ANS Adv Nurs Sci. 1981;3(2):95–113.
22. Andrist LC, Mac Pherson KI. Conceptual models for women's health research: reclaiming menopause as an exemplar of nursing's contributions to feminist scholarship. Annu Rev Nurs Res. 2001;19:29–60.
23. Dennerstein L, Dudley EC, Hopper JL, Guthrie JR, Burger HG. A prospective population-based study of menopausal symptoms. Obstet Gynecol. 2000;96:351–8.
24. Burger HG, Cahir N, Robertson DM, Groome NP, Dudley E, Green A, Dennerstein L. Serum inhibins A and B fall differentially as FSH rises in perimenopausal women. Clin Endocrinol (Oxf). 1998;48(6):809–13.
25. Mitchell ES, Woods NF, Mariella A. Three stages of the menopausal transition from the Seattle Midlife Women's Health Study: toward a more precise definition. Menopause. 2000;7:334–49.
26. Soules MR, Sherman S, Parrott E, Rebar R, Santoro N, Utian W, Woods NF. Executive summary: Stages of Reproductive Aging Workshop (STRAW). Fertil Steril. 2001;76:874–8.
27. Harlow SD, Cain K, Crawford S, Dennerstein L, Little R, Mitchell ES, et al. Evaluation of four proposed bleeding criteria for the onset of late menopausal transition. J Clin Endocrinol Metab. 2006;91:3432–8.
28. Harlow SD, Crawford S, Dennerstein L, Burger HG, Mitchell ES, Sowers MF, ReSTAGE Collaboration. Recommendations from a multi-study evaluation of proposed criteria for staging reproductive aging. Climacteric. 2007;10(2):112–9.
29. Harlow SD, Mitchell ES, Crawford S, Nan B, Little R, Taffe J, ReSTAGE Collaboration. The ReSTAGE Collaboration: defining optimal bleeding criteria for onset of early menopausal transition. Fertil Steril. 2008;89:129–40.
30. Taffe JR, Cain KC, Mitchell ES, Woods NF, Crawford SL, Harlow SD. "Persistence" improves the 60-day amenorrhea marker of entry to late-stage menopausal transition for women aged 40 to 44 years. Menopause. 2010;17:191–3.
31. Randolph J, Zheng H, Sowers MR, Crandall C, Crawford S, Gold EB, Buga M. Change in follicle-stimulating hormone and estradiol across the menopausal transition: effect of age at the final menstrual period. J Clin Endocrinol Metab. 2011;96:746–54.
32. Randolph Jr JF, Sowers M, Gold EB, et al. Reproductive hormones in the early menopausal transition: relationship to ethnicity, body size, and menopausal status. J Clin Endocrinol Metab. 2003;88:1516–22.
33. Sowers MR, Zheng H, McConnell D, Nan B, Harlow SD, Randolph Jr JF. Estradiol rates of change in relation to the final menstrual period in a population-based cohort of women. J Clin Endocrinol Metab. 2008;93(10):3847–52.
34. Randolph Jr JF, Sowers M, Bondarenko I, Gold EB, Greendale GA, Bromberger JT, et al. The relationship of longitudinal change in reproductive hormones and vasomotor symptoms during the menopausal transition. J Clin Endocrinol Metab. 2005;90:6106–12.
35. Burger H, Burger HG, Hale GE, Robertson DM, Dennerstein L. A review of hormonal changes during the menopausal transition: focus on findings from the Melbourne Women's Midlife Health Project. Hum Reprod Update. 2007;13(6):559–65.
36. Sowers MR, Zheng H, Mc Connell D, Nan B, Harlow S, Randolph JF. Follicle stimulating hormone and its rate of change in defining menopause transition stages. J Clin Endocrinol Metab. 2008;93:3958–64.
37. Sowers MR, Eyvazzadeh AD, McConnell D, Yosef M, Jannausch ML, Zhang D, et al. Anti-mullerian hormone and inhibin B in the definition of ovarian aging and the menopause transition. J Clin Endocrinol Metab. 2008;93(9):3478–83.
38. Lasley BL, Santoro N, Randolf JF, Gold EB, Crawford S, Weiss G, et al. The relationship of circulating dehydroepiandrosterone, testosterone, and estradiol to stages of the menopausal transition and ethnicity. J Clin Endocrinol Metab. 2002;87:3760–7.
39. Crawford S, Santoro N, Laughlin GA, Sowers MF, McConnell D, Sutton-Tyrrell K, et al. Circulating dehydroepiandrosterone sulfate concentrations during the menopausal transition. J Clin Endocrinol Metab. 2009;94(8):2945–51.
40. Burger H, Dudley E, Dennerstein J, Cui L, Hoppper J. A prospective longitudinal study of serum testosterone dehydroepianderosterone sulfate and sex hormone binding globulin levels through the menopause transition. J Clin Endocrinol Metab. 2000;85(8):2832–938.
41. Woods N, Carr MC, Tao EY, Taylor HJ, Mitchell ES. Increased urinary cortisol levels during the menopausal transition. Menopause. 2006;13:212–21.
42. Lasley BL, Crawford S, McConnell DS. Adrenal androgens and the menopausal transition. Obstet Gynecol Clin North Am. 2011;38:467–75.
43. Kay M, Voda A, Olivas G, Rios F, Imle M. Ethnography of the menopause-related hot flash. Maturitas. 1982;4:217–27.
44. Freedman RR, Subramanian M. Effects of symptomatic status and the menstrual cycle on hot flash-related thermoregulatory parameters. Menopause. 2005;12:156–9.
45. Freedman RR. Hot flashes: behavioral treatments, mechanisms, and relation to sleep. Am J Med. 2005;118(12B):124–30.
46. Freedman RR. Pathophysiology and treatment of menopausal hot flashes. Semin Reprod Med. 2005;23:117–25.
47. Thurston RC, Sutton-Tyrrell K, Everson-Rose SA, Hess R, Matthews KA. Hot flashes and subclinical cardiovascular disease: findings from the Study of Women's Health Across the Nation Heart Study. Circulation. 2008;118(12):1234–40.
48. Thurston RC, Christie IC, Matthews KA. Hot flashes and cardiac vagal control: a link to cardiovascular risk? Menopause. 2010;17(3):456–61.

49. Woods NF, Smith-DiJulio K, Percival DB, Tao EY, Taylor HJ, Mitchell ES. Symptoms during the menopausal transition and early postmenopause and their relation to endocrine levels over time: observations from the Seattle Midlife Women's Health Study. J Womens Health. 2007;16(5):667–77.
50. Thurston RC, Kuller LH, Edmundowicz D, Matthews KA. History of hot flashes and aortic calcification among postmenopausal women. Menopause. 2010;17(2):256–61.
51. Thurston RC, Sutton-Tyrrell K, Everson-Rose SA, Hess R, Powell LH, Matthews KA. Hot flashes and carotid intima media thickness among midlife women. Menopause. 2011;18:352–8.
52. Thurston RC, Santoro N, Matthews KA. Adiposity and hot flashes in midlife women: a modifying role of age. J Clin Endocrinol Metab. 2011;96:1588–95.
53. Thurston RC, Sowers MR, Chang Y, Sternfeld B, Gold EB, Johnston JM, et al. Adiposity and reporting of vasomotor symptoms among midlife women: the Study of Women's Health Across the Nation. Am J Epidemiol. 2008;167(1):78–85. Epub 2007 Sep 19.
54. Thurston RC, Sowers MR, Sternfeld B, Gold EB, Bromberger J, Chang Y, et al. Gains in body fat and vasomotor symptom reporting over the menopausal transition: the Study of Women's Health Across the Nation. Am J Epidemiol. 2009;170(6):766–74. Epub 2009 Aug 12.
55. Thurston RC, Sowers MR, Sutton-Tyrrell K, Everson-Rose SA, Lewis TT, Edmundowicz D, Matthews KA. Abdominal adiposity and hot flashes among midlife women. Menopause. 2008;15(3):429–34.
56. Thurston RC, Khoudary SR, Sutton-Tyrrell K, Crandall CH, Gold E, Sternfeld B, et al. Are vasomotor symptoms associated with alterations in hemostatic and inflammatory markers? Findings from the Study of Women's Health Across the Nation. Menopause. 2011;15:1044–51.
57. Crandall CJ, Tseng CH, Crawrord SL, Thurston RC, Gold eB, Johnston JM, et al. Association of menopausal vasomotor symptoms with increased bone turnover during the menopausal transition. J Bone Miner Res. 2011;26:840–9.
58. Corwin EJ, Cannon JG. Gonadotropin modulation of interleukin 1 secretion. J Gend Specif Med. 1999;2:30–4.
59. Smith-Di Julio K, Perciva DB, Woods NF, Tao E, Mitchell ES. Hot flash severity in hormone therapy users and nonusers across the menopausal transition. Maturitas. 2007;58(2):191–200.
60. Thurston RC, Bromberger JT, Joffe H, Avis NE, Hess R, Crandall CJ, et al. Beyond frequency: who is most bothered by vasomotor symptoms? Menopause. 2008;15(5):841–7.
61. Williams RE, Kalilani L, DiBenedetti DB, Zhous X, Granger AL, Fehnel SE, et al. Frequency and severity of vasomotor symptoms among peri- and postmenopausal women in the United States. Climacteric. 2008;11:32–43.
62. Williams RE, Kalilani LK, DiBenedetti DB, Zhou X, Fehnel SE, Clark RV. Healthcare seeking and treatment for menopausal symptoms in the United States. Maturitas. 2007;58:348–58.
63. Woods NF, Mitchell ES. Symptoms during the perimenopause: prevalence, severity, trajectory, and significance in women's lives. Am J Med. 2005;118(12B):S14–24.
64. Barnabei VM, Cochrane B, Aragaki A, Nygaard I, Williams RS, McGovern PG, et al. The effects of estrogen plus progestin on menopausal symptoms and treatment effects among participants of the Women's Health Initiative. Obstet Gynecol. 2005;105:1063–73.
65. Col NF, Guthrie JR, Politi M, Dennerstein L. Duration of vasomotor symptoms in middle-aged women: a longitudinal study. Menopause. 2009;16:453–7.
66. Gibson CJ, Thurston RC, Bromberger JT, Kamarck T, Matthews KA. Negative affect and vasomotor symptoms in the Study of Women's Health Across the Nation Daily Hormone Study. Menopause. 2011;18:1270–7.
67. Gold EB, Block G, Crawford S, Lachance L, FitzGerald G, Miracle H, et al. Lifestyle and demographic factors in relation to vasomotor symptoms: baseline results from the Study of Women's Health Across the Nation. Am J Epidemiol. 2004;159:1189–99.
68. Freeman EW, Sammel MD, Lin H, Gracia CR, Kapoor S, Ferdousi T. The role of anxiety and hormonal changes in menopausal hot flashes. Menopause. 2005;12:258–66.
69. Freeman EW, Sammel MD, Oin H, Gracia CR, Pien GW, Nelson DB, et al. Symptoms associated with menopausal transition and reproductive hormones in midlife women. Obstet Gynecol. 2007;110:230–40.
70. Shaver J, Giblin E, Lentz M, Lee K. Sleep patterns and stability in perimenopausal women. Sleep. 1988;11:556–61.
71. Shaver JL, Giblin E, Paulsen V. Sleep quality subtypes in midlife women. Sleep. 1991;14:18–23.
72. Shaver JL, Johnston SK, Lentz MJ, Landis CA. Stress exposure, psychological distress, and physiological stress activation in midlife women with insomnia. Psychosom Med. 2002;64:793–802.
73. Shaver JL, Paulsen VM. Sleep, psychological distress, and somatic symptoms in perimenopausal women. Fam Pract Res. 1993;13:373–84.
74. Woods NF, Mitchell ES. Sleep symptoms during the menopausal transition and early postmenopause: observations from the Seattle Midlife Women's Health Study. Sleep. 2010;33:539–49.
75. Ensrud KE, Stone KL, Blackwell TL, Sawaya GF, Tagliaferri M, Diem SJ, et al. Frequency and severity of hot flashes and sleep disturbance in postmenopausal women with hot flashes. Menopause. 2008;16:1–6.
76. Pien GW, Sammel MD, Freeman EW, Lin H, DeBlasis TL. Predictors of sleep quality in women in the menopausal transition. Sleep. 2008;31:991–9.

77. Kravitz H, Zhao X, Bromberger J, Gold EB, Hall MH, Matthews KA, et al. Sleep disturbance during the menopausal transition in a multi-ethnic community sample of women. Sleep. 2009;31:979–90.

78. Mitchell ES, Woods NF. Pain symptoms during the menopausal and early postmenopause: observations from the Seattle Midlife Women's Health Study. Climacteric. 2010;13:467–78.

79. Kravitz HM, Avery E, Sowers M, Bromberger JT, Owens JF, Matthews KA, et al. Relationships between menopausal and mood symptoms and EEG sleep measures in a multi-ethnic sample of middle-aged women: the SWAN sleep study. Sleep. 2011;34: 1221–32.

80. Campbell JG, Bromberger JT, Buysse DJ, Hall MH, Hardin KA, Kravitz HM, et al. Evaluation of the association of menopausal status with delta and beta EEG activity during sleep. Sleep. 2011;34:1561–8.

81. Woods NF, Mitchell ES. Pathways to depressed mood for midlife women: observations from the Seattle Midlife Women's Health Study. Res Nurs Health. 1997;20:119–29.

82. Woods NF, Mariella A, Mitchell ES. Depressed mood symptoms during the menopausal transition: observations from the Seattle Midlife Women's Health Study. Climacteric. 2006;9:195–203.

83. Woods NF, Smith-DiJulio K, Percival DB, Tao EY, Mariella A, Mitchell ES. Depressed mood during the menopausal transition and early postmenopause: observations from the Seattle Midlife Women's Health Study. Menopause. 2008;15:223–32.

84. Bromberger J, Matthews K, Schott LL, Brockwell S, Avis NE, Kravitz HM, et al. Depressive Symptoms during the menopausal transition: the Study of Women's Health Across the Nation (SWAN). J Affect Disord. 2007;103:267–72.

85. Bromberger JT, Schott LL, Kravitz HM, Sowers M, Avis NE, Gold EB, et al. Longitudinal change in reproductive hormones and depressive symptoms across the menopausal transition: results from the Study of Women's Health Across the Nation (SWAN). Arch Gen Psychiatry. 2010;67:598–607.

86. Cohen L, Soares C, Vitonis A, Otto M, Harlow B. Risk for new onset of depression during the menopausal transition: the Harvard Study of Moods and Cycles. Arch Gen Psychiatry. 2006;63:385–90.

87. Freeman E, Sammel M, Lin H, Nelson D. Associations of hormones and menopausal status with depressed mood in women with no history of depression. Arch Gen Psychiatry. 2006;63:375–82.

88. Avis NE, Crawford S, Longcope R, Stellato C. Longitudinal study of hormone levels and depression among women transitioning through menopause. Climacteric. 2001;4:243–9.

89. Avis NE, Brambilla D, McKinlay SM, Vass K. A longitudinal analysis of the association between menopause and depression: results from the Massachusetts Women's Health Study. Ann Epidemiol. 1994;4: 214–20.

90. Morrison MF, Freeman EW, Lin H, Sammel MD. Higher DHEA-S levels are associated with depressive symptoms during the menopausal transition: results from the PENN ovarian aging study. Arch Womens Ment Health. 2011;14:375–82.

91. Janssen I, Powell LH, Matthews KA, Cursio JF, Hollenberg SM, SuttonTyrell K, et al. Depressive symptoms are related to progression of coronary calcium in midlife women: the Study of Women's Health Across the Nation (SWAN) heart study. Am Heart J. 2011;161:1186–91.

92. Mitchell ES, Woods NF. Cognitive symptoms during the menopausal transition and early postmenopause: observations from the Seattle Midlife Women's Health Study. Climacteric. 2011;14:252–61.

93. Greendale GA, Wight RG, Huang M, Avis N, Gold EB, Joffe H, et al. Menopause-associated symptom and cognitive performance: results from the Study of Women's Health Across the Nation. Am J Epidemiol. 2010;171:1214–24.

94. Greendale GA. Effects of the menopause transition and hormone use on cognitive performance in midlife women. Neurology. 2009;72:1850–7.

95. Luetters C, Huang MH, Seeman T, Buckwalter G, Meyer PM, Avis NE, et al. Menopause transition stage and endogenous estradiol and follicle-stimulating hormone levels are not related to cognitive performance: cross-sectional results from the Study Women's Health across the Nation (SWAN). J Women's Health. 2007;16:331–44.

96. Le Resche L, Popescu A, LeResche L, Truelove EL, Drangsholt MT. Gender differences in pain modulation by diffuse noxious inhibitory controls: a systematic review. Pain. 2010;150(2):309–18.

97. Szoeke CE, Cicuttini FM, Guthrie JR, Dennerstein L. The relationship of reports of aches and joint pains to the menopausal transition: a longitudinal study. Climacteric. 2008;11:55–62.

98. Dugan SA, Everson-Rose SA, Karavolos K, Sternfeld B, Wesley D, Powell LH. The impact of physical activity level on SF-36 Role-physical and bodily pain indices in midlife women. J Phys Act Health. 2009;6:33–42.

99. Dugan SA, Powell LH, Kravitz HM, Everson-Rose SA, Karavolos K, Luborsky J. Musculoskeletal pain and menopausal status. Clin J Pain. 2006;22: 325–31.

100. Woods NF, Smith-DiJulio K, Mitchell ES. Sexual desire during the menopausal transition and early postmenopause: observations from the Seattle Midlife Women's Health Study. J Womens Health. 2010;19:209–18.

101. Avis NE, Zhao X, Johannes CB, Ory M, Brockwell S, Greendale GA. Correlates of sexual function among multi-ethnic middle-aged women: results from the Study of Women's Health Across the Nation (SWAN). Menopause. 2005;12(4):385–98.

102. Dennerstein L, Lehert P, Buirger H. The relative effects of hormones and relationship factors on

102. sexual function of women through the natural menopausal transition. Fertil Steril. 2005;84(1):174–80.
103. Gracia CR, Sammel MD, Freeman EW, Liu L, Hollander L, Nelson DB. Predictors of decreased libido in women during the late reproductive years. Menopause. 2004;11(2):144–50.
104. Carpenter JS. The hot flash related daily interference scale: a tool for assessing the impact of hot flashes on quality of life following breast cancer. J Pain Symptom Manage. 2001;22:9–989.
105. Woods NF, Mitchell ES. Symptom interference with work and relationships during the menopausal transition and early postmenopause: observations from the Seattle Midlife Women's Health Study. Menopause. 2011;18:654–61.
106. Joffe H, White DP, Crawford SL, McCurnin KE, Economou N, Connors S, Hall JE. Adverse effects of induced hot flashes on objectively recorded and subjectively reported sleep: results of a gonadotropin-releasing hormone agonist experimental protocol. Menopause. 2013;20:905–14.
107. Woods NF, Cray L. Editorial: symptom clusters and quality of life. Menopause. 2013;20:5–7.
108. Cray L, Woods NF, Mitchell ES. Symptom clusters during the menopausal transition and early postmenopause: observations from the Seattle Midlife Women's Health Study. Menopause. 2010;17:972–7.
109. Woods NF, Cray L, Herting J, Mitchell ES. Hypothalamic-pituitary-ovarian and hypothalamic-pituitary-adrenal and autonomic nervous system biomarkers and symptom clusters during the menopausal transition and early postmenopause. Menopause. 2014. in press.
110. Avis NE, Brockwell S, Colvin A. A universal menopausal syndrome? Am J Med. 2005;118(suppl 12B):S37–46.
111. Sievert LL. Menopause: a biocultural perspective. New Brunswick: Rutgers University Press; 2006.
112. Seivert LL. Comparisons of symptom experience across country and class. Menopause. 2013;20:594–5.
113. Sievert LL, Obermeyer CM. Symptom clusters at midlife: a four-country comparison of checklist and qualitative responses. Menopause. 2012;19:133–44.
114. Lock M. Encounters with aging: mythologies of menopause in Japan and North America. Berkeley: University of California Press; 1993.
115. Woods NF, Mitchell ES, Percival DB, Smith-DiJulio K. Is the menopausal transition stressful? Observations of perceived stress from the Seattle Midlife Women's Health Study. Menopause. 2009;16(1):90–7.
116. Smith DiJulio K, Mitchell ES, Percival DB, Woods NF. Well-being during the menopausal transition and early postmenopause: a within-stage analysis. Womens Health Issues. 2008;18(4):310–8.
117. Sowers M, Zheng H, Tomey K, Karvonen-Gutierrez C, Jannausch M, Li X, et al. Changes in body composition in women over six years at midlife: ovarian and chronological aging. J Clin Endocrinol Metab. 2007;92(3):895–901.
118. Sowers MR, Wildman RP, Mancuso P, Eyvazzadeh AD, Karvonen-Gutierrez CA, Rillamas-Sun E, et al. Change in adipocytokines and ghrelin with menopause. Maturitas. 2008;20:149–57.
119. Carr MC, Kim KH, Zambon A, Mitchell ES, Woods NF, Casazza CP, et al. Changes in LDL density across the menopausal transition. J Invest Med. 2000;48:245–50. 50:1947–1954.
120. Derby CA, Crawford SL, Pasternak RC, Sowers M, Sternfeld B, Matthews KA. Lipid changes during the menopause transition in relation to age and weight: the Study of Women's Health Across the Nation. Am J Epidemiol. 2009;169(11):1352–61.
121. Wildman RP, Janssen I, Khan UI, Thurston R, Barinas-Mitchell E, El Khoudary SR, et al. Subcutaneous adipose tissue in relation to subclinical atherosclerosis and cardiometabolic risk factors in midlife women. Am J Clin Nutr. 2011;93:719–26.
122. Sutton-Tyrell K, Wildman R, Matthews K, Chae C, Lasley B, Brockwell S, et al. Sex-hormone-binding globulin and the free androgen index are related to cardiovascular risk factors in multiethnic premenopausal and perimenopausal women enrolled in the Study of Women Across the Nation (SWAN). Circulation. 2005;111(10):1242–9.
123. Wildman RP, Mancuso P, Wang C, Kim M, Scherer PE, Sowers MR. Adipocytokine and ghrelin levels in relation to cardiovascular disease risk factors in women at midlife: longitudinal associations. Int J Obes (Lond). 2008;32:740–8.
124. Sowers M, Matthews K, Jannausch M, Randolph J, McConnell D, Sutton-Tyrell K, et al. Hemostatic factors and estrogen during the menopausal transition. J Clin Endocrinol Metab. 2005;90(11):5942–8.
125. Lee CG, Carr MC, Murdoch SJ, Mitchell E, Woods NF, Wener MJ, et al. Adipokines, inflammation, and visceral adiposity across the menopausal transition: a prospective study. J Clin Endocrinol Metab. 2009;94(4):1104–10.
126. Yasui T, Maegawa M, Tomita J, Miyatani Y, Yamada M, Uemura H, et al. Changes in serum cytokine concentrations during the menopausal transition. Maturitas. 2007;56(4):396–403.
127. Torrens J, Sutton-Tyrell K, Zhao X, Mathews K, Brockwell S, Sowers M, et al. Relative androgen excess during the menopausal transition predicts incident metabolic syndrome in midlife women: Study of Women's Health Across the Nation. Menopause. 2009;16:257–64.

Part VI

Menopause and Cosmetic Procedures

Menopause and Cosmeceuticals

32

Estela G. de Nóvoa, Raquel Fávaro,
Thaísa S.T. Silvino, Fernanda C.N. Ribeiro,
Raissa M. Santos, and Adilson Costa

Contents

32.1	Introduction	456
32.2	Retinoids	456
32.3	Antioxidants	457
32.4	Fatty Acids	458
32.5	Anti-glycation	459
32.6	Cosmeceutical Metals and Ions	460
32.6.1	Zinc	460
32.6.2	Copper	460
32.6.3	Silicon	461
32.6.4	Magnesium	461
32.6.5	Iron	461
32.6.6	Selenium	461
32.6.7	Aluminum	461
32.6.8	Titanium	461
32.6.9	Strontium	461
32.6.10	Potassium	462
32.6.11	Silver	462
32.6.12	Lead	462
32.6.13	Mercury	462
32.7	Moisturizers	462
32.7.1	Natural Moisturizing Factor (NMF) and Intercellular Lipids	462
32.7.2	Ion Pumps	463
32.7.3	Aquaporins	463
32.7.4	Classification of Moisturizers	463
32.7.5	New Categories of Moisturizers	464
32.8	Microdermabrasion	465
32.8.1	Microabrasive Cosmeceuticals with Direct Action	465
32.8.2	Microabrasive Cosmeceuticals with Indirect Action	467
32.9	Peptides	467
32.9.1	Signaling Peptides	467
32.9.2	Neurotransmitter Inhibitory Peptides	468
32.9.3	Carrier Peptides	468
32.9.4	Enzyme Inhibitory Peptides	468
32.9.5	Other Peptides with a "Cinderella Effect"	468
32.10	Growth Factors	468
32.10.1	Growth Factors and Their Functions	469
32.11	Sunscreens	469
32.11.1	Sunscreens and Vitamin D	469
32.12	Topical Volumizers and Fillers	470
32.12.1	Cosmeceuticals with Volumizing and Filler Effects	470
32.12.2	Growth Factors	470
32.12.3	Hyaluronic Acid	471
32.12.4	Asiaticoside	471
32.12.5	Dimethylaminoethanol	471
32.12.6	Ubiquinone: Coenzyme Q10	471
32.12.7	Botanical Extract of Commiphora Mukul: Commipheroline®	471

E.G. de Nóvoa, MD (✉) • R. Fávaro, MD
T.S.T. Silvino, MD • A. Costa, MD, MSc, PhD
Department of Dermatology,
Pontifical Catholic University of Campinas,
Av. John Boyd Dunlop, Campinas, São Paulo
13059-900, Brazil
e-mail: dermato@hmcp.puc-campinas.edu.br;
favororaquel@yahoo.com.br;
thastannous@gmail.com;
adilson_costa@hotmail.com

F.C.N. Ribeiro, MD • R.M. Santos, MD
Dermatology Research, KOLderma Clinical
Trials Institute, Campinas, São Paulo Brazil
e-mail: Fernandacnr@hotmail.com;
raissarms@hotmail.com

32.12.8	Tetrahydroxypropyl Ethylenediamine (THPE).........................	471
32.12.9	Hibiscus Extract Rich in Amino Acids: Linefactor®..................................	472
32.13	**Nanocosmeceuticals**	472
32.13.1	Skin Application	472
32.13.2	Photo-Protection	472
32.14	**Thermal Water**.....................................	473
32.15	**Topical Vitamins**...................................	473
32.15.1	Vitamin A..	473
32.15.2	Vitamin B..	474
32.15.3	Panthenol..	475
32.15.4	Vitamin C..	475
32.15.5	Vitamin E..	476
32.16	**Alpha Hydroxy Acids**...........................	476
32.17	**Estrogens**..	476
References...		476

32.1 Introduction

Skin aging is gauged by the combined effects of time (intrinsic aging) and environmental factors (extrinsic aging), by changing the structure intra- and extracellularly [1, 2].

These aforementioned effects are two independent processes, clinically and biologically distinct, which affect the structure and function simultaneously. However, evidence suggests that both present converging molecular and biochemical pathways that lead to skin aging [1, 3, 4].

Unlike young skin, the mature skin presents well-defined clinical and histological changes, especially the thinning of the dermis, the loss of dermal collagen, and the decrease in lipid production, intensified by the effect of cumulative sun exposure and oxidative damage caused by pollution, stress, and smoking. These changes manifest as wrinkles, loss of elasticity, dryness, and texture changes in mature skin [2, 5, 6].

Cosmeceuticals are still the most popular option to improve the appearance of the skin and delay the aging process. These products provide a noninvasive way to mitigate the effects of weather and the environment. They may be defined as topical products which, when coming in contact with the skin, skin appendages, and mucosa, can cause structural and/or functional changes, without having a therapeutic but rather a preventive purpose and not restricted exclusively to beautification [1, 5, 6].

To be effective, cosmeceuticals need to act not only on the horny outer layer of the epidermis but through it, and like any other product for topical use, cosmeceuticals have to respect the principles of dermatology-pharmacokinetics [1, 3, 6].

Although there are many examples of mere cosmetic effects, the most successful manufacturers of cosmeceuticals have been doing research on the aging process and have turned the knowledge so acquired into formulations that may make a difference from a cellular point of view [2, 3, 5].

32.2 Retinoids

In the skin, retinoids (RET) play a crucial regulatory role in the functions of epidermal growth and differentiation. Studies have demonstrated therapeutic benefits, such as cell regeneration, exfoliation, and collagen synthesis [1, 7].

The biological effects of retinoids include improvement of fine wrinkles and acne vulgaris, decrease in roughness, improvement in reducing actinic keratoses, and hyperpigmentation. From a histological perspective, following treatment with RET, effects such as epidermal hyperplasia, stratum corneum compaction, reduction of the granular layer and melanocyte hypertrophy, restoration of cell porosity, increased angiogenesis, formation of new collagen, and skin elasticity normalization may be observed [1, 7, 8].

The improvement in clinical signs of skin aging is attributed to the ability of RET to correct the dermal functions, especially by increasing the production of components of the extracellular matrix (ECM) through fibroblasts. The improvement in skin elasticity associated with the capacity of tissue repair also makes RET suitable for the treatment and prevention of dermal stretch marks. Another important aspect of RET action on the dermis relates to its in vivo ability to reduce the activation of AP-1, induced by exposure to ultraviolet radiation (UVR). Since the overexpression of AP-1 occurs in aged and photoaged skin, and AP-1 is a key mediator in stimulating the activity of metalloproteinase, it is possible that RET, through its role in regulating the action of this protein, is capable of restoring the balance between the production and degradation of the extracellular matrix (ECM) on the skin [7, 8].

Some retinoids have greater impact on topical skin use: retinol (vitamin A), retinyl palmitate, beta carotene, tretinoin, isotretinoin, adapalene, and tazarotene. In this context, we find two major families of retinoids: acids (isotretinoin and tretinoin) and nonacids. The said retinoids act on different receptors, but at the end of the biotransformation process, the nonacids also turn into retinoic acid, activating the same receptor retinoid acid [7, 9].

Tretinoin is considered as the gold standard in the approach to photoaging [1, 8].

Despite the fact that tretinoin has been used in dermatology since the early 1960s, it was only in the 1980s that its importance in the treatment of aging skin was discovered. The efficacy of tretinoin in the treatment of photoaging was first demonstrated by Kligman and his collaborators in 1984, using animal models. For a period of 10 weeks, the authors observed and noted the progress taking place in photoaged mice treated with tretinoin. Significant repair and formation of new collagen in the dermal papilla of these test subjects were observed, which correlated with decreased wrinkles in the human skin [1, 7, 8].

In 1996, Fischer and collaborators found that skin previously treated with topical tretinoin 0.1 % displayed a complete blockage of collagens and the synthesis of gelatinases, thus preventing collagen degradation when exposed to the sun [1, 7].

Clinically, following 3 months of use, a thinned and compact stratum corneum may be observed with the thickness of the epidermis folded double, coupled with a more regular growth pattern, with the disappearance of nuclear atypia and keratoses. In the fourth month, a thickening and regularization of the grenz zone may be detectable (rich in collagen type IV), projecting into the papillary dermis with regeneration of blood capillaries. More than 6 months of use may result in reduction of wrinkles, actinic keratoses, and pigmented actinic lesions. In 48 weeks, no qualitative or quantitative clinical differences may be observed following everyday use of high concentrations. In 70–90 % of the cases, stinging, erythema, desquamation, and xerosis occur and may necessitate limited use [7, 9, 10].

Despite isotretinoin being typically recommended for the treatment of acne, it is viewed as an alternative approach to photoaging, because isotretinoin is a neocollagenous substance that inhibits the functioning of metalloproteinases; however, it is more tolerable than tretinoin [7, 8].

There is no consensus on the use of adapalene in photoaging; however, some studies have demonstrated benefits [7, 8].

Tazarotene, initially employed in the treatment of psoriasis, has recently proved to be a powerful ally in the treatment of photoaging. It displays the ability to be antiproliferative and anti-inflammatory and possesses the normalizing property of keratinocyte differentiation. The latter quality affects its ability to reduce skin roughness, mottled pigmentation, and the appearance of fine wrinkles. However, it has a high irritation potential [7–9].

32.3 Antioxidants

As part of the natural aging process, the endogenous defense mechanisms decrease, while the production of oxygen-reactive species increases [1, 11].

During this process, free radicals form as products of normal human metabolism. In extrinsic aging, the production is stimulated by exogenous factors, such as exposure to ultraviolet radiation (UVR), smoking, alcohol consumption, and pollution. Part of these skin changes is attributable to the production of free radicals. In addition, inflammatory phenomena may contribute to skin aging and the genesis of various nosological processes [12, 13].

The body's defense mechanisms are endogenous, enzymatic, nonenzymatic, and metal chelators with antioxidant activity. Of the enzymatic mechanisms, we may highlight the superoxide

Table 32.1 Classification of antioxidants

Liposoluble	Water soluble	Others
Vitamin E (tocopherol)	Vitamin C	
Idebenone	Green tea	
Lycopene	Silymarin	Selenium
Curcumin	*Coffea arabica* and coffee berry	
	Resveratrol	
	Pomegranate	
	Genistein	
	Polypodium leucotomos	
	Niacinamide	
	Pycnogenol	

dismutase system (SOD), catalase, and glutathione peroxidase; on the other hand, among nonenzymatic mechanisms, we have vitamins E and C, glutathione, and ubiquinone, which protect from and neutralize free radicals (Table 32.1) [1, 13].

The topical use of antioxidants may be effective in the prevention of skin aging. Recent surveys suggest that a combination of different antioxidants has synergistic effects and, thus, better efficacy when compared with the isolated use of an antioxidant [1, 14].

Some of the most effective:

Vitamin E: Prevents spontaneous oxidation of polyunsaturated elements and protects, in functional terms, important cellular structures, likely through inhibiting lipid peroxidation [1, 11, 12].

Coenzyme Q10 (ubiquinone): Research has shown a decline in the rate of coenzyme Q10 (CoQ10) in aged skin compared to young skin [1, 11, 12].

Idebenone (analogous synthetic of coenzyme Q10): Has been proved to be stronger than CoQ10. A study based on topical use on the skin of a compound containing idebenone has delivered positive results toward the improvement of the signs of skin aging [1, 11, 12].

Vitamin C (ascorbic acid): Plays an essential role in the synthesis of collagen and elastin, which may offset the negative effects of UV radiation on the skin. On account of its role in collagen production and the ability to eliminate damage caused by ROS, ascorbic acid has been studied for use in the treatment of the effects of aging. The dermal fibroblasts in the elderly outweigh the reduced proliferative capacity, provided treatment takes place with adequate levels of ascorbic acid [1, 11–13].

Genistein: Is an isoflavone derived from soy, possessing the ability to inhibit oxidative DNA damage caused by UVR [1, 11, 12].

Niacinamide: In addition to its antioxidant activity, it has anti-inflammatory, immunomodulatory, and depigmentation properties. The use of niacinamide results in an improvement of texture and skin tone and reduced fine lines, wrinkles, and hyperpigmentation [1, 11, 12].

32.4 Fatty Acids

With an increase in age, the characteristics of the skin change, and its capacity to combat external aggressions decreases. According to some authors, this condition is driven by changes in lipids that comprise the stratum corneum [1, 15].

Skin aging can induce epidermal lipids and the formation of free fatty acids (FFA), which, as a vicious circle, can further alter the physiological functions forming part of the skin aging process [16, 17].

A recent study analyzed the change in the composition of fatty acids in the epidermis through the process of intrinsic aging and in vivo UV exposure in human skin. The presence of 11,14,17-eicosatrienoic acid (ETA), polyunsaturated omega-3, was found to be significantly reduced in the skin, with a predominance to intrinsic aging [16, 17].

The increase in the content of ETA in the epidermis of photodamaged skin which has been acutely exposed to UV radiation is associated with the increased expression of human elongase-1 and phosphodiesterase A2, which is calcium independent. Thus, it was shown that ETA prevented the expression of MMP-1 after UV irradiation. Inhibition of the synthesis of ETA using, for example, EPTC (S-ethyldipropylthiocarbamate), which inhibits human elongase-1, increased the expression of MMP-1 (promoting degradation of extracellular proteins triggered by UV radiation) and contributed to the photoaging of human skin. Consequently, these results suggest that UV rays increase the levels of ETA as a photo-protective mechanism [1, 15, 16].

Fatty acids have received much attention as permeation enhancers, used to enhance the absorption of drugs and cosmeceuticals through the stratum corneum. Among the fatty acids, linoleic and oleic acids have risen to prominence [16, 17].

Although fatty acids are widely used as absorption promoters, the choice of a perfect fatty acid depends on the active substance to be used, as well as the solvent [1, 16].

32.5 Anti-glycation

The understanding of the aging process involves understanding the changes that occur in molecules and their regeneration capacity. One of the biochemical reactions of this process is the non-enzymatic glycosylation, which is known to discolor and harden foods [1, 15].

Nonenzymatic glycosylation is a reaction of an aldehyde group of glucose with the amino group of a protein, to form a base (a Schiff base). This reaction usually occurs enzymatically; however, in collagen and medium- and long-living proteins, glucose can bind irreversibly without the intervention of enzymes. This spontaneous biochemical aging process contributes to the progressive damage of skin tissue and probably to the malfunction of organs (Fig. 32.1) [18, 19].

The end products of advanced glycation (AGE) damage cells by way of four basic mechanisms:

- Modifications of intracellular structures including those involved in gene transcription [4, 19]
- Interaction with extracellular matrix proteins and signaling changes between the matrix molecules and cells [4, 19]
- Modifications of proteins or blood lipids that can bind to specific receptors, causing the production of inflammatory cytokines and growth factors [4, 19]
- AGE accumulation in the skin [4, 19]

Since endogenous formation of AGE is a slow process, long-lasting proteins, such as collagen, are the proteins most susceptible to the accumulation of AGE [1].

The glycation process is characterized by intra- and intermolecular cross-links, which reduce the possibility of the AGE being removed by catabolic processes, contributing to its accumulation. In collagen proteins, for example, this process contributes to the stiffness and loss of elasticity of the skin tissue. Systemic medications, researched as anti-glycation substances, are as follows: amino guanidine, acetylsalicylic acid, D3P9195, ALT 946, ALT 711, metformin, and angiotensin II receptor blockers [1, 18, 19].

Functional consequences:

- Increased cellular oxidative stress and promotion of inflammatory reactions [1, 4].
- Deactivation of the creatine kinase enzyme responsible for the formation of ATP. The underproduction of ATP causes oxidative DNA damage, cellular senescence, and aging [1, 4].
- Deactivation of protective enzymes, such as catalase, superoxide dismutase, and peroxidase, resulting in a reduction of the antioxidant defense of cells. This can lead to genetic changes, cancer, and premature aging syndromes [1, 4].

Although none of medications listed above has been approved and accredited with a specific anti-AGE indication, although some anti-glycation substances are already in the preclinical and clinical testing phases [1, 18].

Most topical anti-glycation substances available on the market are intended to block the start of the glycation process, interfering in the connection between the carbonyl group of the aldehyde and the amine. The main disadvantage

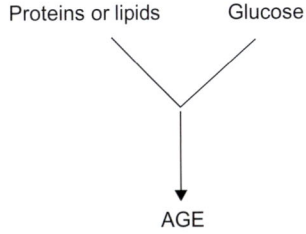

Fig. 32.1 Reaction of glycation (Maillard reaction – 1912)

of this blocking process is the failure/lack of selectivity, which may cause possible interference in certain beneficial processes. Topical anti-glycation cosmeceuticals are as follows: Aldeine, Algisium C, Alistin, Ameliox, Coffee Skin, Dragosine, Trylagen, and Preventhelia [18, 19].

32.6 Cosmeceutical Metals and Ions

The use of metal ions is considered as the oldest medical text registered (about 1500 BC), namely, the Ebers papyrus of ancient Egypt. As an example, calamine (a natural material containing zinc oxide) was prescribed to treat many diseases of the skin and eyes; green minerals based on copper were used for burns and itching [1, 20, 21].

Metal ions are used as beauty products (pigments, colorants) or for skin protection (blocking ultraviolet rays). In direct contact, they not only affect the skin but may cause dermatitis by irritation or allergies if specific concentrations are exceeded [20, 22, 23].

Bioelectricity is one of the fundamental ways for the cells to communicate with each other. The skin uses these bioelectrical signals to activate the process of repair and healing. With aging, these bioelectrical signals decrease and consequently cause a reduction in the production of collagen and elastin. Research has shown that a solution of mineral ions, containing zinc and copper, combined with water can work as a "battery," generating an electric current resulting in the inhibition of c-fos (a component of the AP-1), decreased greasiness, increased cellular adhesion, improved skin barrier structure, increased firmness, organization and repair of skin tissue, reduced skin response to stress, promotion of skin homeostasis, and inhibition of inflammation (Table 32.2) [1, 22, 23].

Table 32.2 Classification of the metals found in nature

Essential metals	Residual metals	Toxic metals
Zinc	Zinc	Mercury
Copper	Lead	Lead
Magnesium	Silver	Arsenic
Selenium	Aluminum	Aluminum
Iron	Iron	
Potassium		
Chrome		
Titanium		
Aluminum		
Strontium		

32.6.1 Zinc

Zinc is an essential chemical element of life. It interferes with the metabolism of proteins and nucleic acids, stimulates the activity of over 100 enzymes, contributes to the proper functioning of the immune system and wound healing, and interferes with perceptions of taste and smell, as well as DNA synthesis [22, 23].

Zinc is used in products such as shampoos and creams for acne [1, 20].

The FDA has included zinc oxide in the list of substances generally recognized as safe for use as nutrients (GRAS). It has been proven that zinc reduces the genetic and cellular damage caused by exposure to light and enhances the strength of skin fibroblasts to oxidative stress [20–22].

Zinc oxide has been used for many years in several lip products, makeup, face powder, etc. [21, 22].

Zinc, in its bioavailable form, helps to improve the healthy appearance of the skin by minimizing fine lines caused by environmental stress, thus normalizing the skin surface [20, 22].

32.6.2 Copper

The number of copper compounds used in personal care products is lower. Copper peptides function to block the enzyme 5-alpha reductase, the enzyme responsible for the conversion of free testosterone into dihydrotestosterone, which in turn is responsible for the process of miniaturization of the hair follicle in androgenetic alopecia. These peptides are effective SOD-mimetic agents which catalyze the destruction reaction of superoxide anion (O2-) and, therefore, prevent this strongly degenerative free radical agent from increasing damage to the skin [1, 21, 22].

Research has also shown that its topical use, combined with vitamin C and zinc, stimulates the production of elastin [13, 20].

The copper-rich moisturizer presents peptides that make the skin firmer, restoring elasticity. It resulted in rapid skin improvement and a reduction of lines and wrinkles [1, 23].

32.6.3 Silicon

Without the presence of silicon in the atmosphere, the existence of life in the universe would be impossible [1, 23].

Studies have demonstrated that the amount of this substance in the human body decreases with age, due to such factors as aging, exposure to ultraviolet rays, and dryness of the fabric used as a substitute for organic silicon [20, 23].

Silicon is kept intact by hydrogen-type bonds of different polysaccharide and polyuronidic chains, including proteins, which are responsible for supporting the skin and also essential for the growth process [21, 22].

32.6.4 Magnesium

Magnesium functioning is linked to calcium. It participates in the production of specific proteins with a genetic code, contributing to the stabilization of the double helix of DNA, the synthesis and use of links with a lot of energy, as well as the synthesis and activity of multiple enzymes. In its biotechnologically bioavailable form, it energizes and tones the skin and works synergistically with zinc to promote natural revitalization. Combined with vitamin C for topical use, it functions to inhibit tyrosinase, thus promoting collagen synthesis, and also possesses anti-free radical properties [1, 20, 23].

32.6.5 Iron

Iron is a remineralizer, responsible for skin color, and an essential nutrient for oxygen metabolism and mitochondrial function. It acts and impacts on skin homeostasis and on damage repair. Iron also participates in the intracellular redox process [1, 23].

The lack of this element manifests as thinning of the epidermis, dryness, and lack of elasticity. In its bioavailable form, it promotes healthy-looking skin as a whole [1, 23].

32.6.6 Selenium

The properties of capturing bioavailable selenium free radicals, biotechnologically, and its increased effectiveness make it an excellent component in formulations for skin protection (such as sunscreens and antioxidants [1, 20].

Selenium helps to neutralize the free radicals formed by UVA and UVB radiation, making it possible to obtain complete and effective cosmetics to minimize the effects caused by solar radiation exposure [21, 22].

32.6.7 Aluminum

Its major use is for the control of perspiration, in formulations such as aluminum chloride hydroxide, aluminum chloride hydroxide allantoin, and AZAG (aluminum zirconium pentachlorohydrex or tetrachlorohydrex) [1, 20, 21].

32.6.8 Titanium

Titanium is widely used in titanium dioxide form by the pharmaceutical and cosmetic industries for the manufacture of makeup products such as compact powder, blushes, shadows, nail polishes, and especially sunblocks [1, 23].

32.6.9 Strontium

Its primary use when applied topically appears to be as an anti-inflammatory and anti-irritant substance [1, 22].

Strontium sulfide is used in shaving products because of its aforementioned specific properties [1, 22].

32.6.10 Potassium

Potassium ion is present at the ends of chromosomes (telomeres) and stabilizes the structure. The hexahydrate ion (equivalent to magnesium) stabilizes the DNA and RNA structures, offsetting the negative charge of the phosphate group [1, 20, 23].

Potassium deficiency in humans can cause acne, constipation, depression, fatigue, growth problems, insomnia, muscle weakness, nervousness, and breathing difficulty. In excess quantity, on the other hand, hyperpotassemia can cause weakness and difficulty to articulate words [21, 23].

Topical potassium in compounds with PCA and glycyrrhizic acid has moisturizing, anti-inflammatory, anti-irritant, and hypoallergenic properties [20, 21, 23].

32.6.11 Silver

Silver is toxic. However, most of the salts it contains are not absorbed and remain in the blood until deposited on the mucous membranes, forming a grayish film [1, 20, 23].

Other silver compounds, such as silver nitrate, have antiseptic properties and are used in solutions for the treatment of irritations of the mouth and throat [1, 20].

32.6.12 Lead

Lead is one of the metals that cause the most poisoning in humans and pollution to the environment. In large doses of contamination, lead seriously affects the central nervous system (CNS) and causes damage to the liver, kidneys, reproductive organs, and gastrointestinal tract [1, 22].

32.6.13 Mercury

Mercury accumulates mainly in the kidneys, bones, liver, spleen, brain, and adipose tissue. Any deposit that is not eliminated in the urine and feces stays in the body and interferes with protein synthesis [20, 22].

Moreover, it has harmful effects on the CNS, increasing the release of several neurotransmitters, and has been connected to multiple sclerosis [20, 21].

32.7 Moisturizers

The skin is the largest organ of the human body and provides humans with contact to the environment. Its functions are perception, thermoregulation, secretion and excretion, metabolism, and protection. It is, therefore, a complex organ that aids in the defense against the adverse effects of the external environment. To perform this task, the integument should be in its normal condition, i.e., intact [1, 24–26].

For the skin to be in its proper condition of operation, two basic processes are required: skin cleansing and moisturizing. Cleansing contributes to removing the external debris, natural skin secretions, and microorganisms. Moisturizing, in turn, guarantees the water content of the epidermis and the epidermal barrier [25, 27].

Natural moisturizing factor (NMF), intercellular lipids, and ion pumps are part of the dynamic mechanisms involved in natural hydration [1, 24].

32.7.1 Natural Moisturizing Factor (NMF) and Intercellular Lipids

The water in the epidermis is not sufficient for hydration if no similar retention factors of the same kind are present, thus preventing its evaporation. Two structures fulfill this role: the NMF and intercellular lipids [1, 27].

The keratinocytic component of the NMF has amino acids derived from filaggrin protein as the main constituent agent. The NMF retains water and ensures the normal appearance of the integument [1, 25].

The intercellular lipids, derived from nucleated keratinocytes and placed on the stratum corneum, are bipolar structures with a "hydrophilic head and hydrophobic tail." They control the permeability and intercellular movement of water and seal the NMF in corneocytes, retaining the intercellular water content [1, 27].

The natural moisturizing factor is composed of amino acids, carboxylic acid, pyrrolidone, lactate, urea, ammonia, uric acid, glucosamine, creatinine, citrate, sodium, potassium, calcium, magnesium, phosphate, chloride, sugars, fatty acids, peptides, and other undefined substances [1, 26].

Intercellular lipids found in the skin include ceramides, cholesterol, fatty acids, cholesterol sulfate, and cholesterol esters [24, 25].

32.7.2 Ion Pumps

Next to amino acids, ionic component is the most important molecular structure of NMF, accounting for 18.5 % of this structure. These trace elements are in constant interaction with each other, balancing electrolytes. This ionic state, as well as its interface with other skin barrier structures, contributes toward establishing a suitable hydration profile [1, 28].

Ions actively participate in maintaining the water content of the intra- and extracellular environment. Of all the ion channels, the Na/K pump is best known and is responsible for maintaining the concentration of these ions [1, 28].

Another very important ion in epidermal hydration is calcium, necessary for keratinocytic differentiation and desmosome stabilization and increasing intercellular cohesion in order to reduce flaking, thereby improving the epidermal barrier function [1, 28].

32.7.3 Aquaporins

Aquaporins are integral membrane proteins. There are currently 13 known species of aquaporins. Aquaporin-3 (AAQP3) stands out for being permeable to water molecules such as glycerol and urea, which are important skin moisturizing agents and known as aquaporins. On the skin, it is located in keratinocytes of the epidermis and represents a permeable channel, controlling skin hydration. The AQP3 levels may be reduced compared to high concentrations of calcium, 1.25 dihydroxyvitamin D, and UV radiation [1, 26].

The topical all-trans retinoic acid stimulates gene expression and the AQP3 protein in epidermal keratinocytes. AQP3 is also expressed in human skin fibroblasts, and normal epidermal growth factors increase its expression and cell migration [24, 26].

The relevance of AQP3 in skin diseases associated with abnormalities in water homeostasis, such as atopic dermatitis, psoriasis, xeroderma, and ichthyosis, still needs to be established and so too its beneficial potential to modulate the function of AQP3 with topical inhibitors or activators. Aquaporin research in the field of skin hydration, however, is pointing toward potential interesting benefits in addressing primary xerosis [24, 26].

32.7.4 Classification of Moisturizers

Moisturizers are classified according to the action mechanism of their compounds. Thus, they can be classified as occlusive, emollients, and humectants (Table 32.3 and Fig. 32.2) [1, 27].

Most frequently, commercially available products use compounds of each of these classes in their formulations. The composition of a moisturizer is the secret to its success [27, 28].

32.7.4.1 Occlusives
These are products rich in occlusive components which slow the evaporation and epidermal loss of water through the formation of a hydrophobic film on the skin surface and interstitium, between the surface keratinocytes. These are usually fatty compounds, more effective when applied to the slightly moist skin. Although greasy, they may present an oil-free profile [1, 27, 28].

32.7.4.2 Humectants
These are products comprised of substances that retain water in the horny outer layer, or draw water from the dermis, or, alternatively, in environments with atmospheric humidity greater than 70 %, draw water from these environments. These compounds are associated with occlusive

Table 32.3 Examples of moisturizers

Occlusive	Humectants	Emollients
Hydrocarbon oils/waxes	Glycerin	Protective emollients
Petrolatum	Honey	Diisopropyl dimer dilinoleate
Mineral oil	Ammonium lactate	Isopropyl isostearate
Paraffin	Urea	Castor beans
Scalene	Propylene	Fat liquors
Silicone derivatives	Sodium pyrrolidone carboxylate (sodium PCA)	Propylene
Dimethicone	Hyaluronic acid	Jojoba oil
Cyclomethicone	Sorbitol (glucitol)	Ceramides
Phospholipids	Panthenol	Octyl octanoate
Fatty alcohols	Polyglycerylmethacrylate	Isopropyl palmitate
Sterile alcohol	Gelatin	Glycol stearate
Lanolin alcohol	Sodium lactate	Lanolin
Lecithin		Cetyl stearate
Sterols		Hexyl dodecanol
Candelia		Oleyl alcohol
Lanolin acid		Soybean sterols
Cholesterol		
Vegetable waxes		
Beeswax		

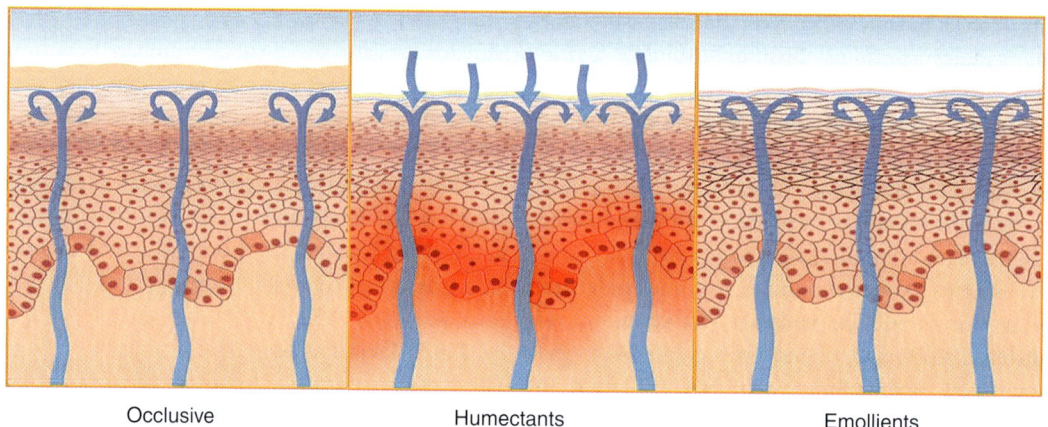

Fig. 32.2 Main types of moisturizers (Reproduced with permission from Costa [1])

compounds. The cosmetic actions of humectants are directly proportional to the concentration used, as well as its adverse effects [1, 27, 28].

32.7.4.3 Emollients

Known as products with "special mechanisms," emollients are rich in compounds capable of filling the inter-corneocytic cracks, retaining water in this layer. Such hydrating capacity is achieved by increasing the cohesion between these cells, increasing the natural "occlusive" capacity of the horny layer of the skin [1, 27, 28].

32.7.5 New Categories of Moisturizers

Some authors establish two new classes of commercial skin moisturizers, namely, protein repairers (e.g., collagen) and barrier restorers (e.g., N-palmitoyl ethanolamine, ceramides, polyunsaturated fatty acids, omega-3 complex, and liposomes). The former are classified as occlusive agents, and the barrier restorers are considered as emollients [1, 27, 28].

32.8 Microdermabrasion

Microdermabrasion is an important process in skin rejuvenation, as it accelerates the process of tissue repair, increasing desquamation of epidermal cells, therefore bringing about cell renewal and elimination of dead skin cells. The reduction of cell cohesion promotes skin softness and facilitates the penetration of antiaging products [1, 25, 29].

Microabrasive agents promote exfoliation, whether physical or chemical, and cell renewal. Silica, microspheres of jojoba, walnut shell powder, and Fiber T1 are physical exfoliants that promote a mechanical exfoliation, facilitating the loss of cell adhesion in the surface stratum corneum. On the other hand, chemical exfoliants decrease the cohesion between the corneocytes by different mechanisms. Good examples are retinoids and hydroxy acids [1, 9, 29].

In addition to these active agents, the pharmaceutical and cosmetic industries have provided new direct microabrasive agents (whose main action is to promote desquamation) and indirect microabrasive agents (which operate in basal keratinocytes or in fibroblasts, thus increasing cell renewal and, secondarily, skin peeling) [1, 29].

32.8.1 Microabrasive Cosmeceuticals with Direct Action

32.8.1.1 Physical
Farmal (Fiber T1)
A compound composed of tapioca fiber extracted by means of physical separation, solvent-free, in a process that preserves within its composition a portion of starch which confers on the skin proper exfoliation with an ultimate sensation of softness. It is recommended for stimulating skin cell renewal following the physical process of exfoliation [1, 29].

Walnut Shell Powder
Walnut's scientific name is *Juglans regia*. Powder can be derived from its crushed shells. Walnut grain is extremely durable, angular, and multifaceted, and its particles are very small. It is considered a mild abrasive [1, 29].

32.8.1.2 Chemicals
Elastocell
Elastocell or lysine carboxymethyl cysteinate is chemically synthesized by virtue of the reaction of cysteinate with monochloroacetic acid, followed by salification with lysine. It acts in the treatment of aging skin through three simultaneous and synergistic mechanisms, keratoplastic, hydration, and tensor effect, demonstrated by in vitro and in vivo studies [1, 29].

Azeloyl Glycine
A dermocosmetic derived from the condensation of azeloyl acid combined with glycine to form the potassium azeloyl diglycinate salt. It has the following properties: anti-keratinization by cytostatic inhibition of keratinocytes; sebum regulation, by reducing free fatty acids through competitive inhibition of 5-alpha reductase; whitening, resulting from the inhibition of tyrosinase; and antiacne through gathering of all anti-keratinization, sebum regulation, anti-inflammatory, and antibacterial effects. It is a bacteriostatic for *Propionibacterium acnes* and a bactericide for *Staphylococcus aureus* and *Streptococcus pyogenes*. It should not be used in association with hydroquinone, kojic or glycolic acid, and alpha hydroxy acids [1, 29].

Biomimetic Peptide/Liposomal Peptide for Biomimetic Peel
Liposomal peptide compound promotes the reduction of cell adhesion between keratinocytes and cellular turnover periods, either by mimicking the peeling process of young skin or producing a biomimetic peel. It promotes skin rejuvenation with hydration and improves the texture of photodamaged skin, smoothes

expression lines and pigmentation irregularities, and also improves brightness and softness [1, 29].

Lanablue

This is a blue/green algae extract (*Aphanizomenon flos-aquae*), found in a rare ecosystem, the Klamath Lake, in south central USA. It has a retinoid-like action, promoting the restructuring of skin surface and smoothing of wrinkles, roughness, and hyperpigmentation. It increases the synthesis of collagen, elastin, and fibronectin and has an anti-free radical and moisturizing action [1, 29].

Vitinoxine

It is composed of galactomannans (sugars, such as glucose, mannose, and galactose); arranged in monosaccharides, disaccharides, or oligosaccharides; and obtained from the enzymatic hydrolysis of alfalfa extract (*Medicago sativa*). It acts on the epidermis, regulating the differentiation of keratinocytes, and on the dermis by stimulating fibroblast proliferation and collagen production, in addition to inhibiting metalloproteinases responsible for collagen degradation [1, 29].

Revinage

This is a botanical derivative extracted from *Bidens pilosa*. In vitro studies demonstrated retinoid-like action by not acting on RAR receptors, but rather by regulating the expression of genes that inhibit transcription factors, demonstrating a 34 % reduction of activated transcription factor activity. It has no effect on cell longevity since it enhances the expression of the sirtuin 6 gene, and also affects the extracellular dermal matrix, by increasing collagen 1. It increases the expression of procollagen, sirtuin 6, and epidermal growth factor receptor genes. It stimulates transformation growth factor-beta (TGF-beta) and functional elastin. It reduces the synthesis of metalloproteinase 1. It also has a depigmentation effect, caused by the reduction of melanin, the inhibition of MSH hormone, and the inhibition of tyrosinase 1-related protein. It also possesses an anti-greasiness effect, by reducing dihydrotestosterone. Furthermore, it controls cell replication through proteins such as P300 (histone). It acts as an antioxidant, through the increase in superoxide dismutase, catalase, and malondialdehyde. It is also an anti-inflammatory agent that reduces mediators, such as cyclooxygenase-2, prostaglandin E2, and leukotriene B4 [1, 29].

Vita-A-Like

It is a purified ingredient from the seed of *Vigna aconitifolia*, a legume rich in carbohydrates, protein, water, lipids, and polyphenols. It has a retinoid-like action, which renews and strengthens the epidermis. It promotes increased cell turnover, as demonstrated by in vitro studies, through the production of hepatocyte growth factor via dermal fibroblasts, inducing the proliferation of keratinocytes and epidermal renewal [1, 29].

N-Acetyl-Glucosamine (NAG)

It is a natural component of glycosaminoglycans, glycolipids, and glycoproteins of the membrane, a precursor of the hyaluronic acid biopolymer. It has exfoliating effects, affecting the adhesion between corneocytes by inducing desquamation and differentiation of the epidermis through the interaction with CD44 receptors in corneocytes, which makes the cross-linking between cells more difficult. Furthermore, it has moisturizing effects and reduces fine lines. Studies have shown that it stimulates the synthesis of hyaluronan in the fibroblasts as a hyaluronic acid precursor [1, 29].

Pumpkin Enzyme

It is a protease obtained from pumpkin fermentation with *Lactobacillus lactis*. The hydrolysis of skin proteins induces exfoliation, softness, and attenuation of fine wrinkles [1, 29].

Renew Zyme

It is also a proteolytic enzyme. It is an active agent of pomegranate (*Punica granatum* L.) with ellagic acid polyphenol as an active component. It promotes cell renewal with skin exfoliation and stimulation of collagen production, preventing wrinkles and expression lines. In addition, it has anti-inflammatory, antioxidant, emollient, antineoplastic, and depigmentation activities [1, 29].

32.8.2 Microabrasive Cosmeceuticals with Indirect Action

32.8.2.1 Structurine
It is an agent derived from white lupine (*Lupinus alba*), is rich in oligosaccharides and glutamine peptides, and has low molecular weight. Effects demonstrated through in vitro studies include stimulation of the synthesis of filaggrin protein, responsible for the formation of corneocytes, and other structural proteins of the skin [1, 29].

32.8.2.2 Glyco-Repair
It is a compound rich in oligo-galactomannans, purified from seeds of the carob tree *Ceratonia siliqua*, which is able to restore the skin barrier and regenerate the natural mechanism of skin cell repair [1, 29].

32.8.2.3 Biocalcium
Biocalcium is the calcium salt of L-pyrrolidone carboxylic acid (L-PCA), a carrier of extracellular calcium into the cell. In vitro and in vivo studies demonstrated that in lower intracellular concentrations, it stimulates the proliferation of keratinocytes, with increased profilaggrin, keratin 10, ceramides, and glycosyl ceramides. It promotes the synthesis and organization of the cornified envelope, causes the synthesis of lipids that participate in the cell cohesion of the skin barrier function, hydrates the skin, and inhibits metalloproteinase 1, reducing the degradation of collagen [1, 29].

32.8.2.4 Pro-collasyl
It is a formulation with high concentrations of water-soluble organic silicon silanetriol, connected to the marine collagen associated with polypeptides from rice. It directly stimulates the fibroblasts and, consequently, increases collagen synthesis, promoting the regulation of cellular metabolism and cellular repair cycle. Deep skin restructuring occurs, with the attenuation of wrinkles and improvement of texture and hydration [1, 29].

32.8.2.5 Algisium C2
This compound derives from organic silicon and a polysaccharide extracted from brown alga. In vitro studies indicated fibroblast proliferation, cytostimulation with increased production of collagen by aged fibroblasts, anti-glycation activity, anti-free radicals, and anti-inflammatory and hydration effects. In vivo studies reinforced its antiaging and moisturizing effects [1, 29].

32.9 Peptides

Both amino acids and peptides improve the texture, turgor, and regularity of the skin surface and achieve antiaging results without the undesirable adverse effects caused by retinoids. At the molecular and functional level, substances belonging to this group of active agents are capable of increasing collagen regeneration and preventing their degradation and interfere with and slow down different stages of the aging process. Among the protein molecules with greater aging activity are the peptides that are divided into signalers, neurotransmitter inhibitors, and enzyme carriers and inhibitors, classified according to their main functional effects (Table 32.4) [1, 30, 31].

Cosmeceutical peptides are generally well tolerated. Due to their molecular weight, the greater presumed adverse effect is the development of allergic contact dermatitis. Although there is little scientific basis to support safe prescription of topical peptides, they appear to offer promising options as cosmeceuticals for skin treatment [1, 32].

32.9.1 Signaling Peptides

They stimulate fibroblasts and collagen or elastin production, reducing the action of collagenase. They also function to increase the amount of glycosaminoglycans, proteoglycans, and fibronectin. On healthy skin, these effects result in the reduction of lines and wrinkles caused by aging, making skin firmer and younger looking [31, 33].

Table 32.4 Examples of peptides

Main signaling peptides	Main neurotransmitter inhibitory peptides	Main enzyme peptides	Peptides with "Cinderella effect"
Glycyl-histidyl-lysine tripeptide	Argireline	Derivatives of soy protein	Tensine
Palmitoyl pentapeptide (Pal-KTTKS)	Vialox pentapeptide-3	Rice-derived peptides (Colhibin)	Raffermine
Valine-glycine-valine-alanine-proline-glycine (VGVAPG) or palmitoyl oligopeptide and palmitoyl tripeptide 3/5	Leuphasyl	Silk protein	Easylift
Tripeptide 10	Syn-Coll peptide		PephaTight
Citrulline			Sesaflash
Pentamid-6			
Aquaporin			

32.9.2 Neurotransmitter Inhibitory Peptides

Different types of botulinum toxin are able to act on cholinergic neurons, causing selective proteolysis of SNARE complex proteins (N-ethylmaleimide-sensitive factor attachment protein receptor), responsible for acetylcholine release and muscle contraction. The neurotransmitter inhibitory peptides inhibit muscle contraction, reducing lines and rhytids secondary to facial movements [31, 33].

32.9.3 Carrier Peptides

They stabilize and transfer metals, such as copper, important for healing and good performance of enzymatic processes. The role of copper in aging entails its action as a cofactor for superoxide dismutase, an important antioxidant enzyme, and lysyl oxidase, linked to the production of collagen and elastin [31, 33].

32.9.4 Enzyme Inhibitory Peptides

Derivatives of soy protein inhibit the action of proteases. This plant derivative is often used as an antiaging agent, skin moisturizer, and sunscreen and in hair products. Peptides derived from rice (Colhibin) inhibit metalloproteinase activity and induce gene expression of hyaluronidase synthetase 2, which are used as antiaging and film-forming agents, as well as in hair conditioners. The silk protein has a high affinity for copper and inhibits lipid peroxidation, tyrosinase activity, and keratinocyte apoptosis [1, 31].

32.9.5 Other Peptides with a "Cinderella Effect"

For some years, there have been cosmeceutical products on the market that produce fast antiaging effects, with short duration. They are proteins with high molecular weight with a film-forming characteristic that cause, as they dry, the film to retract over the skin, providing a tension sensation and making the surface firmer and smoother [1, 31].

32.10 Growth Factors

Recent advances in understanding the role of growth factors in the aging process may provide the opportunity to develop products for specific skin cosmeceuticals. Although it is still unclear how large molecular weight proteins (such as growth factors) penetrate the site of action, the results of multiple clinical studies have demonstrated the beneficial effects of topical use of these substances in order to reduce the signs of skin aging symptoms [1, 34–36].

Studies examined the effectiveness of the combination of growth factors and cytokines, which demonstrated the improvement of skin hydration, roughness, and depigmentation. Apart from the 26 clinical improvements of wrinkles, histological evaluation revealed changes in epidermal thickness, increased density of fibroblasts in the surface dermis, and collagen formation [1, 34–36].

The degree of clinical and histological improvement obtained with non-ablative laser resurfacing is very similar to that observed with the use of topical growth factors, since both appear to involve the same action mechanisms. Topical application of growth factors and cytokines may also work synergistically with retinoic acid and antioxidants [1, 34–36].

32.10.1 Growth Factors and Their Functions

- *TGF-beta (beta 1, beta 2, and beta 3)*: Stimulates the production of collagen and glycosaminoglycan, enhances the synthesis of fibronectin, inhibits matrix degradation, and facilitates cellular chemotaxis [1, 35]
- *PDGF (platelet-derived growth factor)*: Stimulates angiogenesis, promotes wound healing, and removes necrotic tissue [34, 35]
- *GM-CSF (granulocyte and mast cell-stimulating factor)*: Stimulates the proliferation and differentiation of hematopoietic lineage cells, improves the function of monocytes and macrophages, and enhances the leukocyte activity [1, 35]

There are no documented risks associated with the topical application of growth factors, except for potentially allergic reactions in patients with hypersensitivity to these substances [1, 35].

However, theoretical concern has been raised about the possibility of growth factors stimulating the development of melanomas. This theory is based on the findings of a few growth factor receptors, such as VEGF, in various types of melanoma. Another concern in relation to growth factors is the ability to induce the formation of hypertrophic scars [34, 35].

32.11 Sunscreens

Sunscreens are essential in the practice of photo-protection, which also includes the search for shade during hours with maximum ultraviolet (UV) radiation – between 10 am and 4 pm – and the use of protective clothing (wide-brimmed hats and sunglasses). It is a well-documented fact that constant exposure to sunlight is associated with the formation of actinic keratosis and nonmelanoma skin cancer, while intermittent exposure to sunlight is a pertinent factor in the development of melanomas. It has been proved that regular application of sunscreen prevents actinic keratosis and squamous cell carcinoma (SCC). In contrast, there is controversy regarding its effectiveness in preventing basal cell carcinoma (BCC) and melanoma [1, 37–39].

The effects of UVR are well known. UVB radiation is known to cause direct DNA damage, and this overexposure to radiation results in sunburns, carcinogenesis, and immunosuppression. Exposure to UVA initiates the production of reactive oxygen species (ROS), resulting in indirect DNA damage. Clinically, the effects of overexposure to UVA radiation include tanning, accelerated photoaging, photo-carcinogenesis, and photo-immunosuppression. The irradiance of UVA radiation from sunlight on the surface of the Earth is 20 times greater than that of UVB radiation. Since the spectral variation of UVA (320–400 nm) is greater than UVB (290–320 nm), UVA penetrates deeper into the skin throughout the day. Thus, for effective photo-protection, it is essential to use products that offer protection against UVA and UVB [1, 37–39].

32.11.1 Sunscreens and Vitamin D

Adequate serum levels of 25-hydroxyvitamin D [25 (OH) D], ranging between 75 and 100 nmol/L, are demonstrably linked to many beneficial effects on health [27]; specifically these positive effects are observed in relation to dental health, muscle and bone strength, hemodynamic effects, control of diabetes, and other risks of several autoimmune conditions and malignant processes. According to the Institute of Medicine (2010), the data relating to vitamin D and bone health are solid enough to be used as a basis to make recommendations on; however, extraskeletal data are inconclusive. The intake of vitamin D recommended by the Institute of Medicine (IOM) for individuals between 1 and 70 years of age is 600 IU/day. The IOM also advocates that serum levels of 20 ng/ml (50 nmol/L) meet the demand of 97.5 % of the population [38, 39].

The sources of vitamin D include diet and supplements, as well as skin exposure to UVB spectrum sunlight. Certain factors increase the risk of deficiency of 25 (OH) D, including strict photo-protection [38, 39].

However, the regular application of sunscreens does not usually result in vitamin D deficiency, the reason being that, although the conformity assessment of SPF sunscreen requires the use of 2 mg/cm^2, people usually only apply 0.5–1.0 mg/cm^2. Thus, the actual SPF is significantly less than the declared values [38, 39].

Given the notorious effects of UVR on skin malignancies and photoaging, photo-protection should be supported and encouraged by all physicians, coupled with recommendations on the importance of the adequate intake of vitamin D supplements [38, 39].

32.12 Topical Volumizers and Fillers

Some substances may have a filler effect on rhytids and create a volumizing effect on the skin. These substances, in addition to settling on the skin surface, interact, penetrate, and modify the treated skin [1, 40–43].

32.12.1 Cosmeceuticals with Volumizing and Filler Effects

32.12.1.1 Anthraquinone
Morinda citrifolia fruit extract has the ability to stimulate the biosynthesis of type I collagen and glycosaminoglycans in primary cultures of normal human fibroblasts. It has been established that anthraquinone significantly increases the production of C-terminal peptide of type I procollagen and glycosaminoglycans and also reduces the expression of dose-dependent metalloproteinase-1 in human fibroblasts. In addition, a nanoemulsion containing anthraquinone was found to increase procollagen type I in the skin of mice [40, 43].

32.12.1.2 Extract from the Inner Layer of Chestnut
The inner layer/bark of chestnut (*Castanea crenata* S. and Z. *Fafaceae*) has been used as an active antiwrinkle and skin-firming agent in eastern Asia for a long time [17]. An extract containing 70 % ethanol obtained from this layer can increase the expression of adhesion molecules, such as fibronectin, vitronectin, and fibroblasts, conceivably leading to skin-firming and antioxidant effects [1, 40].

32.12.2 Growth Factors

The primary mechanism through which growth factors and cytokines may have effects on the dermal matrix is via penetration though hair follicles, sweat glands, or damaged skin. They interact with cells on the epidermis, such as keratinocytes, to produce signaling cytokines that affect deeper dermal cells, such as fibroblasts. Aged skin is thinner, is more susceptible to skin diseases, and takes longer to recover from the loss of barrier function. Adding lipophilic substances that enhance the penetration by the epidermis or peptides that alter the barrier may increase the absorption of protein by the skin [1, 40].

The epidermal-dermal communication path in the process of wound healing may play a critical role in mediating the effects of the topical application of growth factors and cytokines. Keratinocytes express surface receptors of many growth factors and cytokines, including KGF (FGF7), TGF-B, IL-1, TNF-alpha, EGF, IFN-y, and GM-CSF, which are present in some commercial displays of cosmeceuticals. The penetration of small amounts of these molecules in the viable portion of the epidermis following topical application can induce keratinocytes to produce growth factors such as PDGF, IL-1, TGF-alpha, and TGF-B. A paracrine effect on the proliferation and activation of dermal fibroblasts has been demonstrated, leading to the regeneration and remodeling of dermal extracellular matrix [1, 40, 43].

32.12.3 Hyaluronic Acid

This acid derives from the family of glycosaminoglycans. Through its emollient and humectant properties, hyaluronic acid promotes water retention in the dermis by filling the spaces between scaly keratinocytes and also improves rhytids, distensibility, and suppleness of the skin. The topical use of this substance leads to retention of water in the dermis, with improved elasticity, hydration, and skin turgor, as well as mechanical support of the skin [42, 44].

Under regular skin conditions, hyaluronic acid is found in the dermis and epidermis, but cannot penetrate into the dermis when applied topically [42, 44].

In the skin, the hyaluronic acid can be synthesized by fibroblasts. Consequently, in order to increase the production of hyaluronic acid by dermal fibroblasts, it would first be necessary to increase the content of hyaluronic acid of the skin. In recent years, numerous active agents, such as N-methyl-1-serine, soy extract, Musk T, and PDGF-BB, have been reported/recognized for their ability to promote the synthesis of hyaluronic acid on cultures of human dermal fibroblasts [42, 44].

32.12.4 Asiaticoside

Asiaticoside is a saponin which can be isolated from Asian Centella, a plant that has been used for centuries in some Asian countries, often to improve skin healing [1, 41, 43].

Studies have shown that asiaticoside can increase the synthesis of type I collagen and promote fibroblast proliferation and extracellular matrix synthesis in healing [1, 41, 43].

32.12.5 Dimethylaminoethanol

An analogue of vitamin B and a precursor of acetylcholine, dimethylaminoethanol (DMAE) has numerous applications and is found naturally in marine fish (anchovies, sardines, and salmon). It displays anti-inflammatory effects, increases skin firmness, and improves facial muscle toning. A randomized study with a 3 % DMAE documented efficacy and safety in improving expression lines formed in the frontal and periorbital regions, in addition to increased lip volume [1, 41, 43].

32.12.6 Ubiquinone: Coenzyme Q10

Coenzyme Q10 exerts an antioxidant effect against the action of hydrogen peroxide and UVA in keratinocytes and fibroblasts, protecting them from DNA damage. A German study showed a reduction of photoaging in vivo, reducing the depth of wrinkles and epithelial turnover time [1, 41, 43].

32.12.7 Botanical Extract of Commiphora Mukul: Commipheroline®

This botanical extract is obtained from the Commiphora mukul tree, which belongs to the Burseraceae family. This tree secretes a resin known as "bdellium." The oleoresin is obtained from the incision of the bark of the tree; in this form, it is known as "guggul" and has been used for years in Ayurvedic medicine [1, 41, 43].

Commipheroline® is an active agent obtained from such oleoresin which acts through two synergistic mechanisms: favoring lipogenesis and limiting lipolysis [1, 41, 43].

By increasing the storage of triglycerides, Commipheroline® helps to maintain the skin condition by improving the appearance of rhytids. It can also be used to stimulate the action of antiaging products in concentrations of 0.2–0.6 % [1, 41, 43].

32.12.8 Tetrahydroxypropyl Ethylenediamine (THPE)

The modulation of the size of surface epidermal keratinocytes causes a rapid tightening effect on the skin. THPE® acts through a mechanism which causes keratinocytes to contract, thus leading to a better facial contour after a few minutes of application. The contraction of surface epidermal keratinocytes causes a slight compression, resulting in increased density and tension in the epidermis [1, 43].

32.12.9 Hibiscus Extract Rich in Amino Acids: Linefactor®

Linefactor® is an aqueous plant extract obtained from the seeds of *Hibiscus abelmoschus*. This active agent targets B-FGF or FGF-2 [1, 40].

In addition to its role in the healing process, FGF-2 stimulates cell proliferation, as well as the synthesis of collagen and glycosaminoglycans. However, FGF-2 is very easily degraded when found free on the skin. In young skin, it is connected to heparan sulfate proteoglycan (HSPG), which makes it more stable and favors binding to receptors of fibroblasts [1, 40].

During the aging process, the amount of HSPG decreases and the growth factors are more susceptible to degradation. Linefactor® was formulated to provide a biometric action, similar to proteoglycans with FGF-2. Thus, the protection of growth factors favors a greater contact time with the skin cells, inducing the activation of the synthesis of collagen and GAG [1, 40].

32.13 Nanocosmeceuticals

Nanotechnology-based products provide unique or innovative properties to cosmetic products. By containing nanostructures, they may be defined as nanocosmetics. The best performance of nanocosmetics is attributable to the small size of their particles and their large surface area [1, 45–47].

Nanotechnology in cosmeceutical products covers their application to skin and hair products. In the latter case, they are applied to the hair follicle and its stem [1, 45].

Nanoparticles for cosmeceutical use can be classified into two distinct groups: soluble (labile) and insoluble. Soluble nanoparticles are those comprising of different biodegradable materials capable of eliminating the living organisms. In such a case, both living organisms and the environment do not suffer any impact as a result of the accumulation of this type of material. Some examples are liposomes composed of phospholipids; polymeric nanoparticles, structured with biocompatible and/or biodegradable polymers without oil (nanospheres) or with oily core (nanocapsules); and solid lipid nanoparticles or nanostructured lipid carriers and those only comprising of lipids. All these soluble nanoparticles are employed as safe vehicles, acting as programmed carriers of such cosmetic active agents. Another characteristic of these nanoparticles is their aqueous liquid formulation, providing their establishment in the environment. Thus, dispersion into the air is avoided to ensure their environmental safety before degradation [1, 45–47].

On the other hand, insoluble nanoparticles are those that linger after use or action. The main application of insoluble particles is in photoprotection. The main representatives are nanosized metal oxides, zinc oxide, and titanium dioxide [1, 45].

32.13.1 Skin Application

In general, cosmetic, cosmeceutical, and dermatological products with specific action should have low systemic absorption. This requirement is often technically difficult to achieve, but essential for unintended effects resulting from this absorption to be avoided. Nanotechnology is an important alternative in the development of more selective and safer products. Nanoparticles serve as carrying compartments of substances for cosmetic or dermatological use and may act as a reservoir or barrier to control the delivery and reduction of contact in the case of sensitizing substances [1, 45].

32.13.2 Photo-Protection

The nanotechnology formulations of sunscreens have certain advantages, such as the possibility of improvement in the photostability of organic sunscreens, their retention within the upper layers of the epidermis, the increase of sun protection factor (SPF), and the spectrum of sun protection [1, 45].

32.14 Thermal Water

The sources of thermal water are generally classified into five main categories: bicarbonate, sulfate, sulfite, chloride, and trace elements. They may be cold (below 20 °C), mild (between 20 and 30 °C), or hot (up to approximately 100 °C). There are twelve treatment guidelines for these sources. However, their curative use was considered as completely empirical, and for years, doctors doubted their therapeutic value [1, 48].

Thermal water has been used for many years in spas or sprinkled on the skin, showing good results in patients with chronic inflammatory skin diseases. Recently, some publications have illustrated the action mechanisms of thermal water. It has been established that thermal water, rich in selenium, offers protective action against the short- and long-term deleterious effects of oxygen-reactive generated species, for example, through exposure to ultraviolet light (i.e., antioxidant, immunomodulatory, and anticarcinogenic effects). Moreover, the potential anti-inflammatory and anti-irritant effects justify their use as an active ingredient in topical formulations and/or cosmeceuticals [48, 49].

32.15 Topical Vitamins

Vitamins are essential compounds for the various functions of the human body. Some vitamins may be synthesized, but others are only obtainable through an appropriate diet [1, 3, 50].

Scientific evidence shows that certain vitamins are useful in the prevention and topical treatment of photoaging. They are part of a system of antioxidants that protect the skin from oxidative stress [1, 50].

The topical vitamins A, C, E, and B3 have powerful antioxidant and anti-inflammatory properties, but to achieve maximum effectiveness, the product must be presented in proper formulations. Products containing alpha-tocopherol (vitamin E), L-ascorbic acid (vitamin C), retinol (vitamin A), and niacinamide (vitamin B3) are effective in the treatment of photoaging [30, 50].

Several studies have identified the importance of topical antioxidants as protective agents against skin damage caused by ultraviolet radiation. This protective action only happens when these active agents are used before sun exposure, especially in a routine way. When the topical antioxidant is applied only after exposure to UV radiation, photo-induced injuries, such as cell death and the production of free radicals, may not be avoided, even if such damages are partially addressed [1, 50].

These compounds have also been proved to be effective in the treatment of inflammatory dermatitis, acne, and pigmentation and scarring problems. There is emerging evidence that multivitamin compounds provide additional effects, increasing their efficiency in comparison to individual compounds [1, 50].

32.15.1 Vitamin A

The human epidermis contains significant amounts of vitamin A (retinol), responsible for metabolizing enzymes, nuclear receptors, and a complex system that may become unstructured by the effects of ultraviolet A and B irradiation (UVA and UVB). The action mechanism of UV irradiation can lead to vitamin A deficiency in the skin [10, 50].

Vitamin A cannot be synthesized and is obtained through diet, animal sources (retinoids), and vegetables (carotenoids). A small percentage of retinol in the body is converted into its active form (tretinoin), which passes through an intermediate form, the retinaldehyde [1, 50].

Most of the retinol is converted into retinyl ester, a form of deposit. Retinoids are derivatives (natural or synthetic) of vitamin A. Of the various categories of cosmeceutical products, vitamin A is most often delineated in medical literature, and numerous studies have shown its efficacy in the treatment of aging skin, acne, and many other skin diseases [10, 50].

Some derivatives of vitamin A are used cosmetically, especially retinol, retinaldehyde, and retinyl esters (e.g., acetate, propionate, and retinyl palmitate esters). Through endogenous enzymatic reactions, these forms convert, at the end of the reaction, into trans-retinoic acid, which is the functional form of active vitamin A found in the skin [10, 50].

These substances (retinol, retinaldehyde, and retinyl esters) may be used in cosmeceutical products. However, since they are not biologically active, and until such time as the enzymatic conversion occurs, the effectiveness of the product depends on the format of the retinoid, its proper concentration, its stability in the product, the optimal level of enzymes in the skin, and its ability to convert into retinoic acid [10, 50].

It appears that the functional concentration of topical retinol varies from 0.3 to 4 %, but most cosmeceutical products on the market contain lower levels. Some clinical studies using appropriate methodology show the efficacy of retinol (in low concentrations) and retinyl propionate in the treatment of facial wrinkles and hyperpigmentation. The retinaldehyde concentration of 0.05 % is also clinically effective. The retinyl palmitate and retinyl acetate are not considered effective against photodamage. Retinoids, in general, are better tolerated by the skin compared to retinoic acid [10, 50].

Tretinoin (retinoic acid) can be used in varying concentrations (0.01–0.1 %) and usually has clinical and histological efficacy, but possesses greater irritation potential compared to other forms of presentation of vitamin A [10, 50].

Among the various changes induced, some are relevant for antiaging effect (such as those which lead to the thickening of the epidermis) and increased proliferation and epidermal differentiation in addition to the increased production of epidermal glycosaminoglycans (GAG), hence providing an increase in epidermal hydration and in the production of dermal extracellular matrix (ECM). It stimulates the gene expression of procollagens I and III, leading to increased thickness of the dermis [1, 10].

In addition, retinoids also have inhibitory effects, for example, on the production of basic substance in excess on the photodamaged dermis and on the expression of tyrosinase, an enzyme connected with melanin production [1, 10].

32.15.2 Vitamin B

Niacinamide or nicotinamide (an active form of vitamin B3 or niacin) is part of the group of hydrosoluble vitamins. It is obtained through diet (meat, fish, milk, eggs, and nuts), and nicotinamide deficiency is one of the factors that cause pellagra [1, 50].

There is a downside to using nicotinic acid in topical cosmeceuticals, because its vasodilatation side effect may result in flushing. The same effect is not detected with the use of topical niacinamide [1, 50].

Vitamin B3 has antioxidant properties. It is a precursor of enzymatic cofactors involved in various skin reactions. It is therefore used in a variety of topical cosmeceutical products. Although the exact biochemical mode of action is not well understood, several studies describe their cosmetic benefits and possible mechanisms [1, 50].

Below are some of their cosmetic effects:
- Improvement of the skin barrier, reducing transepidermal water loss, due to the increased production of lipid barrier (increase of ceramides) [1, 41]
- Reduction of the size of follicular ostia and improvement of the texture, by reducing the production of sebum [1, 41]
- Reduction of erythema based on their anti-inflammatory properties [1, 41]
- Improvement of fine lines, based on increased collagen production and reduction of the excessive production of GAG in the dermis [1, 41]
- Reduction of pigmentation by inhibiting the transfer of melanosomes to keratinocytes [1, 41]

There are numerous studies describing the beneficial effects of niacinamide in the topical treatment of acne and photodamaged skin. It should be noted, however, that its effectiveness is about one-third to one-fifth of the effectiveness of tretinoin at 0.025 %. In the treatment of skin rejuvenation, a study with adequate methodology, using 5 % niacinamide, revealed a statistically significant reduction of facial pigmentation after 8 weeks. Some authors describe an improvement of the skin texture based on an increased speed of epidermal turnover, working with a mild exfoliating action. These findings were described using nicotinamide in concentrations of 2.5 % and 3.5 %, supported by statistically significant results [1, 50].

Improvement in reduction of fine wrinkles, blemishes, and skin erythema and the elasticity of the face has also been detected with the use of 5 % nicotinamide, 2 times/day for 12 weeks. In the treatment of photodamaged skin, the effectiveness of nicotinamide has been compared to that of clindamycin 1 % gel used for acne treatment [1, 50].

32.15.3 Panthenol

Panthenol, or provitamin B5, is also known as pantothenol panthenyl and alcohol; D-panthenol is its active form. It is well tolerated by the facial skin and has moisturizing function, associated with the improvement in skin texture and elasticity [1, 50].

By improving the skin barrier, it protects the skin against irritation, in addition to providing anti-inflammatory and antipruritic effects. It can be used to reduce the irritating effects of other products such as tretinoin [1, 50].

32.15.4 Vitamin C

As the skin ages, the dermis becomes thin and its collagen content decreases. These changes are accelerated in a chronic manner as a result of UV exposure. UV radiation induces the formation of free radicals. Based on its action on the biosynthesis of collagen and on the reduction of free radicals, vitamin C or L-ascorbic acid (AA) may be used, as an alternative, through the skin [1, 30, 50].

Vitamin C acts as a depigmentation agent, by virtue of it being an antioxidant and inhibitor of tyrosine. Its anti-inflammatory effect is also described based on the reduction of erythema associated with postoperative laser procedures (resurfacing) [1, 30, 50].

L-ascorbic acid is vital for the functioning of cells, and this is particularly evident in the tissue during the formation of collagen, acting as a cofactor for essential enzymes in the biosynthesis of collagen [1, 30, 50].

The topical use of vitamin C is not a new concept, and several of its properties, such as antioxidant and powerful stimulator of collagen production, are well known; however, its instability has always made adherence to the treatment more difficult [30, 50].

Topical L-ascorbic acid is the most effective presentation of vitamin C and one of the few presentations that is stable and can actually penetrate into the dermis. Therefore, in order to function effectively, the pH of the formulation has to be lower than 3.5. The maximum absorption for percutaneous absorption is 20 %. Higher concentrations curiously worsen the absorption. Esters of vitamin C are more stable, but less likely to penetrate into the dermis [30, 50].

Owing to its anti-inflammatory properties, vitamin C becomes an attractive active agent for the treatment of various inflammatory conditions such as eczema and follow-up application of CO_2 laser treatment [1, 30, 50].

A clinical study evaluating the use of vitamin C in photodamaged skin concluded that topical vitamin C at 5 %, applied 2 times/day for 180 consecutive days, may significantly improve the appearance of photodamaged skin characterized by the recovery of its clinical features (brightness, texture, and loss of pigmentation) and growth of collagen and elastic fibers in the dermis. The combination of vitamins C and E is synergistic, especially in relation to sun protection, inhibiting not only the acute damage caused by UV radiation (such as erythema) but also the chronic effects of radiation, such as photodamage and skin cancer [30, 50].

Thus, topical vitamin C is an important and beneficial active agent in the treatment of photoaging and other inflammatory dermatoses, provided it meets the requirements of stability, concentration, pH, and permeability [30, 50].

32.15.5 Vitamin E

Natural vitamin E is a liposoluble antioxidant present in plasma membranes and tissues. Like vitamin C, it has to be obtained through diet (vegetables and vegetable oils, seeds, grains, nuts, and some meats). In the skin, vitamin E is especially abundant in the stratum corneum, delivered by sebum. Vitamin E is depleted with skin aging and topical application provides benefits to the patient. It protects cell membranes from peroxidation [1, 50].

Its biologically active form, known as alpha-tocopherol, inhibits the activity of protein kinase C (which increases with aging in fibroblasts) and inhibits the production of collagenase [1, 50].

Vitamin E has the potential to prevent and improve skin damage caused by free radicals, in particular those caused by UV radiation (such as burns, photoaging, and skin cancer). In vitro studies have shown that alpha-tocopherol reduces the number of sunburn cells and marks of photo-oxidative damage on the skin. With an effect similar to that of vitamin C, it reduces erythema and edema. Although this formulation is difficult to stabilize, the combination of vitamins A and C with vitamin E increases the photo-protection effects [1, 50].

32.16 Alpha Hydroxy Acids

They are a group of hydrophilic organic acids used as moisturizers, exfoliants, and keratolytics. These include the following acids: glycolic, lactic, citric, pyruvic, malic, and tartaric acids. Glycolic acid and lactic acid are the acids most often employed [1, 51, 52].

The use of ammonium lactate at 12 % and lactic acid at 5 % or 12 %, in addition to providing epidermal effects, may lead to increased thickness of the dermis, improving the smoothness of the skin and wrinkles [51, 52].

Glycolic acid is used in cosmeceutical products in concentrations up to 10 %. There is some evidence of its effect in the increase of the extracellular matrix in order to improve the quality of elastic fibers and increase the density of dermal collagen [7], with clinical improvement of fine lines and hyperpigmentation [1, 51].

32.17 Estrogens

Through specific receptors, estrogens stimulate the synthesis of transforming growth factor (TGF-β) and keratinocyte proliferation. They produce an increase in the thickness of the epidermis, the layer of glycosaminoglycans and lipids, and maintain skin hydration by reducing transepidermal water loss [53–56].

Some reports have also shown increased synthesis of elastic fibers following the use of creams containing estradiol [53, 55, 57, 58].

However, it is not known whether the use of topical estrogens on the face would be beneficial to mitigate the effects of skin aging. Further studies still need to be conducted to establish the minimum dose for such beneficial effects without causing systemic damage [55, 56, 58].

In a study conducted to evaluate the use of estradiol 0.01 % gel on the face for 24 weeks, an increase in the concentration of hyaluronic acid in the dermis without associated systemic effects was confirmed [58].

References

1. Costa A. O Conceito de Cosmecêutico. In: Costa A, editor. Tratado Internacional de Cosmecêuticos. Rio de Janeiro: Guanabara Koogan; 2012. p. 3–6.
2. Giacomoni PU. Advancement in skin aging: the future cosmeceuticals. Clin Dermatol. 2008;26:364–6.
3. Binic I, Lazarevic V, Ljubenovic M, Mojsa J, Sokolovic D. Skin ageing: natural weapons and strategies. Evid Based Complement Alternat Med. 2013; 2013:1–10.
4. Bhawan J, Andersen W, Lee J, Labadie R, Solares G. Photoaging versus intrinsic aging: a morphologic assessment of facial skin. J Cutan Pathol. 1995;22:154–9.
5. Bruce S. Cosmeceuticals for the attenuation of extrinsic and intrinsic dermal aging. J Drug Dermatol. 2008;7(2 Suppl):17–22.

6. Tsai TC, Hantash BM. Cosmeceutical agents: a comprehensive review of the literature. Clin Med Dermatol. 2008;1:1–20.
7. Mukherjee S, Date A, Patravale V, Korting HC, Roeder A, Weindl G. Retinoids in the treatment of skin aging: an overview of clinical efficacy and safety. Clin Interv Aging. 2006;1(4):327–48.
8. Kligman AM, Grove GL, Hirose R, Leyden JJ. Topical tretinoin for photoaged skin. J Am Acad Dermatol. 1986;15:836–59.
9. Sorg O, Kuenzli S, Kaya G, Saurat JH. Proposed mechanisms of action for retinoid derivatives in the treatment of skin aging. J Cosmet Dermatol. 2005;4:237–44.
10. Bhawan J, Gonzalez-Serva A, Nehal K, Labadie R, Lufrano L, Thorne EG, et al. Effects of tretinoin on photodamaged skin. A histologic study. Arch Dermatol. 1991;127:666–72.
11. Baumann L, Allemann IB. Antioxidants. In: Cosmetic dermatology. 2nd ed. New York: McGraw-Hill; 2009. p. 292–305.
12. Baumann LSA. Refresher o antioxidants. Skin Allergy News. 2004;35(5):31.
13. Cabelli DE, Bielski BH. Kinetics and mechanism for the oxidation of ascorbic acid/ascorbate by H02/02 radicals: a pulse radiolysis and stopped flow photolysis study. J Phys Chem. 1983;87:1805.
14. Nelson D, Cox M. Lehninger principles of biochemistry. 4th ed. New York: W.H. Freeman; 2005.
15. Berg JM, Tymoczko JL, Stryer L. Bioquimica. 6th ed. Rio de Janeiro: Guanabara Koogan; 2008.
16. Fujji M, Hori N, Shiozawa K, Wakabayashi K, Kawahara E, Matsumoto M. Effect of fatty acid esters on permeation of ketoprofen through hairless rat skin. In J Pharm. 2000;205(1-2):117–25.
17. Kim EJ, Kim M-K, Jin X-J, Oh J-H, Kim JE, Chung JH. Skin aging and photoaging alter fatty acids composition, including 11,14,17-eicosatrienoic acid, in the epidermis of human skin. J Korean Med Sci. 2010;25:980–3.
18. Danby FW. Nutrition and aging skin: sugar and glycation. Clin Dermatol. 2010;28:409–11.
19. Holt S. Specific anti-aging factors for natural clinicians. Townsend Lett. 2008.
20. Albergoni V. Physiological properties of copper and zinc. In: Rainsford K, Milanino R, editors. Cooper and zinc in inflammatory and degenerative diseases. Philadelphia: Wolters Kluwer; 1998. p. 7–17.
21. Chantalat J, Bruning E, Sun Y, et al. Biomimetic signaling technology generated by a bi-mineral complex reduces signs of photo-aging in the eye area. J Am Acad Dermatol. 2010;62:AB 59, Abstract P1624.
22. Dreno B. Oligoelements et peau. Dermatol Pratique. 1996;182(1):1–3.
23. Idson B. Trace minerals in cosmetics, part 1. Drug Cosmet Ind. 1990;146:18–20, 88.
24. Hara M, Ma T, Verkman AS. Selectively reduced glycerol in skin of aquaporin-3-deficient mice may account for impaired skin hydration, elasticity, and barrier recovery. J Biol Chem. 2002;277:46616–21.
25. Addor FAS, Aoki V. Barreira cutânea na dermatite atópica. An Bras Dermatol. 2010;85(2):184–94.
26. Hara-Chikuma M, Verkman AS. Roles of aquaporin-3 in epidermis. J Invest Dermatol. 2008;128:2145–51.
27. Addor FAS, Curi T. Hidratação em dermatologia. In: Lupi P, Belo J, Cunha PR, editors. Rotinas em diagnóstico e tratamento da sociedade brasileira de dermatologia. Rio de Janeiro: Guanabara Koogan; 2010. p. 265–7.
28. Heald P, Burton CS, Callaway L. Moisturizing the skin. N C Med. 1993;44(4):234.
29. Briden ME, Green BA. Topical exfoliation-clinical effects and formulating considerations. In: Draelos ZD, Thaman LA, editors. Cosmetic formulation of skin care products. New York: Taylor&Francis; 2006. p. 237–50.
30. Abdulghani AA, Sheer A, Shirin S, et al. Effects of topical creams containing vitamin C, a copper-binding peptide cream and melatonin compared with tretinoin on the ultrastructure of normal skin. Dis Manag. 1998;1:136–41.
31. Cullander C, Guy RH. Routes of delivery: case studies. Transdermal delivery of peptides and proteins. Adv Drug Deliv Rev. 1992;8:291–329.
32. Kamoun A, Landreau JM, Godeau G, Wallach J, Duchesnay A, Pellat B, et al. Growth stimulation of human skin fibroblasts by elastin-derived peptides. Cell Adhes Commun. 1995;3:273–81.
33. Falla TJ, Zhang L. Efficacy of hexapeptide-7 on menopausal skin. J Drugs Dermatol. 2010;9(1):49–54.
34. Gold MH, Goldman MP, Biron J. Efficacy of novel skin cream containing mixture of human growth factors and cytokines for skin rejuvenation. J Drugs Dermatol. 2007;6:197–201.
35. Bullard KM, Longaker MT, Lorenz HP. Fetal wound healing: current biology. World J Surg. 2003;27:54–61.
36. Fitzpatrick RE. Endogenous growth factors as cosmeceuticals. In: Draelos DD, Dover JS, Alam M, editors. Cosmeceuticals. Philadelphia: Elsevier Saunders; 2005. p. 133–8.
37. Butler ST, Fosko SW. Increased prevalence of left-sided skin cancers. J Am Acad Dermatol. 2010;63(6):1006–10.
38. Hexsel CL, Bangert SD, Hebert AA, Lim HW. Current sunscreen issues: 2007 food and drug administration sunscreen labelling recommendations and combination sunscreen/insect repellent products. J Am Acad Dermatol. 2008;59(2):316–23.
39. Kullavanijaya P, Lim HW. Photoprotection. J Am Acad Dermatol. 2005;52(6):937–58.
40. Agostini T. Ácido hialurônico; principio ativo de produtos cosméticos. Updated 2010. 25 Oct; Cited 31 Mar 2011. Available from: http://www.webartigos.com.
41. Bergstrom KG. Beyond tretinoin: cosmeceuticals for aging skin. J Drugs Dermatol. 2009;8(7):674–7.
42. Masson F. Acide hyaluronique et hydratation cutanée. Ann Dermatol. 2010;137(1):523–5.
43. Nugent CG. Novas formulações em cosmecêuticos transdérmicos. In: Draelos ZD, Dover JS, Alam M,

editors. Cosmecêuticos. Rio de Janeiro: Elsevier; 2005. p. 229–33.
44. Patriarca MT, de Moraes AR B, Nader HB, Petri V, Martins JR, Gomes RC, et al. Hyaluronic acid concentration in postmenopausal facial skin after topical estradiol and genistein treatment: a double-blind, randomized clinical trial of efficacy. Menopause. 2013;20(3):336–41.
45. Beck RCR, Guterres SS, Pohlmann AR, editors. Nanocosmetics and nanomedicines: new approaches for skin care. Berlin: Springer; 2011.
46. Pohlmann AR, et al. Structural model of polymeric nanospheres containing indomethacin ethyl ester and in vivo antiedematogenic activity. Int J Nanotechnol. 2007;4:454–66.
47. Subbiah MTR. Application of nutrigenomics in skin health: nutraceutical or cosmeceutical? J Clin Aesthet Dermatol. 2010;3(1):44–6.
48. Bacle I, Megs S, Lauze C, Macleod P, Dupuy P. Sensory analysis of four medical spa spring waters containing various mineral concentrations. Int J Dermatol. 1999;38:784–6.
49. Staquet MJ, Peguet-Navarro J, Latourre F, Schmitt D, Rougier A. In vitro effects of a spa water on the migratory and stimulatory capacities of human epidermal langerhans cells. Eur J Dermatol. 1997;7:339–42.
50. Manela-Azulay M, Bagatin E. Cosmeceuticals vitamins. Clin Dermatol. 2009;27:469–74.
51. Bernstein EF, Lee J, Brown DB, Yu R, Van Scott E. Glycolic acid treatment increases type I collagen mRNA and hyaluronic acid content of human skin. Dermatol Surg. 2001;27(5):429–3.
52. Ditre CM, Griffin TD, Murphy GF, Schmitt D, Rougier A. Effects of α-hydroxy acids on photoaged skin: a pilot clinical, histologic, and ultrastructural study. J Am Acad Dermatol. 1996;34:187–5.
53. Callens A, Vaillant L, Lecomte P, Berson M, Gall Y, Lorette G. Does hormonal skin aging exist? A study of the influence of different hormone therapy regimens on the skin of postmenopausal women using non-invasive measurement techniques. Dermatology. 1996;193:289–94.
54. Brincat M, Versi E, Moniz CF, Magos A, de Trafford J, Studd JW. Skin collagen changes in postmenopausal women receiving different regimens of estrogen therapy. Obstet Gynecol. 1987;70:123–7.
55. Neder L, Medeiros SF. Estradiol tópico não interfere na expressão da enzima metaloproteinase-1 em células da pele fotoexposta. An Bras Dermatol. 2012;87(1): 70–5.
56. Archer DF. Postmenopausal skin and estrogen. Gynecol Endocrinol. 2012;28(2):2–6.
57. Schmidt JB, Binder M, Demschik G, Bieglmayer C, Reiner A. Treatment of skin aging with topical estrogens. Int J Dermatol. 1996;35:669–74.
58. Son ED, Lee JY, Lee S, Kim MS, Lee BG, Chang IS, et al. Topical application of 17-estradiol increases extracellular matrix protein synthesis by stimulating TGF signaling in aged human skin in vivo. J Invest Dermatol. 2005;124:1149–61.

Cosmetic Procedures in Menopause

Renan Lage, Maria da Glória Samartin Sasseron, Elisa Moraes, Erica B. Botero, Lissa S. De Matos, and Adilson Costa

Contents

33.1	**Introduction**	479
33.2	**Approach to the Cosmetic Patient**	479
33.3	**Aging and Menopause**	480
33.4	**Cosmetic Procedures in Menopause**	481
33.4.1	Chemical Peels	481
33.4.2	Botulinum Toxin	484
33.4.3	Filling	486
33.4.4	Laser	489
33.5	**Summary**	491
References		491

R. Lage, MD (✉) • M. da Glória Samartin Sasseron
E. Moraes, MD • E.B. Botero, MD
L.S. De Matos, MD • A. Costa, MD, MSc, PhD
Department of Dermatology, Pontifical Catholic University of Campinas,
Av. John Boyd Dunlop, Campinas, São Paulo 13059-900, Brazil
e-mail: renanmedxxxv@yahoo.com.br;
ronigloria@andradas-net.com.br;
ELISAMORAES36@YAHOO.COM.BR;
erica_botero@hotmail.com;
lissasm@gmail.com;
adilson_costa@hotmail.com

33.1 Introduction

Modern western society is obsessed with achieving youth and beauty. Since the latter half of the twentieth century, there has been an increasing focus on the body and face as a means of self-expression and identity. However, the desire for external/outward beauty is not a uniquely late twentieth-century phenomenon. Well-documented beauty practices date as far back as Cleopatra's milk bath, the use of kohl to darken and enhance the eyes, vegetable dyes on the cheeks and lips and hair adornments. Historically, people often had to endure extreme discomfort and risk, in order to conform to culturally imposed modes of beauty [1].

33.2 Approach to the Cosmetic Patient

The skin of menopausal women is likely to undergo structural changes [2]. To remain intact, this organ depends mainly on estradiol, which is produced by the ovaries. As the production of this hormone reduces by one-half at the end of the hormonal cycle, a decrease occurs in the amount of fibroblasts, which are responsible for the production of collagen and elastin fibres that form the tissues for skin support. The change causes a reduction of blood flow through the vessels and decreases the water retention capacity of cells and also slows the activity of sebaceous and sweat glands, which produce sebum to protect the epidermis as a natural filter. Without the same hydration and moisture, the skin becomes dry, wrinkled and saggy, thin and brittle and more susceptible to abrasions and the effects of sun exposure. These changes are the reasons why patients in menopause are responsible for much of the demand for cosmetic procedures [2].

Cosmetic patient care involves specific nuances. In most cases, the demand is not related to pathological physical changes, but rather to changes affecting the patient psychologically. Therefore, the medical principle "to do no harm" should be preserved because we are dealing with non-pathological conditions.

Physical appearance has been linked to increased success in the workplace and social environment, increased job security and self-esteem. Therefore, when dealing with the physical appearance of someone, physicians are also responsible for an improvement in the quality of life [1].

The pre-procedure evaluation is of utmost importance. This is when the doctor not only defines procedures to be performed but also advises the patient about the risks and clinical response that are expected to occur with the physical changes.

The beauty concepts imposed by the society and perceived by the patient are important factors to be considered in the evaluation. These perceptions may vary according to gender, age, culture and origin. However, some beauty perceptions remain over time and may be considered as universal. Changes in the face are considered to be the most important aspect, and even more than facial symmetry, skin appearance is considered to be of higher importance to most patients.

To ensure good postoperative results and patient satisfaction, physicians have to understand the personal desires, in association with a proper assessment of what is possible based on age, skin type and changes found, always providing guidance and documenting all inquiries. As a first approach, the ideal is to ask what patients would like to improve in their appearance. We may find that we are often surprised by generic answers, coupled with high expectations. Therefore, physicians should prioritise and inform whether these requests are feasible [3].

33.3 Aging and Menopause

As people age, their concerns about appearance increasingly focus on their faces. For example, in a study conducted in 1994, 24 women, ages 29–75, were interviewed, and half of them had undergone some form of cosmetic surgery. The younger women were mostly concerned about the shape and appearance of their bodies, while the older women were worried about their faces. The older women disliked wrinkles and drooping skin and had undergone facelifts, chemical peels and chin tucks [3].

Skin aging is a process influenced by environmental, genetic and hormonal factors and can be described in terms of structural and functional changes. The structural changes include thinning, dryness, slight scaliness, fine wrinkling, looseness or loss of elasticity, irregular and mottled pigmentation, hair loss, colour changes and decreased perspiration. The functional changes include reduced barrier function, reduced wound healing ability, reduced immunological responsiveness, reduced thermoregulatory ability and increased risk of skin cancer [3].

The effects of postmenopausal oestrogen deficiency are thought to include atrophy, decreased collagen and water content, decreased sebaceous secretions, loss of elasticity and manifestations of androgen excess. It is really difficult to distinguish between the changes that occur specifically with age and those occurring as a result of oestrogen deprivation [4].

Collagen atrophy is a major factor in skin aging. With age, partial degeneration of collagen occurs, and there is also a significant decline in the dermal quantity of collagen [4].

Collagen aging occurs as a result of progressive cross-linking between the collagen molecules. A larger proportion of the cross-links between collagen molecules become irreducible, while there is a decline in the number of undeveloped and reducible cross-links. There is a reduction in the number of fibroblasts that synthesise collagen and vessels that supply the skin. This contributes to an increase in looseness, making wrinkles more evident [5].

Elastin fibres are closely linked and interwoven with the collagen fibrils so that they can recoil after transient stretching, preventing overstretching. Young women with premature menopause were shown to have experienced accelerated degenerative changes in dermal elastic fibres [6].

Transepidermal water loss may occur with age. Glycosaminoglycans have a high water-binding capability and are essential for normal skin hydration [6]. During the aging process, there is also a decrease in the production of glycosaminoglycans in the connective tissue. There is also a higher intracellular concentration of protocollagen lysyl-hydroxyproline transferase, which is an enzyme responsible for collagen breakdown [7]. The loss of connective tissue in skin aging results in increased distensibility and loss of tonicity, leading to a progressive deepening of facial creases and wrinkling.

Another important factor that contributes to the aging process in the face is the loss of bone mass. During menopause, bone turnover increases and may remain high for up to 25 years after the last menstrual period [8]. The changes observed in the midface skeleton include the lower orbital rim remodels and loses anterior projection, the midface loses vertical height and the pyriform aperture recesses posteriorly. Woodward et al. observed these results in a review of consecutive facial CT scans of 50 females and 50 males. Their analyses demonstrated that the angles of the pyriform process and the lower orbital rim retruded with age, while the anterior lower eyelid fat pads appeared to become more prominent [9].

Changes in the subcutaneous and deep cheek fat over time contribute to the pathogenesis of midfacial aging. Recent studies have sought to define the fat compartments of the face and describe their clinical importance. Superficial midfacial fat pads include the medial, middle and lateral cheek fat compartments. The deep medial fat pad underlies the superficial middle fat pad. Inflation of the deep medial fat pad with saline in cadavers has been shown to eliminate the V deformity, reduce the size of the nasolabial fold and diminish the appearance of the tear trough. Based on this finding and other anatomical observations, the authors have proposed that volume loss in the deep midfacial fat compartment may be one of the primary determinants of the morphologic appearance of the aging midface [10, 11].

With all these biological changes, Dermas and Braun (2001) outline the signs of the aging face:
- A lined forehead
- Drooping brows, with a hooded appearance toward the lateral upper lid
- Loss of cheek roundness and deep nasolabial folds secondary to loss of subcutaneous fat
- Sagging neck lines resulting from loss of platysma muscle tone
- Loss of chin definition, from submental fat deposit
- Drooping of the nasal tissue
- Wrinkling of the skin around the mouth, with thinning of the lips

There are many different kinds of procedures to correct all these signs of aging.

33.4 Cosmetic Procedures in Menopause

33.4.1 Chemical Peels

Exfoliation of the skin has been used for centuries by many cultures. The first known reports come from the Egyptian civilisation. The skin with sun damage was considered a sign of lower social status, and women made use of many substances such as alabaster, oils, salts, baths with fermented milk (due to the presence of lactic acid) and wine (rich in tartaric acid) to improve their skin appearance.

The medical use of chemical peels dates back to 1882, when Unna described the properties of salicylic acid, resorcinol, phenol and trichloroacetic acid (ATA), which are products still used today [12, 13].

A chemical peel involves the application of caustic agents that cause a controlled destruction of parts of the epidermis and/or dermis, followed by the regeneration of tissues. To be considered an "ideal" peel, it has to be able to promote minor necrosis and induce greater formation of possible new tissues. Peels are recommended for the treatment of wrinkles, melanosis, actinic keratosis, melasma and postinflammatory hyperpigmentation. They are also used in the treatment of acne and its sequelae, stretch marks and keratosis pilaris (changes less common in menopause) [12, 13].

Technically, they may be divided into superficial, medium and deep peels [14]. The most suitable peels for patients with marked degree of photo-aging, sagging skin, pigmented lesions resulting from long-time sun exposure and primary changes in menopause are medium and deep peels.

Rating:
1. Superficial peels penetrate in a part or all of the epidermis.
2. Medium peels penetrate the epidermis and a part or all of the papillary dermis.
3. Deep peels reach the reticular dermis.

33.4.1.1 Main Agents [13]

Resorcin Paste: found in concentrations of 30 %, 40 % or 50 % and is suitable for residual hyperpigmentation, acne scars, large pores and melasma. It is considered a very effective superficial agent.

The paste should be applied all over the area to be treated and left in contact with the skin for 15–30 min. In about 2 days, the patient's skin starts to peel, and this process may continue for up to 1 week.

Jessner's Solution: peeling agent consisting of 14 % resorcinol, 14 % salicylic acid and 14 % lactic acid in an alcohol base (95 % ethanol).

It may be used with a superficial peeling action when applied alone and with medium action when combined with trichloroacetic acid (20–30 %). This is a widely used procedure for the treatment of the skin with skin wrinkles and sun damage.

Glycolic Acid: acid recommended in the treatment of light photo-aging and superficial wrinkles in the face and extrafacial areas. Slight flaking may occur.

5-Fluorouracil: typically used in a 5 % concentration cream for the treatment of actinic keratosis. In the 1990s, a fluor-hydroxy pulse peel was described with which 5-FU was combined with a previous application of Jessner's solution and 70 % glycolic acid. The 5-FU was applied with gloved hands and remained on the skin for 24 h until it could be removed at home. The treatment is performed in 8 weekly or fortnightly pulses and offers good efficacy, tolerability and low cost.

Salicylic Acid: used in a solution of 20 % or 30 % ethanol, with superficial effects. Treatment suitable for fine wrinkles, providing improvement in skin appearance.

Tretinoin: used to treat photo-aging and also applied before and after chemical peels.

Trichloroacetic Acid (*ATA*): used since 1962 as an agent in photo-aging chemical peels. A versatile, efficient and low-cost agent, with no toxicity. Available in various concentrations (10–90 %), it may be used separately or in combination with other agents. It does not need to be diluted, neutralised or removed. Widely used to treat moderate to advanced photo-aging (Figs. 33.1 and 33.2) [14].

Phenol: single agent capable of inducing a deep peel. It may be applied all over the face and is recommended for advanced photo-aging, as well as for the elderly and people with skin types I to III.

It is normally used for localised treatment of perioral and periocular regions. Some complications may include hypopigmentation, skin

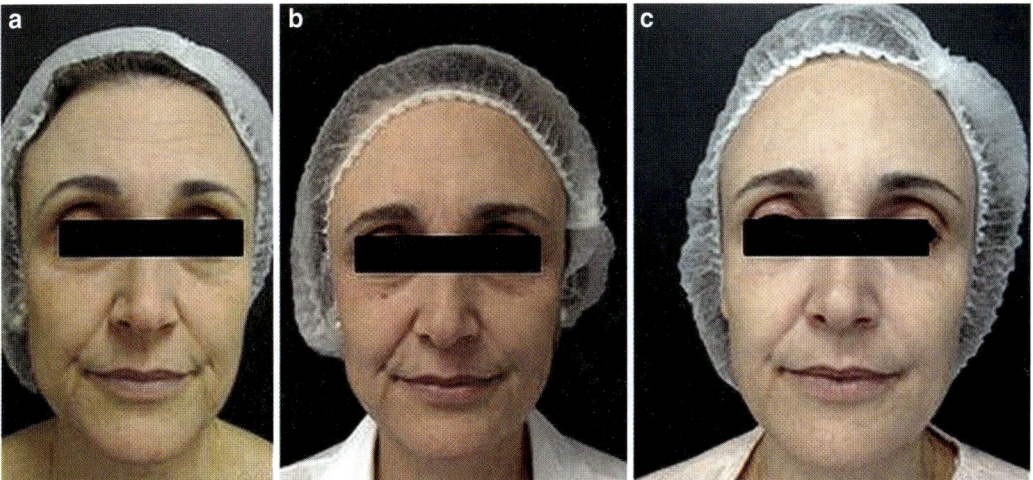

Fig. 33.1 (**a**) Pre-procedure. (**b**) Seven days postoperative radiofrequency in lower eyelid. (**c**) Thirty days postoperative radiofrequency plus treatment with hyaluronic acid dermal filler

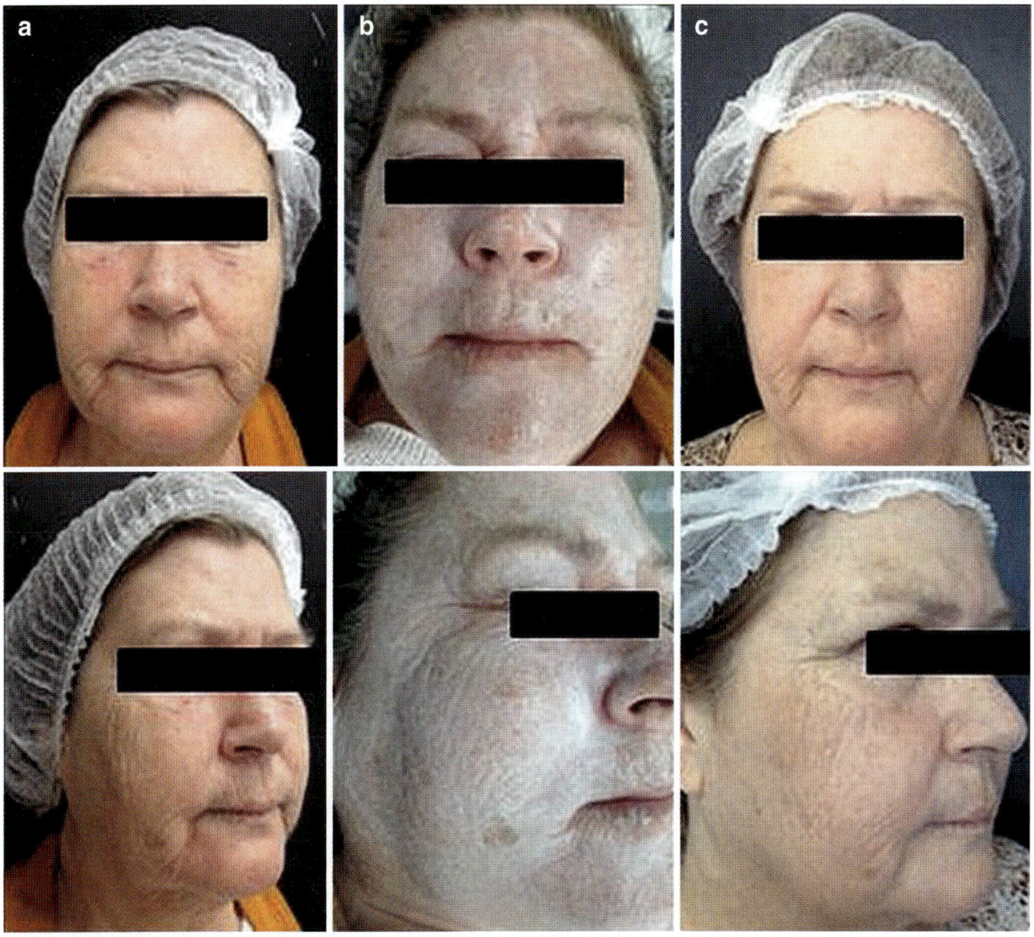

Fig. 33.2 (**a**) Pre-procedure. (**b**) Immediately postoperative Jessner's solution + ATA 25 % peeling. (**c**) Thirty days postoperative Jessner's solution + ATA 25 % peeling

atrophy, cardiac arrhythmias, renal and laryngeal oedema, exacerbation of concomitant disease and toxic shock syndrome. Therefore, before exposing a patient to such a procedure, laboratory tests (general, liver function, kidney function), in association with heart evaluation, preferably through ECG, are mandatory. During the procedure, patients' renal and heart functions should be monitored [13–15].

Antimicrobial prophylaxis is recommended to prevent viral and bacterial infections.

Results are excellent and long lasting.

33.4.1.2 Skin Preparation Before Peels

To obtain better clinical response, at least a 4-week regular and continuous preparation is necessary prior to the performance of chemical peels.

The use of sunscreen is essential [13], in association with topical tretinoin (in any of its concentrations), hydroquinone, adapalene, tazarotene, kojic acid and alpha hydroxy acids. Selecting the most suitable product is based on skin evaluation and condition [16, 17].

33.4.1.3 Application Techniques

Cleaning the skin is essential before the agent of choice may be applied, in order to remove any oiliness that could hinder the absorption of the product [15].

Acetone is still the most used product, which may also be used in an alcohol-based solution, in equal parts.

The chemical agent may be applied with gauze, cotton swabs, brushes and even gloved hands.

33.4.1.4 Contraindications
- Inadequate photoprotection
- Pregnancy
- Stress and neurotic excoriations
- Use of oral isotretinoin for less than 6 months (medium and deep peel)
- Impaired healing or formation of keloids
- History of postinflammatory hyperpigmentation
- Difficulty understanding
- Unrealistic expectations [14]

33.4.1.5 Major Complications

Medium peels are procedures that require care in the postoperative period. In the first few hours, a rash may appear and also be associated with an oedema during the first days following the procedure, presenting an appearance of "sunburned" skin. In these cases, the use of cold compresses and topical nonsteroidal anti-inflammatory drugs is recommended. The patient should be advised on the scaling, hygiene and use of moisturisers. Uneven pigmentation, prolonged erythema, changes in healing and scarring are possible complications [15].

Medium or deep peels performed carelessly or too intensively may generate unsightly and disfiguring scars. Experience and prudence are required to perform these procedures [13].

The most used type of deep peel is phenol, a substance that has cardiotoxic, hepatotoxic and nephrotoxic effects. There are reports of acute renal dysfunction or exacerbation of chronic renal failure after the performance of phenol peels, as well as the emergence of cardiac arrhythmias or worsening of any pre-existing arrhythmia. Intravenous hydration should be performed both during and after the procedure, in order to prevent renal toxicity.

The use of derivatives of petrolatum helps to maintain hydration and prevent crusting. Reepithelialisation begins after 3 days and is complete in about 1–2 weeks. In some cases erythema can persist for 3 months [13].

33.4.1.6 Post-peeling Guidelines
- Keep photoprotection.
- Proper hygiene.
- After medium and deep peels: avoid intense exercise and sweating; never handle scales or crusts. Patients should not engage in intense activities for 1 week.
- Apply topical corticosteroids in case of pruritus, eczematous lesions or prolonged erythema.
- Periodic revaluations related to each procedure.

33.4.2 Botulinum Toxin

In dermatology, the main indications for botulinum toxin are treatment of dynamic wrinkles of the face [18] and neck, lifting the tip of the nose, correcting gummy smile and treatment of axillary, plantar and palmar hyperhidrosis. The use of the toxin can be isolated or combined with other aesthetic treatments aimed to prevent facial aging, such as peels, fillers, lasers and others.

Currently, the toxin is a well-known substance, and there is no doubt of its safety and efficacy. Some issues such as dilution, diffusion, duration and effects still remain moot. Botulinum toxin is a neurotoxin produced by a Gram-positive anaerobic bacterium, *Clostridium botulinum* [12]. The toxin molecule consists of a single polypeptide chain having a heavy chain (110 kD) that has affinity with the endplate responsible for the internalisation of the toxin, while the light chain (50 kD) blocks the release of acetylcholine-dependent calcium [12].

The action of botulinum toxin occurs selectively in cholinergic motor nerve endings, inhibiting the release of the neurotransmitter acetylcholine in the presynapse of the neuromuscular junction, causing a dose-dependent reduction of muscle contraction which results in a flaccid paralysis. The effect starts within 48–72 h or a maximum of 1–2 weeks and may last for 4–6 months [13].

Seven different types of toxins are produced: A, B, C1, C2, E, F and G. The different types are classified according to their cellular target, potency and duration of action, and only serotypes A and B are commercially available.

33.4.2.1 Presentation
Four types of botulinum toxin are available on the market. Botox® was the pioneer product on the market and offers a wide variety of indications, both cosmetic and therapeutic, and is available in 100U. Dysport®, a product already approved for use in 65 countries, differs from Botox® in the process of purification of the toxin. While Botox® is purified by repeated precipitation and redissolution, Dysport® is purified by a column separation method, which can lead to certain changes in the multiprotein complex formed around the toxin. Despite these constitutional differences, clinical applications and efficacy are similar. Xeomin® is the only BTX-A which does not have the multiprotein complex in its structure, bearing no differences in relation to Botox® as to strength, safety and efficacy. Prosigne® is a BTX-A of Chinese origin, with efficacy, safety and tolerability similar to Botox® for the treatment of cervical dystonia [18].

33.4.2.2 Indications
Botulinum toxin carries a lock endplate and is therefore indicated for use in the muscle plane and for the treatment of dynamic wrinkles. The classic applications of the toxin include forehead, glabellar and lateral orbital wrinkles [18]. Among the nonclassical indications for the application of toxin is the treatment of perioral, nasal, chin, cheekbones, neck and presternal wrinkles and lines.

33.4.2.3 Contraindications
Contraindications of use include [18]:
- Pregnancy and breastfeeding
- Presence of infection around the injection area
- Neuromuscular diseases, such as myasthenia gravis, Bell's palsy and Eaton Lambert syndrome
- Hypersensitivity to the components of the formula – botulinum toxin and human albumin
- Concomitant use of antibiotic amino glycosides, polymyxin, tetracycline, penicillamine, cyclosporine, calcium channel antagonists and local anaesthetics
- Immunosuppression
- Collagen diseases
- Diabetes
- Alcoholism
- Coagulation disorders or treatment with anticoagulants

Special attention should be given to patients' expectations. Unrealistic expectations about the outcome of the procedure, as well as marked skin aging with excessive sagging, may be considered certain contraindications of the procedure.

Every patient should be examined because the anatomy of the facial region may vary considerably.

33.4.2.4 Applications of Botulinum Toxin [18]

Upper third of the face:

- Glabella: wrinkles of the glabellar area are formed by the action of the procerus and corrugator muscles. To evaluate this area, ask the patient to pull the eyebrows down and closer together. The product is injected in two to three points in each corrugator and one to two points in the procerus.
- Wrinkles in the lateral area of the eyes: wrinkles in the lateral area of the eyes are formed by contraction of the orbicularis oculi muscle. Three to four lateral points can be injected in the indicated area.
- Forehead: wrinkles on the forehead are formed through contraction of the frontal muscle. The patient is asked to raise the eyebrows, i.e. to make a face of surprise so that this area may be evaluated. The product may be injected in several equidistant points in this area.

Middle third of the face:

- Wrinkles at the top and side areas of the nose: these wrinkles are caused by contraction of nasal muscles and the medial portion of the orbicularis. These wrinkles can be corrected by applying 1 to 2U of toxin above the nasofacial groove. Intradermal application is recommended, with the needle directed from the side to the upper part of the nose.

Lower third of the face:

- Diminishment of chin skin's "orange peel" appearance: the muscles connected to chin wrinkles are the depressors of the lower lip, the depressors of the angles of the mouth and the mentalis muscle. Appearance improvement in the chin area can be achieved by injecting 3–5 U in the midline of the chin, near the edge of the mandible.
- Correction of depression of labial commissures: the product is injected in the depressor muscle of the angle of mouth, at a point in the lower extension of the nasolabial folds, near the mandibular arch.
- Perioral line wrinkles: these wrinkles can be treated with injections in the midline of the oral orbicularis muscle, near the vermilion border. The injection points should be parallel to the wrinkles, one in each quadrant. This procedure should be performed carefully, always based on small doses, given the risk of paresis and lip incompetence.
- Nasolabial or nasogenian folds: these folds can be reduced by injection of the product in the levator muscle of the upper lip. The product should be injected in points parallel to the folds.
- Correction of "Chinese moustache": the product is injected in the depressor muscle of the angle of the mouth.

Neck:

Treatment of the platysma muscle, which is responsible for the horizontal and vertical lines. About 1–3 U of the toxin may be injected in each point of the muscle, 1–2 cm apart from each other and from the mandibular border. Horizontal neck lines may also be treated by intradermal injection of 1–2 U per point, at a distance of 1.5–2 cm from the wrinkle.

33.4.3 Filling

The use of fillers has become, in recent decades, one of the main procedures performed by dermatologists. Based on the obvious aging population and the increased life expectancy, people's interest in improving general appearance has grown exponentially, justifying the increasing demand for minimally invasive procedures.

In youth, we consider that the shape of the face should be an inverted triangle, in which the base is formed by the union of the cheeks and the chin. A youthful face is characterised by convex areas that reflect light. In the aged face, we find concave areas that create shadows and a deposition of fat combined with sagging and individual features, such as obesity and photo-aging, which change the inverted triangle face pattern [19].

The initial use of filling techniques for the face occurred in 1893, when autologous fat was used for tissue increase. In 1958, researchers at Harvard Medical School showed that a solid collagen gel could be produced in the laboratory. In the early 1970s, a group at Stanford University began a process that resulted in the release of an injectable collagen (Zyderm). Shortly after, the bovine collagen-based fillers (Zyplast, Zyderm II) came. In 1996, the first fillers based on hyaluronic acid were launched.

- Currently, there is a great demand for ideal facial fillers with the following characteristics:
- Non-allergenic
- Approved by the health authorities
- Noncarcinogenic/non-teratogenic
- Non-migrating
- Minimum inflammation
- No visible skin changes (undetectable)
- Reproducible
- Durable
- Stable
- Good cost/benefit
- Easy to apply
- Easy to store
- Short recovery time

There is no ideal filler. Hyaluronic acid is the implant with properties that most closely match the characteristics of an ideal filler [16, 19].

To perform the necessary procedure, minimal knowledge of the facial anatomy is required (vessels, nerve endings and muscles) in order to avoid adverse reactions and complications [16]. One should be careful with local necrosis, which is rare, but may occur with any implants. This is caused by blood compression or obstruction of the filler or by direct injury of a vessel. The most common area is the glabella. The initial clinical sign is the appearance of painless whitening spots near the area being filled. If this occurs, the procedure should be immediately stopped; the area should be massaged and treated with warm compresses.

33.4.3.1 Types of Fillers Available

Bovine Collagen: Zyderm and Zyplast have been the only fillers approved for cosmetic use in the United States for over 20 years. They present a short duration of 3 months, on average, and have a low incidence of allergic reactions. Double skin tests are required prior to the first application, although this does not guarantee that the patient will not have any reaction later.

Poly (L-Lactic Acid) Microsphere: synthetic material used since 1954. This material has been safely used in sutures (Vicryl, Dexon); in absorbable pins in orthopaedic, neurological and craniofacial surgeries; and as drug carriers. Although it usually causes allergies, it does not contain animal proteins. Commercially known as Sculptra, it has been used to remodel the face contour. Its effect takes about 1 month to start and peaks one year after the first application.

Poly (*Methyl Methacrylate*) (*PMMA*): PMMA microspheres combined with bovine collagen form Artecoll. Once injected, the particles may not be broken down by enzymes. Thus, when implanted incorrectly or in an exaggerated manner, they may only be surgically removed at the risk of unsightly scars. Foreign body reactions may occur.

Hyaluronic Acid: this product is currently used most because it is the closest substance to an ideal filler. This is a highly hydrophilic substance, with a short half-life of only 1–2 days. To have greater durability, its molecules should be cross-linked to prevent them from degrading quickly. It may be a natural product, when extracted from rooster combs (Hylaform), or synthetic, when synthesised by fermentation of the bacterium *Streptococcus equi* (Restylane, Juvederm 24, Perfecta, among others). According to the number of gel particles per millilitre, the products will have greater or lesser durability, thus determining at what level they may be implanted in the skin.

Calcium Hydroxyapatite: hydroxyapatite is a hard, crystalline mineral composed of calcium, phosphate and hydroxide ions, which is the major constituent of mature bone. As it is an inorganic salt found in ordinary tissue, it has excellent biocompatibility. Hydroxyapatite has been used for more than 15 years as an agent in reconstructive orthopaedic surgery, according to studies. It is formulated as microspheres that form a scaffold to which fibroblasts anchor to produce new collagen. Radiesse is the only product currently available in the USA that uses hydroxyapatite. It is manufactured as an aqueous gel solution that contains these microsphere fragments of calcium hydroxyapatite. The gel (composed of cellulose, glycerine and water) provides immediate augmentation effects and must be degraded by macrophages to release the hydroxyapatite. This process usually takes 2–3 months, at which time new collagen synthesis begins and attaches to the scaffold, which withstands degradation by macrophages that is 1–2 years. Thus, this filler is not permanent and has both immediate and gradual results.

Fillers Not Approved for Use in the USA: Aquamid is a gel containing 2.5 % nonabsorbable cross-linked polyacrylamide that is currently available in Europe, Australia, South America and the Middle East for the correction of nasolabial folds, mouth corners, perioral wrinkles, and glabellar frown line and contouring of chin, cheek and vermillion borders. It is not FDA approved for use in the USA. It is a permanent filler with a half-life in the human body of more than 20 years [14, 15].

33.4.3.2 Contraindications

Fillers are contraindicated only in patients with autoimmune diseases under immunosuppressive therapy or with locoregional skin infections.

33.4.3.3 Complications

There are few adverse effects, which may be transient or delayed [17]. Transient effects may include redness, swelling, pain and bruising. Delayed effects may include the late formation of foreign body granulomas.

Special attention should be given to application in the glabellar region, which may lead to blindness due to the installation of retrograde blood flow into the cavernous sinus [20, 21].

33.4.3.4 Techniques

The decision on how deep the product should be applied involves the type of product and the desired correction in the patient's skin. In general, the deeper the damage, the deeper the distribution of the filler should be [16].

In general, most seasoned injectors favour a "zone" approach rather than filling the single rhytid. This addresses the volume depletion in other areas that may accentuate folds for which patients seek treatment (Fig. 33.3).

There is no universal acceptance on the proper implantation technique of fillers [16]. Common techniques include linear threading, serial puncture, fanning, crosshatching and depot injection. Pain and risk of vessel puncture can be minimised with smaller calibre needles. Retrograde injection may also reduce risk of injection into a vessel [21].

Linear Threading

With a linear threading technique, the area to be filled is punctured with the needle and advanced to the end position for the field to be augmented. The needle should be kept parallel to the skin and filler deposited within the same plane throughout injection. While the needle is withdrawn, slow constant pressure is applied to the plunger to deposit filler at an even rate. For deep defects, a layered approach can be adopted, where successive threading is placed at multiple depths. The amount of filler injected depends on the location, depth and type of filler used.

Serial Puncture

With this technique, microdroplets are deposited with successive injections placed 2–10 mm apart. The skin can be tented up with the needle inserted to ease the deposition of microdroplets. This method has been described to be effective for silicone injection.

33.4.3.5 Fanning/Crosshatching

Techniques such as fanning and crosshatching involve several linear passes of injection next to one another to augment larger areas of tissue. This technique is more commonly used to correct cheek concavity using agents that require deep dermal or subdermal deposition, such as PLLA or calcium hydroxyapatite. With deeper deposition, the needle can be oriented with the bevel facing up during this technique, in con-

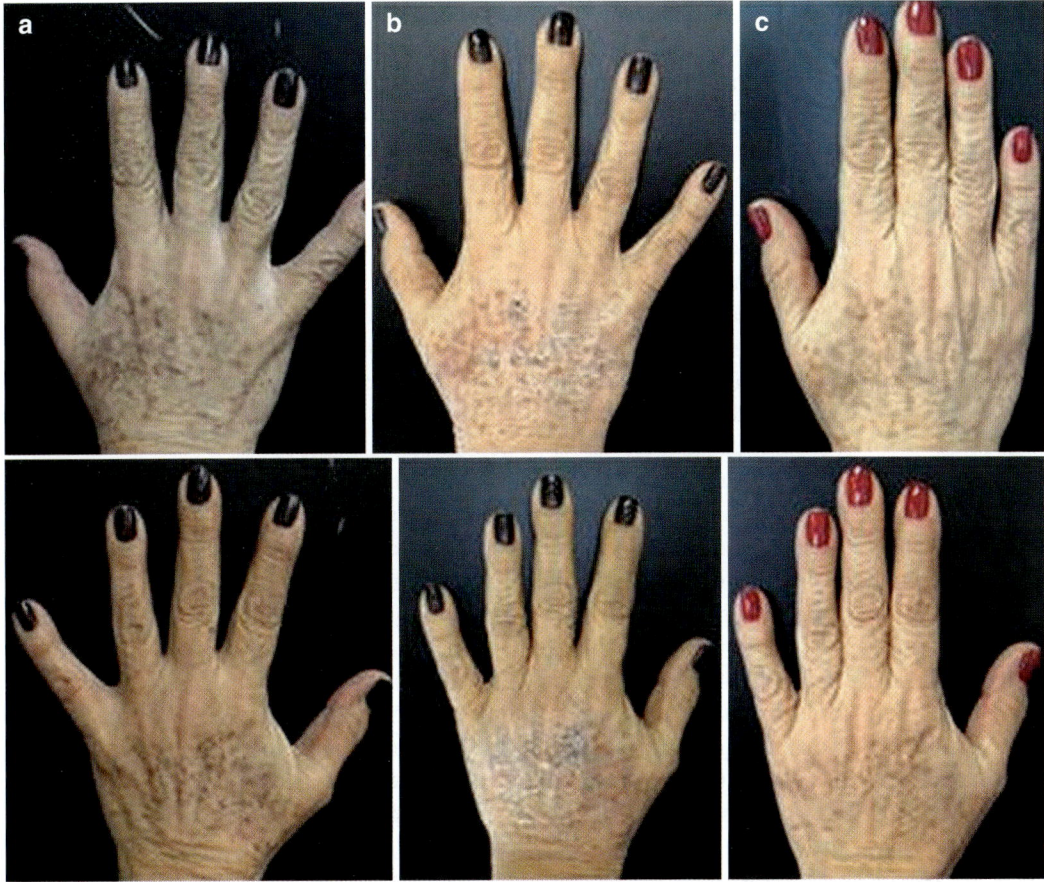

Fig. 33.3 (**a**) Pre-procedure. (**b**) Seven days postoperative of ATA 25 % past. (**c**) Thirty days postoperative with ATA 25 % past

trast to a downward facing bevel in more superficially placed product. After advancing the needle, the filler is deposited with each withdrawal. It may be helpful to outline the area to be injected prior to the procedure for more accurate results. It is key that the distribution of product be uniform [15].

33.4.4 Laser

Lasers stimulate molecules of a homogeneous surface [22, 23]. To start the treatment of a patient with multiple lesions, it is necessary to know the basic operation of the apparatus; therefore, knowledge of chromophores is key.

Each component of the skin lesions or the skin itself will have an individual characteristic and an individual response to different wavelengths. Water, melanin and haemoglobin absorb the light emitted in different ways, and from such absorption, we may have a photothermal, photochemical or photomechanical response that will determine the clinical response to the lesion or abnormality found.

In general, the longer the wavelength used, the greater the skin penetration will be. Radiation penetration may also be influenced by the size of the power source. The larger the source, the greater the light penetration will be. In other words, as source size increases, the energy used shall be increased to avoid loss of effectiveness in the concentration of light on the skin.

The resulting energy is measured in joules (J), and the most widely used parameter is J/cm^2 (fluency). The higher the flow, the higher the possibility of thermal damage in the treatment area [14, 15].

33.4.4.1 Types of Laser
Ablative
CO2 and erbium lasers are available for us. They may be used for cutting, steaming and dermal remodelling purposes [23].

In the cutting mode, the CO2 laser may be used for haemostasis and sterilisation during surgical procedures. Its use in dermatologic surgeries requires precision and refined techniques.

In the steaming mode, the CO2 and erbium lasers, as the name implies, are used to steam and destroy various types of lesions such as viral warts, condylomas, verrucous nevus, xanthelasma and sebaceous hyperplasia, among others.

Its main use with menopausal women is for dermal remodelling in the treatment of wrinkles. It is an aggressive, but effective, treatment, usually showing significant improvement with just a few sessions.

Its use in pulsed mode promotes the evaporation of thin layers of the skin with each pulse. Thus, a part of the epidermis and dermis is removed through successive ablations. A thermal damage halo is formed around the steamed area, capable of inducing shortening and formation of new collagen fibres, which are responsible for the results obtained with the procedure.

The erbium laser presents less tissue damage than that observed with the CO2 laser and is generally safer, although more sessions are required to achieve the desired effects.

The most common side effects are prolonged erythema (up to 3 months), milium formation, infections (bacterial and viral), dyschromias and scars [14, 15, 22, 23].

Non-ablative
This type of laser is recommended for the treatment of vascular and pigmented lesions, without causing damage to nearby structures in the target tissue [23].

When using non-ablative lasers, one must be concerned about the epidermal melanin layer as it acts as a protective barrier to the penetration of certain wavelengths. Especially in patients with skin types IV–VI and tanned skin, the possibility of increased temperature on the skin may cause adverse effects such as superficial burns and formation of vesicles, dyschromias and scarring.

In order to minimise thermal damage to the epidermis and reduce patient discomfort, some techniques may be used for cooling the epidermis, such as the use of cold packs, cold compresses (prior to laser application) and cooled or variable laser tips, capable of reducing the temperature of the skin [23].

The devices may be used for different purposes, such as stimulation of collagen synthesis, as well as correction of pigmented and melanocytic lesions.

The devices most commonly used for the treatment of aging skin (fine wrinkles) are Nd:YAG (1,340 nm), diode (1,420 nm) and erbium (1,540 nm). Their action mechanism is based on the stimulation of collagen production, secondary to the increase of local temperature, without ablation or tissue necrosis. The results are less aggressive than with the ablative techniques, ranging from moderate to mild, after several treatment sessions.

For vascular lesions as telangiectasias, nevi, and poikiloderma of Civatte, the most commonly used equipment is KTP (532 nm) dye laser (585, 595 and 600 nm) and Nd:YAG (532 and 1064 nm).

On the other hand, for melanocytic lesions such as lentigines, solar melanosis, freckles, periorbital hyperpigmentation and postinflammatory pigmentation, the most commonly used equipment is ruby (694 nm), alexandrite (755 nm), Nd:YAG (532 and 1,064 nm) and KTP (532 nm) [14, 15].

IPL (Intense Pulsed Light)
This technology has been used more and more, given its versatility and lower cost, as compared with lasers. Its actions come from the use of polychromatic electromagnetic radiation (wavelength range 400–1200 nm). It may be used to treat vascular and pigmented lesions, in addition to hair removal and non-ablative rejuvenation.

For best results in rejuvenation, maximum power may be used, without causing side effects.

Epidermolysis and protein denaturation, with the formation of dermal fibrosis, are the main effects. Thus, in addition to erythema and oedema, blisters and crusts may appear, with consequent dyschromias and scarring (rare). Therefore, in order to prevent the occurrence of adverse events, the epidermis should be protected through cooling [14].

33.5 Summary

As explained throughout this chapter, we may conclude that the cosmetic approach to menopausal patients should be global, considering all specific anatomic aspects of skin aging during menopause. During treatment, the patient should be made aware of the results that may be actually achieved, as well as any possible complications arising from the relevant procedure. Should the doctor and patient agree, treatment may be started, always in strict compliance with the limits of the product or equipment to be used and the real possibility of response to the patient's aesthetic complaints.

References

1. Honigman R, Castle DJ. Aging and cosmetic enhancement. Clin Inter Aging. 2006;1(2):115–9.
2. Archer DF. Postmenopausal estrogen and skin. Gynaecol Endocrinol. 2012;28(s2):2–6.
3. Goodman M. Social, psychological and developmental factors in women's receptivity to cosmetic surgery. J Aging Stud. 1994;8:375–96.
4. Calleja-Agius J, Brincat M. The effect of menopause on the skin and other connective tissues. Gynaecol Endocrinol. 2012;28(4):273–7.
5. Castelo-Branco C, Duran M, González-Merlo J. Skin collagen changes related to age and hormone replacement therapy. Maturitas. 1992;15(2):113–9.
6. Bolognia JL, Braverman IM, Rousseau ME, Sarrel PM. Skin changes in menopause. Maturitas. 1989;11:295–304.
7. Anttinen H, Orava S, Ryhanen L, Kivirikko KI. Assay of Protocollagen lysyl hydroxylase activity in the skin of human subjects and changes in the activity with age. Clin Chim Acta. 1973;47:289–94.
8. Takahashi M, Kushida K, Hoshino H, Ohishi T, Inoue T. Biochemical markers of bone turnover not decline after menopause in healthy women. Br J Obstet Gynaecol. 1999;106:427–31.
9. Richard MJ, Morris C, Deen BF, Gray L, Woodward JA. Analysis of the anatomic changes of the aging facial skeleton using computer-assisted tomography. Ophthal Plast Reconstr Surg. 2009;25(5):382–6.
10. Rohrich RJ, Pessa JE. The fat compartments of the face: anatomy and clinical implications for cosmetic surgery. Plast Reconstr Surg. 2007;119(7):2219–27.
11. Rohrich RJ, Pessa JE, Ristow B. The youthful cheek and the deep medial fat compartment. Plast Reconstr Surg. 2008;121(6):2107–12.
12. Rotta O. Dermatology: clinical, surgical and cosmetic interest. Cap 82: 655–660, Cap 88: 689–696, Cap 89: 697–700. São Paulo: Editora Manole; 2009.
13. Yokomizo VMR, Benemond TMH, Chisaki C, Benemond PH. Chemical peels: review and practical application. Cosmet Dermatol Surg. 2013;5(1):58–68.
14. Kede MPV, Sabatovich O. Aesthetic dermatology. 1st ed. São Paulo: Editora Athenaeum; 2004. p. 563–72.
15. Murad A, Gladstone HB, Tung RC. Cosmetic dermatology. Philadelphia: Elsevier; 2009, Peels Chapter 5, 81–101; Fillers Chapter 4, 59–79; Laser Chapter 7, 113–130.
16. Monteiro E, Parada MOB. Dermal fillers – Part 1, RBM. 2010;67, Special Dermatology, Indexado LILACS: S0034-72642010004700002.
17. Gadelha AR, Costa BMI. Dermatologic surgery in office. 2nd ed. São Paulo: Editora Atheneu; 2009. p. 557–65.
18. Carruthers J. Carruthers botulinum toxin products overview. Skin Therapy Lett. 2008;13(6):1–4.
19. Monteiro E. Facial aging: volume loss and hyaluronic acid, RBM. 2010;67(8), Indexado LILACS: S0034-72642010005000007.
20. Antonio CR, Antonio JR, Garcia AC, Correia AA. Fill in the glabellar region, dissecting the reasons for the high incidence of complications and blindness. Cosmet Dermatol Surg. 2012;4(2):111–3.
21. Crocco EI, Alves RO, Alessi C. Adverse events of hyaluronic acid injectable. Cosmet Dermatol Surg. 2012;4(3):259–26.
22. Niwa ABM, Macéa JM, Birth DS, Torezan L, Osorio NES. Erbium at 2,940 nm fractionated treatment of cutaneous photoaging of the face-evaluation after 15 months. Cosmet Dermatol Surg. 2010; 2(1):34–8.
23. Costa FB, El Ammar ABPC, Campos VB, Kalil CLPV. Complications with the use of lasers. Part II: laser ablative fractional and not fractional and non-ablative fractional laser. Cosmet Dermatol Surg. 2011;3(2):135–46.

Part VII

Menopause and Global Considerations

Menopause: Cross-Cultural Considerations

34

Paula R. DeCola

Contents

34.1	**Biological Construct**	496
34.2	**Cultural Construct**	496
34.3	**Influencing Factors**	496
34.4	**Other Possible Confounding/Contributing Factors**	497
34.5	**Cross-Cultural Findings Real or Artifact**	498
34.6	**Age of Onset**	498
34.6.1	North America and Europe	498
34.7	**Geographical or Cultural Expression of Symptomatology**	500
34.7.1	Vasomotor Symptoms	500
34.7.2	Vaginal Atrophy	502
34.8	**Attitudes and Symptom Experience: Cultural Implications**	503
34.9	**Across Countries Weight Gain Associations with Menopause**	504
34.10	**Summary**	504
References		505

The intersection of sex and gender plays a vital role in the process of aging as well as with specific conditions associated with the aging process. In terms of menopause, the gender or sociocultural aspects of the experience are purported to be uniquely reflected in the variation of symptoms presented by women in different countries cultures and geographies. This hints at the important interplay between biology, sociology, ethnicity, and culture.

According to the UNFPA report, "Aging in the Twenty-First Century" one in nine persons in the world is aged 60 years or over, and this is projected to increase to one in five by 2050 [1]. This demographic phenomenon is affecting low- and high-income countries alike. Further, there is a disproportion in the ratio of men to women as we age, and this is well documented within the above 60 population. In 2012, for every 100 women aged 60, there were 84 men [1]. The World Health Organization has estimated that in 2030, there will be around 1.2 billion postmenopausal women, with 47 million women entering this stage of life every year [2]. As more women live longer, the management of the menopause transition and women's healthcare post the reproductive years will become increasingly important on a global basis. However, few countries are presently addressing the specific healthcare needs associated with this increased life expectancy in terms of health policy or provision of care.

P.R. DeCola, RN MSc
External Medical Affairs, Pfizer Inc,
219 East 42nd Street, New York, NY 10017, USA
e-mail: paula.decola@pfizer.com

34.1 Biological Construct

It has been acknowledged that menopause is not an event but rather a process that starts and ends gradually over time. There are different classifications which are used to define menopause status and the various shifts from a biological perspective. These include length of cycle along with a monotropic rise in follicle-stimulating hormone (FSH), characteristics of bleeding, and FSH rates of change. These types of parameters help mark the transition from ovarian function to failure. Yet, in terms of defining natural menopause, there is general agreement that it occurs once a woman is without menses for 1 year. Soules et al. support this definition and further characterize stages subsequent to menopause the first of which is characterized by further ovarian hormone drop-off and accelerated bone loss [3].

Garcia et al. [4] noted that often subtle changes in bleeding patterns provide an indication of the earliest hormonal changes associated with the menopause transition as well as the symptoms associated with this transition [4]. These initial indicators could be useful signs for clinicians and be used as the impetus for patient education. This education could be focused on the menopause transition, as well as on healthy lifestyles and behavior change. This could support assuaging menopausal symptoms as well as support the prevention of some of the more common comorbid conditions associated with aging and this transition.

34.2 Cultural Construct

There is growing support that suggests that in addition to biological aspects of menopause, cultural components also exist. This can account, at least in part, for the range and frequency differences of menopausal symptoms seen globally. Indeed, women's attitudes regarding menopause are multidimensional [5]. Some women in certain societies can dread aging; they may associate it with failing attractiveness as well as other negative self-perceptions [6]. The effects of culture on menopause symptom expression may also be attributable to acculturation. The result could, in part, account for the differing prevalence of symptoms seen within an ethnic group depending on an individual's country of residence and not necessarily their country of origin [7]. Further, cultural differences in aspects such as the meaning of menopause and an individual's attitude toward menopause could play a role in accounting for these variations [8]. This includes whether menopause is thought of as a natural event or a medical condition [8].

34.3 Influencing Factors

There has also been a relationship shown between women's overall health status and the extent of her distress by and perception of symptoms related to this transition [9]. Additionally, there are a number of other factors that have been associated with the prevalence of menopausal symptoms as well as the degree of burden experienced due to their presence. These include a number of lifestyle as well as environmental factors.

The results of the United States based Study of Women's Health Across the Nation (SWAN) found that certain characteristics were independently associated with earlier natural menopause; these included women with lower number of years in schooling; history of heart disease; active cigarette smoking; marital status of separated, widowed or divorced; and current unemployment. Later natural age of menopause was associated with prior use of contraceptives, Japanese ethnicity, and parity [10].

Smoking has been identified in a number of studies as being associated with an earlier age of onset of menopause [10–13]. Hayatbakhsha et al. [11] also report that women who quit smoking have a lower chance of early onset menopause than current smokers. In a systemic review of studies on this topic, in 2008, the evidence of this association is not clear in terms of the duration of smoking and the quantity of cigarettes smoked [14].

A 2009 review [15] on the effects of exercise on menopausal symptoms referred to a number of observational studies and noted that the relationship between physical activity and fewer menopausal symptoms is inconclusive, while a number of clinical studies have shown that physically active women report fewer menopausal symptoms [16–19].

Diet is another factor implicated in effecting menopause. Nagata et al. [20] found that a high intake of polyunsaturated fat was associated with earlier onset of menopause and was not able to confirm previous findings that an inverse association between green and yellow vegetable intake and the age of natural menopause exists. Nagel et al. [21] reported that high intake of carbohydrates was associated with an earlier menopause while higher intake of protein and total fat was associated with a delay in the onset of natural menopause. A literature search on various factors' effect on age at natural menopause reported that although few studies have been conducted on the effects of diet on age of natural menopause, the existing data supports that the high intake of calories, fruits, and proteins delay age at natural menopause and further reported that moderate alcohol consumption also delays the age of natural menopause; alcohol has also been implicated in the presence of hot flashes [22].

On a related topic to diet, the effects of body mass index on menopause analyzed from the Study of Women's Health Across the Nation (SWAN) shows luteal activity in premenopausal and early perimenopausal women is strongly affected by body size [23]. Further, the study reported that women with higher BMIs (greater than 25 kg/m^2) were more likely to have longer total cycle length, a shorter luteal phase, and lower overall gonadotropin and luteal phase progesterone metabolites. The authors suggested that these findings imply that women with the higher BMIs may have an increased likelihood of chronic cycle dysfunction [23]. Further, Davis et al. confirmed the results of prior studies showing that the greater the BMI, the later the age at menopause and cited the Penn Ovarian Aging Study which indicated a positive association between BMI and the likelihood of transitioning from pre- to perimenopause but not from peri- to postmenopause [24].

In terms of environment, a woman's work while associated with increased self-esteem has also been reported to have a negative impact on menopausal women [25–28]. Studies have reported that certain working environments have increased the intensity of a woman's symptoms [27, 29–31]. A study of Egyptian females working in a government faculty of medicine reported that poor working conditions related to factors such as ventilation, humidity, and temperature were perceived to play a role in aggravating their menopausal symptoms [27]. Similar findings were reported in a study involving female police officers [30]. Reynolds reported that menopausal women were affected by their work conditions in a few ways including when they were required to work in enclosed spaces or with a new client [31].

34.4 Other Possible Confounding/Contributing Factors

The effect of family history on the onset of menopause in terms of timing, experience, and expressed symptoms has been widely discussed. It has been known that women inherit factors for the number of oocytes [32]. The burgeoning field of epigenetics further highlights the effects of environment including the intrauterine environment on gene expression and therefore most likely on the ovarian store. Indeed, as noted earlier, there are a number of parameters that have been reported to affect the ovarian store, these includes factors such as smoking [10–13], physical activity [15–19], and diet [20–22].

The effect of environment on familial concordance has been raised in a few studies that have focused on twins [33]. A large study undertaken in the United Kingdom which included 2,060 individuals who were first-degree relatives in the age of 31–90 showed women whose mother or non-twin sister had an early menopause had an increased risk of early menopause [33]. The study also noted that women had an increased rate of late menopause if their mother or non-twin sister had a late menopause. Morris et al. [33] reported that both shared environment and hereditary factors contributed to these findings.

34.5 Cross-Cultural Findings Real or Artifact

Although there is significant support for cross-cultural research, concerns have also been registered. One concern is that some publications report cross-cultural findings from disparate research studies, while another relates to the sweeping generalizations made from studies with relatively small numbers of participants. Other studies use symptom lists that have originated from the United States and Europe and are employed unaltered within countries with greatly differing cultures and perspectives. Additionally, symptom checklists are subjective assessments; therefore, the effects of culture can independently influence responses. This is particularly possible with aspects such as symptom tolerance, perspectives on aging, as well as health attitudes. Indeed, even the effects of a health system on women's experience of menopause and their perception of therapeutic interventions are potential confounders.

Therefore, assessing whether menopause is associated with similar mental and physical symptoms or whether there are significant cross-cultural deviations can be difficult to ascertain. However, assessing cross-cultural manifestations is important in terms of determining whether there is a common set of conditions for menopause on a global basis. And there is a significant amount of research devoted to studying the differences in genes, cultures, and environments. The North American Menopause Society has been supportive of cross-cultural research [34]. Therefore, in order to assess if there are true cross-cultural differences, it is important to assess outcomes using statistical assessments that involve controlling for various variables.

34.6 Age of Onset

Inherently, one of the least subjective criteria to assess across cultures is the age of final menstrual period, although this criteria has also been called into suspicion. It is seen by some to be subject to methodological assessment differences across studies. Further, these evaluations are frequently self-reported and as such are believed to be subject to underestimation [35].

Nonetheless, based on reports from differing types of studies, the age of natural menopause appears to occur at an earlier age within regions that are comprised of countries with lower- to middle-income economies. There appears to be both an east to west and north to south difference. Women in Europe and North America tend to be older than the age documented for women in most of the countries within Asia and Latin America. Further, a trend appears to be present, based on a limited number of studies with relatively small sample sizes, that women from within the Middle East and Africa have a natural age of menopause that is comparable to that of Asian and Latin American women. In fact, women within Africa and the Middle East appear, as a whole, to have the earliest natural age of menopause globally; refer to Table 34.1. Moreover, differences in the age of menopause onset were noted within subregions, across countries, and based on ethnic or racial background, as well as based on country of origin. Additional details on these phenomena are described below.

34.6.1 North America and Europe

34.6.1.1 North America

Within North America, the median age of natural menopause reported in the Study of Women's Health Across the Nation (SWAN) was 52.54 years [36]. The study assessed 3,302 from across the United States and included 5 ethnic/racial groups. A similar finding was reported in a study looking at the median age of menopause for women in the United States (US) and Spain, the finding for the United States was 52.6 years [37]. While within Canada, the average age of menopause has been cited as being 51 years [7].

Regional differences were also identified within the United States. In a cross-sectional survey of 22,484 women, after controlling for covariates, it was noted that women from the Southern part of the United States reported menopause 10.8 months earlier than Northeastern women, 8.4 months earlier than midwestern women, and 6.0 months earlier than western

Table 34.1 Age of natural menopause

Continent	Country	First author	Number of subjects	Age range	Mean age	Median age
Europe	Europe	Dratva [41]	5,288	30–60		54
North America	United States	Gold [36]	3,302	40–55		52.54
Asia 1	Japan	Yasui [48]	24,152	>40		52.1
Asia 2	Thai	Chompootweep [53]	2,375	45–59	49.5	
Asia 3	China	Yang [49]	9,939	40–65	48.9	
Asia 4	India	Kriplani [50]	350		46.7	48
Africa	Nigeria	Olaolorun [61]	1,189	40–60		50
Latin America	Latin America	Blumel [45]	17,150	40–59		48.6
Middle East 1	United Arab Emirates	Benera [58]	450	>45		48
Middle East 2	Iran	Delavar [57]	1,397	45–63	47.7	

women ($p<0.05$) [38]. The cause for this effect is not known.

In terms of racial differences from within the United States, Gold et al. [10] reported no difference between Caucasian and African American women in terms of menopause onset, yet within this report, they cite two earlier studies that demonstrated that African American women had an earlier onset of menopause by 6–12 months in comparison to Caucasian women. McKnight et al. [38] in 2011 found similar findings to Gold in that no racial difference in age at menopause was shown between black and Caucasian women after covariates were controlled for in a cross-sectional survey of 22,484 women in the United States [37]. A study of 17,070 women aged 35–55 years found African American women had earlier onset of natural menopause, and this was strongly associated with smoking and inversely associated with body mass index and oral contraceptive use [39].

Henderson et al. [40] reported that Japanese American women experienced late natural menopause in comparison to women of Latin heritage as well as Caucasian women in the United States. Additionally, Latin women living in the United States, but born outside of the United States, had earlier onset of menopause then women born in the United States with Latin heritage [40].

European women had a median age of natural menopause of 54 years based on a study of 5,288 women randomly selected in nine European countries between 1998 and 2002 [40]. The later age of menopause across Europe has been noted in a number of other studies [41–44]. As was seen within the United States, there are geographical variations within Europe; Southern Europe in general has an earlier age of natural menopause compared to Northern Europe [41]. In fact, the study indicated that there was also variation across countries and that the age of natural menopause was shifting toward later ages [41].

34.6.1.2 Latin America

Latin American women have an earlier age of menopause than those within Europe and North America. In a study involving 17,150 healthy women surveyed from 15 Latin American countries, the median age of menopause was reported as 48.6 years and the mean age was 49.4 ± 5.5 [45]. The onset ranged from 53 years in Cartagena de Indias (Colombia) to 43.8 years in Asuncion (Paraguay) [45]. Further it was found that women living at or above 2,000 m and those with lower levels of education were more prone to an earlier menopause [45]. In a survey of 4,548 women across all regions in Mexico, the mean age at menopause was 47.9 ± 3.82 years [46], while the median age at menopause was reported to be 50 years in a study comprising 4,056 women in seven cities within Latin America and the Caribbean [47].

34.6.1.3 Asia

There is great diversity among the various countries comprising Asia. Yet the mean and median age of menopause in Asia is fairly consistently reported. The exception to this is Japan. In fact Japanese women have one of the latest median ages of natural menopause, comparable to women in the west. This is evidenced within the Japan Nurses' Health Study, in which a cross-sectional analysis revealed a median natural age of menopause of 52.1 years [48]. This as noted is in contrast with the general trend in Asia wherein the natural age of menopause is comparatively early in relation to that seen in the west.

A cross-sectional study conducted in China including a total of 9,939 women reported 48.9 years as the mean age of natural menopause [49]. While a series of studies involving women in India closely mirrored the age reported in China with an average age at menopause calculated as 48.0 [50], and at 48.7 for two other studies [51, 52]. Further, a study of Thai women in Bangkok reported an average age of menopause of 49.5 ± 3.6 [53], and a study in Singapore reported a mean age of 49 years among 2,354 women [7].

34.6.1.4 Middle East
Studies within the Middle East revealed a median age of menopause that is somewhat comparable to Asia in that on average it is on the younger side of the age range continuum. This includes a median age of 50 reported in a study including 858 Saudi Arabian women of which 391 were postmenopausal [54], a median age of natural menopause of 49.3 years for 298 women in Lebanon [55], and a median age of 50 based on a study of 143 women in Jordan [56]. The mean age recalled by a sample of 1, 397 women in Iran was 47.7 ± 4.9 years [57]. While a study involving a sample of 450 United Arab Emirates women aged 45 years and above, the median age of natural menopause was 48 years [58].

34.6.1.5 Africa
Relatively few studies were found that evaluated menopause in African women. However, two studies, one in Ghana and one conducted in Nigeria reported a median age of 50.2 years [59, 60]. Further, a cross-sectional community-based study with a total of 1,189 Nigerian women reported the median age of menopause as 48 years [61]. Lastly, a small community-based study in Nigeria among 273 menopausal women reported a mean age at menopause as 51.41 ± 3.26 years [62].

34.7 Geographical or Cultural Expression of Symptomatology

There is an ongoing controversy as to whether there are universal menopausal symptoms. There are a number studies from North America and Europe that report relatively high numbers of menopausal symptoms in comparison to studies that have been conducted in Asia. As well, there appears to be differing perspectives in the experience of menopause across cultures. For example, women in Japan see menopause as an event which is not considered to be a negative experience, while about half of American women believe menopause is a disagreeable event [63]. However, irrespective of country, it has been reported that the majority of women pass through menopause with no or very little symptoms of discomfort [64]. Differences in FSH, estradiol, and luteinizing hormone have been shown across populations; however, the clinical significance of these findings is currently unclear [65]. Yet, these findings provide some rudimentary indication in favor of the existence of cross-cultural differences.

34.7.1 Vasomotor Symptoms

There are varying rates of vasomotor symptoms, such as hot flash, hot flush, and night sweats, reported in the literature. These differences are shown across geographic areas and ethnic categories; refer to Fig. 34.1. It has been suggested that menopausal status may also have a role in the expression of these differences: premenopausal women appear to have the lowest rates, while perimenopausal women experience the highest rates of this symptom cluster [66].

34.7.1.1 North America and Europe
Vasomotor symptoms are commonly reported within North America and Europe. The North American Menopause Society [67] notes that about 55 % of women report experiencing hot flashes. Freeman et al. [65] cite results from prior

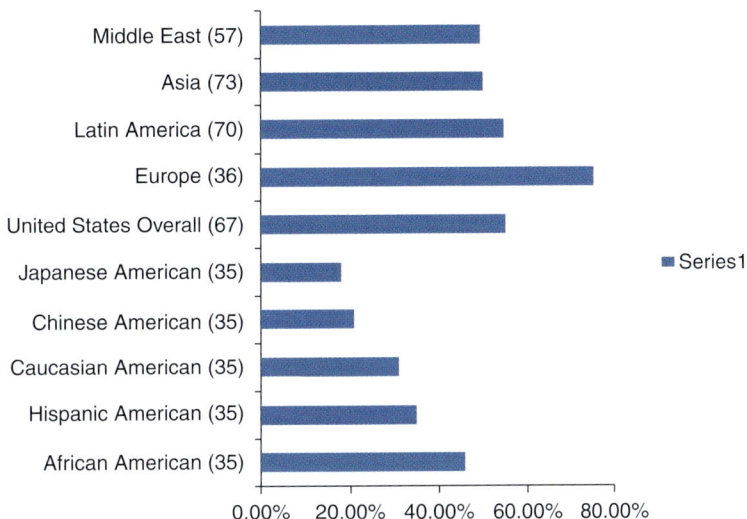

Fig. 34.1 Percentage of vasomotor symptoms by region (US by race/ethnicity)

analyses of the Study of Women's Health Across the Nation (SWAN) that revealed African American women had the highest rates of vasomotor symptoms; this included both hot flushes and night sweats. African American women had these symptoms at a rate of 46 %, followed by Hispanic (35 %), Caucasian (31 %), Chinese (21 %), and Japanese (18 %) [65]. The publication further reports that another analysis of the SWAN data noted that African American women had the highest reported prevalence of night sweats and that the group with the lowest proportion of premenopausal women had the highest prevalence of hot flushes or night sweats [65]. While studies conducted in Europe also show high rates of night sweats in fact up to three fourths of the women in these studies experienced hot flashes [35]. Yet, there are country differences, for example, Dutch women reported the symptoms at a rate of 80 % and women within Britain reported these symptoms at a rate of about 54 % [68].

34.7.1.2 Latin America

Latin America is reported to have high rates of severe menopause transition symptoms. In terms of the rate of vasomotor symptoms, a range between 50 and 68.9 % has been noted in the literature [69]. A 2011 Blumel et al. paper [69] found that 54.5 % of 8,373 women from 16 Latin American countries reported vasomotor symptoms and that these symptoms persisted into late postmenopause. It was also reported from this same study that the vasomotor symptoms negatively affected quality of life [69].

34.7.1.3 Asia

Asian countries are reported to have relatively low rates of vasomotor symptoms ranging from 10 % to 20 % in countries such as Hong Kong, [70] India, Indonesia, and Thailand [64]. In Japan, rates of vasomotor symptoms range from 12 to 25.7 % [71]. When reviewing two multinational studies based in Asia, the ranking of the most common symptoms tended to differ from those seen in the west. The most common symptoms, reported in the Pan-American Study, representing 11 countries from the region were not those related to vasomotor symptoms, but rather were body and joint aches (86.3 %) and memory problems (80.1 %) [72]. In fact hot flushes were reported at a rate as low as 5 %, based on responses from women within Indonesia [72]. In the Asian Menopause Survey, the most common symptoms were sleeplessness (61.7 %), irritability (60 %), followed by migraines (55.9 %), while hot flashes were reported at a rate of 49.9 % [73]. Barber [65] suggests that symptom ranking may differ between Eastern and western women and further notes that Asian women are less aware of treatment options than their western counterparts.

34.7.1.4 Middle East

Studies within the Middle East vary in terms of reported rates of vasomotor symptoms but have been noted to be in keeping with western rates. Sallam et al. [74] reported in a study of 200 Egyptian women who experienced hot flashes that the rate was 87.7 %. Further, a cross-sectional study of 450 women in Egypt noted that 90.7 % experienced hot flashes [75] and a study involving 143 women in Southern Jordan showed a rate of 62 % [56]. A cross-sectional survey conducted in Libya reported vasomotor symptoms at a rate of 76.6 % [76]. In contrast, a study within Iran reported a rate of 49.3 % in a sampling of 1,397 women [57] and a study within the United Arab Emirates noted a vasomotor symptom rate of 40 % [58].

34.7.1.5 Africa

There is limited information found regarding African women; however, two studies from within Africa reported relatively similar findings. A prospective survey involving 152 women in Akosombo District in Ghana reported hot flash rates of around 57 % [59]. A cross-sectional survey in Nigeria involving 186 women noted hot flashes were experienced by 58.1 % of the respondents and that this symptom was viewed as the most problematic one [77]. A second study in Nigeria among 273 women reported a similar rate of 57 % [62].

34.7.2 Vaginal Atrophy

Vaginal atrophy is experienced, at rate reported to be as high as about half of all postmenopausal women. This cluster of symptoms often negatively affects quality of life [78]. Symptoms of vaginal atrophy include vaginal dryness, itching, burning or soreness, as well as dyspareunia. Additionally, urinary tract symptoms can also be present in some women including nocturia, dysuria, urgency, frequency, and incontinence which includes leaking urine and recurrent urinary tract infection [79]. Sexual dysfunction is also associated with vaginal atrophy, and this cluster of symptoms is believed to be linked to a reduction in estrogen [78, 79].

34.7.2.1 North America and Europe

The prevalence of vaginal atrophy within the United States has been reported as being as high as 51 % (80) in contrast to a reported rate in Canada of 34 % [81]. Interesting, however, is that only 24 % of women in the United States attribute their symptoms to menopause [82]. Further, in a survey conducted within North America, 60 % of women over 45 years of age who had used hormone therapy in the past or who had never used hormone therapy had vaginal atrophy complaints and the majority (90 %) of these women considered these to be problematic [83]. Yet, multiple studies found that relatively low numbers of women (25 %) seek medical consultation for this type of symptom [81].

The international online survey, Vaginal Health: Insights Views and Attitudes (VIVA) included 3,250 postmenopausal women (last menses was more than 12 months before entry) between the ages of 55 and 65 [80]. This included women from Canada, Denmark, Finland, Norway, Sweden, United Kingdom, and the United States and concentrated on assessing perceptions about vaginal distress. Almost half of the respondents (45 %) reported having a symptom related to vaginal atrophy with the lowest rate being reported in Sweden (38 %) and the highest in the United States (51 %) [80].

Another survey (CLOSER) that was conducted in Canada, Denmark, Finland, France, Italy, Norway, United Kingdom, and the United States reported that more than half of the North American respondents avoided sexual intimacy due to vaginal symptoms [78]. Additionally, half of the surveyed women responded that their clinician had not initiated a discussion of postmenopausal vaginal wellness [78]. There were country differences present with regard to this point; on the higher end were women from the United Kingdom (60 %), Canada (59 %), United States (56 %), and Norway (53 %), and on the lower end were women from Sweden (35 %) and Finland (33 %) [78].

34.7.2.2 Latin America

The Collaborative Group for Research of the Climacteric in Latin America (REDLINC) assessed sexual dysfunction in 7,243 women aged 40–59 year of age. The survey was conducted in 11 Latin American countries and sexual function was assessed using the Female Sexual Function Index (FSFI) [84]. The FSFI is comprised of 6 domains: desire, arousal, orgasm, pain, lubrication, and satisfaction [84]. Of the 5,391 women who were sexually active, 56.8 % of the respondents reported sexual dysfunction and the prevalence of sexual dysfunction varied per center; it ranged from 21 to 98.5 %. The sexual dysfunction domains with the highest scores also varied by center [84]. Desire was the domain with the highest score across sites and vaginal dryness was the factor most associated with sexual dysfunction [84]. In a cross-sectional survey among 125 Native-American Bolivian women, the chief complaint was loss of libido, and this symptom was reported by 51 % of the respondents, followed by genital itching 40.8 % and dyspareunia 40 % [85].

34.7.2.3 Asia

Overall, the highest rates of symptom complaints reported by women within the pan-Asia menopause study were not related to vaginal atrophy, but rather related to muscle and joint pains. These occurred on average at a rate of 86.3 % and ranged from 76 % in Korea to 96 % in Vietnam [72]. In contrast vaginal atrophy symptoms were reported at the following lower rates: vaginal dryness 55.7 %, vaginal itching 39.7 %, dysuria 37.4 %, and painful intercourse 29.9 % [72].

In a cross-sectional study of 1,000 postmenopausal women from China, Malaysia, Taiwan, Thailand, and Hong Kong, most women (66 %) reported no reductions in sexual function [73]. Yet, symptoms of vaginal atrophy were on average reported by 37.4 % of the women. The countries with the higher rates were Hong Kong 51 %, Taiwan 47.9 %, and Thailand 45 %, and those reporting lower rates included China 31 % and Malaysia 29.6 % [73]. Further, awareness of hormone therapy (HT) was low; over 30 % of women were not able to mention one benefit of this treatment [73].

34.7.2.4 Middle East

Research on vaginal atrophy within the Middle East was not readily identified. Gynecological matters, by virtue of cultural mores, remain a private and somewhat of a shameful matter [86]. Yet, in a retrospective study conducted in Iran, a statistical increase in urinary frequency was identified for women entering menopause, and a statistically significant increase of complaints of dry vagina were identified postmenopause [57]. Further, a cross-sectional study of 450 Egyptian women aged 50–59 years of age noted that 89.1 % of participants reported decreased sexual desire [75].

34.7.2.5 Africa

Lastly, within Africa a study in Nigeria revealed urinary frequency at a rate of 38.7 % and vaginal dryness and discomfort or discharge at a rate of 35.5 % [77]. A South African study involving structured interviews with 102 women in Durban found the women experienced a number of vaginal and urinary complaints related to atrophy, such as painful sex 43 %, dry vagina 51 %, loss of libido 41 %, pruritus 32 %, dysuria 39 %, and urinary frequency 40 % [87].

34.8 Attitudes and Symptom Experience: Cultural Implications

There appears to be some relationship between a woman's attitudes toward menopause and their experience of symptoms. Avis and McKinlay [88] in 1991 reported from the Massachusetts Women's Health Study that women with negative attitudes toward menopause prior to the transition reported higher frequencies of hot flashes. Ayers et al. [9] note in their review of 13 studies that pre- and perimenopausal women as well as younger women had the most negative attitudes toward menopause. This seems to align with the perception that the perimenopausal transition is most fraught with physiological changes. Another explanation is that women ultimately adapt to the symptoms over time. Further, countries such as the United States, whose culture and healthcare system tends to "medicalize" menopause rather than view it as a life course process, have higher frequencies of "negative symptoms" [9]. As well, there is evidence that supports the notion that the more negative a woman's attitude is to the transition, with or without the existence of comorbid mood disorder, the greater the number of menopause-related symptoms [9].

Obermeyer 2000 [35] points out that the prior mental and general health status of a woman is a good predictor of mental health during the menopause transition. As well, it is noted that various cultures place both positive and negative perspectives on aging as well as on menopause complicating the ability to assess this parameter.

Yet, a study conducted in Qatar assessing the menopause experience of Qatari Arab and non-Qatari Arab women reported that religious beliefs and culture are intimately linked to their experience of menopause [86]. It was also reported to be linked to the participants' perspective that western women undoubtedly experience menopause differently from Qatari women due to this aspect [86].

Gupta et al. [89] report on studies which indicate that women who have migrated from another country tend to retain the menopausal symptom profile of their native country [89]. Yet, in a study of women from the Indian subcontinent within the United Kingdom, Gupta notes that the UK Asian women experience of menopause is more aligned to the Caucasian women in the United Kingdom than those experienced by women in Delhi [89]. This is most notable with respect to vasomotor symptoms.

Another attitudinal factor that affects both the frequency and the level of distress of vasomotor symptoms is women's sense of their level of control. This is inversely related, in that more perceived control is associated with less distress and reported rates of frequency [90–93].

34.9 Across Countries Weight Gain Associations with Menopause

High-, middle-, and low-income countries around the globe share the phenomena of a rising level of obesity. The overall incline in obesity as well as rates of overweight women has been largely attributed to lifestyle behaviors. Yet, it has been shown that women carry the greater burden of this disease [94]. Davis et al. [24] reported, based on a literature review, that weight gain cannot be attributed to menopause alone; however, the transition is associated with increases in total body fat and abdominal fat increases [24]. In general there is a steady 0.5 kg annual weight gain seen in women postmenopause [24].

The analysis also shows that body weight does have an effect on the menopause transition. As previously noted, increased weight has been associated with a later age of natural menopause onset. There have been longitudinal studies that have indicated that the higher the basal metabolic index, the later the age of natural menopause [95]. There is also support for the finding that as weight increases, menopausal symptoms also increase. Therefore, obesity is an independent risk factor for increased reporting of severe symptoms [96, 97]. Yet, Thurston et al. report based on a sub-cohort of women from the Study of Women's Health that women with higher basal metabolic indices and waist circumferences experienced fewer hot flashes [98].

34.10 Summary

As the average age of women extends past 80 years, most females will spend about one third of their lives postmenopause. It has been estimated that almost 80 % of women report at least one symptom associated with menopause, such as hot flushes or sleep or mood disturbances [99]. Yet, it can be difficult to discern menopause symptoms from those associated with the aging process. This complicates the ability to determine if there are common menopause symptoms across populations. Another complication is the recognition that certain mood disturbances such as depression, a condition associated with menopause, can involve somatization. It has been suggested that somatic complaints may be culturally mediated. Therefore, somatic symptoms may account for some aspect of the cross-cultural menopausal differences seen on a geographic, ethnic, or other subpopulation basis [100]. Culture by definition refers to elements such as one's beliefs, values, and attitudes and one's behaviors acquired through social learning. All of these factors are indeed plausible influencers on how an individual can interpret, internalize, and communicate symptoms and health.

Symptom clustering, which identifies correlations among symptoms, done through the use of statistical analysis, has given us some additional insight into the menopause transition. Sievert and Obermeyer 2012 found that indeed there are associations between somatic and emotional symptoms, and these vary across countries [100]. Further, they suggest that this supports the notion that culturally relevant psychosocial distress may be presented through somatic symptoms.

Cross-cultural differences are present in terms of the geographic or ethnic trends toward an earlier or later age of menopause. There are implications for these trends. Studies demonstrate that early menopause is positively associated with coronary heart disease as well as stroke [101, 102]. As well, studies have shown that earlier menopause has been shown to be associated with early onset osteoporosis [103]. Further, a Norwegian study of 19,731 women found an inverse relationship between age at menopause and the all-cause mortality rate ($p = 0.003$) [104]. Conversely, later menopause is positively associated with superior cognitive functioning later in life, but this study also demonstrated that there was a greater risk of endometrial and breast cancer [105].

In the end, this assessment of cross-cultural differences clearly calls for the need for more rigorous studies designed specifically to determine if cross-cultural differences do exist and there are a core set of symptoms associated with menopause on a global basis. The review seems to support the notion that there are symptoms that do traverse geographic and cultural boundaries. While, as noted above, some may be somatic, there are others that are well linked to hormonal changes; this includes vasomotor and vaginal atrophy symptoms. However, Avis et al. [106] concluded, based on a factor analysis of various studies that a single symptom pattern consisting of somatic, psychological, and menopausal symptoms does not appear to be present [106].

This review of literature did evoke some fundamental points regarding quality of life, access to healthcare, health literacy, and gender equity. Culture does seem to influence health literacy in terms of the level of knowledge regarding menopausal symptoms, the ability to articulate the benefits and risks associated with treatment options, as well as the ability to access to care. As with many healthcare matters, there seems to be a socioeconomic gradient that exists, higher wealth being associated with higher health literacy, access to care, and general health.

The north and west versus the south and east divide is defined by income, access to care, and approach to the menopause transition. The former having a more medicalized approach aligned with greater access to care, with the latter characterized by less access to care, yet a tendency to organically accept the transition as part of the cycle of life as well as often not seeking symptom relief.

As the postmenopausal time extends to one third of women's life, it is critically important that quality of life issues are adequately addressed. The symptoms associated with menopause and the aging process itself affects quality of life including sexual health. This fosters the need to address individual health from a holistic perspective. Additionally, there appears to be adequate evidence to suggest the need for care to be provided with the relevant cultural context and competency. The value of different interventions needs to be weighed with safety, efficacy, cost-effectiveness, and quality of life in mind. An imperative exists, fueled by gender equity, which states that the health of women must be of paramount importance, not only during their reproductive years but also as they pass from the point of ovarian function to the point of the final menstrual period.

References

1. United Nations and Help Age International Aging in the twenty first century. UNFPA: New York; 2012.
2. World Health Organization. Research on the menopause in 1990's. Geneva: World Health Organization; 1996.

3. Soules MR, Sherman S, Parrott E, Rebar R, Santoro N, Utian W, Woods N. Executive summary: stages of reproductive aging workshop (STRAW). Climacteric. 2001;4:267–72.
4. Garcia CR, Sammel MD, Freeman EW, Lin H, Langan E, Kapoor S, Nelson D. Defining menopause status: creation of a new definition to identify the early changes of the menopausal transition. Menopause. 2005;12(2):128–35.
5. Woods NF, Saver B, Taylor T. Attitudes toward menopause and hormone therapy among women with access to health care. Menopause. 1998;5(3): 178–88.
6. Kowalcek I, Rotte D, Banz C, Diedrich K. Women's attitude and perceptions towards menopause in different cultures: cross-cultural comparison of pre-menopausal and post-menopausal women in Germany and Papua New Guinea. Maturitas. 2005;51(3): 227–35.
7. Palacios S, Henderson VW, Sisles N, Tan D, Villaseca P. Age of menopause and impact of climacteric symptoms by geographical region. Climacteric. 2010;13(5):419–28.
8. Avis NE, Crawford S. Cultural differences in symptoms and attitudes toward menopause. Menopause Manage. 2008;17(3):8–13.
9. Ayers B, Forshaw M, Hunter M. The impact of attitudes towards the menopause on women's symptom experience: a systematic review. Maturitas. 2010; 6(S1):28–36.
10. Gold EB, Bromberger J, Crawford S, Samuels S, Greendale GA, Harlow SD, Skurnick J. Factors associated with age at natural menopause in a multiethnic sample of midlife women. Am J Epidemiol. 2001; 153(9):865–74.
11. Hayatbakhsha R, Clavarinob A, Williams GM, Sinac M, Najmana JM. Cigarette smoking and age of menopause: a large prospective study. Maturitas. 2012;72(4):346–52.
12. Sammel MD, Freeman EW, Liu Z, Lin H, Guo W. Factors that influence entry into stages of the menopausal transition. Menopause. 2009;16(6): 1218–27. 16.
13. Harlow BL, Signorello LB. Factors associated with early menopause. Maturitas. 2000;35(1):3–9.
14. Parente RC, Faerstein E, Celestea RK, Wernecka GL. The relationship between smoking and age at the menopause: a systematic review. Maturitas. 2008;6(4): 287–98. 1.
15. Daley AJ, Stokes-Lampard H, MacArthur C. Exercise to reduce vasomotor and other menopausal symptoms: a review. Maturitas. 2009;63(3):176–80.
16. Moilanen J, Aalto AM, Hemminki E, Raitanen J, Luoto R. Prevalence of menopause symptoms and their association with lifestyle among Finnish middle-aged women. Maturitas. 2010;67(4):368–74.
17. Kemmler W, Lauber D, Weineck J, Hensen J, Kalender W, Engelke K. Benefits of 2 years of intense exercise on bone density, physical fitness, and blood lipids in early postmenopausal osteopenic women: results of the Erlangen Fitness Osteoporosis Prevention Study (EFOPS). Arch Intern Med. 2004;164(10):1084–91.
18. Wildman RP, Schott LL, Brockwell S, Kuller LH, Sutton-Tyrrell K. A dietary and exercise intervention slows menopause-associated progression of subclinical atherosclerosis as measured by intima-media thickness of the carotid arteries. J Am Coll Cardiol. 2004;44(3):579–85.
19. Wallace BA, Cumming RG. Systematic review of randomized trials of the effect of exercise on bone mass in pre- and postmenopausal women. Calcif Tissue Int. 2000;67(1):10–8.
20. Nagata C, Wada K, Nakamura K, Tamai Y, Tsuji U, Shimizu H. Association of physical activity and diet with the onset of menopause in Japanese women. Menopause. 2012;19(1):75–81.
21. Nagel G, Altenburg H-P, Nieters A, Boffetta P, Linseisen J. Reproductive and dietary determinants of the age at menopause in EPIC-Heidelberg. Maturitas. 2005;52:337–47.
22. Sapre S, Thakur R. Lifestyle and dietary factors determine age at natural menopause. J Midlife Health. 2014;5(1):3–5.
23. Santoro N, Lasley B, McConnell D, Allsworth J, Crawford S, Gold EB, et al. Body size and ethnicity are associated with menstrual, cycle alterations in women in the early menopausal transition: the study of women's health across the nation (SWAN) daily hormone study. J Clin Endocrinol Metab. 2004;89(6): 2622–31.
24. Davis SR, Castelo-Branco C, Chedraui P, Lumsden MA, Nappi RE, Shah D, Villaseca P. Understanding weight gain at menopause. Climacteric. 2012;15(5):419–29.
25. Whiteley J, Wagner JS, Bushmakin A, Kopenhafer L, Dibonaventura M, Racketa J. The impact of the severity of vasomotor symptoms on health status, resource use, and productivity. Menopause. 2013; 20(5):518.
26. Geukes M, van Aalst MP, Nauta MCE, Oosterhof H. The impact of menopausal symptoms on work ability. Menopause. 2012;19(3):278–82.
27. Hammam RAM, Abbas RA, Hunter MS. Menopause and work – the experience of middle-aged female teaching staff in an Egyptian governmental faculty of medicine. Maturitas. 2012;71(3):294–300.
28. Williams RE, Levine KB, Kalilani L, Lewis J, Clark RV. Menopause-specific questionnaire assessment in US population-based study shows negative impact on health-related quality of life. Maturitas. 2009;62(2): 153–9.
29. Paul J. Health and safety and the menopause: working through the change. London: Trades Union Congress; 2003.
30. Griffith A, Cox S, Griffith R Wong Y. Police officers; ageing, work and health- a research report on the experience of ageing at work, with particular reference to the menopause, and its impact on the well-being of women police officers aged 40+.

Gravesend: British Association of women in Policing; 2006. Available fomr INSERT HTTTP.
31. Reynolds F. Distress end coping with hot flushes at work implications for counselors in occupational settings. Counseling Psychology quarterly, 1999;12(4): 353–61.
32. Leidy LE. Biological Aspects of menopause: across the lifespan. Annu Rev Anthropol. 1994;23:231–53.
33. Morris DH, Jones ME, Schoemaker MJ, Ashworth A, Swerdlow AJ. Familial concordance for age at menarche: analyses from the breakthrough generations study. Paediatr Perinat Epidemiol. 2011;25(3): 306–11.
34. Utian WH. The menopause in perspective from positions to patches. Ann N Y Acad Sci. 1990;592:1–7.
35. Obermeyer CM. Menopause across cultures: a review of the evidence. Menopause. 2007;3:184–92.
36. Gold EB, Crawford SL, Avis NE, Crandall CJ, Matthews KA, Waetjen LE, et al. Factors related to age at natural menopause: longitudinal analyses from SWAN. Am J Epidemiol. 2013;178(1):70–83.
37. Reynolds RF, Obermeyer CM. Age at natural menopause in Spain and the United States: results from the DAMES project. Am J Hum Biol. 2005;17(3): 331–40.
38. McKnight KK, Wellons MF, Sites CK, Roth DL, Szychowski JM, Halalnych JH, et al. Racial and regional differences in age at menopause in the United States: findings from the Reasons for Geographic and Racial Differences in Stroke (REGARDS) study. Am J Obstet. 2011;205:353e1–8.
39. Palmer JR, Rosenberg L, Wise LA, Horton NJ, Adams-Campbell LL. Onset of natural menopause in African American women. J Public Health. 2003;93: 299–306.
40. Henderson KD, Bernstein L, Henderson B, Kolonel L, Pike MC. Predictors of the timing of natural menopause in the multiethnic cohort study. Am J Epidemiol. 2008;167(11):1287–94.
41. Dratva J, Go'mez Real F, Schindler C, Ackermann-Liebrich U, Gerbase MW, Probst-Hensch NM, et al. Is age at menopause increasing across Europe? Menopause. 2009;16(2):385–94.
42. Gudmundsdottir SL, Flanders WD, Augestad LB. Physical activity and age at menopause: the Nord-Trøndelag population-based health study. Climacteric. 2013;16:438–46.
43. Thomas F, Renaud F, Benefice E, de Meeus T, Guegan JF. International variability of ages at menarche and menopause: patterns and main determinants. Hum Biol. 2001;73:271–90.
44. Meschia M, Pansini F, Modena AB, de Aloysio D, Gambacciani M, Parazzini F, et al. Determinants of age at menopause in Italy: results from a large cross-sectional study. Maturitas. 2000;34:119–25.
45. Blumel JE, Chedraui P, Calle A, Bocanera R, Depiano E, Figueroa-Casas P, et al. Age at menopause in Latin America. Menopause. 2006;13(4):706–12.
46. Legorreta D, JA M, Hernández I, Salinas C, Hernández-Bueno JA. Age at menopause, motives for consultation and symptoms reported by 40–59-year-old Mexican women. Climacteric. 2013;16(4):417–25.
47. VeLez MP, Alvarado B, Lord C, Zunzunegui MV. Life course socioeconomic adversity and age at natural menopause in women from Latin America and the Caribbean. Menopause. 2010;17(3):552–9.
48. Yasui T, Hayashi K, Mizunuma H, Kubota T, Aso T, Matsuma Y, et al. Factors associated with premature ovarian failure, early menopause and earlier onset of menopause in Japanese women. Maturitas. 2012; 72(3):249–55.
49. Haines CJ, Pan P, Zhang Q, Sun Y, Hong S, Tian F, et al. Menopausal symptoms in southern China. Climacteric. 2008;11(4):329–36.
50. Kriplani A, Banerjee K. An overview of age of onset of menopause in northern India. Maturitas. 2005;52: 199–204.
51. Kakkar VK, Kaur D, Chopra K, Kaur A, Kaur IP. Assessment of the variation in menopausal symptoms with age, education and working/non-working status in north-indian sub population using menopause rating scale (MRS). Maturitas. 2007;57:306–14.
52. Bairy L, Adiga S, Bhat P, Bhat R. Prevalence of menopausal symptoms and quality of life after menopause in women from South India. Aust New Zeal J Obstet Gynaecol. 2009;49:106–9.
53. Chompootweep S, Tankeyoon K, Yamaral P, Poomsuwan P, Dusitsin K. The menopausal age and climacteric complaints in Thai women in Bangkok. Maturitas. 1993;17:52–62.
54. Greer W, Sandridge AL, Chehabeddine RS. The frequency distribution of age at natural menopause among Saudi Arabian women. Maturitas. 2003;46:263–72.
55. Reynolds RF, Obermeyer CF. Age at natural menopause in Beirut, Lebanon: the role of reproductive and lifestyle factors. Ann Hum Biol. 2001;28(1):21–9.
56. Shakhatreh FMN, Mas'ad D. Menopausal symptoms and health problems in women aged 50–65 years in Southern Jordan. Climacteric. 2006;9:305–11.
57. Delavar MA, Hajahmadi M. Age at menopause symptoms at midlife in a community in Babol, Iran. Menopause. 2011;18(11):1213–8.
58. Bener A, Rizkb DE, Ezimokhaib M, Hassan M, Micallef R, Sawaya M. Consanguinity and the age of menopause in the United Arab Emirates. Int J Gynaecol Obstet. 1998;60(2):155–60.
59. Kwawukume EY, Ghosh TS, Wilson JB. Menopausal age of Ghanaian women. Int J Gynaecol Obstet. 1993;40(2):151–5.
60. Okonofua FE, Lawal A, Bamgbose JK. Features of menopause and menopausal age in Nigerian women. Int J Gynaecol Obstet. 1990;31(4):341–5.
61. OlaOlorun F, Lawoyin T. Age at menopause and factors associated with attainment of menopause in an urban community in Ibadan, Nigeria. Climacteric. 2009;12:352–63.
62. Adanikin AI. Adaption to menopause in Southwest Nigeria. Int J Gynaecol Obstet. 2013;122(1):85.
63. Anderson D, Yoshizawa T, Gollschewski S, Atogami F, Courtney M. Menopause in Australia and Japan: effects

64. Lock M. Symptom reporting at menopause: a review of cross cultural findings. J Br Menopause Soc. 2002;8(4):132–6.
65. Baber RJ. East is east and west is west: perspectives on the menopause in Asia and the west. Climacteric. 2014;17:23–8.
66. Freeman EW, Sherif K. Prevalence of hot flushes and night sweats around the world: a systematic review. Climacteric. 2007;10:197–214.
67. North American Menopause Society. Treatment of menopause-associated vasomotor symptoms: position statement of the North American Menopause Society. Menopause. 2004;11:11–33.
68. Sethi K, Pitkin J. British –Asian women's views on and attitudes toward menopause and hormone replacement. Climacteric. 2000;3(4):248–53.
69. Blumel JE, Chedraui P, Baron G, Belzares E, Bencosme A, Calle A, et al. A large multinational study of vasomotor symptom prevalence, duration, and impact on quality of life in middle-aged women. Menopause. 2011;18(7):778–85.
70. Lam PM, Leung TN, Haines C, Chung TK. Climacteric symptoms and knowledge about hormone replacement therapy among Hong Kong Chinese women aged 40–60 years. Maturitas. 2003;45:99–107.
71. Brown DE, Sievert LL, Morrison LA, Reza AM, Mills BA. Do Japanese American women really have fewer hot flashes than European Americans? The Hilo women's health study. Menopause. 2009;16(5):870–6.
72. Haines CJ, Xing SM, Park KH, Holinka CF, Ausmanas MK. Prevalence of menopausal symptoms in different ethnic groups of Asian women and responsiveness to therapy with three doses of conjugated estrogens/medroxyprogesterone acetate: The Pan-Asia Menopause (PAM) study. Maturitas. 2005;52:264–76.
73. Huang K-E, Xu L, Jaisamrarn U. The Asian menopause survey. Maturitas. 2010;65:276–83.
74. Sallam H, Galal AF, Rashed A. Menopause in Egypt: Past and present perspectives. Climacteric. 2006;9:421–9.
75. Loutfy I, Aziz A, Daddous NI, Hassan MHA. Women's experience of menopause: a community based study in Alexandria. Egypt East Mediterr Health J. 2006;12(S2):S93–106.
76. Taber YA, ben Emhemed HM, Tawati AM. Menopausal age, related factors and climacteric symptoms in Libyan women. Climacteric. 2013;16:179–84.
77. Agwu UM, Umeora OUJ, Ejikeme BN. Patterns of menopausal symptoms and adaptive ability in a rural population in south-east Nigeria. J Obstet Gynaecol. 2008;28(2):217–21.
78. Simon JA, Nappi RE, Kingsberg SA, Maamari R, Brown V. The CLOSER (Clarifying vaginal atrophy's impact on sex and relationships) survey: implications of vaginal discomfort in postmenopausal women and in male partners. Menopause. 2013;10(9):2232–41.
79. Nappi R, Davi SR. The use of hormone therapy for the maintenance of urogynecological and sexual health post WHI. Climacteric. 2012;15(3):267–74.
80. Nappi RE, Kokot-Kierepa M. Vaginal Health: Insights, Views and Attitudes (VIVA) results from an international survey. Climacteric. 2002;15:36–44.
81. Nappi RE, Kokot-Kierepa M. Women's voices in the menopause: results from an international survey on vaginal atrophy. Maturitas. 2010;67:233–8.
82. Kingsberg SA, Wysocki S, Magnus L, Krychman ML. Vulvar and vaginal atrophy in postmenopausal women: findings from the REVIVE Survey. Int Soc Sex Med. 2013;10:1790–9.
83. Santoro N, Komi J. Prevalence and impact of vaginal symptoms among postmenopausal women. J Sex Med. 2009;6(21):33–42.
84. Blümel JE, Chedraui P, Baron G, Belzares E, Bencosme A, Calle A, et al. Sexual dysfunction in middle-aged women: a multicenter Latin American study using the Female Sexual Function Index. Menopause. 2009;16(6):1139–48.
85. Castelo-Branco C, Palacios S, Mostajo D, Tobar C, von Helde S. Menopausal transitions in Movima women, a Bolivian native-American. Maturitas. 2005;51(4):380–5.
86. Murphy MM, Verjee MA, Bener A, Gerber LM. The hopeless age? A qualitative exploration of the experience of menopause in Arab women in Qatar. Climacteric. 2013;16:550–4.
87. Mashiloane CD, Bagratee J, Moodley J. Awareness of and attitudes toward menopause and hormone replacement therapy in an African community. Int J Gynecol Obstet. 2002;76(1):91–3.
88. Avis NE, McKinlay SM. A longitudinal analysis of women's attitudes toward the menopause: results from the Massachusetts health study. Maturitas. 1991;13(1):65–79.
89. Gupta P, Sturdee DW, Papitsch-Clark A. Mid-age health in women from the Indian subcontinent (MAHWIS): general health and the experience of menopause in women. Climacteric. 2009;121:26–37.
90. Kandiah J, Amend V. An exploratory study on perceived relationship of alcohol, caffeine, and physical activity on hot flashes in menopausal women. Health. 2010;2(9):989–96.
91. Shaw CR. The perimenopausal hot flash: epidemiology, physiology, and treatment. Nurs Pract. 1997;22(3):55–6.
92. Reynolds FA. Perceived control over menopausal hot flushes: exploring the correlates of a standardized measure. Maturitas. 1997;27(3):215–21.
93. Pimenta F, Leal I, Maroco J, Ramos C. Perceived control, lifestyle, health, socio-demographic factors and menopause: impact on hot flashes and night sweats. Maturitas. 2011;69(4):338–42.
94. WHO. Obesity and Overweight fact sheet. Geneva: World Health Organization; 2013.
95. Akahoshi M, Soda M, Nakashima E, Tominga T, Ichimarry S, Scto S, Yano K. The effects of the body mass index on age at menopause. International Journal of obesity and the lated Metobolic Disorders. 2002;26:961–8.

96. Fernández-Alonso AM, Cuadros JL, Chedraui P, Mendoza M, Cuadros AM, FR P-L. Obesity is related to increased menopausal symptoms among Spanish women. Menopause Int. 2010;16:105–10.
97. Van der Chedraui P, Hidalgo L, Chavez D, Morocho N, Alvarado M, Huc A. Menopausal symptoms and associated risk factors among postmenopausal women screened for the metabolic syndrome. Arch Gynecol Obstet. 2007;275(3):161–8.
98. Thurston RC, Santoro N, Matthews KA. Adiposity and hot flashes in midlife women: a modifying role of age. J Clin Endocrinol Metab. 2011;96(10):E1588–95.
99. Greenblum CA, Rowe MA, Neff DF, Greenblum JS. Midlife women: symptoms associated with menopausal transition and early postmenopause and quality of life. Menopause. 2013;20(1):22–7.
100. Sievert LL, Obermeyer CM. Symptom cluster at midlife: a four country comparison of checklist and qualitative responses. Menopause. 2012;19(2):133–44.
101. Wellons M, Ouyang P, Schreiner PJ, Herrington DM, Vaidya D. Early menopause predicts future coronary heart disease and stroke: the multi-ethnic study of atherosclerosis. Menopause. 2012;19(10):1081–7.
102. Astma F, Bartelink ML, Grobbee DE, van der Schouw YT. Postmenopausal-status and early menopause risk factors for cardiovascular disease: a meta-analysis. Menopause. 2006;13(2):265–79.
103. Gallagher JC. Effect of early menopause on bone mineral density and fractures. Menopause. 2007;14(3PtS):567–76.
104. Jacobsen BK, Heuch I, Kvale G. Age at natural menopause and all-cause mortality: a 37 year follow-up of 19,731 Norwegian women. Am J Epidemiol. 2003;157(10):923–9.
105. McLay RN, Maki PM, Lykestsos CG. Nulliparity and late menopause are associated with decreased cognitive with decreased cognitive decline. Neuropsychiatr Clin Neurosci. 2003;15(2):161–7.
106. Avis NE, Brockwell S, Colvin A. A universal menopausal syndrome? Am J Med. 2005;19(S12B):37–46.

Printing and Binding: Stürtz GmbH, Würzburg